W9-BES-201

HEALTHCARE ETHICS

A Theological Analysis

Benedict M. Ashley, OP, PhD. STL

Kevin D. O'Rourke, OP, JCD, STL

The Catholic Health Association of the United States
St. Louis, MO

Imprimatur:
    Msgr. Maurice F. Byrne
    Vice Chancellor of St. Louis
    May 8, 1989

Library of Congress Cataloging-in-Publication Data

Ashley, Benedict M.
    Healthcare ethics: a theological analysis / Benedict M. Ashley, Kevin D. O'Rourke. — 3rd ed.
        p.   cm.
    Rev. ed. of: Health care ethics, 2nd ed. c1982.
    Bibliography: p.
    Includes index.
    ISBN 0-87125-158-2
    1. Medical ethics. 2. Medicine—Religious aspects—Catholic Church. 3. Christian ethics—Catholic authors. 4. Pastoral medicine—Catholic Church. I. O'Rourke, Kevin D. II. Ashley, Benedict M. Health care ethics. III. Title.
    [DNLM: 1. Ethics, Medical. 2. Pastoral Care. 3. Religion and Medicine. W 50 A817h]
R724.A74   1989
241'.642—dc19
DNLM/DLC
for Library of Congress   89-916
                                                                        CIP

CONTENTS

Preface xi
Introduction xiii
     Purpose of the Book xiii
     Outline and Method xiii
     Christian Values xiv
     Particular Issues xv
     Pastoral Care xvi

PART 1 THE HEALTH SEEKER 1

Chapter 1 On Being Fully Human 2
    Overview 2
    1.1 Health is for Persons 2
        To Be a Person 4
    1.2 Personal Health in Community 6
    1.3 Politics of Personhood 9
        Christian Ethical Consensus 9
        A Wide Consensus 10
        Individualism and Human Rights 13
    1.4 Priorities in Needs and Values 16
    1.5 Principle of Human Dignity in Community 19

Chapter 2 Health and Disease 20
    Overview 20
    2.1 Concepts of Health and Disease 20
        Concepts of Health 20
        Concepts of Disease 25
        Organismic Theory 27
        Sociologists' View of Health and Illness 29
    2.2 Biological Health and Biologism 31
    2.3 The Higher Levels of Health 34
    2.4 Principle of Totality and Integrity 36
        Integrity of the Person 36
        Totality of the Person 37
        Totality and Integrity 41

Chapter 3 Personal Responsibility for Health 44
    Overview 44
    3.1 The Person and Healing 44
        Affirmation of Life 47
    3.2 Preventive Medicine and Lifestyle 49
    3.3 Principle of Stewardship and Creativity 51
        Scientific Doubts 52

3.4 Principle of Prudent Conscience and Informed Consent 54
Need for Truth 54
Certitude in Ethical Decision 56
Solving Doubts 57
Guidance by the Spirit 59
Developing Doctrine 60
A Well-Formed Conscience 64
Moral Decision in an Immoral World 66
Informed Consent 68
3.5 Patient's Rights 70
Choosing a Physician 70
Protection of Rights 72

PART 2 THE HEALING PROFESSION 75

Chapter 4 The Healthcare Profession 76
Overview 76
4.1 Professions: Depersonalizing Trends 76
Personalistic Concept of a Profession 78
Physicians and Patients with AIDS 80
Healthcare Counseling 81
4.2 Traditional Ideals of the Medical Profession 83
Priest or Scientist? 83
The Christian Physician 86
4.3 Medical Education and Its Biases 88
Biases 90

Chapter 5 Personalizing the Healthcare Profession 94
Overview 94
5.1 The Counseling Relationship 94
Models of Professional-Patient Relations 94
Psychotherapeutic Methods 96
Medical Model 98
Healthcare Fees 100
5.2 Principle of Professional Communication 102
Listening and Truth Telling 102
Confidentiality 103
5.3 Peer Relations and Professional Discipline 107
Calling to Account 109

Chapter 6 Social Organization of Healthcare 112
Overview 112
6.1 Organizational Models and Principle of Subsidiarity 112
Models 112
Centralization 114
A New Model 115

Common Good 116
Subsidiarity 119
Functionalism 122
6.2 Limits to Healthcare 126
6.3 The Hospital as Community 127
Cure and Care 127
A Healing Community 129
6.4 The Health Team 131
Physicians and Co-Workers 131
Nurses, Social Workers, and Patient Advocates 133
6.5 The Catholic Hospital and Long Term Care Facility 136
Catholic Identity 136
6.6 Ethics Committees and Mission Effectiveness Committees 138
Purpose 139
Mission Effectiveness Committees 140
6.7 Healthcare, Ethics, and Public Policy 142
Evaluation 143

PART 3 BIOETHICAL DECISION MAKING 145

Chapter 7 The Logic of Bioethical Decisions 146
Overview 146
7.1 The Logic of Bioethical Debate 146
Ethical Pluralism 146
Deontological Versus Teleological Ethical Methodologies 147
7.2 Deontological (Duty) Methodologies 149
Emotivism 149
Religious Legalism 151
Positivism 152
Formalism 153
Existentialism 154
7.3 Teleological (Means-End) Methodologies 154
Teleology and Natural Law 154
Utilitarianism 155
Situationism 156
Proportionalism 158
7.4 Prudential Personalism 159
Criteria of Morality 159
Jesus as Model 161
Basic Common Needs 162
7.5 An Evaluation of Ethical Methodologies 164
Prudential Personalism Versus Proportionalism 164
Ontic Values and Disvalues 166
Physicalism 168
Application of Methodologies 169
Summary 171

Chapter 8   Norms of Christian Decision Making in Bioethics 173
    Overview 173
    8.1   Is There a Christian Ethics? 173
          What Is An Ethical Principle? 175
    8.2   Norms of Christian Faith 176
          Principle of Well-Formed Conscience 177
          Principle of Free and Informed Consent 179
          Principle of Moral Discrimination 179
          Relation of Act to Goal 181
          Moral Discernment 183
          Principle of Double Effect 184
          Principle of Legitimate Cooperation 188
          Principle of Professional Communication 190
    8.3   Norms of Christian Love 191
          Motivation 191
          Principle of Human Dignity in Community 192
          Principle of Common Good, Subsidiarity, and Functionalism 193
          Principle of Totality and Integrity 194
    8.4   Norms of Christian Hope 196
          Principle of Growth through Suffering 197
          Principle of Personalized Sexuality 199
          Principle of Stewardship and Creativity 201
    8.5   Coordination of the Principles 203

PART 4   DIFFICULT BIOETHICAL DECISIONS 205

Chapter 9   Medical Limits: Abortion, Triage, and Research Involving Human
          Subjects 206
    Overview 206
    9.1   Deciding Who Is the Human Subject of Medical Therapy 206
          Biography 209
          Puzzles 211
          Advocacy of Personhood 213
    9.2   Abortion 214
          Traditional Views 214
          Woman's Right to Decide 220
          Conclusions 224
    9.3   The Law and Personhood 225
          The Supreme Court Decision 226
          Pluralism 228
    9.4   Triage and the Limit to Extending Care 231
    9.5   Experimentation or Research on Human Subjects 234
          Potential Difficulties 234
          Principles of Research on Human Subjects 236
          Proxy or Vicarious Consent 239
          Psychological Experimentation 242
    Conclusion 243

Chapter 10   Sexuality and Reproduction 244
    Overview 244
    10.1   Principle of Personalized Sexuality 244
                Inseparable Values 246
                Reasons for Christian View 247
                Technology and Values 249
                Personalized Sexuality 252
    10.2   Controversy on Contraception 253
                Attempt to Find a Solution 256
                Search for Consensus 258
                Theological Factors 259
                Reasons for Dissent 260
                "Open to the Transmission of Life" 263
                An Obvious Question 264
    10.3   Responsible Parenthood Through Natural Family Planning 267
                Modern Methods 269
                Advantages of Natural Family Planning 270
    10.4   Sterilization and Other Methods of Contraception 271
                Sterilization 271
                Directive 20 273
                Alleged Reasons 275
                Hospital Policy 275
                Material Cooperation 276
                Other Contraceptive Methods 278
    10.5   Artificial Insemination and In Vitro Fertilization 280
                In Vitro Fertilization with Embryo Transfer 280
                Theological Evaluation 281
                Surrogate Motherhood 283
                Reaction to Church Teaching 284
                Assisted Procreation 284
    10.6   Treatment of Rape Victims 286
                Antifertility Treatment 288
    10.7   Pastoral Approach to Medical Sexual Problems 290
                Pastoral Implications of *Humanae Vitae* 290
                Some Objections 292
                A Development Approach 294
                Synod of Bishops 297
                Education for a Sexual Future 298

Chapter 11   Reconstructing Human Beings 301
    Overview 301
    11.1   Modifying the Human Body 302
    11.2   Organ Transplantation 304
                Other Issues 308
    11.3   Sexual Reassignment 313
                Reasons to the Contrary 314

11.4   Genetic Intervention 316
        Gift or Order 316
        Complex Forms of Intervention 317
11.5   Genetic Screening and Counseling 320
        Genetic Counseling 323
        Parental Responsibility 325

Chapter 12   Psychotherapy and Behavior Modification 328
   Overview 328
   12.1   The Concept of Mental Illness 328
   12.2   Psychotherapeutic Methods and Goals 332
        Methods 332
        Goals 334
   12.3   Ethical Problems of Psychotherapy 338
        Punishment 338
        Risks 340
        Value Systems 342
   12.4   Behavior Control 345
        Ethical Guidelines 349
   12.5   Addiction or Chemical Dependency 351
   12.6   Sex Therapy and Research 355
        Therapy 355
        Christian Principles 356
        Research 358

Chapter 13   Suffering and Death 359
   Overview 359
   13.1   Mystery of Death 359
   13.2   Fear of Death 361
   13.3   Defining Death 364
        Brain Death Criteria 366
        Partial Brain Death 367
   13.4   Truth Telling to the Dying 368
   13.5   Care for the Corpse or Cadaver 371
        Autopsy 373
   13.6   Euthanasia and Suicide 374
        Other Opinions 375
        Rejecting a Distinction 378
   13.7   Allowing to Die 380
        Who Decides 384
        Pain 386
        Pastoral Norms 387

PART 5 PASTORAL MINISTRY IN HEALTHCARE 389

Chapter 14 Pastoral Care and Ethical Decisions 390
    Overview 390
    14.1 Religious Ministry and the Healthcare Team 390
            Need for Pastoral Healthcare 390
    14.2 Ministry to the Hospital Staff 394
    14.3 Spiritual Counseling in Healthcare 396
            Trust 396
            Discernment 399
    14.4 Celebrating the Healing Process 401
            Word and Sacrament 401
            Anointing the Sick and Reconciliation 402
            Baptism and Eucharist 405
    14.5 Ethical Counseling and Pastoral Care 408
            Respecting the Patient's Value System 408
            Subjective and Objective Morality 410
            Christian Discernment 412
Bibliography 415
Name Index 471
Subject Index 485

PREFACE

Because of new developments in medical ethics, in response to requests from those who have found our work useful, and in an effort to improve our presentation, we offer this third edition of *Healthcare Ethics*. The present literature on medical ethics is so vast, no one can claim mastery of it all. In an effort to be current and somewhat comprehensive, the bibliography has been thoroughly revised; however, significant citations from previous editions have been retained. Thus we hope to present contemporary sources of the developments in medical ethics, retaining continuity with the recent past. For most of the topics discussed, we have cited authors having various points of view. Some of them confirm our own arguments, whereas others differ. Consequently, the citation of an author is not intended to mean that the article or book always confirms our own statements, nor that the author's data or analysis has been incorporated into our own text, but rather to enter into dialogue with other authors and to provide the reader with additional resources on the topic. Fortunately, much of the contemporary writing on medical ethics is catalogued by, and available at, the National Reference Center for Bioethics Literature at Georgetown University, Washington, DC. The able and generous staff at this facility, especially Patricia Milmoe McCarrick, aided considerably in the revision of this work.

We have rewritten certain topics that our readers wished clarified or for which new data and further reflection led us to somewhat different conclusions. The sections on the right to healthcare and the need for universal health insurance have been modified in light of the changed political situation, yet the ethical principles supporting our positions remain firm. Chapter 7, The Logic of Bioethical Decisions, has been revised for the sake of clarity, and Chapter 8, Norms of Christian Decision Making in Bioethics, has been revised in view of the continuing debate among Catholic theologians on exceptionless moral norms. Because of new developments in medicine, continued reflection, and dialogue with others, we have rewritten the sections on conscience, health insurance, ethics committees, federal commissions on bioethics, identity of Catholic healthcare facilities, abortion, research, contraception, sterilization, rape, in vitro fertilization, organ transplants, brain death, euthanasia, allowing to die, and genetic engineering. In addition, we have added sections on AIDS in various places throughout the text, hoping to cover the pertinent ethical issues arising from AIDS in their proper context. Our discussion of ethical issues in the social organization of healthcare psychotherapy has profited from further study and the observations of our colleagues. We believe that the social and professional problems in medicine are more acute than when the first two editions were published. Thus we believe the first six chapters of the text, which address these issues, are even more significant than they were originally.

In writing this book and preparing the second and third editions, we have received help from several people and support and encouragement from many others. Though we cannot possibly name all those who have contributed, we do wish to publicly thank those who were directly involved. First of all, we are grateful to our past and present colleagues at the St. Louis University School of

Medicine, The Catholic Health Association, the Institute of Religion, and Aquinas Institute of Theology for their fraternal support and intellectual stimulation. We are grateful also to the readers of the original edition: John Doyle, PhD; Richard Fox, PhD; William May, STD; Edward Spillane, PhD; Maria Rieckelman, MM, MD; Thomas Hilgers, MD; Thomas F. O'Meara, OP, STD; and Dennis R. Zusy, OP, PhD. We are equally grateful to the readers of the second edition: Rodney M. Coe, PhD; Anita Pepper, PhD; Dermott Smith, MD; Thomas Hilgers, MD; Hanna Klaus, MD; Girgis Mikhail, MD; Patricia Monteleone, MD; Carmelo Sgarlata, MD; and Dennis R. Zusy, OP, PhD.

The readers of this thoroughly revised third edition were: Philip Boyle, OP, STL; Rodney Coe, PhD; Coy Fitch, MD; Peggy Donovan, RN, BSN; William Stoneman, MD; Alberto Galofre, MD; Manual Comas, MD; Larry Lewis, MD; Val Willman, MD; James Monteleone, MD; Noreen D'Souza, MD; Kenneth Smith, MD; Betty Diehl, MD; Arthur Baue, MD; Alice Kitchen, MD; Dermott Smith, MD; and Albert Moraczewski, OP, PhD. During the course of this revision, Donna Callis, administrative assistant at the Center for Health Care Ethics, managed the revision with grace and patience.

Naturally, we take responsibility for all mistakes, overstatements, or understatements that might be contained in this book. But we also acknowledge wholeheartedly that the book would never have been completed without the help and support of the above-mentioned people.

Benedict Ashley, OP, PhD, STM
Kevin O'Rourke, OP, JCD, STM

INTRODUCTION

PURPOSE OF THE BOOK

Modern medicine has unprecedented power to heal human beings of physical and mental disease, to keep them healthy, and even to improve the human race. This power can be used to humanize life or to dehumanize and destroy it. It can be used justly to benefit all, or it can be used to benefit the few at the expense of the many. How to use such power is a question of values and, therefore, of individual and group decisions that are not merely technical but ethical.

Two reasons have induced us to add to the already extensive literature on medical-ethical and bioethical topics. First, too much of this literature focuses on a few controversial but sometimes minor topics, while neglecting the broader and major issues affecting human health and the healthcare professions. Second, we want to assist Christian, and especially Catholic, healthcare professionals and healthcare facilities faced with the difficult and often puzzling responsibility of giving witness to a long tradition of humanistic healthcare, while working with other professionals and government agencies committed to diverse value systems.

OUTLINE AND METHOD

We believe each person bears primary responsibility for personal health and the right to retain ultimate control over personal health. We also believe each person has the right to the help and care of the community in achieving personal health as well as the reciprocal obligation to assist other members of the community in the same search. Thus Part 1 of this book deals with the dignity of the human person in community and his or her right to health and the responsibility for it.

Part 2 deals with the responsibilities of the community, of the government, and particularly of the healthcare profession to assist persons in the search for health.

We use the broad term *healthcare* profession rather than *medical* profession because this book addresses not only physicians but all those engaged in serving others in their search for health. If sometimes we devote more attention to physicians than to other members of the health team, it is only because physicians are more visible and their responsibilities more clearly defined by professional traditions. What we say of them the reader should apply to other health team members, the respective differences having been considered.

Because of its emphasis on the individual's primary responsibility for health, this book can also help the general public understand their own rights and responsibilities in relation to the healthcare profession, which exists only to serve them.

After dealing with the mutual relations between the health seeker and the healthcare professional, we turn in Parts 3 and 4 to the process of ethical decision making, which involves both health seeker and professional.

Too often today, bioethical controversies are confused and frustrating because the participants do not define the value systems to which they are committed. Scientifically educated healthcare professionals know how to deal with facts, but often they are untrained in any method of dealing with values. Consequently, Part 3 deals with the logic of ethical decision making, showing that currently many such logics do not necessarily contradict one another, but are often very one-sided.

Two traditions of medical ethics are used in the United States, the deontological and teleological (Pellegrino and Thomasma, 1988). These traditions are represented by two pioneers of medical ethics, Paul Ramsey (1970, 1977, 1988) and Joseph Fletcher (1954, 1982). They oppose each other on most issues because Ramsey works from a deontological ethics (duty ethics) of abstract, universal, rational rules of moral obligation, whereas Fletcher works from a *teleological* (means-ends utilitarian, consequentialist, situationist) ethics, which emphasizes pragmatic decisions in unique contexts. To escape this polarization of ethical debate, we propose what we call *prudential personalism*. As with teleological ethics, it is prudential because it makes intelligent practical decisions about the means to meet concrete human needs; but as in deontological ethics, it rejects a merely pragmatic, utilitarian calculation of consequences as an adequate method of moral decision by human persons. This ethics is not a deontology, however, but a personalism. Rather than basing ethical decisions on axiomatic rules, prudential personalism bases such decisions on principles derived from our experience of the needs of human persons as they share in the historically developing human community.

It is not enough, however, to choose a logic or formal procedure for ethical decision making; such decisions must be made in the context of some specific value system. Many assume today that the theological value systems of the various religions—Catholic, Protestant, Jewish, and so forth—will always be pitted against each other in polemics that have no rational solution. Many also assume that if there is to be any public debate and consensus, it must be in terms of a neutral, philosophical, secular, and humanistic value system.

CHRISTIAN VALUES

We take a different view, and in Part 2 we propose a system of values or ethical principles frankly Christian and Roman Catholic (not denying room for pluralism even here). We believe that every human being has some type of value system that is either religious or equivalent to a religion. To label one of these as neutral or humanistic is, from the outset, to give it a privileged position, which can only frustrate honest debate and any effort to achieve some measure of sincere cooperation in a pluralistic society. For a long time in the United States, the Protestant value system was taken as self-evident, and all efforts of Jews and Catholics to defend their own value systems were rejected as an intrusion of a private religion on public civil debate. Today the academic community and the media assume that humanism is self-evident (just as Marxism is assumed to be self-evident in some countries), and any effort to speak up in the name of a "religious" value system is decried as an imposition.

Catholics reason ethically in terms of a value system rooted in a view of reality contained in the Christian Gospel, interpreted by the Church in its life of faith and authoritatively formulated by the pope and the bishops (Vatican II, 1964a). Catholics believe this Gospel with the commitment of faith, and they accept its ordinary formulation and application by the pope and bishops with "religious assent" (Vatican II, 1964a), even when this lacks the final authority of solemn definition. This commitment to authoritative teaching, as well as respect for a long tradition of Catholic theological reflection, however, cannot exempt educated Catholics from listening honestly to other systems of belief, nor from comparing beliefs with the discoveries of science and history and with the personal experience of life (Vatican II, 1965c). For the Catholic, therefore, faith and reason are complementary, not contradictory, sources of truth and value.

Testing of belief affects the way Catholics understand and apply their fundamental convictions. Catholics who are professionals in any field have a serious responsibility to accept the teaching of the Church but also a responsibility to contribute to its development and application. The same must be said of those who adhere to other beliefs and value systems; they also have an obligation to be open to dialogue undertaken in a truth-seeking spirit. None of us has the right to say to another, "You are biased because you are committed to the truth." Each of us seeks the truth through a belief and value system in which we think and, if we are honest, in which we seek to deepen, broaden, and make more realistic. Since the Second Vatican Council, Catholics have experienced how fruitful such an ecumenical approach can be, not so much for conversion of others as for a convergence of insight. In this book we attempt to follow that method, which requires both an openness to the opinions of others and a deepening of our own Christian and Catholic identity.

PARTICULAR ISSUES

Part 4 applies this method of seeking truth to major controversial issues ranging from birth to death. This requires engaging in a type of ecumenism internal to the Catholic community since its introduction by the Second Vatican Council, namely, theological pluralism within a Catholic framework. Today the Catholic ethical system is not viewed as complete and absolutely fixed, but as essentially historical and dynamic in character. At any given historical moment there exists in the Catholic community an authoritative moral teaching that provides a firm basis for any ethical discussion. In medical ethics, remarkably, this teaching developed even before the Second Vatican Council (1963-1965) in the writings of Pope Pius XII (died 1958), who was keenly aware of such issues. The United States Catholic Conference has applied some of these teachings to healthcare in the *Ethical and Religious Directives for Catholic Health Facilities* (1971). Because we hope that our book will be useful to those working in such facilities, we give due recognition to the pastoral guidance of the Second Vatican Council and to the teaching of the popes and bishops, especially as expressed in the *Directives*.

Nevertheless, at any given moment in the history of the Catholic Church, developing moral understanding is in response to current problems. This development is not always well-balanced or even healthy. Catholics may learn by pragmatic needs from the value systems of others, but we may also lose much in the process. A frequently cited example of this is the distortion suffered by Christian sexual ethics from the influence of Stoicism when it was the popular value system of the Roman Empire (Noonan, 1965).

In this process of development there is no easy way to distinguish progress from retrogression; neither conservatives nor liberals have any guarantee that they are automatically in the right. Consequently, along with an exposition of the authoritative position of the pastors of the Roman Catholic Church, we have included various interpretations of such positions and of proposals for their refinement and revision made by committed Catholic theologians. We hope that in doing so we are in line with the intellectual independence, combined with respect for authority and tradition, that seems to us one of the chief features of a Catholic and Christian value system.

Because our ethical discussion of concrete issues is presented within the Catholic value system, we have subtitled this book *A Theological Analysis*. We define *analysis* in this case as an effort to solve concrete ethical problems in terms of principles rooted in Sacred Scripture and tested by the experience of individuals and communities motivated by faith. We believe these principles are discovered most effectively when we employ every form of insight available to us: historical and personal experience, scientific discovery, philosophical reflection, and the Gospel light shining in Scripture and in the living tradition of the Christian community.

PASTORAL CARE

Such an analysis leads us to complete the book with a discussion of healthcare precisely as it is a Christian ministry. This final Part 5 shows that in a healthcare team that aims at healing the total human person, spiritual ministry must play an integral part. The chaplain in any healthcare facility or the pastoral care department has the essential function of assisting healthcare to take on a fully human and Christian vitality. This cannot be achieved if the chaplain and the department monopolize this ministry, but only if they can convince all members of the healthcare team that as Christian professionals, they are also engaged in a Christian ministry. Physicians, nurses, administrators, and the variety of auxiliaries in a Catholic healthcare facility are gifted with talents and professional competence through which they truly minister the healing power of Jesus Christ present to our suffering and hoping world.

Part 1

THE HEALTH SEEKER

The first concern of medical ethics should be the persons who seek health rather than the professionals or institutions that provide it. Thus, Part 1 of this book deals with *The Health Seeker*.

Chapter 1 examines the quest to be fully human, because the search for health is only one aspect of that search for complete humanness with which all ethics is concerned. Chapter 2 develops the notion of health that is rooted in the natural desire to be fully human. Chapter 3 concludes that although each person has the primary responsibility for his or her own health, it can be achieved only with the help and care of the community.

CHAPTER 1

On Being Fully Human

OVERVIEW

This chapter argues that the basic principle of healthcare ethics is the dignity of the human person (1.1). However, the human person can be healthy and whole only in a human community, because to be a person is to be capable of interpersonal relations (1.2). By implication, an ethics of health must also be a politics of health; that is, a community must establish values, norms, and standards to help its members achieve health. There are many competing ethical systems in the United States and in the world. For many this seems to make a workable medical ethics impossible. Even in pluralistic societies, however, progress can be made toward ethical consensus (1.3). The chief obstacle to forming such a consensus is not disagreement about the human values to be sought, but a disagreement about priorities among these values. Thus, to resolve some of the ethical conflicts in the field of healthcare, a hierarchy of values must be established (1.4). Chapter 1 concludes with a formulation of the basic Principle of Human Dignity in Community, on which the ethical arguments of this entire book rest (1.5).

1.1   HEALTH IS FOR PERSONS

Ethics concerns the needs and values of human persons. Health is a vital human need; nothing is more human, more personal. Health is and always has been one of the main preoccupations of the human community. To develop an ethics of human healthcare, therefore, we must have an accurate notion of what it means to be human (Chapter 1), as well as an accurate notion of health (Chapter 2).

Concern about human health goes beyond physical well-being. In 1958 the World Health Organization (WHO) declared: "Health is a state of complete physical, mental, and social well-being and not merely the absence of disease or infirmity." That definition has been widely accepted and criticized (Callahan,

1973b; Gillon, 1986c), but at least it has advanced the notion that human health is not limited to physical concerns.

Today it is no longer easy to explain what the term *human* means. We live in a technological age in an artificial environment, and we view the world through scientific eyes. To understand the *human* being, we need to recover a sense of our own humanity, our difference from the machine and even from the world of nature, which has become subject to scientific probing and technological manipulation (ITEST, 1984). In trying to determine what makes human beings different from animals, plants, and the dust of the earth and stars, we need not isolate or alienate human beings from the natural world of physics or biology. Rather, we must try to locate ourselves in the universe of things to which we are related in countless ways and yet in which we sometimes feel so alone, both as human beings and as an individual being who asks, Who am I?

Perhaps the best way to approximate a working definition of the human person in the ethical context of this book is to begin with the notion of human need. The human being is not definable as a static entity, but as a dynamic system of needs (Maslow, 1970). Human beings have many of the same needs as plants and animals, but we experience these needs in a distinctive way. Animals experience need when they hunger, thirst, gasp for air, or pursue a mate. Human beings not only feel such needs, but we also have at least some understanding of why we have them. We also devise alternative ways of satisfying these needs, puzzle over what we need most, and even create needs never experienced by human beings in the past.

To ascertain which human needs and capacities are genetically determined and common to the whole human species and which have been created by human culture is not easy. Sociobiologists such as Edward Wilson and Charles Lumsden (1981) argue that the evolution of the human species from its primate ancestors verifies to some degree the biological origin and survival of human behavioral tendencies. Nevertheless, even sociobiologists recognize that the evolution of the remarkable human brain has given humankind the capacity to break through the largely fixed and genetically determined types of behavior characteristics of even our closest primate relatives. Human beings have the need and the capacity to use symbols, invent tools, communicate by speech with its variety of invented languages, and create and modify social and political systems in a manner only faintly foreshadowed in the behavior of other animals (Griffin, 1984).

This need and capacity to develop a diversity of cultural patterns, however, masks the genetically inherent and common needs and capacities that might serve to define human nature. Anthropology and history have found it difficult to verify cross-cultural universals; also, we do not have recourse to the behavior of so-called primitive peoples because their cultural history is as long as ours. Even the study of infant behavior yields only equivocal results, since infants behave only in response to the culture into which they are born.

Nevertheless, the very difficulty we experience in trying to separate human nature from human culture gives us a clue. What defines us as human beings is precisely this limited but real transcendence of rigid biological determinism. We are indeed bodily, biological, animal beings with inherent needs for food, shelter, and reproduction, but we also have the types of brain and intelligence that make it possible and necessary to choose from a vast range of ways to satisfy these needs. Culture is only the expression of our nature, which is to be intelligently free. This embodied intelligent freedom defines us as human and gives unity and continuity to the human family across time and space.

To Be a Person

To have this need and capacity for intelligent freedom is to be a *person*. The reason ordinary language does not apply the term *person* to an animal, even a pet, is because human beings do not experience animals as self-conscious autonomous beings. Animals do not talk back. This is why some philosophers today want to broaden the definition of person to include not only "intelligence" and "freedom" but also "ability to communicate," "to care," and "to be called forth." Note, however, that in ordinary usage the terms *person* and *personality* are not identical. A person has a personality; that is, persons are the kinds of beings that understand and feel for each other in a human, freely intelligent manner. It is this *expression* of personhood that is personality.

Medical ethics is confronted by the obvious fact that many human beings hardly seem to be persons as we have just defined that term—the infant; the seriously defective, the senile, and the unconscious human being; and even ourselves when we are asleep. Is medical ethics concerned with those who are not fully persons? Certainly such human beings exhibit little that can be called personality, since their behavior seems to be only at the animal or even the plant level. We sometimes say of a comatose, brain-damaged victim of an accident, "He is now in a vegetative state."

Such difficulties highlight that in the human organism, intelligent freedom is intimately linked to the central nervous system and more precisely to the frontal lobes of the cerebral cortex. When the normal functioning of this relatively small but extremely complex part of a human being is inhibited, that person ceases to be actively, intelligently free. He or she sinks back into the deterministic reflexes or physiological reactions of the animal or vegetative level of functioning. As long as the higher brain centers function, however, a human being manifests a personality even when the rest of the body is largely destroyed. Such a person seems to need little from the rest of the body except a supply of oxygenated and nutritive blood to bring energy to the brain and carry away its wastes. Theoretically, at least, someday a living and conscious brain may be able to exist without a body at all. Will the human person in his or her own unique individuality still be present, still be actively self-aware, and possess intelligent freedom?

Some ethicists recently have proposed a distinction between being *human* and being a *person* (Engelhardt, 1986a; Tauer, 1985). They define "person" as a self-conscious, free, moral agent; thus infants or victims of senility, although human (i.e., biologically members of the human species), are not, at least in a proper sense, persons. Engelhardt (1977) goes so far as to entitle one essay,

"Some Persons Are Humans, Some Humans Are Persons, and the World Is What We Persons Make of It." Does this imply that "moral agents" are free to grant personal status or to deny it to their inferiors—a position that elites have always found very convenient in justifying their neglect or oppression of the powerless?

Such a view is very difficult to reconcile with any scientific account of the unity of human nature and does violence to ordinary language. According to our ordinary use of language, to be a human person does not require that here and now one is functioning as an intelligent, free, moral agent, but to have that *innate power* to develop such capacities and to exercise them more or less effectively under favorable and appropriate conditions. We are actually persons, in the sense of having human rights, even when we are not actually, but only potentially, moral agents.

The static view that humanhood is separate from personhood fails to recognize that a human person is not a pure intelligence as is an angel—as Plato and philosophical idealism have always contended—but a *bodily being*, evolving out of the natural world it shares yet never separated from it. Consequently, human self-awareness and freedom emerge only at high points of a very complex process, much of which is subconscious and dependent on bodily development and function. When a human organism is conceived, his or her uniqueness is genetically determined by a novel combination of traits. At that moment, a unique human body comes into being and is continuously identifiable. In refutation of idealistic conceptions of the human person as a "self-conscious mind," recent philosophy insists that bodily identity is necessary to the notion of the human person (Echstein, 1970). Even the medieval scholastics who argued for the survival of the human soul did not consider it a complete human person. They believed the soul received its identity from its relation to the body it would receive again at the resurrection. The whole life process involves a development of this unique body-mind in constant interaction with its environment.

Every individual has a *biography* that consists in mature actualization of intelligent freedom and the manifestation of a unique personality. This life story passes through many phases of fetal and infant development before the brain can function at higher levels. Even during adult life, persons function with intelligent freedom only at certain times and in certain relations to their environment. Much of the adult's life is taken up with routine—sleep, eating, relaxation—when intelligence is working at a level below that of creative freedom. Yet this same person carries on the total process of living in all its phases. Getting sick and getting well are both parts of this continuous, struggling process of living development. Thus defining human personhood as "embodied intelligent freedom" presupposes a life process that goes on at many levels of activity, but that is more clearly manifest and definable by its maximum, its high point of integration. Medical ethics must always take into account that the person who needs help in a particular crisis of illness is a being who exists not merely here and now, but who also has a history and a future.

The term *personality*, as typically used, also emphasizes the individuality of each member of the human race. Because the essence of human nature is embodied intelligent freedom, each human being transcends the commonalities

5

of this nature and attains a unique biography of personal choices. To be truly human, I must also be truly *myself*. I must live out my life, taking responsibility for its ultimate direction. Such is a reasonable interpretation of the paradoxical view of some existentialist philosophers who say, "Man has no nature, but only a history." Individual differences between one human being and another are immense, resulting in a vast range of personalities. Even monozygotic twins, who are genetically very similar, are still able to live personal lives and have distinct biographies. Twins can disagree, can go separate ways. No doubt if someday science produces human clones—a test-tube production of several individuals of the same species—these human beings would each still have a life to live and would live it in a unique way.

This account of what it is to be a human person leads to a preliminary formulation of the goal of healthcare:

> The goal of healthcare is to contribute to the full development of human persons, that is, *to help human beings become intelligently free*. Healthcare fails whenever it tends to depersonalize its clients by ignoring or restricting this freedom.

1.2   PERSONAL HEALTH IN COMMUNITY

Every ethical problem about healthcare ultimately may be reduced to the conception of what it is to be human and to actualize personhood. However, this must not lead to the error of individualism (so influential in American culture), which conceives the person in isolation, continually defending himself or herself against the encroachments of society (Bellah, 1986). What then is the relation of human person to human community?

The classical definition "man is a rational animal" makes sense only if the terms animal and rational are understood as tags for a vast, ever-increasing body of information gathered by the behavioral sciences and the humanistic disciplines. *Animal* refers to man's evolutionary origin and complex physiochemico-biological structure. *Rational* describes very complex human behavior at peak moments that rises to a freedom that transcends the instinctive life of animals. To say "man is a rational animal" is to say men and women of every race belong to a single, interacting human community that is not only able to eat, drink, and procreate, but also to think scientifically and creatively, to debate and make political decisions, and to make love personally. Aristotle suggested this by saying "man is a *political* animal" (*Politics* 1, 1253a), giving the word *political* a much broader connotation than it has today.

Thus the notion of person cannot be satisfactorily defined except in relation to its correlative—the notion of society or community. John Walgrave (1965), speaking in phenomenological terms, has written:

> That which is proper to a person and finds its fulfillment in personality cannot be defined exclusively as "self-possession." A complete definition should read "self-possession with an objectively directed project of life." The closedness of self-possession has meaning only through openness to objective

life. That to which the activities of the objective project of life are directed is ultimately the personal world in which being real finds its proper realization. In this way we ultimately arrive at "personal community" as the unitary formula which defines the objective of the activity making a person. This activity itself can be summed up in the word "love." Love then, which creates the personal community, is the proper perfection of personality (pp. 114-115).

No human person can exist apart from a human community. Each of us has parents, and no one of us can develop either physically or psychologically without constant interhuman relationships. The human brain cannot develop fully without language, and language is a cultural, social creation (Johanson, 1981). Even if in the future persons are produced in a test tube, they will be the product of a technological community and will be able to develop only within it.

The correlation of person and community is not merely superficial. People need a community not merely because it supplies them with certain instrumental needs (food, housing, clothing, defense), but because their personalities can be fulfilled only in the act of communication and sharing. If personhood is embodied intelligent freedom, it can be fulfilled only in the free act of knowing and loving. In the whole universe the most complex, varied, integrated, and beautiful beings are persons; only in them can the desire to know and love find full play. All science's efforts to understand the universe culminate in exploring the mystery of human persons, who, with their complexity, freedom, and potential for intercommunication, are the highest outcome of the evolutionary process.

Our knowledge of each other, however, cannot be achieved by simple observation in the way we can study a rock, a tree, or a dog. To know *you*, to understand you intimately, I must form a specifically human relation with you, whether as an enemy, a master, a slave—or better—a co-worker, a lover, or a friend. Such knowledge also involves feeling, even love. I must freely reveal myself to you if you are freely to reveal yourself to me. This means that a healthcare professional cannot understand a patient or diagnose his or her ailment as if the patient were a thing, because he or she is a person whose whole mode of health or sickness is *relational*.

For Christians this correlation of person and community has a still deeper significance for two reasons (Kiesling, 1986):

1. The Christian God is a personal God, a trinity of persons who totally share one single being, life, knowledge, and love. Thus the ultimate reality is a community of persons that sets the pattern for all other realities, including our human reality.
2. The Christian God has created each unique human person for himself or herself, that is, with the intention of drawing each of us to share in our own eternal, trinitarian life. "This fellowship of ours is with the Father and his Son, Jesus Christ" (1 Jn 1:3).

Consequently, the Christian healthcare professional, in his or her effort to heal another human being, is a minister of God helping that patient to share more fully in the everlasting community of the Father, Son, and Holy Spirit.

This emphasis on the intimate relation of person to community, however, should not lead us into the exaggeration of those who argue that personhood is *conferred* on the individual by the community not through reason of some inherent right, but on the basis of conditions set by the community. Thus the philosopher Ronald M. Green (1974), using a "social contract" theory similar to that of John Rawls (1971), argues, "The issue of abortion...comes down to the question of whether rational agents could find it rational in the circumstances of moral choice to confer rights on the fetus and, if so, the nature and extent of these rights" (p. 62). The geneticist Joshua Lederberg (1967) locates the beginning of human personhood around the first year of life, because "at this point only does [a person] enter into a cultural tradition which has been the special attribute of man by which he is set apart from the rest of the species." The philosopher and medical ethicist H.T. Engelhardt, Jr. (1986b) argues:

> Not all humans are persons. Fetuses, infants, the profoundly mentally retarded and the hopelessly comatose provide examples of human nonpersons. Such entities are member of the human species.... They do not have standing in the moral community.... One speaks of persons in order to identify entities one can warrant blame and praise.... For this reason it is nonsensical to speak of respecting the autonomy of fetuses, infants, or profoundly retarded adults who have never been rational (pp. 107-108).

The significance of this theory of imputed personhood for the abortion debate is discussed in Chapter 9. As an explanation of the relation of person to community, it fails to take into account that the human person has a capacity and openness to knowledge and love of other persons. Consequently, human personhood is based on innate capacities, not on acceptance of others. Personhood is never completely actualized in this earthly life but is always in a process of growth, which consists primarily in the deepening of communal relations.

Community, in its turn, exists to assist each of its member-persons in this process of growth. Thus, as soon as a unique human organism is conceived, he or she begins this actualizing process and has a right to help from the human community to complete this process. The community, therefore, does not confer on or impute personhood to the sleeping, un-self-conscious infant or fetus, but rather responds to its silent demand to live and grow.

By extension, the hospital or other care facility is a human community dedicated to the healthcare of human persons. The healthcare facility does not confer the power to get well on the patients; this power is inherent in their capacity for personal life. These patients include not only the self-conscious one, but also the comatose or senile person, the child, the infant, and the unborn person. Each is a human organism in the process of living out a human life. Each has an ethical claim on the healthcare community for help (which has limits) in his or her growth and struggle to actualize the inherent capacity for knowledge, love, and human relationship, which depend so intimately on physical health. The very purpose and meaning of the healthcare community, as of every human community, is to help its members grow in personhood.

Similar to the theories of imputation as a source of personhood is the attempt of Joseph Fletcher (1974, 1979) to enumerate "indicators of humanhood," because along with the biological criterion of "neocortical function," he selects "self-awareness," "euphoria" (as found in a retarded but happy child), and "human relationships." Such signs certainly indicate stages in the process of the actualization of a person, but they do not necessarily mark the beginning of that process. Also they do not indicate when a person with rights first exists and demands the care of the community (Iglesias, 1984a).

1.3 POLITICS OF PERSONHOOD

Christian Ethical Consensus

The intrinsic relation of persons to community implies that there is a *political* aspect to all human events. Therefore the ethics of the human person in community must also be *politics;* that is, it must take into account the ways by which human persons develop value systems socially, sometimes through debate and often through conflict. To develop the politics of healthcare means to discern priorities and to develop policies based on those priorities. If we do not realistically face up to this political aspect of ethics, we will find ourselves each defending his or her own subjective ethical stance in endless and fruitless polemics. Today it has become all too apparent that health is a profoundly political issue—not merely in terms of the argument over "socialized medicine," but in the sense that the problems of poverty, food, population, and pollution are national and international health problems (Navarro, 1986).

In light of the many political decisions regarding healthcare, many Christians are tempted to despair and withdraw from ethical controversy. In the pluralistic world of today, how is ethical debate even possible, let alone practical consensus? Warring value systems appear to be irreconcilable. Only political power will prevail; today, however, Christians are bitterly opposed by their fellow Christians and are often accused of politicizing religious differences and imposing sectarian morality on the public. In the health field, this disagreement among Christians is very sharp in matters such as contraception, sterilization, abortion, in vitro fertilization, and euthanasia.

Nevertheless, withdrawal by Christians from ethical debate was not countenanced by the Second Vatican Council (1965c), which recognized the fact of pluralism, renounced any policy of religious imperialism, and proposed an ecumenical approach to differences in faith and value systems. First, Catholics must be convinced that they form a single faith community with all others who acknowledge Jesus as Lord, ordinarily signified by baptism. Within this community, of course, are great differences of opinion on certain ethical questions as a result of the historical divergence and isolation of one church from another. Such differences should not, however, overshadow the profound agreement among Christians that Jesus Christ, portrayed for them in the Scriptures and the living history of his faithful followers, is the norm of ethical personhood and communal life.

We have subtitled this book *A Theological Analysis* precisely because for us the ultimate ethical norm is not a set of ethical rules but Jesus Christ—God become truly human. Therefore he is our model of what it is to be human, as well as the source of grace that empowers us to overcome our sinful inhumanity and become truly human. Thus, in a search for consensus with all those of goodwill, we can honestly join with humanists to make the world more human; we can also join with fellow Christians in prayer, meditation, fraternal dialogue, and cooperation. To lose hope in the possibility of this union of heart and mind in Christ (1 Co 1:10) is to lose hope in Jesus as Savior of all humanity.

Care for the sick, as well as the sinful, was one of Jesus' first concerns. He healed before he preached, and he went out to the lepers, the most neglected members of the community. If Christians embrace this concern for the bodily needs of the alienated, the experience of charity will sweep away many of the one-sided views that divide us. It was no accident that the source of the recent upsurge in the ecumenical spirit was the common opposition of Christians of every denomination to the tyranny of the totalitarian governments of Hitler, Mussolini, and Stalin.

A Wide Consensus

The Second Vatican Council (1965a, c) insisted that this spirit of dialogue must extend beyond the Christian family to other religions. Judaism and Islam believe in the same personal God as do Christians and also have the same fundamental convictions about the dignity of the human person in relation to God (Vaporis, 1986). In the history of healthcare, Jews and Muslims made fundamental contributions which have become part of the tradition of Christian healthcare (Galdston, 1981; Ullmann, 1978).

The Eastern religions of India and China are beginning to influence American life. At first sight, however, their outlook might appear incompatible with the Christian emphasis on the dignity of the human person in relation to a personal God, since they teach that the individual, after a series of reincarnations, is absorbed into the unity of the Absolute. Closer study, however, reveals that this Absolute is not subpersonal, nor impersonal, but superpersonal. Thus it becomes possible for monotheists to join with believers in these Eastern religions in a common search for authentic spiritual selfhood (Thundy, 1985). Americans are beginning to appreciate how much these religions, with their meditative disciplines, can contribute to personal integration and total health.

In addition, the *nature religions* of native Americans and others have taught an appreciation of our relation to nature in its mysterious wisdom and cosmic rhythm. Modern medicine is beginning to learn from the ecological experience of such peoples (L. Moore, 1987). We cannot return to Eden, but woe to us if we forget it.

Thus Christians can learn much from other world religions about ethical dialogue and the pursuit of true health (Feldman, 1986a). Today, however, these religious systems of values seem to be receding before the worldwide advance of secularization that dominates both the First World of the democracies and the Second World of the Marxists, both of which are competing for the domination of the Third World of underdeveloped peoples (John Paul II, 1987a). Moreover, this secularized view of humankind seems more congenial to the science and technology on which modern medicine is based than are the older religious views of man. In response to this situation, however, the Second Vatican Council has indicated that dialogue with nonbelievers should be sought (Vatican II, 1965a).

The Christian is inclined to judge the agnostic world view of humanism that prevails in the democratic countries and the atheistic world view of the Marxists as absolutely contradictory to Christianity. Tracing the origin of these new world philosophies, however, reveals that they are sociologically equivalent to the older world religions (D'Arcy, 1969; V. Smart, 1984). The religious wars that resulted from the breakdown of Christian unity in the sixteenth and seventeenth centuries and the shock of discovering other ethically admirable religions of the New World and Asia led to a religious vacuum in Europe. Out of this arose the new philosophy of humanism (the Enlightenment, sometimes called secular to distinguish it from the older Christian humanism), which enthusiastically accepted the rise of science and technology as a more efficient means to solve human problems than prayer, ritual, and traditional dogmas (MacIntyre, 1981).

Thus, according to the well-known *Humanist Manifesto* (1933), signed by a group of distinguished American thinkers under the leadership of our most famous American philosopher, John Dewey:

> Religion consists of those actions, purposes, and experiences which are humanly significant. Nothing human is alien to religion. It includes labor, art, science, philosophy, love, friendship, recreation—all that is in its degree expressive of intelligently satisfying human living.... Religious humanism considers the complete realization of human personality to be the end of man's life and seeks its fulfillment and development in the here and now. This is the explanation of the humanist's social passion (p. 13).

Thus humanism rejects the notion of an afterlife for human beings and their dependence on a God or an Absolute, but it does so precisely in the interest of human dignity (Kurtz, 1983). Believing that the older religions tend to excuse human beings from full responsibility to create a good society here and now, this humanist position has been reaffirmed by an international group in the *Paris Statement of 1966* and, in the United States, in the *Humanist Manifesto II* (1973).

Where humanism is not dominant, Marxism has become the contemporary equivalent of a religious system of values. Although Marxism shares many values with humanism, it has an even more materialistic conception of humanity, according to which human beings emerge from nature by a struggle to control and refashion it (even their own nature) to suit their purposes. Historically, the human community has spent much of its energies in an internal class struggle of people against people. Marxists believe that today is the threshold of an age when this class struggle will be dissipated by the rise to power of the productive members of society, so that humankind will at last be free to apply all its energies to the conquest of nature through the use of scientific technology (Fromm, 1975).

> The humanistic Marxist Milan Prucha (1965) writes: Man is not the universal purpose of the world which religious illusion believes him to be. Man came

into existence in a certain part of the universe, under certain favorable conditions, as a partial product of the development of matter. He must, therefore, assert himself through his practical activity against the world as a whole; rooted in the world, he must carry into it a meaning given by human existential needs (p. 140).

Marx comprehends the essence of man as the result of specific human activity, in accordance with his concept of practical materialism. Man as a natural being creates social reality. This is a new reality, in which the being of each individual achieves its content only in relation to other individuals, in relation to the social entity (p. 144).

Many Catholics are under the impression that the Catholic Church, because it opposes communism, favors capitalism. They are unacquainted with the fully developed social teaching of recent popes (John Paul II, 1987a; Paul VI, 1967) which must be considered in any Catholic approach to today's ethical problems, including those in the medical field. This Catholic teaching attempts to transcend the capitalist-communist impasse, based in both camps on a materialistic conception of society. The popes urge us to work for a world community based on spiritual goals and economic cooperation. They link human health and world poverty as the most fundamental ethical problems of our time, which are often ignored in the United States by bioethics, whereas much is made over secondary problems such as eugenics and heart transplants.

The Second Vatican Council (1965c) has emphasized that Christians have much to learn from the humanist's emphasis on human beings' responsibility to use reason, science, and technology to solve human problems. The otherworldly view of religion rightly deserves the accusation that religion is often an "opiate of the people," when it should be a challenge to use the talents given us by God to overcome poverty, disease, and injustice. For this reason, Catholic healthcare professionals should strive to heal any schizoid dualism in their own thinking between their religious view of life and an enlightened scientific view of the world. Christians cannot accept agnostic and sometimes mechanistic and materialistic interpretations of scientific findings (Ehrenfeld, 1978), but they can and should join enthusiastically in the advance of scientific research and its application to the solution of human problems of health.

Catholic liberation theologians (Boff, 1986; Gutierrez, 1977) have taken a further step by arguing that Catholics can learn something from the Marxist criticism of capitalism. They point out that when Jesus announced the coming of the Kingdom of God, he was not talking merely about a temporal reality but was declaring the fulfillment of Old Testament prophetic demands for justice to the poor and oppressed. The Kingdom of God begins here on earth with social justice (John Paul II, 1980a), and no one will gain heaven who has neglected to work for social justice on earth (Viviano, 1988). Jesus declared in the Parable of the Sheep and the Goats (Mt 25:31-46), "I was hungry and you never gave me food.... Insofar as you neglected to do this to one of the least of these, you neglected to do it to me"; in the Parable of Lazarus and the Rich Man (Lk 16:19-31), Jesus taught the same lesson. Consequently, a genuine Christian ethics cannot be written from the viewpoint of the status quo, which in a sinful world tends to reflect the materialistic spirit of domination and possessiveness. Such ethics must view the world from the side of oppressed persons whose needs have been ignored and neglected. Thus Jesus pointed to his preaching of the Gospel to the poor as the best sign of the authenticity of his own mission (Mt 11:5). Therefore a Christian politics of healthcare must be based on advocacy for the rights of neglected persons.

Why is the conflict between the individualism of capitalism and the collectivism of communism so unresolvable? Christian theology ascribes this conflict to a profound misunderstanding of the relation of person to community. The notion of *personal* is often confused with the notion of *private*. Thus it appears that to favor the community is to *sacrifice* the person to the collective. This is true if the community is based on a sharing of material goods. Such goods can be shared among individuals only by dividing them up and giving to each a private share. What one gets, the other loses, and vice versa. This is the way it works in modern societies based primarily on the sharing of material goods such as economic production and military power. Consequently, those who oppose selfish individualism sometimes turn to communism, wherein the person is sacrificed to the society.

Christian politics, however, aims at the sharing of *spiritual* goods: truth and love. Material goods should be distributed so as to promote spiritual sharing, but they are not the primary basis of community. When spiritual goods are shared, no one loses, but each gains, possessing them more perfectly. Only in such spiritual sharing is profound community between human persons possible. Thus the common good is not opposed to the personal good; rather, it is the deepest heart of the personal good of each person. Private goods are actually *less* personal than this common good.

This theory may sound impractical until we realize that scientific truth is a spiritual good. Is it not true that today scientists across the world are united in the advancement and sharing of scientific research, yet they are deeply divided by the politics of their countries' quests for economic and military power?

Therefore a Christian politics today will aim at overcoming world conflict by witnessing to spiritual values and subordinating material ones as instruments for attaining spiritual community. This is why dialogue in an ecumenical spirit has to be the greatest political strategy of the Christian. Healthcare is directed at the body; as a healing process, however, it is directed to a spiritual goal, the appreciation of persons in their intelligent freedom.

Individualism and Human Rights

Now it should be clear why Catholic theology perceives that extreme form of humanism, sometimes called *radical individualism,* as the greatest danger to the development of an ethical consensus in a pluralistic society. Typical humanism has a strong concern for social justice, but radical individualism rejects the belief that community as such is a moral value. This ethic—proposed by Hobbes in the seventeenth century, supported in more moderate form by Locke, and given a new form by Nietzsche in the nineteenth century—has had a profound effect on

American society from Emerson to its diverse advocates among psychotherapists (Szasz, 1977, 1987) on the left and libertarians such as Ayn Rand (1967), George Gilder (1982), and Robert Nozick (1981).

The ethic of radical individualism is summed up in the principle, "I have a right to live my own life as long as I don't hurt anybody else"; "hurt" meaning direct harm by bodily injury or damage or theft of private property (Bloom, 1987). According to this ethic, society exists only as a means to protect one individual from another, so as to leave each to pursue his or her private purposes. Moreover, any claim of one human being on another that is not contractual goes beyond the right to be let alone and is therefore unethical. Ethical behavior becomes the consistent pursuit of self-interest within a minimal code of law and contract enforcement. Proponents of this ethic often argue (1) that people really act this way and therefore other ethics are hypocritical and (2) that this system of laissez faire actually produces more economic prosperity and human progress than do collectivist and altruistic ethics.

For laissez faire capitalists to argue, however, that they have a right to amass a fortune because it is "good for society" is itself hypocritical, since their real belief is that they have a right to their own lives no matter what the social consequences as long as they do not provoke those more powerful than themselves to destroy them.

This extreme form of individualism is perhaps best labeled *privatism*, and it was also the ethic of some of the counterculturists of the 1960s. Although they were in revolt against the aggressive money-making privatism of their parents, counterculturists had learned privatism's basic attitudes, which they reinterpreted in terms of freedom and love, that is, as an individualistic search for selfish pleasure and irresponsibility.

Privatism seems still to be growing in American society in the 1980s (Bellah, 1986). It is the most difficult value system to deal with, even for a Christian who has the will to try to find some point of contact. However, even here the individualists deserve their due. When Rand (1967) attacks altruism and proposes the new selfishness, she obviously supposes that Christians teach an altruistic ethics in which the person is called on to sacrifice his or her self-fulfillment to the community. She rightly sees this as unreal and sentimental. What she does not realize is that to Catholics the command "Love thy neighbor as thyself" (Mk 12:31) implies that we must *love ourselves* before we can love anyone else. Selfishness is not repudiated because it seeks the good of the self, but because it denies the self access to those goods that can be achieved only by sharing with other persons. Thus Catholics can agree with radical individualists that each person has as his or her first moral duty to seek genuine self-fulfillment. This is not sinful selfishness, but a duty to the God who made human beings so they could make good use of their gifts.

Furthermore, Christians should take up the challenge to show by hard-headed, realistic, and rational arguments that this self-fulfillment demands that people not isolate themselves in sinful selfishness, but become open to community, where this self-fulfillment lies. In this way Christians can learn something from privatism about good healthcare; namely, that (as Chapter 2 argues in detail) each person has the primary responsibility for the care of his or her own health, a responsibility that cannot be passed on to the healthcare profession or to society.

The rise of recent "conservative" movements that seek to defend traditional Christian family life and a legitimate patriotism but confuse these values with a privatism and nationalism indifferent or antagonistic to social justice (Fitzgerald, 1986) presents a difficult ecumenical problem. Unfortunately, "liberal" Christians have sometimes compounded this confusion in their zeal for social justice by seeming to reject domestic virtue and sober patriotism (as these are commended in the Scriptures) and to adopt very different attitudes derived from humanism or Marxism. To overcome these confusions, Christians must demonstrate how the Gospel inseparably unites the virtues of private and social life, loyalty to one's country, and a still greater loyalty to the whole human family.

This ecumenical search for ethical consensus has its solid legal and political foundations in the United Nations' *Universal Declaration of Human Rights* (1948), signed by almost all the countries of the world and supported by all the major religions as well as by humanists and Marxists. Catholics have been urged by the Pontifical Commission on Peace and Justice (1973), by Pope Paul VI (1974), and Pope John Paul II (1988) to support the Declaration as a sound (although not complete) basis for modern ethics. It begins with a fundamental statement that formulates the very notion of person and community for which we have just argued:

> Article 1: All human beings are born free and equal in dignity and rights. They are endowed with reason and conscience and should act towards one another in a spirit of brotherhood.

Here "reason and conscience" are equivalent to "intelligent freedom" and "brotherhood" to "community," in terms of which we have defined the human person. The Declaration then effectively concretizes this abstract principle by enumerating 29 basic human rights. Among these are the following, which should serve as a magna charta for a modern healthcare ethics:

> Article 3: Everyone has the right to life, liberty, and security of person.
>
> Article 22: Everyone, as a member of society, has the right to social security and is entitled to realization, through national effort and international cooperation and in accordance with the organization and resources of each state, of the economic, social, and cultural rights indispensable for his dignity, and the free development of his personality.
>
> Article 25: (1) Everyone has the right to a standard of living adequate for the health and well-being of himself and of his family, including food, clothing, housing, and medical care and necessary social services, and the right to security in the event of unemployment, sickness, disability, widowhood, old age, or other lack of livelihood in circumstances beyond his control....(3) Motherhood and child-hood are entitled to special care and assistance. All children, whether born in or out of wedlock, shall enjoy the same social protection.

According to Article 2, all these rights apply to all human beings "without distinction of any kind, such as race, color, sex, language, religion, political or other opinion, national or social origin, property, birth, or other status." Moreover, Article 29 (1) asserts, "Everyone has duties to the community in which alone the free and full development of his personality is possible."

Of course, Christians are far from having fulfilled their obligations under the *Declaration* in the United States, let alone in the whole world. Nevertheless, it stands as a proof that in the twentieth century a basic consensus already exists on the fundamental ethical values on which world community must be based. The aim of this book is to take that consensus very seriously without, however, glossing over the profound differences that continue to divide the Christian and the secular communities and that challenge us to further research and dialogue.

1.4 PRIORITIES IN NEEDS AND VALUES

The fact that the nations of the world are at least nominally agreed on a list of human rights or values is an important step toward increasing ethical consensus, but it is only a first step. This is unfortunate, since the adoption of the *Universal Declaration* has shown the diversity in the interpretations of many of these rights. When carefully examined, this diversity reveals that ethics must not only list agreed-on values, but must also deal with the question of priorities. What is the "hierarchy of values"? Some will reply that this question of emphases and priorities is a wholly subjective matter about which rational discussion is impossible. Whether this is the case can be decided only if the concept of value and its relation to objective facts are examined more closely.

We have already argued that ethics has to do with the satisfaction of the *needs* of human persons in their lives as intelligently free social beings. We have now to ask more precisely, What are these needs? Are some needs more basic than others? The general answer is that human needs are satisfied by human values, and the most basic needs by the most basic values, but the term value is vague. It was originally used in economics but has been extended in usage to cover a spectrum of analogical meanings (Perry, 1980). A given human value, however, is always correlative to a human need; that is, it is desired to satisfy the need. On the other hand, a negative value is inimical to show human need, and a neutral value neither satisfies nor obstructs a need. A value, therefore, can be something so trivial as a cup of water to satisfy thirst or so sublime as the truth of Plato's philosophy to satisfy thirst for meaning in the cosmos. A behavioral test for a value is the human reaction to it, that is, whether the value is rejected or accepted. Human debate about whether something is desirable or undesirable, acceptable or unacceptable, is clear evidence that what is in question is some value or a conflict of values.

In the twentieth century British and American ethicists have conducted a long and rather tedious debate about the relation between facts and values (Hancock, 1974; Rachels, 1986). This controversy arose because scientists today take great pains to formulate scientific statements in value-free language. This model, however, if followed in ethical and political discussions, is self-defeating.

Ethical and political talk deals not merely with the description of facts, but with how these facts are to be changed for the better.

This long controversy is still not over, but it has led to some points of agreement. First, ethical debate clearly cannot be divorced from all reference to facts; for example, every bioethical debate depends on an accurate knowledge of the medical facts (Thomasma, 1984). Second, the debaters must give good reasons for their ethical positions in terms of these certified facts (Hare, 1952, 1987). That is, it is irrelevant in bioethical debate merely to talk about how one *feels* about abortion; there must also be reference to its consequences for those involved. Third, in all ethical discussions people refer to evident human needs (for example, it is good to be able to see and walk, bad to be blind and crippled), so that serious ethical issues arise when it is a question of blinding or mutilating a human being (B. Brody, 1983a). Fourth, ultimately ethical debates return to questions about value systems, that is, to the religious or philosophical view of the meaning and value of human life as a whole.

Chapters 7 and 8 take a definite stand on this facts-value issue. At this point, suffice it to say that ethical values are rooted in the value of human persons and in the concern to meet their basic needs in the human community in balanced and consistent ways.

Others have devised even more elaborate lists of natural needs (Grisez, 1983), but some, such as Gordon Allport (1937, 1961), have objected to all such classifications as too heavily based on the notion of instincts. For Allport, the innate tendencies of human beings are so broad, require so elaborate a set of cultural conditions to develop, and develop so much in the context of an individual personality with a personal biography that he wishes to avoid the notion of need or instinct altogether. Allport speaks only of the development, differentiation, and integration of a personality in interaction with natural and social environments. However, Allport cannot avoid discussing different *tendencies* of the human organism in the effort to adjust to or control his or her environment. We consider these *tendencies* to be similar to natural *needs*.

Thus we can distinguish at least the following dimensions of personality, or levels of need (B. Ashley, 1972; Maslow, 1970; Vaillant, 1977):

1. The *biological dimension* (Maslow's physiological needs). Human persons share with all living organisms the need to maintain themselves homeostatically in a dynamic relation with their environment, to grow and mature to full biological development as individuals, and to continue the species through reproduction. This is the level usually dealt with by biologists and physicians.

2. The *psychological dimension* (Maslow's safety needs, as well as belonging-ness and love needs in their more emotional aspects). Human persons are psychic organisms who sense, imagine, and feel. This is the level of need generally dealt with by experimental psychologists and psycho-therapists.

3. The *social dimension* (Maslow's esteem needs, as well as the belongingness and love needs in their more developed aspects). This is the level of human free choice within the limits of an existing culture. Social

17

dimension comprises the need of the individual both for self-control and for social relations beyond those determined by the family. This is the level dealt with by lawyers, political leaders, and clergy acting as moral counselors.

4. The *spiritual or creative dimension* (Maslow's need for self-actualization, including needs to know and understand, to contemplate, and to create). Although many refer to this level of need as the spiritual, we add the word *creative* because many people confine the meaning of *spiritual* to our relationship to God. This is the level of commitment, creativity, and transcendence at which persons not only live within a culture, but criticize it, transcend it, and contribute to it. This dimension includes all activity with a creative element—in art or science or political innovation—in addition to religious activity as it extends to ultimate, cosmic meaning. This is the level dealt with by the inspiring teacher and spiritual guide.

Each of these levels contains a complex of natural and cultural needs; the cultural needs are rooted in the natural needs but greatly expand them. It cannot be emphasized too strongly that these four levels of needs are not stories in a building but *dimensions* that can no more be separated from one another than the length, breadth, and height of a cube. Every human act or event has *all* four dimensions. A human spiritual activity, whether the creative activity of a scientist or artist or the graced acts of faith, hope, or love, is at the same time a biological, psychological, and social event. Reciprocally, human biological acts or events, whether eating, sexual activities, or simple physical movement, are not only psychological events but uniquely human social and spiritual events.

Moreover, the reciprocity between these levels of the organization and function of the human personality are hierarchically ordered. Thus spiritual activities are the deepest, most central, and most integrating; biological activities are the least unified and the most peripheral; and psychological and social activities have intermediate positions. At the same time, the higher activities in this hierarchy are rooted in and dependent on the lower ones in a network of interrelations. Nevertheless, each level has a certain genuine autonomy and differentiation in its structure and modes of functioning, so it is necessary (as Chapter 2 demonstrates) that each be served respectively by the different professions of medicine, psychotherapy, ethical counseling, and spiritual direction, using different healing and helping techniques.

The ethical problem persons face is to plan their lives and engage in political decision in such a way that *all* these needs are satisfied to some degree in an integrated and consistent manner. This obviously requires the adjustment of priorities in regard to both aims and objectives and adjustment of the practical steps to be taken. This activity also demands the subordination, and even sacrifice, of less important needs to greater ones. The exact mix or proportion will depend on both the culture and the individual.

Thus health as a value cannot be understood ethically in isolation from the whole hierarchy of values of which it is a part.

1.5   PRINCIPLE OF HUMAN DIGNITY IN COMMUNITY

This section examines the *humanity* of the health seeker. It is humanity that differentiates human health from mere animal or vegetative health and from the functioning of a well-oiled machine. This discussion of humanity can be summed up in four statements:

1. Healthcare must serve human persons. Human health is the physical and psychological well-being of a living organism of the human species, distinguished from other animals by his or her personhood; that is, the organism's capacity for intellectual freedom, which can be actualized only in a truly human community. Such a community must be based primarily on the sharing of human values—the communication of truth and love—and only instrumentally on material values.

2. Since human health can be achieved only in a human community, an ethics of healthcare is also a politics. In modern pluralistic society, a politics of ethics demands an effort to increase moral consensus in regard to values and priorities through worldwide ecumenical dialogue among all those who hold diverse value systems, religious or secular. The existing basis of such a consensus is the United Nations' *Universal Declaration of Human Rights* (1948), based on the principle of human dignity.

3. The *Principle of Human Dignity in Community* can be formulated as follows: all ethical decisions, including those in healthcare, should satisfy both the innate and the cultural needs (biological, psychological, social, spiritual) of every human person as a member of the world community and some national community.

4. The specific Christian contribution to the development of this ethical consensus is its vision of authentic human dignity, as revealed in Jesus Christ, and its confident hope, based on the grace of Christ that this consensus can be practically achieved.

CHAPTER 2

Health and Disease

OVERVIEW

Chapter 1 asserts that the natural and cultural needs of the human person are the basis on which Christian ethics can seek agreement with other ethical systems. Health is the aspect of human need with which this book is concerned. Thus the concept of human health and disease that this chapter develops is grounded in the multidimensional character of the human person in community. Since health is the ultimate goal of all healthcare, this concept of health and the human right to achieve it serves as the groundwork on which we develop an ethics of healthcare.

First, this chapter deals with the concept of the person as multidimensional (2.1) and then with the various types of health—biological (2.2), psychological, ethical and social, and spiritual (2.3)—and how they are interrelated in total or integral health. Finally, 2.4 explains the Principle of Totality and Integrity, which summarizes the foregoing discussion and has many applications in concrete medical decisions, such as those concerning the transplanting of human organs.

2.1 CONCEPTS OF HEALTH AND DISEASE

Concepts of Health

The word *health* is related etymologically to the Anglo-Saxon word from which are derived not only *healing* but also *holiness* and *wholeness* (Erde, 1979; Vaux, 1978). The root of that word denotes "completeness," a whole that has all its parts. Such a whole can be considered statically as a *structure* with all its parts—each properly proportioned and all parts in their places. Thus a crippled person lacks wholeness or health because some part of his or her anatomy is missing or deformed. However, health can also be considered dynamically as a *functional* whole, in which all necessary functions are present and acting cooperatively and harmoniously. Thus some sicknesses do not involve any lack of a part or organ or its deformity, but rather a dysfunction; that is, some needed function is suppressed or there is a lack of harmonious balance between functions, as in diabetes or hyperthyroidism.

Since the goal of medicine is fostering and restoring health, the medical profession should certainly be able to explain what health is. One has only to ask the average medical student or student nurse to define health, however, to discover that their medical education is lacking in this area. Medical schools and nursing schools assume that students will glean an adequate notion of health simply from dealing with sick and healthy patients. No doubt this sometimes happens, but such an unexamined presupposition can be dangerous. For a medical professional to be working devotedly toward a goal that is vague and ill-defined is as absurd as for a cancer research team to be looking for a cure without trying first to understand the nature of the disease.

Henrik Blum (1974, 1983; Gish, 1984), in an effort to formulate a health planning guide, proposes no less than eight definitions of health, each with experience-tested advantages and disadvantages, and then adds a ninth definition of his own. In summary these are:

1. According to the *medical model,* "health is freedom from superimposed or unnatural influences." This concept has encouraged medicine to seek the causes of disease but has prolonged the dying process and discouraged preventive medicine.

2. The *preventive* or *public health model* also views health as freedom from superimposed disease, and disease is something against which barriers can be raised or whose invasion can be detected early and minimized so that function can be restored. This concept also fails to consider sufficiently the social factors of disease.

3. The *humanitarian* or *well-being model* (e.g., that of the World Health Organization [WHO]) places "man at the center of its concerns" and works for the survival of infants and mothers, the alleviation of malnutrition and cruel treatment, the ready availability of healthcare, and the provision of a safe and pleasant environment. This concept, too, has tended to prolong hopeless suffering and to substitute charity to the needy for justice in defense of the human right to adequate healthcare.

4. The *economic model* views disease in terms of factors that might prevent entry into the work force, cause the loss of effective workers and homemakers, prevent the education of productive workers, cause losses from low-productive performance, and affect cost-benefit ratios and thus lower the gross national product of a country. Such a concept has spurred on practical efforts to raise the standard of health in many countries, but it also opens the way to extermination (calculated neglect) of persons who are poor risks and poor producers.

5. The *super biological systems model* defines disease "as a natural phenomenon, and health as adaptation to environmental demands to the degree to which the individual is capable." This view stresses normal growth, development, and functioning at physiological, psychological, and sociological levels. This model has promoted scientific research but has

21

emphasized the cure of degenerative disease in adults rather than better health for those who still have a life to lead.

6. The *philosophical model* and the similar *mental health model* regard health as "the pursuit of the maximal capacity for self-realization or self-fulfillment." This concept has led to a deeper, more humane notion of healthful living, but it is open to interpretation in a selfish, individualistic sense and to neglect of less-gifted and educated groups in society.

7. The *ecological* or *species-survival model* displaces human beings from the center of things. It views human health as dependent on humankind's capacity to maintain the ecological balance of nature or to shift it cautiously to our own advantage as a species without destroying it. This view has not yet been time-tested; it promises greater respect for limited resources, however, but also may lead to defense of the social status quo in favor of the developed nations.

8. The *Third World model* emphasizes the survival of the victims of modern technology. It views disease as the result of social oppression by the advanced countries. Health is the result of a social liberation in which underdeveloped people will achieve greater productivity, learn to control population growth without genocide, and maintain religious values in the face of secularism. This concept focuses on the need for universal social justice, but it tends toward a kind of irrationalism.

9. Blum synthesizes the preceding concepts into a working definition for a *health planning model:*

> Health consists of the capacity of an organism (1) to maintain a balance appropriate to its age and social needs, in which it is reasonably free of gross dissatisfaction, discomfort, disease or disability; and (2) to behave in ways which promote the survival of the species as well as the self-fulfillment or enjoyment of the individual (p. 93).

Briefly, "health is the state of being in which an individual does the best with the capacities he has, and acts in ways that maximize his capacities" (p. 93). Blum contends that this can be measured in terms of eight parameters: (1) prematurity of death, (2) departure from physiological norms, (3) discomfort, (4) disability to function, (5) internal satisfaction, (6) external satisfaction, (7) positive health, and (8) capacity to participate in social activities.

Blum's discussion is appropriate to his immediate practical purpose, but it does not provide a fundamental concept of health that might unify all these diverse aspects. For this we must seek further.

In the actual practice of medicine today, *health* is most frequently defined (McDowell and Newell, 1987) in terms of standard physiological parameters—the vital signs, various chemicals in the blood, electroneurological readings, and so forth—as well as by gross anatomy and histology. Moreover, a complete physical examination and diagnosis of health by means of physiological tests and computerized calculations is anticipated and is partly practical already. Health, therefore, will soon be defined by a model of what is normal.

Such a model will raise some problems, however (Bakken, 1985). First, an exact, universal definition of human health in these terms obviously is impossible, and only a *range* of normal values can be achieved. In the case of some values, such as temperature, this range is large, but in all cases what is identifiably healthy for one individual does not necessarily indicate a state of health for another person. How can the model of normality be determined? *Normal* is not identical with *average,* since most persons today conceivably are not very healthy. The normal, therefore, is an *ideal* (N. Brown, 1985). How can such an ideal be determined in a way that is not arbitrary but that has a sound empirical basis?

This question prompts the notion of health as *optimal functioning* (Mershey, 1986). Clearly, health in the structural sense of absence of anatomical lesion or deformity is the same as optimal functioning because as the axiom states: *structure is for function.* The absence of a functionless part (e.g., the appendix) is not a defect of health but an advantage. Moreover, the deformity of an organ ultimately must be judged in terms of whether it is capable of optimal function. Even appearance can be considered one aspect of function because physical beauty has a social function. Thus a human being is healthy if he or she can function optimally. This implies that each organ and organ system is functioning well and that all are functioning together to form a single life process, of which the diverse functions are harmoniously interrelated yet differentiated phases.

This concept of health is a consequence of the basic concept of a human being as an *organism* (etymologically "a complex of instruments" or organs), that is, a *living whole composed of functionally differentiated parts.* A human being is thus a dynamic or *open system.* A system is a "complex of interacting elements" (Bertalanffy, 1968). A living system is dynamic or open, that is, capable of maintaining *homeostasis* (dynamic stability) in relation to its environment by regulating the input and output of matter and energy.

As Ludwig von Bertalanffy shows, the characteristics and behavior of the whole complex cannot be reduced to the characteristics and behavior of the parts, since the parts do not exist or act separately but in mutual interrelation and interaction. Moreover, in more complex systems there are several *levels* of organization in *hierarchical order,* so that the higher levels of function include the lower levels but cannot be reduced to them. The fallacy of reductionism is attempting to explain these higher levels of functioning simply in terms of lower levels or to explain the system merely in terms of its parts. To avoid reductionism, the interrelation and interaction of the parts and the levels of organization in the whole must be considered fully. The whole of the organism is not some mystical or extraneous entity added to the parts of the system; it is precisely the structural and functional interrelation and interaction of the parts.

Obviously, a definition of health in terms of optimal functioning of an open system must include the output of that system. A living thing cannot maintain itself in static existence; it must interact with the environment. This is especially obvious because living individuals must also reproduce to maintain the species, but it is also clear that living things modify the environment in their own interests. Thus animals build shelters and nests, fertilize plants on which they feed, and rid their environment of enemies. In fact, the present earth environment is largely the product of living things that have modified both the soil and the atmosphere in ways favorable to life (Birch, 1981).

In the case of human beings, a further step must be taken. Because they are cultural as well as natural beings, human beings' interaction with the environment is highly creative. They modify the environment with conscious purpose, so that civilization is the production of a city, that is, an increasingly man-made environment. Today people are beginning to think about living in an environment almost entirely artificial, for example, on the moon or even on constructed satellites, where nothing will be natural except the basic raw materials from which the total environment will be humanly constructed.

Still more interestingly, human creativity is not limited to interaction with an external environment. Man creates not only external things, but also mental and emotional symbols; these fulfill certain needs that cannot be fulfilled by what is merely objective, that is, outside conscience (Cassirer, 1953). Ultimately, human beings need to assimilate the whole order of the external environment. Thus scientists are constantly striving to recreate, as it were, the entire external cosmos in the form of symbols. The great importance of this human life process, from a personalistic point of view, is that such symbols provide communication between persons in the form of language. Human society is ultimately this communication by which we all come to live in the same symbol universe.

This internalization of the environment, however, does not nullify interaction with the external environment. Scientific knowledge can be increased only by experimentation, and communication can be accomplished only through languages, which require an external medium. Moreover, scientific advance is also technological advance. To learn more about the world, we often have to change it. Developing a human culture breaks down the barrier between mind and matter, between the internal and the external. Thus the human organism as a system is progressively opening up to include other human persons and the entire cosmos, as scientific visionaries such as Alfred North Whitehead (1929) and Pierre Teilhard de Chardin (1964) have so vividly shown.

In view of this concept of human functioning, human health as optimal functioning means not only an internal harmony and consistency of function within the organism, but also the capacity of the organism to maintain itself in its environment. With the human race especially, this means extending itself creatively to produce an ever-expanding culture. This is why the WHO, in the definition given in 1.1, insists, "Health is a state of complete physical, mental, and social well-being and not merely the absence of disease or infirmity."

Blum ends his discussion (summarized earlier in this chapter) with the brief formula, "Health is the state of being in which an individual does the best with the capacities he has, and acts in ways that maximize his capacities." Similarly, Rodney Coe (1978) defines disease as "the subjective evaluation by the individual that something is wrong with him *as an individual* and usually first noted in terms of a reduced ability to perform social roles" (p. 144). John Freymann (1974), in view of the reduction of acute disease in present times, urges health be redefined as "the presence of social function, that is, the ability to cope with and control one's environment to the maximum extent possible within the constraints of nature and circumstance" (p. 383). Optimal human functioning, however, is something more than the ability to cope with one's environment. Furthermore, an individual's capabilities are themselves open to improvement in view of the fundamental human capacity for intelligent freedom and creativity. Thus, to be precise, a definition of health must also be open, that is, be constantly revised in view of a deepening and enriching vision of human capacities for culture.

In 1.4 the levels of human needs are placed in a hierarchical order from primary physical needs to higher or cultural needs according to Maslow's scheme of five needs, or more conveniently, the four levels of *biological, psychological, social,* and *spiritual* or creative needs. Health in the broad sense of the WHO definition is thus "optimal functioning of the human organism to meet biological, psychological, social, and spiritual needs." However, the healthcare professions are concerned with health in the narrower sense of optimal functioning at the biological and psychological levels, *yet in the context of the integration of all four levels* (Pellegrino and Thomasma, 1988). Thus, although physicians specialize in biological or psychological functions, they must never neglect or ignore the social and spiritual needs of their patients if they wish to be truly concerned about health.

Concepts of Disease

Given this concept of health as structural and functional wholeness of the human organism in relation to the self and to the environment—a wholeness that extends even to the social and spiritual, to holiness—the notion of disease can also be more precisely defined (Bakken, 1985; Boorse, 1981). The WHO definition maintains that disease and infirmity are not the exact contrary of health. Health, as we have defined it, is optimal functioning. For an organism to fall short of optimal functioning without actually being diseased or infirm is possible, since an organism can be healthy in a narrow sense without actually being used to its full capacity. However, without optimal functioning, the failure to function soon leads to dysfunction. A man can be healthy in this narrow sense and still be lazy and half alive through lack of full use of his capacity for living, but he will not stay healthy even in this minimal way for long because his faculties will atrophy.

The terms *disease, illness, sickness, malady, ailment, disorder, complaint,* and many more synonyms have different connotations (Clouser et al., 1981; Margolis, 1986). Some seem to be more subjective; that is, they designate the feelings of the victim (e.g., illness, sickness, complaint); whereas others are more objective (disease, malady, ailment, disorder) (Boorse, 1981). This distinction can be questioned, however, since *disease* comes from *dis-ease,* implying a subjective sense. This book uses the term in its broad sense as the opposite of health.

In the history of medicine, as Owsei Temkin has shown (1963; Lain-Entralgo, 1970), the pendulum has constantly swung between two concepts of disease: the ontological and the physiological. The *ontological concept* regards diseases as separate entities (devils, contagions, morbific matters, bacteria, genetic defects, neuroses, psychoses), which can be classified and named as are plants and animals. The organism constantly fights to throw off such diseases as alien invaders that disturb its homeostasis. Those who think in this way tend to diagnose diseases in terms of clearly classified and labeled entities and to treat them by seeking specific remedies (e.g., specific drugs, specific surgical procedures).

The opposite of the ontological concept, the *physiological concept* views disease as a breakdown of the internal harmony of the organic system because of hyperfunctioning or hypofunctioning of an organ. Thus dysfunction opens the organism to attack by external agents such as bacteria, but the bacteria are not the primary cause of the disease. If the organism were functioning properly, it would resist such bacteria. Classifying or labeling diseases is dangerous, therefore, because disease is essentially the condition of an *individual* who is internally maladjusted. The advocates of this position thus tend to emphasize regimen or life-style and to use drugs and surgery secondarily to assist in the adjustment of the individual organism.

As Temkin and Lain-Entralgo show, the central tradition of medicine (usually identified with that of Hippocrates, the Greek "Father of Medicine") has always tried to reconcile these two extreme positions. In view of the account given of the organism as a dynamic system, such a reconciliation should not be too difficult. The physiologists are correct in thinking of health first as an internal homeostasis or harmony within the organism and disease as an imbalance. The organism as a system is constantly adjusting by means of feedback to changes in the environment. These minor fluctuations are not diseases; rather, they are health itself.

If the system fluctuates beyond a certain range, however, it cannot recover homeostasis without a major readjustment. This may be possible through the internal vital powers, but only at the cost of a period of sickness in which many normal functions must be minimized while the organism uses all its energies to readjust. Such a disease is acute illness. Also, the organism may readjust but at the cost of permanent diminishing of function or suppression of some functions. Then the disease becomes chronic, or permanent crippling or handicap results.

Finally, the adjustment may be greater than the organism can achieve, and death results. Death may be the result of acute disease or aging. Some researchers have hypothesized that aging may result from natural physiological processes that have been genetically programmed as a result of evolutionary selection—the removal of mature organisms after they have had time to reproduce in order to provide more living space for the next generation to mature and reproduce in its turn (Engelhardt, 1979). As yet this hypothesis has not been confirmed. More probably, aging is the gradual debilitation of a living system exposed to repeated disease and trauma. Thus aging is simply an application of the second law of thermodynamics (the law of increasing entropy) to living systems.

From this point of view, death is always the result of disease. Therefore death cannot be said to be natural if *natural* is meant, as the Greeks meant, the optimal function or health of the organism. Physiologically speaking, the organism seems to be made to live forever, always recovering from any malfunction. Thus death is caused by injuries inflicted on the organism from the environment, not from any intrinsic tendency. A homeostatic system, by definition, is one that maintains itself perpetually when not disturbed.

Organismic Theory

Now we move to the other side of the picture. The organism is an open system that constantly interacts with the environment. This is where the ontological theory of disease has relevance. The organism is homeostatic, but limits exist to its power of self-maintenance. Consequently, when the environment is altered beyond a certain normal range, the organism is unable to survive, Thus, when the oxygen content of the air, the temperature, or the number of bacteria in the environment greatly changes, the human organism undergoes stress, then disorganization, and finally death. Therefore diseases can be classified according to various external agents that tax the capacity of the organism to maintain itself. Diseases can be viewed as entities such as plague, pollution, or radiation sickness, that affect all the individual organisms in a given area. From this point of view, disease and death are natural in the sense that the terrestrial environment is a part of the evolutionary process from which no individual, but only the species, is protected. The species itself ultimately yields to the rise of new species. Without disease and death, natural evolution cannot continue.

This organismic theory of health and disease has been central to Western medicine, but it has had strong competition from the mechanistic theory, which dates back to the Greek Democritus. Even today the thinking of many biologists and medical educators is influenced by the mechanistic theory (Wilson and Lumsden, 1981). This theory of health does not deny that an organism is an open system, but it tends to view it in reductionist terms. For a mechanist, the parts seem to be more significant and more practically controllable than the whole. The whole is too complex either to understand or to manage, and its relational character seems tenuous and abstract. One can see and touch the parts, but to mechanists, relations seem to be only mental constructs. Mechanists are more comfortable with anatomy or structure than with function or process. They tend to reduce process to quantitative measurements of results. Their diagnoses tend toward ontologistic views in which disease is the result of alien bacteria, organic lesions, and so forth. In treatment they incline toward a mechanical adjustment of parts by surgery or use of specific drugs. This attitude is encouraged today by three factors: (1) the specialization in medicine, which emphasizes the treatment of particular organs or organ systems rather than the whole patient; (2) the increasing use of a multiplicity of drugs, of complex surgery, and of various measuring devices in diagnosis; and (3) the theoretical success of molecular biology, which promises to give an account of the whole human organism in terms of its ultimate atomic parts.

Maintaining an organismic view in no way denies the mechanistic view; rather, it includes this view. The notion of dynamic system necessarily includes a detailed analysis of the parts, the interacting elements. To posit vitalistic or holistic forces apart from the interaction of the parts is unscientific (Sinha, 1983). An organismic view, however, insists that the relations among the parts are just as real, just as scientifically observable and intelligible, as the interrelated parts. Moreover, the parts themselves cannot be observed or understood in isolation but only in the context of the system in which they exist. The eye or the kidney, the cell, and even the macromolecular gene cannot be understood except in the context of the whole organism of which they are parts. Medical specialization, therefore, can never be separated from a medical understanding of the whole person, nor can health or disease be defined except in terms of the whole and its parts.

One of the factors that has contributed to mechanistic prejudices in medicine has been the fear of teleology (see 1.4). A homeostatic system necessarily introduces the notion of ends and means, since such a system tends to constantly achieve a normal state that is the end or, in Greek, *telos*—namely, optimal functioning. The various vital processes thus are means tending to an end or goal. They have direction or inherent tendency. This is precisely what the Greeks meant by *nature*. The nature of a thing is its goal-directed tendency. For a living thing, such goal-directedness is its tendency to develop embryologically into a mature, fully differentiated organism—to carry on the various vital functions in an optimal manner, to reproduce itself, to maintain itself in the environment, and to modify the environment and itself in a life-enhancing, or creative, way (Nagel, 1979).

The mechanist is uncomfortable with these concepts because they seem to introduce purpose into the natural world and to imply some type of psychic dimension even in plants and minerals. Moreover, the mechanist argues that such thinking has been fruitless in scientific research, since science does not deal with purposes but with agents that produce results according to fixed laws. In particular, the theory of evolution, which has been so successful in modern biology, seems to explain all living things purely in terms of agent-causes, that is, the natural selection (without any guiding purpose) of those things most able to reproduce in a given environment.

The fallacy of this mechanistic rejection of teleology is twofold: (1) the supposition that purpose necessarily implies consciousness in that which tends to a goal and (2) the supposition that the identification of an agent-cause is a sufficient explanation of a process. Teleology simply implies that inherent in agent-causes are tendencies to produce directed or goal-oriented actions and processes. Bertalanffy (1968) and others have shown that homeostatic systems necessarily involve directed and purposeful tendencies controlled by feedback mechanisms. As Bertalanffy states:

> ... teleological behavior directed towards a characteristic final state or goal is not something off limits for natural science and an anthropomorphic misconception of process which, in themselves, are undirected and accidental. Rather it is a form of behaviour which can well be defined in scientific terms and for which the necessary conditions and possible mechanisms can be indicated (p. 46).

In medicine particularly, some have actually wanted to eliminate the term *health* altogether on the grounds that it is normative—a value term rather than a scientific value-free term. Once teleology is admitted, however, then the *goal* becomes the norm or value from which the means to the goal are also evaluated. Having defined human health as optimal functioning and having understood this as the satisfaction of innate and cultural needs, or the realization of potentialities, we have defined a norm by which the means to health can be discriminated from what tends toward disease and death, that is, the suppressing or disuse of functions.

Sociologists' View of Health and Illness

Recently, however, a very powerful criticism has been raised against all such definitions of *health* and *disease* by the sociologist Eliot Freidson in his book *Profession of Medicine: A Study of the Sociology of Applied Knowledge* (1971) (see also Fabrega, 1980). Beginning with Talcott Parsons (1951), sociologists have been studying the medical profession as the typical profession and have been trying to specify not so much its technical as its *social* function (Aiken, 1986). Eliot Freidson, basing his ideas on the sociology of knowledge of Peter Berger and Thomas Luckmann (1966), develops a theory he calls "the social construction of illness." He grants that some physical disorders (and perhaps some mental ones) are unambiguously, and objectively, "illness," such as a broken leg or smallpox. He emphasizes, however, that these disorders are only a small part of what society considers to be illness and with which the medical profession deals. The actual definition of *health* and *disease* in any society is a "social construction" produced by many variable factors and essentially dependent on how society, the medical profession, and the patient behave toward certain phenomena.

Furthermore, Freidson (1971), Conrad and Kern (1981), and other authors emphasize that the tendency in the United States today is to assign the term *illness* to more and more phenomena previously given other labels:

> The medical mode of response to deviance is thus being applied to more and more behaviour in our society, much of which has been responded to in quite different ways in the past. In our day, what has been called crime, lunacy, degeneracy, sin, and even poverty in the past is now being called illness, and social policy has been moving toward adopting a perspective appropriate to the imputation of illness. Chains have been struck off and everywhere health professionalism has been raised to legitimate the claim that the proper management of deviance is "treatment" in the hands of responsible and skilled professionals. The labels of sin and crime being removed, what is done to the deviant is likely to be said to be done for his own good, done to help him rather than punish him, even though the treatment itself may constitute a deprivation under ordinary circumstances. His own opinions about his treatment are discounted because he is said to be a layman who lacks the special knowledge and detachment that would qualify him to have his voice heard (pp. 249-250).

If the sociologists are correct, it seems extremely unjust for a society thus arbitrarily to label persons sick because they do not conform to average behavior in that society. Consequently, some people today are demanding that society cease to label any behavior sick or abnormal unless it is obviously dangerous to others. Thus the psychoanalyst Thomas Szasz, whom Freidson quotes with approval, argues that drug addiction and alcoholism should be treated not as diseases but as personal preferences that, if they do any harm, harm only the addict. Similarly, the American Psychiatric Association has removed homosexuality from its list of mental illnesses to avoid stigmatizing the homosexual, whose behavioral tendencies should simply be considered personal preferences (R. Bayer, 1987; Marmoc, 1980).

This approach of Freidson, Szasz, and others, although undoubtedly very useful in uncovering the social processes by which definitions of health and normality are constructed in different cultures, prompts the question of whether all definitions of health are simply cultural artifacts. Obviously, this question raises a broad epistemological issue about *cultural relativism*. Even Freidson, however, admits that some conditions (e.g., broken bones) can be determined as abnormal by objective criteria that are transcultural. His real point is that such definitions are too readily used to cover other conditions that are only *analogously* diseases.

Analogy is a necessary mode of thought and dangerous only when it is not recognized as such. This book deliberately extends the term *health* from its strict medical application at the biological level to the other dimensions of human personality. This seems necessary to do justice to the wholeness of the human person, who can be sick in many different but closely interrelated ways. At the same time, we have tried to avoid the pitfalls pointed out by Freidson and Szasz by clearly distinguishing the different analogical uses of health and disease in the four dimensions of human personality and to indicate the different criteria of normality appropriate to each.

The application of such varied criteria is not always easy or unambiguous or free from arbitrary social construction (Armstrong, 1980). With due respect for the cautions of the sociologists of knowledge, however, we hope to improve constantly our transcultural statements of these criteria.

The theologian Paul Tillich (1967) has remarked that human beings, as illusion prone as they are, can easily mistake for genuine health what he calls "unhealthy health." Of the unhealthy health, Tillich says:

> ... (it) comes about if healing under one dimension is successful but does not take into consideration the other dimensions in which health is lacking or even imperiled by the particular healing. Successful surgery may produce a psychological trauma; effective drugs may calm down an uneasy conscience and preserve a moral deficiency; the well-trained, athletic body may contain a neurotic personality; the healed patient of the analyst may be sick through lack of an ultimate meaning of his life, the conformist's average life may be sick through inhibited self-alteration; the converted Christian may suffer under repressions which produce fanaticism and may explode in lawless forms; the same society may produce psychological and biological disruptions by the desire for creative insanity (p. 11).

Authentic health, therefore, must be multidimensional.

2.2 BIOLOGICAL HEALTH AND BIOLOGISM

This book cannot present even a sketch of the biological level of human functioning so well known to healthcare professionals. Biological and medical science are constantly making new discoveries about the tissues, organs, and secretions that constitute the human body—their chemical composition, structure, functional interrelations, and control of their differentiation, development, and modification through the environment and individual biography.

The important question for healthcare ethics is how this biological level of functioning can be considered truly human and personal, as having profound moral and spiritual significance. Dualistic theories of the human being have been present in all cultures throughout human history. According to these theories, body and soul are in essential conflict with each other (i.e., the biological and psychological levels of human functioning versus the ethical and spiritual levels). Generally, the body is regarded as the negative factor and the soul as the positive factor.

Underestimating the plausibility of this dualistic anthropology would be a mistake. The body is frequently experienced as a burden, as something negative, for two reasons.

First, a great part of biological functioning is voluntary and deterministic. People cannot voluntarily control much of what goes on inside them. Even with medical advances, biological life is veiled in mystery. Often uncontrollable, such life becomes deranged and fails human purposes. People find themselves weary and exhausted, unable to do what they would like to do. Suffering from pain and disease, people are painfully conscious that eventually the body becomes subject to age and ultimate failure in death. Thus the body appears as a burden, a liability.

Second, the basic biological drives are urgent, constant, and inescapable—the need for sleep, the fear of insecurity, the demands of hunger and thirst, and the tension of sexual desire. They are so insistent that people feel them as compulsions, limiting their freedom and sometimes overwhelming them against their will.

Since the dignity of human personhood consists essentially in self-understanding and freedom, we find it profoundly humiliating to be the helpless victims of our own bodies, with their limited energies, liability to pain, and their urgent and deterministic demands that arise from unconscious depths and disorganize our self-possession and freedom of action. Our bodies seem to drag us down to the animal level of unfree, instinctive, and blind action. In all religious mythologies this pull is often typified in the fear of sexuality as a regression to the primitive chaos (Neumann, 1964). The sex drive has always seemed especially mysterious; it subordinates the freedom of the individual to the imperious needs of the species. People feel severely disturbed at times by sexual passion, reduced to the level of the animal in heat, and deluded by a promise of pleasure that is very brief, and that may be followed by pregnancy, childbirth, and family responsibility. Thus the woman, whose biological functioning is more profoundly determined than the man's by the processes of menstruation, pregnancy, childbirth, and nursing and who in the human species is the more attractive or

31

stimulating partner for sexual activity, is in most cultures mistakenly regarded as somehow negative in contrast to the positive male, who is freer of such biological limitations for other activities (Richardson, 1971).

Thus it is understandable that dualism is so widespread (H. Lewis, 1982). Dualism is essential to certain religious systems (Buddhism, Gnosticism, Manicheism) and has affected all them (the Neo-Platonic influences in Jewish, Christian, and Muslim theologies). In the extreme form (Manicheism), the body is thought of as intrinsically evil (Runciman, 1982). In more moderate forms, the body is simply thought of as negative. One might think that such dualistic views are no longer common, since modern society emphasizes the value of sensual pleasure, the dependence of psychic functions on the body, and the equality of male and female.

Today, however, dualism is reappearing under new forms. Thus some sociobiologists (Greene, 1983) have interpreted the theory of evolution to imply that, in relation to the present environment, the human body is archaic and outmoded. This body was formed by evolution for a primitive environment where human beings had to be highly aggressive and very fertile to survive. Thus the body is not badly adapted to modern artificial culture, in which aggressive drives lead to war and antisocial violence, and excessive sexual drives and fertility lead to overpopulation and neurosis. This view has also been supported by Sigmund Freud's belief that a basic antipathy exists between the demands of civilization and the human being's basic drives and results in the liability to severe neuroses. To this Freud also added the notion of the death wish, an innate tendency of human beings to regress to the primitive and to ultimate extinction of the individual in the universal rhythm of nature (Freud, 1920).

Armed with these ideas, and especially since overpopulation is an increasing threat, many modern theorists are convinced that the biological level of human life is a threat to human freedom (Oakley, 1981) and must be brought under radical control. Many think of the poor and the people of the Third World as primitives—living an instinctive, almost animal life and reproducing "recklessly" as do rabbits. They also think of the traditional feminine role of the mother and housewife as having this limited, unfree, and subhuman character. They therefore propose that the truly human life for men and women should be similar to what upper-class men have always enjoyed, in which biological activities, especially sexuality, are reduced to simple entertainment to be used or not used at will.

From such discussions, one can easily conclude that the facts of human biology as such have no moral significance but derive their moral meaning from the context of culture as a product of human invention and choice. Consequently, many theologians today (C. Curran, 1984; Kosnik, 1977; J. McNeill, 1976) claim that traditional moral theologians went too far when they attempted to establish moral norms on the basis of a distinction between behavior that is natural and behavior that is unnatural for human beings considered as biological organisms. Such faulty arguments, they say, can be rejected as vitiated by the "fallacy of biologism" or "physicalism." On the other hand, defenders of such traditional positions (e.g., Grisez, 1983; W.E. May, 1983) emphasize the opposite danger of a new dualism in which the animal and the rational aspects of human beings are seen as unrelated or even inimical.

It is fallacious to argue that the moral character of human behavior can be settled simply by asking biologists what is natural or unnatural to animals or even to human beings. The important distinction between the moral and the physical specifications of an act are discussed in 8.1. The morality of any act must be considered in the context of the activity of the human person as a whole, since the biological level of function is only one level of the total system. Conversely, however, this consideration means that the moral or social meaning of a human act cannot be indifferent or neutral to its biological character. Every human act is an act of the whole person, involving spiritual, social, psychological, and biological dimensions. Every human biological function has human (and therefore spiritual and social significance) and, conversely, even the most spiritual activities involve the body and must respect the structure and functioning of the body.

A sounder approach to this whole issue can be found in the Aristotelian tradition, which, in opposition to Platonic dualism, stressed the unity of the human person, of which body and soul are only complementary aspects. Theologians of all the great monotheistic religions (Judaism, Christianity, Islam) have insisted that this unity is a necessary implication of the doctrine of the creation of the human person by God and of the resurrection of the body. These theologians also have rejected the notion of reincarnation found in polytheistic religions because it seems to imply that the human person is a purely spiritual being and the body only its prison or a garment to be changed. Christianity goes even further by insisting on the Incarnation (through which God becomes truly a human being in bodily existence) and on the Indwelling of the Holy Spirit in the human body as its temple, through which believers become members of the Body of Christ. This same principle leads to the sacramental concept of the human body by which the basic biological functions become signs of spiritual events; birth is reenacted in Baptism, eating and drinking in the Eucharist, and sexual union in the Sacrament of Matrimony.

Christian theology, however, recognizes a certain measure of truth in body-soul dualism that can be reconciled with the fundamental unity of the human person. The human person is a complex unity in which conflicts can arise, so that the integration and self-individuation of any man or woman can be achieved only by discipline and a sane asceticism. Such asceticism, however, does not imply that the human body in its biological functions is evil or of little value, but rather that it shares in the spiritual dignity of the total person and therefore needs to be integrated with the other dimensions of human personality (Van Kaam, 1985). Thus the body cannot be suppressed or ruthlessly sacrificed to higher values or even trivialized as of no moral significance. Instead, Catholic theology has always been concerned to find a middle way between the dualistic extremes of asceticism and antinomianism and to respect the intrinsic teleology of bodily structures and basic biological functions.

2.3   THE HIGHER LEVELS OF HEALTH

The development of modern psychotherapy and of psychosomatic medicine leaves no doubt that, although mental health is intimately connected with physical health, it is not identical with physical health. Chapter 12 states more precisely what this differentiation and interdependence are. It suffices at this point to grant that such a difference exists, since mental disease is not describable in terms of physiological malfunction but in terms of impairment in the characteristic human ability to deal with the environment by *symbolic* activity and communication.

Human beings far surpass animals in the capacity to use symbols (images, feelings, words) that stand for realities but that can be combined and ordered in many ways different from the relatively fixed order of real things. The images and concepts by which a human being represents the world do so only imperfectly, but they can be verified and refined by the use of them as tools to change the world. Physical disease, especially dysfunctions of the central nervous system, can impair this symbolic activity, but it also can be disturbed by social and educational factors within the symbolic realm itself. For example, a physiologically healthy child can acquire prejudiced ways of perceiving reality and neurotic ways of reacting to it emotionally through his or her social environment. This environment cannot be adequately described as just bodies in time and space; it must also be described as a symbolic communication system.

At this level of symbolic or psychic activity, however, there are also differentiated levels of health and disease that are too often lumped together. To reduce human psychic health to emotional adjustment and maturity is a typical fallacy today that can be termed *psychologism*. Psychologism assumes that a physically healthy person who also is free of mental illnesses, which are considered the proper competency of psychotherapy, is totally healthy (Vitz, 1977).

As Chapter 12 shows, psychotherapy has the modest goal of helping patients acquire that degree of self-understanding and emotional integration that will free them from unconscious psychological determinisms that interfere with daily practical life. Psychologically healthy persons are "in touch with their feelings." They perceive the world of ordinary activity as most people do, without manifestly absurd illusions or projections. They are free to choose between practical alternatives and do not have unrealistic expectations. They are responsible for the consequences of their actions.

At this point of freedom from psychological determination, a whole new level of human activity opens up: the level of free, responsible, moral activity. Psychotic persons are incapable of *moral* action (at least within the area of the psychosis), whereas neurotic persons are severely limited in their freedom and responsibility. Only the free man or woman is a person fully capable of either moral good or evil. Don Browning (1983) pointed out that problems of ethical counseling are often confused with those of psychological counseling. Many clergy today seem to have abandoned their traditional role of helping people make ethical decisions and have become amateur psychotherapists. Chapters 7 and 8 define more precisely the ways in which moral or ethical health differs from psychological health because of the centrality of freedom and responsibility at the ethical level of human functioning.

It is also possible to fall into the fallacy of moralism (Haan et al., 1985). This error reduces human failure to questions of right and wrong, attributes either mental or physical disease to the victims' sins, and attempts to heal them by moral exhortations. The reaction of many people to the AIDS epidemic follows this pattern of thought. A more subtle form of this same fallacy is the assumption that the highest wholeness in the human personality is achieved at the level of practical ethical life. Some people identify the good person with the responsible, prudent, decent man or woman.

This fallacy ignores the deepest and most central fact of the human personality—the aspect that is spiritual, intuitive, and creative. Some psychotherapists of the Jungian and existentialist schools do concern themselves with this level, but only to free such activity from neurotic and psychotic impediments. To deal with this spiritual level of human existence in its own terms is the task of neither the psychologist nor the moralist, but of the philosopher, theologian, and spiritual guide as Chapter 14 shows. Spiritual health and disease, therefore, cannot be reduced simply to moral or psychological terms.

Even at this spiritual level it is possible to fall into the fallacy of what the philosopher Jacques Maritain (1929) called "angelicism"—treating human persons as bodiless angels, or pure souls, as Plato and Descartes conceived the true human self. Human problems cannot be treated in purely spiritual terms, in which the lower levels of functioning, human physiology, human symbolic activity, and human practical responsibility are ignored. Today it seems that this fallacy has influenced those mystical and religious enthusiasts who attempt to heal all bodily, psychological, and moral ills by purely spiritual means.

Thus trying to understand the fullness of human health requires being on guard against those reductionist fallacies that ignore health's many dimensions. For example, to determine whether alcoholism is a sickness without reductionism or arbitrary social construction, alcoholism must first be defined in behavioral terms and then four questions asked. First, is it a biological disease in terms of biological criteria, for example, a change in physiology that puts a strain on biological homeostasis? Second, is alcoholism a psychological disease in terms of psychological criteria, for example, a persistent emotional conflict that restricts the victim's capacity for intelligent free choice? Third, is it a moral disease in terms of social criteria, for example, free choice of behavior that is contradictory to the full actualization of the person in community? Fourth, is alcoholism a spiritual disease by spiritual criteria, for example, closure to intuition, creativity, and commitment? Moreover, how are these different levels of functioning interrelated? The terms *disease* and *health* are used at each of these levels in very different but analogous ways.

2.4   PRINCIPLE OF TOTALITY AND INTEGRITY

Integrity of the Person

In summary, human nature is an open system with several hierarchical orders of functioning. The term *integrity* indicates that in a perfect whole, each part must be fully differentiated and developed. Furthermore, each part must be fitted into the whole and harmonized with it by correct interrelations and interactions with the other parts of the whole. Integrity is lacking when a part is suppressed or unduly inhibited in function or when, on the other hand, one part is hypertrophied to the injury of others.

In a hierarchical order, some parts are said to be higher because they are necessary to the unification and integration of the whole in the performance of its most complex and specific functions (e.g., the central nervous system), and other parts are said to be lower because their functions are more integrated than integrating. The lower parts, however, may be essential for the higher parts to function at all (e.g., liver, kidneys). According to Maslow's theory (1970; see 1.4) of the hierarchy of human needs, the lower needs must be met before the higher needs can be, since lower functions are related to higher functions as means to ends. An end cannot be achieved without the means, but the end *measures* and integrates the means into a whole system. Since the means are relative to the end, however, the means cannot be skipped but can be limited or restricted so that they truly serve the end rather than overpower it.

This concept is expressed in the saying, "He lives to eat, but should eat to live," which means engaging in higher activities ("living") requires eating. Consequently, eating is integral to human life. However, eating is a lower activity, a means, not an end. When eating becomes an end, an absolute not measured by something higher, it destroys the integrity of human functioning.

It would be a mistake, however, to think that only the higher values in this hierarchy are human personal values. People share biological and psychological needs with other animals, whereas they share social and spiritual needs only with other human persons. Nevertheless, all these needs and their correlative values, whether generically animal or specifically human, are *equally* needs and values of the human person, none of which can be destroyed without destroying personhood. People are human not only because they need love, but also because they need food (Pius XII, 1952).

Equally to be avoided today is the widespread error that since human sexuality and other bodily needs are truly human, they differ *totally* in their meaning from animal needs. We do not assert our human identity by denying that we are truly animals with animal needs. A correct understanding of the human person demands a full appreciation of the *mutual* interdependence of all the various dimensions of human personality, all of which are essential to human personhood.

This hierarchical yet interdependent ordering of the four levels of human functioning holds also for any subsystem within each level. At the biological level, the human body is divided into organ systems and these into organs, each having specific functions. The organ systems are usually enumerated as follows: (1) nervous, (2) endocrine, (3) skeletal and muscular, (4) integumentary (skin), (5) alimentary, (6) respiratory, (7) circulatory, (8) excretory, and (9) reproductive. These systems are interrelated in very complex ways and not in any simple, linear hierarchy. However, the nervous system (with the intimately related endocrine system) is obviously the one that coordinates the others and is the most directly involved in the psychological and higher functions. Also, the reproductive system has a special importance because (1) it is directly involved in the evolutionary process by which the human species came to be and is continued and (2) it is the source of the family and thus of the communal character of the human person.

Greater unification of function occurs at the psychic level of personality. Psychic life, however, is also composite. The external senses clearly are differentiated by their organs. Other psychological functions have some type of localization in various parts of the brain, although they also involve other centers and the endocrine system as well. Furthermore, as depth psychology has shown, the field of awareness itself is differentiated into an unconscious, a subconscious, a superego, an ego, and so forth. Although some Catholic moral theologians (C. Curran, 1984) suppose that the so-called faculty psychology traditional in Christian anthropology is obsolete, it still remains valid in the light of modern empirical psychology when properly understood in terms of differentiated functions (emotions) and is very helpful in understanding psychic integration.

At the rational and ethical levels, still greater integration and unification of functions into the self-aware, conscious, free, self-controlling subject or person take place. Even at this level, what have been traditionally called the reason and the will are differentiated as distinct but ultimately correlative functions. Only at the spiritual level do the intellect and will come together in the "still point" (Aloming, 1982) or top of the mind or heart (in the biblical, metaphorical sense) of the human person, in which peak experiences (Frager and Fadiman, 1985) and basic decisions, commitments, and fundamental options take place to complete the total integration of the person.

Totality of the Person

An important ethical question arising from this concept of the human person as an open hierarchical system is whether it is permissible in some circumstances to sacrifice one part or function in the interests of another or of the whole. In medical ethics this is a recurrent problem, such as in surgery, sterilization, and organ transplantation. Traditionally, such cases were covered by the Principle of Totality, simply stated by Thomas Aquinas (1976 ed.) as follows:

> Since any member is part of the whole human body, it exists for the sake of the whole as the imperfect for the sake of the perfect. Hence, a member of the human body is to be disposed of according as it may profit the whole. *Per se*, the member of the human body is useful for the welfare of the whole body; *per accidens* however it can happen that it is harmful, for example, when a diseased member is injurious to the whole body. If, therefore, a member is healthy and continuing in its natural state, it cannot be cut off to the detriment of the whole (II-II,q.65,a.1,c.).

Aquinas applied this principle not only to the individual person considered as a substantial whole, but also by analogy to the community, considered as a whole made up of many distinct but interrelated substances (persons). Thus he defended capital punishment when undertaken by public authority for the sake of the common good, that is, the sacrifice of one member of the community for the good of the whole community (van der Haag and Conrad, 1983). However, in modern times the experience of the totalitarianism of the Nazi and the Stalinist regimes led Pius XII (1952) to stress that this wider interpretation of the principle is only analogical, since the human body and the body politic are very different forms of totalities:

> The community is the great medium ordained by nature and by God to regulate the exchanges by which mutual needs are met, to help each one to develop his personality according to his individual social capacity. The community, considered as a whole, is not a physical unity which subsists in itself. Its individual members are not integrated parts of it. The physical organism of living beings, of plants, animals, or men, possesses as a whole a unity which subsists in itself. Each of the members, for example, the hand, the foot, the heart, the eye, is an integrating part, destined by its whole being to be a part of one complete organism. Outside the organism it has not of its own nature, any meaning, any purpose; its being is wholly absorbed in the complete organism with which it is linked.

> A quite different state of affairs obtains in the moral community and in each organism of a purely moral character. The whole has not here a unity which subsists in itself, but a simple unity of purpose and of action. In the community the individuals are only collaborators and instruments for the realization of the ends of the community.

> What follows with regard to the physical organism? The master, the person who uses this organism, which possesses a subsisting unity, can dispose directly and immediately of the integrating parts, the members and the organs, within the framework of their natural finality. Likewise he can intervene, when and as far as the well-being of the whole demands, to paralyze, destroy, mutilate, separate its members. In contrast, however, when the whole does not possess a unity except of finality and of action, its head, that is to say, in the present case the public authority, retains without doubt a direct authority, and the right to impose its demands on the activity of the parts, but in no case can it dispose directly of its physical being. Moreover, every direct injury attempted against its essential being by public authority is a departure from that sphere of activity which rightly belongs to it (n. 371).

In this discussion Pius XII in one respect widened the Principle of Totality by making it clear that it applied not only to the sacrifice of a diseased organ, but also to that of a healthy organ for the good of the whole body; for example, the removal of healthy testes to suppress the production of hormones that might stimulate the growth of cancer elsewhere in the body (O'Donnell, 1976). Nevertheless, Pius XII clearly intended to restrict the principle to the individual, so that theologians abandoned this principle as a justification for transplantation of organs from one person to another and developed a new justification on the basis of charity. McFadden (1967) has emphasized that the principle is to be understood not in terms of a *part* as a physical part, but rather as a *function*. Thus this principle is not required to justify the cutting of hair or toenails, the removal of (apparently) nonfunctional organs such as the appendix and tonsils (even when they are healthy), and blood transfusions and skin grafts.

Haring (1973), although he accepts Pius XII's restriction of the principle to the individual, interprets the term *whole* not to mean the "whole body," but the "whole person." He writes (his italics):

> The traditional use of the Principle of Totality justified intervention in view of physical health and functioning. Medical ethics for the future must rest on an all-embracing concept of "totality"; *the dignity and well-being of a man as a person in all his essential relationships to God, to his fellowmen, and to the world around him* (p. 62).

Haring goes on to insist that this includes the call from God for human beings to perfect their own nature:

> Each intervention or medical provision that helps or enhances the wholeness of the human person is right—be it a plastic heart or any other fantastic feat. If, for instance, genetic engineering can eliminate the XYY chromosomal anomaly and thus protect humanity from the heavy burden of dangerous criminal tendencies in a number of people, why should we object to it (p. 64)?

Haring is correct in thinking that it is not possible simply to speak of the good of the body, since the body itself is only a part of the person and any substantial part is entirely relative to the substantial whole. In the words of Pius XII already quoted: "Outside the organism it has not of its own nature, any meaning, any purpose; its being is wholly absorbed in the complete organism with which it is linked" (n. 371). If such is true of an organ of the body, it is also true itself as a substantial part of the person, the ensouled organism.

Although his examples are questionable, Haring is also correct in stating that God wills not only that persons care for their bodies, but also that they perfect them, even by new medical technologies, as Chapter 3 explains. Haring's extended definition of "totality," however, is excessive. Looking at the person "in all his essential relationships to God, to his fellowmen, and the world around him," seems to move back into an analogical sense of "whole," since this will include the social and even the cosmic whole.

Consequently, it seems necessary to reformulate the Principle of Totality in a way that not only applies to the good of the whole person, but also clarifies what this good is. Haring is correct in saying that this human good is relational. *Person* is correlative to *community*, as 1.2 shows. But what is it that opens the human being to community?

One could say that a person's highest, most personal powers are at the spiritual level and perhaps also at the social and psychological levels. Consequently, one could argue that any part of the body at the biological level might be sacrificed to contribute to a person's higher functioning. Thus (to enter the world of science fiction) one could also argue that in the future it may be desirable to use medical technology to reduce the human person to a brain floating in a nutritive and protective bath and communicating with other brains electronically. Such a brain would still be a person, capable of "all his essential relationships to God, to his fellowmen, and to the world around him," if these relations are defined in terms of knowledge, love, free choice, communication, and action on matter. Furthermore, such brain-persons could reproduce artificially by some asexual, test-tube process, or to go a step further, might be maintained in deathless perpetuity.

Would this transformation of the human person into a brain-person be for the *good* of the person—a perfecting of human nature—or an impoverishment? Intuitively, most people would probably call it impoverishment. The sound reason for this insight is provided by the foregoing analysis of the complex, hierarchical, mutually dependent structure of human nature as a dynamic system. Human nature cannot be reduced merely to its highest functions, as the Platonists reduced the self to a simple, spiritual soul for which the body was a mere container or instrument. Rather, the human person is a series of interactive integrity (Ramsey, 1975).

The validity of this intuition is even clearer considering the historical, evolutionary character of human nature. Precisely because human nature is an organic bodily system with many levels of functioning, it was fittingly produced by an evolutionary process. Its wholeness consists in the interdependence of higher and lower spiritual and bodily functions. Consequently, the lower functions cannot be sacrificed to the higher functions without qualification. This sacrifice might be to the advantage of the higher functions but not to the good of one part, even if that part is the highest.

To be a perfect human being, therefore, is not merely to have the higher level functions but to have *all* the basic human functions in a harmonious order. This order requires the subordination of the lower functions to the higher functions but also forbids their total sacrifice, since the higher functions depend also on the lower. Also, this dependence cannot be simply supplied by some means external to the person. For example, the ability to produce babies in test tubes does not of itself justify the elimination of the reproductive power of human persons as no longer necessary. The possibility of intravenous feeding does not justify the elimination of the human alimentary system. Human perfection requires that the human person reproduce and eat in a human manner. Such substitutions of external means of life may be justified temporarily out of necessity, but they are not perfections of human nature.

Human bodily functions contribute to higher functions not merely by supplying what is needed for physiological brain functions; they also supply part of the human experience essential to human intelligence and freedom. Bodily feelings (movement, eating, sexuality, manipulation of the environment) develop self-awareness and relation to the community. Thus, if a child were conceived in a test tube and gestated in an artificial womb and then raised in a laboratory, it is doubtful that he or she would have essential human experiences (Rennie, 1985).

Some find it very inconsistent that the Roman Catholic Church disapproves sterilization as a suppression of a basic human function, but lauds the practice of celibacy. Chapters 8 and 10 deal with the question more fully, but here one should note the important distinction between the ethical obligation to preserve basic human capacities (unless forced to sacrifice one to preserve the life of the whole) and the obligation to use one of these capacities in a particular way. Celibate persons do not castrate themselves; they freely choose not to use their sexual powers genitally. This choice does not mean that they fail to return interest on the gift committed to them by their Creator, who made them men and women. Rather, they choose to use their human sexuality in such a way as to learn to love and serve a community wider than the family. This entails sacrifice, it is true, but sacrifice of secondary values rather than of essential values necessary for the complete development of their personhood (K. Clark, 1986; Kiesling, 1977).

Totality and Integrity

The foregoing discussion of totality and integrity can be summarized as follows:
1. Primarily, human health is not merely a matter of organs, but also of capacities to function humanly.
2. In general, any particular human functional capacity can be sacrificed when necessary for the good of the whole person, that is, so that the person may better exercise all other human functions.
3. Secondary functions can always be sacrificed for more basic ones. For example, a finger can be removed to save the use of the hand, since the capacity of action given by one finger is secondary in relation to the capacity given by the hand as a whole.
4. Primary or basic functional capacities, however, cannot be sacrificed even to more important capacities except when it is the only way to preserve the life of the whole person. For example, the capacity for emotional feeling cannot be sacrificed to the power of scientific thinking. To think more effectively, the capacity to think *humanly* cannot be sacrificed. The popular myth of the "mad scientist" is a symbol of human intelligence become self-destructive.

Why then is it sometimes permissible to sacrifice one of these basic human capacities to preserve life? The answer is because in this case it is not a question of sacrificing one basic capacity for another, nor for the better functioning of all other human capacities, but of sacrificing one function so that the whole person should continue to function at all. Only in such extreme necessity does integrity yield to the good of the totality.

It is not always easy to decide which human functions are secondary, which are basic, or which are higher and lower. Nevertheless, ethics must seek to make such discriminations in view of the human system in its many dimensions and levels of organization. If this effort is not made, either human values will be reduced to a single supreme value to which all others can be ruthlessly sacrificed, as the Greek dualists did, or human values will be treated simply as equal items to be added and subtracted in the quantitative manner of utilitarianism. In either case, the multidimensional concept of the human person developed in Chapter 1 will be destroyed.

Thus the good of the whole person requires that all the basic aspects of human personality be simultaneously respected, even when it is necessary to subordinate or even sacrifice in some measure a lower to a higher function. Consequently, we propose the following revised version of the Principle of Totality and name it the *Principle of Totality and Integrity:*

> Except to save life itself, the fundamental functional capacities that constitute the human person should not be destroyed, but preserved, developed, and used for the good of the whole person and of the community.

The significance of this principle is that on the one hand it permits some human values to be given priority over others, but on the other hand it rules out destruction of the fundamental integrity of the person for some partial set of values, except in the most extreme choice between life and death. In striving to reconcile the different values of life, some values must sometimes be subordinated to others. The fundamental values that make us human must not be neglected or abandoned, however, even when some fundamental function must be sacrificed to preserve the whole person as far as possible without losing the whole person. The Christian foundation for this principle is faith in the wisdom of the Creator, who has given persons the gift of human nature, as the Psalmist says (139:13-14):

> Truly you have formed my inmost being; you knit me in my mother's womb. I give you thanks that I am fearfully, wonderfully made; wonderful are your works.

Christians recall God's own respect for the body of his Son, for although he permitted Jesus' death, he inspired the prophets to declare, "Break not one of his bones" (Jn 19:36) and "Nor will you suffer your faithful one to undergo corruption" (Ac 2:27).

Today many discuss whether there is a "right to health" and whether this is the same or different than the "right to healthcare" (Childress, 1984; Boyle, 1986). These questions are considered in Chapter 6. Certainly it must be granted that the right to health by no means relieves persons of the responsibility to care for their own health, as Chapter 3 shows. The right to health also does not give anyone an unqualified claim to the resources of healthcare, since these are necessarily limited and must be distributed to all in some just way. Nevertheless, these qualifications of the right to health do not deny that it is a basic and inalienable right of human persons, as Jesus indicated in the Parable of the Good Samaritan, who recognized that right in the wounded stranger and "was moved with pity at the sight. He approached him and dressed his wounds, pouring in oil and wine" (Lk 11:33b-34).

Thus the right to health possessed by each human person, or the right of quality of life, implies that each person, because of his or her inherent dignity as a person, has the right to the help and care of the community in achieving this multidimensional health, which includes biological and psychological health, the proper concern of the healthcare profession. This right to human wholeness and integrity does not imply, however, that life is not worth living for those who cannot achieve this goal in its fullness. No one fully achieves this goal, and many human beings fall far short of it, especially because the community does not provide them with the help they need or support the scientific research necessary to find ways to supply that help effectively.

CHAPTER 3

Personal Responsibility For Health

OVERVIEW

Chapter 1 points out that the human community is responsible for the full personal development of every one of its members. Chapter 2 explains further that this responsibility includes biological health, as well as the higher levels of human functioning that depend on it. However, the primary responsibility for a person's health rests on that individual, not the community. In this chapter, after considering the need of each person to take responsibility for his or her health (3.1), we explain the implications of this responsibility for daily life (3.2), and the meaning of stewardship (3.3). Having discussed some of the goals pertaining to the pursuit of health, we then outline the elements required for good decision making (informed conscience) and discuss the meaning of informed consent (3.4). Finally, we delineate the rights of patients insofar as physicians and health facilities are concerned (3.5).

3.1 THE PERSON AND HEALING

Biological health concerns what is most individual and private to me, namely, my own body. My body, by its very materiality, its space-time limitations, is mine and mine alone. It identifies me as *not* anybody else. Someone can share a room with me, a table, a bed, even my clothes, but that person cannot truly share my body. Sexual partners exchange the right to use each other's bodies sexually (in biblical language, they become "one flesh," Mk 10:8), but even this intimate union has its limits. Ultimately, it is by reason of my body that I am alone in myself, but it is also by reason of my body that I am in the world of things and persons (B. Ashley, 1985; Shalom, 1985).

My body is profoundly subjective not only because I possess it as my own and know it as myself, but because it is incommunicable. Much of what occurs in my body is hidden even from me; even what I know of it, I know for the most part in a thoroughly subjective way such that I cannot express it. When I consult a physician, 1 experience the difficulty of relating how I feel. Bodily feelings are vivid, yet so vague and so hard to put into words. I am left frustrated and stammering because no one else can really know how I feel. I am the only final judge of whether I really feel well. When no medical test reveals anything wrong with me, but I do not feel well, then I *am* not well.

Even if my sickness is not physiological but imaginary, that imaginary sickness is real at the psychological level and is a psychological illness. At that level, the criterion of health for the psychotherapist is how the client really feels about himself or herself—it is the depth feelings underlying the surface feelings. At the higher ethical and spiritual levels, health also depends on an individual's own conscience, or spiritual discernment. Thus no one but the person ultimately can judge his or her own interior well-being.

Furthermore, this subjectivity is true not only of diagnosis, but also of treatment. The psychotherapist constantly has to remind the client: "No one, ultimately, can help you if you refuse to help yourself." Even the ethical and spiritual counselor must say, "God will help you by his grace, but you must open yourself to that grace." Does not Jesus say in Revelations 3:20: "Here I stand, knocking at the door. If anyone hears me calling and opens the door, I will enter his house and have supper with him, and he with me"?

Healing is a living process that must occur within the organism. Near the end of life patients may be unconscious and purely passive to the surgery, medication, and injections thrust on them, but these treatments seldom result in healing. Convalescence is an active process on the part of patients, and staying well is clearly something that they alone must do. No physician or nurse can make patients take pills, stick to a diet, or take necessary rest and exercise.

In a profound way the will to life and health is the fundamental element in all healing, and this will to life must be intelligent, that is, a realistic search for the means to health. A noted surgeon once said that he dreaded operating on patients who doubted their chances of recovery because in his experience such patients did *not* recover. Most physicians and nurses seem to believe that the patient's fighting spirit is a critical factor in recovering health (Cousins, 1984).

Therefore, whether in working to prevent sickness, to maintain optimal health, to assist recovery from disease, or to rehabilitate oneself after a crippling trauma, a person must make a personal commitment to life and health. It might seem that no special commitment needs to be made, since everyone has an instinct to live. No doubt the need to live, to grow, and to function well is innate; it is the very teleology of any organism. In the human person, however, whose inmost depth of being is not instinctive but free, this commitment is not a given; rather, it must be freely made by the person. Are there not persons who make the opposite commitment to suicide in open or hidden form?

Karl Menninger, in his book *Man Against Himself* (1938), has shown that suicide is only the last step of an intensifying process of self-destruction, of hatred turned away from external objects and toward the self. Clinically, patients who attempt suicide often have a long previous record of psychosomatic illnesses, such as hypertension or ulcers, and of "accidents." Unconsciously, they have been self-committed to death rather than to life. Menninger also believes that religious asceticism, whether Oriental or Christian, is sometimes only a mask for self-hatred.

Menninger and other neo-Freudians cite such clinical evidence in trying to interpret Freud's paradoxical theory of the death wish as the instinctive opposite of the libido, or pleasure principle. Freud (1920) believed that the death wish causes the human organism to regress into more primitive, compulsively repetitive, and ultimately passive types of behavior and that it is a "return to the bliss of the womb," the tomb of eternal night. Menninger is less paradoxical when he interprets this instinct simply as the *aggressive* component of human behavior. He postulates that the pleasure principle leads people to seek satisfactions, and therefore the aggressive principle drives people to seek the destruction of every painful limitation on these strivings for pleasure. When these two principles are not working harmoniously for the organism, aggression may be turned on the self and thus become a death wish.

In sadomasochistic behavior, aggressive action and pain are invested with erotic overtones such that suffering and causing to suffer become intensely pleasurable. In self-hatred, satisfaction is sought through self-pity and the craving for attention and care from others. Some patients seem to enjoy being sick or at least to enjoy constant complaining, obscure ailments, medication, and even painful procedures. A life otherwise empty is at least filled with the drama of disease and therapy.

This commitment to death means that everything associated with the medical profession becomes attractive to some persons and symbolizes their own unconscious drives. They often seduce medical professionals into satisfying their morbid needs. Physicians and nurses may be tempted to pander to these seductions, both because of financial gain and because it is flattering to be needed. In the home, such a neurotic person may induce the whole family to build its life around "tender loving care." One can only wonder whether the tremendous preoccupation of modern American society with the drama of medicine, as displayed on television and in novels, is not evidence that this neurosis has become social as well as individual.

The same sadomasochistic seductions appear in the social and spiritual arenas of politics and religion. Jesus attacked the legalism of some of the Pharisees of his time because these people, who were both political and religious guides, had imposed a moralistic scrupulosity that expressed self-destructive guilt. Puritan and Victorian morality exhibited similar tendencies. In the spiritual sphere, such seductions are reflected in extreme dualistic asceticism with its hatred of the body, the self, and the world. Psychotherapists often are antireligious because they have been so shocked by the way in which moralistic religion seems to have maimed some of their patients (Tancredi and Slaby, 1981).

Neurosis, however, is a counterfeit normality, and it is absurd to blame either medicine or religion as such for these aberrations, however widespread. Surgeons are not usually sadists, although sadism is unconsciously present in a few surgeons and leads to needless surgery. The clergy are not moral sadists, although unconscious sadism may be found in moralistic sermons, unsound ascetical practices, and aberrant rituals.

Affirmation of Life

The commitment to life, which overcomes such commitments to death, is an affirmation of the value not only of pleasure, but also of freedom, intelligence, creativity, and love. As Yahweh says through Moses:

> I call heaven and earth today to witness against you: I have set before you life and death, the blessing and the curse. Choose life, then, that you and your descendants may live, by loving the Lord, your God, heeding his voice, and holding fast to him. For that will mean life for you, a long life for you to live on the land which the Lord swore he would give to your fathers Abraham, Isaac, and Jacob (Dt 30:19-20).

Such a commitment to life has to proceed from the spiritual level, although it is ordinarily manifest at lower levels as well. This deep commitment can be so blocked that persons profoundly dedicated to life in their spiritual center can yet suffer from an unconscious will to death at the psychological level (Lepp, 1966).

The Old Testament presents the Jewish view as profoundly life affirming. It constantly emphasizes the idea that God gives his friends health, security, children, and long life and that God has created men and women for life and wishes to prolong it for them. Faced by the fact that just persons often suffer persecution and martyrdom, the last books of the Old Testament affirm that God will raise his friends from the dead to everlasting life (see 2 M 7:27-29). Jesus approved by saying, "God is God of the living, not of the dead" (Mk 12:27). St. Paul also teaches (Rm 5:12 ff.) that death (and by implication disease and aging) is somehow a consequence of sin (see Ws 1:13-15). Thus disease, aging, and death are not willed by God but only permitted by him as a punishment, the inevitable consequence of the sin of the human race, which has committed itself to death rather than to life. St. Paul joyfully affirms that in Christ all may be born again to everlasting life.

This promise of life should not be understood in merely other-worldly terms. In preaching the Kingdom of God, Jesus taught us to pray for that kingdom to "come on earth...as it is in heaven" (Mt 6:10), and he revealed God's will for us by his miracles of physical healing and restoration to life, even of the dying and dead. Healthcare professionals, in the face of human suffering, often experience a great longing to be able to extinguish pain, restore vigorous life, and close the door to death. They can be sure this compassionate yearning to fight for life and against death is a revelation in their own hearts of God's care for them. "If you, with all your sins, know how to give your children what is good, how much more will your heavenly Father give good things to anyone who asks him!" (Mt 7:11).

When Jesus prayed in the garden, "O, Father, you have the power to do all things. Take this cup away from me. But let it be as you would have it, not as I" (Mk 14:36), he was affirming his own commitment to life. He was also expressing his willingness, however, to endure death if the Father in his transcendent wisdom knew that only through death could doubting men and women be convinced that God and his Son truly love them for their own sake and not for the sake of honor or power.

Thus a sound theology teaches that the Father and Christ desire only life, a desire that is fulfilled in the Resurrection. Following Jesus, who as St. Paul says, was "never anything but 'Yes'" (2 Co 1:20), Christians must always affirm life while being willing to endure the evil of death: (1) as witnesses to others that faith, hope, and love cannot be overcome by the fear and despair of death and (2) as sharers in Jesus' experience of death, by which we learn to be as unselfish, trustful, and hopeful as he was. The Christian, however, endures death serenely not because death is good, but because resurrection and eternal life are good and destroy death forever.

Also, when Christians feel as St. Paul did in prison, when he longed "to be dissolved and to be with Christ" (Ph 1:23), they are not rejecting life but longing to be freed of the barriers that constrict the fullness of life. A Christian can long for death as an inevitable crisis that has to be lived through to achieve full health and life, not as a Freudian regression to the peace of the womb.

Thus it is essential to realize that Christian healthcare should never be directed to the passive acceptance of disease or death, as if these in themselves were somehow spiritual goods. Even a distinguished medical historian such as Henry Sigerist (1960a) errs in thinking that Christianity thought of sickness as sacred. The evidence he cites only proves that Christian thinking is often distorted by the false sadomasochistic notions dating from pre-Christian times or imposed by neurotic abuses of religious symbols. In authentic Christian belief, every individual has a responsibility to choose life and to fight for it. Christians must fight for a full and abundant life and must accept disease and death only as inevitable incidents in the battle, but not as its final outcome (John Paul II, 1980b). Christian acceptance or resignation is not acquiescence, but rather a strategy by which good can be brought out of evil. Sometimes the enemy can be defeated only by patience, turning these evils into opportunities for growth and learning; however, sickness and death should always be perceived as enemies. Christians should stand with St. Paul in condemning death as the ultimate evil: "and the last enemy to be destroyed is death" (1 Co 15:26), especially if *death* is understood as the destruction of the human whole, that is, physical, psychological, moral, and above all, spiritual death.

Spiritual death is nothing more than the commitment to this total death. Deliberately turning from the love of God and neighbor toward a false self-sufficiency is spiritual suicide. This self-sufficiency is so contradictory to the very nature of all persons, to their expansion into community, that this refusal to ask for any help can only end in prideful despair. Physical suicide probably seldom has this character of total death, since usually it seems to be an attempt to escape to some better life or at least to peace and sleep. Spiritual suicide is possible, however, if a person shuts off all others and considers himself or herself entirely self-sufficient.

The person who has made a spiritual commitment to life will strive to achieve wholeness in every dimension of personality. Some are so deceived by dualism that they do not realize that spiritual wholeness requires the care of lower human functions. Thus mystics have neglected social development, moral people have neglected psychological and physical health, and those concerned about psychological health have not perceived its intimate connection with both social and biological health. A true understanding of the commitment to life, however, leads to a balanced concern for the whole personality, a respect for the Principle of Totality and Integrity (2.4).

3.2 PREVENTIVE MEDICINE AND LIFESTYLE

Personal responsibility for health is often thought of as just going to a physician, but this is only a part of it (Engelhardt, 1980; Sider and Clements, 1984). The famous ancient dictum attributed to Hippocrates was that the physician should prescribe "regimen, medicine, and surgery" in that order, meaning by *regimen* the person's lifestyle of diet, rest, and exercise (Edelstein, 1967). Today medical technology is largely in the curative stage rather than the preventive stage (Galdston, 1981). In the future perhaps the emphasis will shift from the hospital to a center for teaching persons how to improve their lifestyles (Lappe, 1985).

A look at current lifestyles in terms of physiological and psychological norms is appalling in view of the extremely unhealthy kinds of lives many people lead. Advances in preventive medicine have mainly taken the form of ridding the environment of infectious diseases and disease carriers. Very few advances have been made to remove environmental pollutants. Civilized human beings, especially those in the twentieth century, seem to be subjecting themselves to more and more unknowns while relying on medicine and surgery to remedy the harm done (Spiro, 1986).

First, modern life often leaves insufficient time for *rest*, not merely in the sense of lack of sleep, but also in the sense of too much stress. People might seem to have more leisure because machines have relieved them of much hard, servile labor. However, this relief is more than offset by the strange routine of urban life that forces us, for example, to spend hours a day driving to and from work in the hazards of traffic. Clearly, as individuals, people are powerless to escape this system, but within it they do have some freedom to make choices that will gradually give their lives greater simplicity and more natural rhythm, free of excessive competition and the drive for success.

Reduced stress also will contribute to moral and spiritual health by making room for a contemplative atmosphere, for service rather than for ambition for power, for solitude and silence, as well as for more time to give to persons and less to things. In the past men and women suffered from the burden of manual work, from fear of enemies, from disease and hunger, but there remained something of the natural rhythm of effort and rest. Today these natural rhythms are often broken up by artificial pressures and hectic overstimulation. As Rordorf (1982) and Kiesling (1970) note, Jewish and Christian cultural traditions were profoundly shaped by the divine command to keep holy the day of rest and reflection (Ex 20:3-12; Mk 2:27).

A stressful life can lead to addiction, the enslavement of human beings to the pursuit of intense pleasure, or anesthesia as an escape from the pain of life (see 12.5). Not only is this addiction to be found in hard drugs, but also in smoking, alcohol, and tranquilizers (Milkman and Schaffer, 1984). It is found in milder form in the common addiction to overeating and in a particularly corrosive way in the anxious twentieth-century pursuit of sexual pleasure. In moderation, none of these things is unhealthy, but in addictive form they become obsessive and destructive (Van Kamm, 1983). The U.S. population suffers from many physical and psychological illnesses as a result of these addictions. Venereal disease is not a negligible problem; however, sexual addiction may have more serious consequences at the psychological and social levels because it promotes a selfish hedonism that stands in the way of true interpersonal love or loyalty and subverts the human social order traditionally based on the family (Carnes, 1983).

Finally, many persons today lack proper physical exercise. Although sports are highly cultivated, they are more watched than played by the average man and woman. The average person does little manual work and seldom walks or dances.

To assume personal responsibility for health, therefore, requires a scientifically based knowledge of hygiene, good diet, rest, exercise, and moderation. These cannot be imposed from without. People need to design their lives to meet personal requirements, which differ greatly. To be healthy, one's lifestyle must express one's true personality, not a false one or a resignation to being half alive (Elinson, 1984).

The problems of mental health are similar. Today people are overstimulated by sensation and passive imagination but impoverished in active imagination, reflection, and meditation. They receive much input, much information, but often little integration of symbols and feelings. They live at the top of their heads, out of touch with their feelings.

Concerning spiritual life, many persons today live without clear commitments or goals and suffer from the emptiness, meaninglessness, and absurdity of life in loneliness, never seeking deep-level communication with others (R. May, 1983). A deceptive kind of pseudohealth is sometimes observed in the comfortable, modern personality whose life is filled with satisfactions when whole anxieties have been alleviated by psychotherapy (Rieff, 1968). As in the past, when religion was sometimes the opiate of the people, concealing the symptoms of acute misery with illusory consolations, so also the illusory secular "happiness" lived by today's "beautiful people" often conceals spiritual emptiness.

To be healthy, therefore, requires the courage to criticize the accepted norms of modern life and face the ethical dilemmas produced by modern technology. Perhaps it is futile even to talk about a natural way of life, as counterculturists do. Has that point in human history arrived when nature must be replaced with a fabricated world, even with human beings who have fabricated themselves?

Although each person has a fundamental responsibility for his or her health, some factors detrimental to health are often beyond personal control (Goodman and Goodman, 1986; Starr, 1981). For example, workers in an asbestos factory cannot protect themselves from asbestos. Thus society often has a role in establishing a healthy environment for those who cannot help themselves, especially the poor. Chapter 6 examines this social responsibility.

3.3 PRINCIPLE OF STEWARDSHIP AND CREATIVITY

"Be fruitful and multiply; fill the earth and subdue it. Have dominion over the fish of the sea, the birds of the air, and all living things on earth" (Gn 1:28). Some ecological enthusiasts have placed on this one verse the blame for the technological ravagement of the natural environment. In the next chapter of Genesis, however, another tradition reports, "The Lord God took the man and settled him into the Garden of Eden to cultivate and care for it" (2:15). Thus, although humankind is lord of lesser creatures, nevertheless its dominion over them, and over itself, is only a *stewardship* for which human beings remain responsible to the One Lord (Hendry, 1980).

Classical theology based Christian ethics on the conviction that God endowed all human beings with one common nature, which remains essentially the same throughout all history, from Adam and Eve to the Last Judgment. Human beings are stewards of this nature, as they are of the world in which God has placed them. By studying the God-given structure and dynamics of this nature, it is possible, so theologians in the past thought, to formulate unchanging moral norms binding for every time and culture. Stewardship demanded that human beings abide by these norms lest they destroy the garden of the world and the temple of their own bodies, which were given them to "cultivate and care for."

Today this traditional concept of stewardship is often criticized as follows:

First, since theologians generally accept the view that the Creator produced the human race by an evolutionary process, they have to take into account the fact that human beings are not finished masterpieces but rather a work in progress. Thus it is no insult to God's creative wisdom for people to suppose that they can further perfect the world and even their own bodies. Indeed, it is to God's praise that he has generously called them to be co-workers with him in his creative task.

Second, human behavior is the result of natural instinct and of culture and social determinism. Human nature exists not in the abstract but in the flux of human history and of individual biographies, where it seems subject to endless variations. How, then, can a universal definition of human nature that is more than an empty commonplace be formulated?

Third, with the rise of modern technology, for the first time in history human beings have achieved a real dominion over nature. In principle, at least, the discovery of the deoxyribonucleic acid (DNA) molecule opens the way for producing life and controlling evolution. Moreover, scientists are acquiring mastery of the building blocks out of which all material things are made and may soon tap the sources of energy that will make it possible to reconstruct the world.

The ethical implication of these discoveries seems to be that ethical norms can no longer be based on human nature because that nature itself becomes a matter of people's choosing (Francoeur, 1976). People may be able to select from among various models of human nature the ones they prefer to construct, just as they do between various models of houses. The prophecy of Karl Marx (1844) that humankind will become its own creator seems to be coming true. Perhaps human beings can even learn to reverse the aging process and make themselves immortal. Then they will no longer be stewards but creators.

Scientific Doubts

Of course the biblical story of the Tower of Babel (Gn 11:1-9) and the Greek myth of Prometheus stealing fire from the gods are evidence that this dream is not new. Before people totally succumb to it, they should take into account certain doubts expressed by scientists themselves. First, it must be noted that these predictions of unlimited human dominion over nature are less convincing now than they were a few years ago when atomic fission and the genetic code were discovered. The ecological crisis has revealed that modern technology in its present form has its limits (Hare, 1987; Rescher, 1980). Every technological advance exacts its price in environmental pollution and depletion of energy resources. Moreover, since evolution has adapted human nature very nicely to its primitive environment, neither that nature nor that environment can be altered without serious risks. Humankind always has to proceed strategically, trying to gain a little more than is lost (Lappe, 1987).

Again, the proposals for genetic engineering, which Chapter 11 discusses from an ethical viewpoint, are still largely theoretical (Esbjornson, 1984; Office of Technology Assessment, 1982). Science has grasped certain basic principles of life, but these principles operate in life systems that are bafflingly complex. The details will be unraveled painfully by long and often frustrating research, as the slow progress in understanding cancer exemplifies.

Furthermore, one ultimate limiting factor is still very little understood. Since human creative intelligence depends on the human brain, any alterations of body structure that might injure the brain will be disastrously self-defeating. Can the human brain be significantly improved? So far as is known, the human brain is the most complex system in the universe. To build it would require far more information than to construct any other system, even the most complex computers so far invented. The brain is relatively very small, however, and unlike a computer it is capable of self-development and some self-repair. As human beings think, they constantly restructure brain circuitry at the synaptic level (G. Edelman, 1987; Facklam and Facklam, 1982; Rosenfield, 1987).

Perhaps, although some speculate about its future (Cruchland, 1984), the human brain is already near the limit of evolution. Thus any kind of improvement that can be made in the rest of the human body must be limited by the requirements of the brain. No doubt people could be turned into brain-persons by replacing most of the other body systems with artificial organs to support the life of the brain. The brain could be fed with information and be allowed to transmit its orders electronically. However, this would eliminate much of the imaginative and affective life that plays so important a part in motivation and interpersonal relations. Would people want, for example, to eliminate sexual reproduction and reduce sex to orgasms produced by direct stimulation of pleasure centers in the brain? This would indeed make one-dimensional men or women (Marcuse, 1964, 1972). Thus the Principle of Totality and Integrity discussed in 2.4 warns of the ethical limits to human self-creation.

Although such warnings are in order, it would be wrong to conclude, as do such modern critics of technology as Jacques Ellul (1980), that modern technology is the temptation of the Serpent, a sin of pride and rebellion against the Creator. God would not have endowed human beings with creative intelligence and freedom if he did not want them to share in his creative action. They are divinely called not merely to preserve the old, but to produce the new. In the *Pastoral Constitution on the Church in the Modern World* (1965c), the Second Vatican Council teaches that technology is a gift of God that requires stewardship as do any other of his gifts.

In its account of God's dominion, classical theology was too greatly influenced by the Old Testament image of the monarch God jealous of his supreme dignity and power. In the New Testament perspective, God is best revealed in Christ, who "though he was in the form of God, did not deem equality with God something to be grasped at, but rather he emptied himself and took the form of a servant" (Ph 2:6-7). Thus God is not jealous of his power but calls persons to share in his work of making all things new (Rv 21:5). Such cooperation is not merely filling in details in a finished "plan of God." Rather, he has called human beings to use their initiative and originality in completing his work.

In creative activity, however, people have to respect their own limits and the limits of the materials with which they must work. These limits are not set by God out of any concern for his own authority. God himself is "limited" by his own wisdom and love, which forbid him to do what is contradictory to his own nature. Human beings are far more limited by the fact that their share in God's knowledge and love is finite. No matter how they may progress in science, freedom, and power, they dare not contradict their own human nature without destroying themselves.

At any given moment in history, people's limits are set by their knowledge. Once they understand some aspect of nature well, they can freely choose to improve nature and surpass it. When they lack that understanding, however, their efforts to improve on nature may prove disastrous. The evils of modern technology are not the result of creative use of knowledge, but of rash exploitation of a nature little understood. Above all, people have failed to understand themselves, their authentic needs and potentialities. To acquire the knowledge they need, research and experimentation, with all the risks involved, are necessary, but even here they must proceed with reverence for the persons and the environment that are at risk.

As a result of these considerations, the *Principle of Stewardship and Creativity* can be formulated as follows:

> The gifts of multidimensional human nature and its natural environment should be used with profound respect for their intrinsic teleology. The gift of human creativity especially should be used to cultivate that nature and environment, with a care set by the limits of human beings' actual knowledge and the risks of destroying these gifts.

3.4 PRINCIPLE OF PRUDENT CONSCIENCE AND INFORMED CONSENT

Need for Truth

Given the limits of human development just mentioned, modern medicine constantly involves both technological and ethical judgments. Modern medical practice must ask not only, "Can it be done?" but also, "Ought we do what can be done?" The sociologist Freidson, in his book *Profession of Medicine* (1971), and several ethicists and physicians (Lappe 1987; Pellegrino and Thomasma, 1988) have shown from different points of view that the claim of healthcare professionals to make autonomous professional decisions about medical matters is invalid. Their professional knowledge making them experts about the techniques of medicine does not imply that they are experts in the *use* of these techniques, since this use involves social, political, and moral issues about which they are not necessarily well-informed.

Thus Freidson and others argue that individuals who seek the services of a medical professional cannot simply delegate to that professional those concrete decisions about their health on the grounds that the physician knows best. For a woman to consent to a tubal ligation because the physician advises it is to take the advice of someone who has special competence in medicine but not in ethics. On the other hand, neither is the individual competent to decide such a question on her own unless she has adequate information about the medical aspects of the decision. There is thus a certain dilemma in medical decisions: Who has the knowledge of both the ethical norms and the medical facts to make a wise decision? And how are these norms and facts to be related to each other (John Fletcher, 1983a)? This dilemma requires a discussion of the problem of a well-formed conscience.

Christian theology has always insisted that when it comes to concrete ethical decisions, each normal individual has the capacity and the responsibility to judge and to act on his or her own judgment. This responsibility cannot be delegated to anyone else or to any institution—not to custom, the law, advisers, or even civil or religious leaders. The capacity to make practical judgments in matters involving ethical issues is called *conscience*. The Second Vatican Council (1965b) stated:

> For the human being has in his or her heart a law inscribed by God. A person's dignity lies in observing this law, and by it he or she will be judged. Conscience is the person's most secret core and sanctuary. There the person is alone with God whose voice echoes in the person's depths. By conscience, in a wonderful way, that law is made known which is fulfilled in the love of God and one's neighbor. Through loyalty to conscience, Christians are joined to others in the search for truth and for the right solution to so many moral problems which arise both in the life of individuals and from social relationships. Hence, the more a correct conscience prevails, the more do persons and groups turn aside from blind choice and try to be guided by the objective standards of moral conduct (n. 16).

Thus people have the responsibility to form a good conscience and to follow it; that is, (1) to obtain as much relevant information as possible about a situation and (2) to make and carry out a decision in accordance with this information. Sin is either failure to take proper steps to form a good conscience or failure to follow the conscience after forming it rightly.

Thus, in any bioethical question, people have the responsibility (1) to learn the facts about the medical condition and other circumstances of the persons involved, (2) to determine in accord with an objective value system the needs and rights of the people involved, and (3) to come to a concrete, personal decision despite disagreement or pressures from others.

Persons who lack the information necessary to make a wise decision in bioethical matters will only make a good decision by chance. If such persons decide wrongly, however, they will have to suffer the consequences of the mistake, no matter how sincerely it may have been made. When people act without proper information, but the lack of information is not caused by their own negligence, such persons are said to be *invincibly* ignorant. Although their ignorance may result in harm to themselves or to others, they are not morally responsible for the harm.

On the other hand, persons who have deliberately failed to seek the information they know is necessary for a realistic decision are said to be *vincibly* ignorant and are morally responsible for the consequences of decisions hampered by this ignorance. This can happen either through neglect (crass ignorance), self-deception (affected ignorance), or willful resolve to ignore the facts (malicious ignorance). Such avoidable ignorance does not excuse people morally for bad decisions. This principle is clearly recognized by decisions of courts in malpractice suits whereby physicians are held responsible for mistakes in judgment they could have avoided. All healthcare professionals have the obligation to obtain the information they need through initial and continuing education, personal study, careful examination of the patient, and consultation with other professionals and perhaps even with the patient's family. This obligation applies not only to medical knowledge, but also to relevant legal and ethical knowledge.

Ignorance is not the only cause of poor judgments. Ethicists point out that people are prevented from *using* the knowledge they may actually possess by various emotional factors. Thus fear, force, unthinking routine, neurotic compulsions, and prejudices may cloud judgment and limit freedom to select among all available alternatives. Modern psychology and social psychology emphasize these limitations on human freedom and realistic choice. They have explained how social background, family training, professional education, and social position can limit perceptions of reality and thus impede moral decision making. In addition, theology recognizes the limitation of our freedom under the name of *original sin*. According to current understanding, this is not merely one remote sin of Adam and Eve, but also the whole burden of human sin from the beginning of history, built into culture and its institutions, even into religious institutions (not to mention healthcare institutions) (Rahner, 1975). People suffer from the effects of this burden and have their freedom restricted by it, but they do not become personally guilty of this sin until they begin to realize this blindness and enslavement and accept their chains rather than struggle to be free of them.

Thus all medical professionals need to take a tip from the psychoanalysts and realize that if they are to be psychologically free to make truly ethical and helpful decisions, they must have insight into their own prejudices, biases, and unconscious motives. All physicians need to be alert to their own tendencies to dominate helpless persons, to take sadistic pleasure in their power over the human body, and to avoid facing their own feelings of tenderness or fear of death. All these emotions are perfectly human; when disciplined, they actually contribute to ethical sensitivity and good judgment. When they are unconscious, neurotic, and self-serving, however, such emotions can lead to unwise judgments. Thus an informed conscience must be supported by a good will and healthy, disciplined emotions. To think that cold-blooded, scientific objectivity will lead to ethically wise decisions is an illusion, just as it is an illusion to think that sentimentality is enough. An emotive ethics contains an important measure of truth, but it is not adequate (see Chapter 7).

Does having full information before making a decision definitely determine what the decision is to be? If it did, then there would be no such thing as *freedom*. Human beings are free not simply because they are relieved from any external coercion, but for two other reasons as well. First, usually there are many alternative means to a goal, some of which are clearly inappropriate, but many are often appropriate, each with its advantages and disadvantages. Second, people can reconsider their informed judgments of conscience because these judgments may involve difficulty, and they can form another judgment of conscience that is less onerous but also less informed. Thus morality always involves a choice, and that choice is not always between a clear-cut good or bad line of action. The choice may be between two good lines of action; moreover, it may be between two objective evils, one of which may appear good to a particular person because it involves less evil.

Since knowledge of the factors involved in any decision seldom results in a determinant judgment that this or that action is best without qualification, it might seem that a rational decision is impossible. However, knowledge is not the only factor involved in a decision of conscience; there is also will supported by feeling (emotion and affection). Our decision will be ethically good only if we have a good will (supported, if possible, by healthy emotions) that inclines us to follow our best information and ethical insight, even if they are not rationally conclusive. Thus an informed conscience needs knowledge of the facts and of the law, but it also requires an affection for what will truly satisfy our needs in an integral manner. This element of affection is unappreciated by many contemporary ethicists who seek to turn ethical decisions into rational balancing acts (Engelhardt, 1986b).

Certitude in Ethical Decision

An informed conscience can still be mistaken about the *objective* goodness of an action because of invincible ignorance. The history of medicine is filled with disturbing episodes in which medical professionals followed a line of treatment and care in accordance with the best knowledge available at the time that turned out to be disastrously mistaken (E. Flannery, 1986). Does this mean that they acted unethically? By no means, but they and the patients nevertheless had to bear the tragic consequences. The same is true of ethical norms, and people should not be unduly disturbed when they find that a rule of conduct that once seemed sound later turns out to be inadequate for the protection of human rights. Thus in recent years the norms for informed consent for medical-ethical experimentation on human subjects (see 9.5) have become much stricter (John Fletcher, 1983a; Jonsen, 1984). Some people have the mistaken impression that progress in civilization means an easier, more liberal morality. In fact, the more knowledgeable people become about human needs, the more careful they are likely to be about the protection of human rights and therefore more likely to propose more precise ethical norms.

As a result, as many healthcare professionals today know only too well, ethical decisions may involve anguish of conscience. People may be faced with the realization (1) that although they have tried to get adequate information, they still do not have all the facts or the clear understanding of values that they really need to make a decision that will be objectively correct, and (2) that even when they have acquired the best knowledge available, the best alternative may remain very unclear because every alternative has advantages and disadvantages. Given such uncertainty, many people try to pass the buck to someone else. By doing so, however, they do not escape responsibility; instead, they assume responsibility for the decision made by the other person, whose judgment may be even less trustworthy than their own. Such uncertainty also causes many to think that in practical matters, an ethical decision is ultimately nothing but a leap in the dark.

This is not the case. People are always obliged to act with *moral* certitude. There may and usually does remain a theoretical or objective doubt as to whether what they decide will actually work out for the best, but there must be no practical doubt. Their conscience must be certain that for them here and now the best thing to do is A rather than B. Otherwise, they would be acting blindly rather than on the basis of goodwill to follow the best information available. Surgeons most often act on moral certitude, knowing that it is theoretically possible that the surgery will not be successful because of reasons that cannot be anticipated.

How can people come to such a practical or moral certitude that here and now this is what they ought to do? After they have formed their conscience as well as possible in the time and place in which they are situated, it will probably become clear that at least some alternatives are excluded as clearly inappropriate means to ethical goals. Among those possibilities that remain, some may be attractive, but people may still not be sure whether they are right or wrong.

Solving Doubts

The great medieval theologians taught that in such doubts people are to choose that course of action that, as far as they can discover, will more probably be the most effective means to achieve their legitimate goals. To act otherwise would be unreasonable and therefore unethical. Thus a person faced with doubts should opt for the course of action that best seems to satisfy his or her integrated human needs. In the seventeenth and eighteenth centuries, however, a more legalistic approach to morality came into vogue. Moralists tended to adopt the methods employed by lawyers who solved doubtful cases by recourse to general legal rules or what moralists called "reflex principles" (Grisez, 1983), such as "A doubtful law does not bind," and "The accused is to be held innocent until proved guilty." Eventually this legal mode of reasoning developed into the system called *probabilism.*

According to probabilism, persons who are in doubt about whether a law exists forbidding a course of action they would like to take, or about whether a law applies in their case, are free to act as they prefer provided that (1) their doubts rest on solidly probable reasons and (2) there is no risk of serious damage to others or to themselves. Proponents of the system argued that all reflex principles can be reduced to a single principle: "In doubt, the presumption is in favor of the existing situation"; that is, people are free to continue their ordinary way of conduct unless new information or a clearer duty demands a change.

Although probabilism was bitterly opposed by some Catholic and Protestant theologians on the grounds that it fostered a legalism and laxity to which the corruption of human nature by original sin makes people liable, probabilism was finally accepted by most Catholic theologians. The legalism on which it rests, however, is still in question. This legalism weakened moral theology in the Catholic Church for many years because it justified a minimalist approach to the moral life.

In the recent past most Catholic healthcare professionals used a very simple method of arriving at this required moral certitude in bioethical questions. They had only to ask what the Catholic position was on abortion, sterilization, and so forth. The answer was easily supplied by the Catholic chaplain, who referred to a standard manual on Catholic medical ethics.

This strict dependence on official teaching often had the disadvantage of leading medical professionals into a merely mechanical method of decision making. Although the answers they arrived at were often right, they seldom understood the reasons why. Morality for many became a set of rules rather than a well-reasoned understanding of the actions that benefit or harm the human person (O'Rourke and Boyle, 1989). Even worse, the tendency developed to consider as unethical only those things explicitly condemned by the Church. The "everyday ethics" of the medical profession, such as the right to informed consent or the responsibility to avoid unnecessary tests and procedures, were overlooked. Some Catholic healthcare professionals became almost schizophrenic in the way they separated their Catholic principles and their professional practices, without attempting to make any intellectual reconciliation of the two.

This reliance on authority had the advantage of fostering the development of uniform policy in Catholic healthcare facilities, giving the individual physician or nurse the security of a quiet conscience. Unfortunately, however, many healthcare professionals were not prepared for an exposure to secular and humanistic values. As with many laypeople, many Catholic healthcare professionals were convinced the Church was behind the times in regard to its teaching on sexuality and marriage. For this reason, some Catholic healthcare professionals of the present generation are as dogmatic in challenging the teaching of the Church concerning bioethics as a previous generation was dogmatic in affirming the teaching of the Church on bioethics.

Many Catholic healthcare professionals probably wish that a simple way of achieving peace of conscience were still available, since they believe they do not have the time to study the teaching of the Church on their own. Moreover, since the call of the Church for Catholics to become involved in the modern world in 1963, and especially since the controversy over Paul VI's encyclical *Humanae Vitae* (1968), peace of conscience among Catholic healthcare professionals has been greatly disturbed. For some, the changed circumstances have meant a crisis of conscience; for others, they have meant rebellion, confusion, or bitter feelings of betrayal. Occasionally, conservative Catholics recriminate their liberal colleagues saying, "If he doesn't accept the pope's teaching, why doesn't he get out of the Church?" Some have left the Church, either because they felt they could not dissent and remain sincere Catholics or, at the other extreme, because they were disgusted with a Church too weak to expel dissenters. Understanding more clearly the nature of Christian morality, the formation of conscience, and the various forms of Church teaching, is the responsibility of any sincere Catholic. The following explanation of Church teaching and formation of conscience is, of necessity, highly simplified and can be supplemented from current authors (Granfield, 1987; Grisez, 1983; W. Smith, 1987; F. Sullivan, 1983).

Guidance by the Spirit

The Christian community of Church is founded on faith in Jesus Christ. Jesus is known only because the good news about him is preached and witnessed. Such witness, however, requires that the teaching authority *(Magisterium)* of Christ and his apostles be continued. The power of the Holy Spirit guarantees that this witness of and in the Christian community will not fail (i.e., it is *infallible* until Christ comes again: Mt 28:18-20; Jn 16:4-16; Jn 17:9-26).

In nineteenth-century theology this magisterium (teaching role) was usually considered the exclusive work of the pope and bishops. They alone seemed to have had the right to teach actively, whereas the other members of the Church were merely passive hearers and learners. The Second Vatican Council (1964a) however, reminded Catholics that Christ's threefold mission as priest, shepherd, and teacher is shared in appropriate ways by *all* members of the Church. Thus, although not all Christians have a special gift of teaching (1 Co 12:29; 1 Tm 1:7), by their baptism and confirmation all Christians participate somehow *actively* in teaching and witnessing the faith (Congar, 1977; O'Meara, 1983). For example, Christian parents have an important share in the active magisterium when they pass on their faith to their children.

This common witness to the faith *(sensus fidelium)* that flows from living a Christian life is not mere public opinion. When pollsters report that a majority of U.S. Catholics do or do not favor abortion or racial discrimination, this is not the sensus fidelium. To discover that faith witness would require finding out what truths relevant to abortion or racism Catholics believe God has or has not *revealed* to his people. The sensus fidelium, therefore, is not human opinion, but the witness of the Christian community to the apostolic faith they have received and by which they live.

A special form of this discernment process is the witness given by those in the community who are especially dedicated to contemplation and intense prayer, which the Bible often refers to as the gift of prophecy (1 Co 14:1-5; Ac 21:9) and which helps the community grow in depth and purity of faith and in the liveliness of hope. Thus Paul VI honored St. Teresa of Avila and St. Catherine of Siena as "Doctors (teachers) of the Church." Also, we should not forget that Christian artists such as Fra Angelico or Michelangelo, scientists such as Teilhard de Chardin or Jerome Lejeune, and philosophers such as Jacques Maritain or Gabriel Marcel help us by their human disciplines to express the faith in its full splendor.

In the Middle Ages, theologians were recognized as playing a special role in the magisterium (Congar, 1967, 1977). Today, some suppose a good Catholic theologian should be content only to explain and defend the pronouncements of the bishops and pope. It is generally admitted, however, that the teaching mission of the Church will be weakened if theologians do not have the freedom to express their honest, well-formed opinions (Theological Commission, 1976).

Developing Doctrine

Sometimes this freedom to express well-founded opinions is called "the right to dissent," (Curran and McCormick, 1988) but more properly it should be called "the right of responsible analysis or criticism" (Ratzinger, 1984b, 1987). The charism of the theologian is to witness to the faith by responsible, scholarly analysis of teaching that involves not only defending official formulations of the faith, but also pointing out defects and proposing hypotheses for the improvement of such formulations—hypotheses that sometimes may seem very daring and novel. Thus Pope John Paul II, in *Familiaris Consortio* (1981b), petitioned theologians to perform this service to clarify the teaching of the Church on marriage. Theologians, as responsible members of the Christian community, have the duty to use their gifts to build up the faith of the community (Ep 4:11-13) by communicating to the public not only their criticisms and difficulties, but also the positive, constructive results of their researches (Theological Commission, 1976). The charism of criticism, analysis, or dissent, that theologians enjoy extends to the ordinary teaching of the Church insofar as its theory is concerned (W. Smith, 1987). The charism does not extend to the determination of authentic pastoral instruction because this is the charism of the bishops and the Holy Father (National Conference of Catholic Bishops, 1978). The right of dissent has been exaggerated in post-Vatican II times because it has been interpreted in accord with political dissent (John Paul II, 1985).

Pastoral ministry makes a very special contribution to the Church's teaching effort (Dulles, 1988). This ministry is not limited to the ordained but is carried on by many men and women whose experience in applying the faith to actual life is essential if the Gospel is to be effectively preached to the poor and to children (Mt 11:5; 18:5-14). For example, religious sisters and brothers probably have contributed more to the active magisterium in the United States than have the ordained clergy (John Paul II, 1987b).

Finally, a special leadership responsibility falls on the bishops, together with their priests and deacons in local churches, and on the pope for the whole Church to unify all these different witnessing voices, to express their consensus in clear terms suited to the times, and to link this to the tradition of the Christian community throughout the world in its historical development. Without such unifying leadership, the spiritual riches of faith and insight contributed by the members of the Church would be dissipated, and the community would be divided in its faith and life. Thus, whereas the role of theologians is primarily critical and analytical, the role of bishops is primarily pastoral and synthesizing (Theological Commission, 1976).

In particular, bishops have the hard task of reconciling partial and extreme views within the Church that might lead to heresy or schism. They can do this best not by condemnation but by wise emphasis on those principal truths and values that keep a straggling flock moving toward its goal. In moral matters, prudent bishops do not burden the freedom of individual consciences by insistence on secondary issues (1 Co 10:23-33), since they recognize that the members of the Church are at many different levels of moral development. Rather, such bishops constantly emphasize the primary goals of Christian life.

Sometimes, however, bishops and popes are confronted with dangerous crises in the life of the community in which, as leaders and pastors, they have the painful duty of using their authority "to bind and to loose" (Mt 16:19; 18:18), to protect the community from disruption, and to strengthen its public witness. This is why in extreme cases a bishop may have to resort, as did St. Paul (1 Co 5:1-13), to excommunication or exclusion from Christian life of those who "will not hear the Church" (Mt 18:17), observing, however, all the care for justice, which today is called "due process."

As so far described, this work of the Magisterium is said to be "ordinary." This ordinary teaching, even as it is authoritatively formulated in the pronouncements of the bishops and pope, is obviously a combination of many different elements of unequal value. How, then, does it share in the infallibility guaranteed to the Christian community by the Holy Spirit's guidance? Immersed in the culture of their own times, most Christians seldom stop to reflect or discriminate the Gospel substance from traditions and opinions that are merely accidental aspects of their faith. Mature Christians, however, do sense that some matters of religious thought and practice are essential to and definitive of Christian commitment, whereas other matters are more or less peripheral and transitory.

Unfortunately, since the Reformation, polemics between the churches have led to a type of religious instruction for Catholics that gives them the impression that loyalty demands equal adherence to every item of traditional Catholicism. Such faulty instruction is largely responsible for the present polarization within the Church between liberals and conservatives. This polarization is forcing Catholics to discriminate between the unfailing Gospel in its inspired tradition and various human traditions that are passing away with the changes of time and the worldwide extension of the Church to include non-European cultures (e.g., communion in hand, form of marriage).

Clearly, the ordinary teaching of the Church, along with such merely human traditions, must also include the whole revealed truth of Scripture and tradition; otherwise the Word of God would not be unfailingly transmitted from one generation to another. Thus, doctrinal minimalists who call into doubt everything in this ordinary teaching on the grounds that it is not "defined *de fide*" run the risk of eliminating much of the richness of the Christian community's faith witness. On the other hand, doctrinal rigorists who identify every traditional belief or practice with the Word of God—who treat anyone who criticizes any pronouncement of a local bishop, a Roman congregation, or a pope as disobedient and disloyal to authority—run the risk of a great shock when they discover that through the years the Church has modified some statements on which it had not come to a definitive and infallible judgment. For example, the Church has modified its teaching on the relationship of Church and state in our era and on ensoulment of the human person.

It is necessary, therefore, to distinguish between those elements of the ordinary teaching of the Church that are the infallible Word of God and those that are simply human, perhaps even erroneous, opinion. To make this distinction requires each person, according to his or her gifts and situation, to engage in prayer, study, and reflection so as to note the signs by which God makes himself known to the Christian community. Taken one by one, these signs may not be completely convincing, but their convergence can lead to a secure conviction that this is the Word of God. These convergent signs are simply the different kinds of witness to the faith already enumerated. When the Scriptures, the faithful, the prophetic contemplatives, the theologians, and the legitimate pastors of the Church, each in their own proper role, give a concurrent witness, a Christian knows that to reject that witness would be to resist the Holy Spirit.

For example, one should consider the witness provided by the Second Vatican Council to the great truths of the Gospel by the pope and bishops in dialogue with theologians and representatives of religious orders, its reception by the vast majority of Catholics, and its general approval by the other Christian churches. This witness provided a secure sign of the Word of God and the presence of the Holy Spirit for all except a few rigorists alarmed by changes in nonessential matters. Nevertheless, the Council did not go beyond the level of the ordinary magisterium by defining new dogmas.

Such ordinary teaching authority is all that Protestants generally recognize in their churches. The Orthodox and Roman Catholic Churches, however, also believe that, when necessary, an ecumenical council of the bishops has the authority to issue a definitive judgment (*extraordinary magisterium*) on a disputed question of faith. Generally, the Orthodox believe that the ecumenicity of such councils must be confirmed by the acceptance of the whole church. Roman Catholics, on the other hand, believe that the Lord, by establishing St. Peter as the chief of his apostles (Mt 16:13-20; Jn 21:15-17), indicated the solution to this need of Church for definitive teaching on questions of faith and morals.

Confirming the teaching of the First Vatican Council on this matter, the Second Vatican Council (1964a) says of the infallible authority of such extraordinary teaching:

> This infallibility, however, with which the divine redeemer wished to endow his Church in defining doctrine pertaining to faith and morals, is co-extensive with the deposit of revelation, which must be religiously guarded and loyally and courageously expounded. The Roman Pontiff, head of the college of bishops, enjoys this infallibility in virtue of his office, when, as supreme pastor and teacher of all the faithful—who confirms his brethren in the faith (see Lk 22:32)—he proclaims in absolute decision a doctrine pertaining to faith or morals. For that reason his definitions are rightly said to be irreformable by their very nature and not by reason of the assent of the Church, inasmuch as they were made with the assistance of the Holy Spirit promised to him in the person of blessed Peter himself; and as a consequence they are in no way in need of the approval of others, and do not admit of appeal to any other tribunal. For in such a case the Roman Pontiff does not utter a pronouncement as a private person, but rather does he expound and defend the teaching of the Catholic faith as the supreme teacher of the universal Church, in whom the Church's charism of infallibility is present in a singular way. The infallibility promised to the Church is also present in the body of bishops when, together with Peter's successor, they exercise the supreme teaching office. Now, the assent of the Church can never be lacking to such definitions on account of the same Holy Spirit's influence, through which Christ's whole body is maintained in the unity of faith and makes progress in it (n. 25).

Although the power to make such definitive judgments extends to the moral teaching with which this book is concerned, it is not easy to point out any such definitive statements of the extraordinary magisterium on concrete ethical questions. However, perhaps some general moral principles have been so defined, for example, the teaching of the Church in regard to contraception (Ford and Grisez, 1978). We should not conclude, therefore, that the Gospel teaches nothing certain about Christian conduct. The correct inference is that to know God's will about what to do or not to do in order to follow Christ, it is necessary to take into account all forms of Christian witness, among which the pastoral documents of the Church provide firm guidance. This ordinary teaching, as expressed in such pastoral documents, may be infallibly certain when confirmed by the convergence of other witnesses, such as liturgical practice or ecumenical witness. However, ordinary teaching is not equivalent to a definitive judgment by the extraordinary teaching authority (F. Sullivan, 1983), and thus in some respects it may be subject to modification.

Even very traditional Catholics need not feel insecure in this situation, since they will find that the main lines of Christian moral life are clear (National Conference of Catholic Bishops, 1976). Also, even in particular issues, there is usually a course of action that enjoys such great probability of correctness that individuals may be quite safe in following it. Moreover, the more important teachings of the ordinary Magisterium of the Church may be ascertained by "the character of the document, from frequent repetition, of the same doctrine or from the manner of speaking" (Vatican II, 1964a). Some matters in everyone's life and in every age of the Church, however, are moral dilemmas about which people must pray earnestly for the Holy Spirit's guidance to make courageous personal and communal decisions. Those who demand greater certainty than this and cry out for the pope to settle every moral question with an infallible definition are exhibiting scrupulous consciences weakened either by neurosis or by lack of real faith in Christ's promise to guide them by the constant presence of his Holy Spirit.

A Well-Formed Conscience

Thus Catholic healthcare professionals need not think that they are sinking into a theological morass in medical-moral matters. They need only keep in mind that two different levels of moral certitude exist: (1) the level of principles and value priorities and (2) the level of concrete application of these principles to particular problems of moral decision. At the level of principles and values, Jesus Christ has given Christians ample guidance on "the weightier matters of the law, justice, and mercy, and good faith" (Mt 23:23); these are clearly expressed in the ordinary teaching of the Church (Vatican II, 1964a). If professionals study the official pastoral documents of the popes and bishops in a spirit of faith, prayer, and reflection, they will discover the chief ethical values at which to aim in making practical medical decisions. The clearer their understanding and appreciation of these values, the surer will be their moral judgment. Without such understanding, mere mechanical obedience to laws and rules will not yield prudent decisions.

The second level of concrete application of ethical principles is a complex and difficult area where official Church teaching can be of great help, but where perfect clarity or undebatable certitude would not be expected. Healthcare professionals are well aware that the clarity and high probability of scientific laws are not to be expected in the application of these laws to particular medical decisions. It is painful to have to make a life-and-death medical decision without being sure how the principles in the medical textbook fit the particular case, but such decisions have to be made every day. In the same way, moral decisions cannot be made simply by referring to theological textbooks or to official Church documents.

In fact, at the level of detailed application of basic moral principles, conscientious Catholics may discover that the pastoral guidance provided by the pope, the bishops, and their priests seems inadequate to the problems with which the laity have to deal. This occurs either because these guidelines do not touch the precise problems the laity struggle with or because, in dealing with such issues, this pastoral guidance seems to ignore experiences, objective facts, and special insights coming from other sources.

In such situations, loyal Catholics may find themselves faced with the question of whether they should publicly criticize the adequacy of official Church teaching. We have already argued that theologians have the duty to carry on such criticism in a responsible and constructive way; so also do other Catholics whose special expertise or experience gives them the right to contribute to the development of magisterial positions. This criticism, however, should be founded on objective argument concerned with the nature or meaning of the teaching. Simply because a teaching is difficult to follow does not imply that the teaching is deficient.

Given this right to discuss authoritative but not definitive pastoral teaching in the spirit of constructive criticism, is there also the right for a Catholic to *act* contrary to such official teaching? Since Catholics are always morally obliged to follow a prudent, informed conscience, unquestionably they not only have such a right but a duty to act on their own best judgment, even when in a particular instance this departs from official teaching. Those who find themselves conscientiously obliged to act this way, however, have to assume the responsibility for the consequences of their action. Putting oneself in opposition to the teaching of the Church should never be done lightly. Also, it is not fair for people, who believe in conscience that they cannot follow the teaching of the Church, to call on the pastors of the community to confirm and approve their judgments of conscience in conflict with the Magisterium. When one does not take others' advice and counsel, one cannot justly blame them for refusing to approve one's stand.

The situation of a Catholic healthcare facility, however, is quite different from that of individual theologians carrying on scholarly debate and from that of individual Catholics forming their personal conscience. A facility supported and approved officially by the local Church has the responsibility of bearing a public witness to Catholic teaching as interpreted by the local bishop. Therefore its policies need to be correlated with authoritative pastoral teaching. In the United States such teaching is proposed in the *Ethical and Religious Directives for Catholic Health Facilities,* issued by the U.S. Catholic Conference (USCC) with the approval of the National Conference of Catholic Bishops (NCCB), as promulgated and interpreted by the local bishops (USCC, 1971).

Because the pastoral guidance of the Church at the level of concrete application leaves considerable room for individual and institutional judgment, the effort of Christians to acquire and act on a well-formed conscience involves some risk and conflict. Thus a vital factor in such efforts is self-criticism or maturity of moral judgment. People have to be aware of their own biases, narrowness of experience and outlook, and half-conscious motivation. Consciences have their own psychological and spiritual pathologies, as do emotions, and have often been weakened or distorted by defective ethical education.

Some persons have a *rigid* conscience; that is, they demand a clear set of laws that they can apply almost mechanically to concrete situations. Without such security, they feel heavily burdened. Some physicians, for example, who are disturbed by present ethical debate in the Catholic Church, suffer from this pathology. More extreme is the scrupulous person who not only demands excessive certitude, but also can never achieve it, no matter how clear the rules. Such persons constantly beg for reassurance from such external authority concerning what is right or wrong and are tortured by neurotic guilt that is not based on any real guilt. This neurotic guilt can be so compulsive that it interferes with rational ethical judgment. Both these pathologies may require psychotherapy and spiritual reeducation. Persons who begin to realize that their conscience is seriously rigid or scrupulous have an obligation to seek help, since such pathologies tend to be progressive (D. Brown, 1981).

On the other hand, some persons have lax, insensitive, *callous* consciences. At the extreme are those psychopaths who seem incapable of keeping in mind the possible consequences of their actions for others or even for themselves. However, a callous conscience is also found in cynical persons who have been so scandalized by the hypocrisy of others and so weary of their guilt over their own frequent sins that they no longer bother to try to inform their conscience. More common among healthcare professionals are those whose moral sensitivity has been hardened by the routine of suffering. Many people also have a tendency to avoid moral responsibility by shifting decisions to others or by blundering ahead into action without making a firm decision. They act *in doubt*, swayed by popular opinion, by the last person they talked to, or by the mood of the moment. For these reasons, the study of medical ethics and regular, orderly discussions with others about ethical issues are necessary for ethical balance and decisiveness.

Moral Decision in an Immoral World

Despite efforts to come to principled moral decisions by which to live in peace of conscience, people may occasionally find themselves with a *perplexed* conscience. This state is not necessarily pathological but rather the result of the human condition in a sinful world wherein finding one's way is not always easy. Some Protestant moralists who stress the total depravity of human nature argue that since persons' actions are distorted by their sinful condition no matter what they do, they should "sin bravely" (to use a paradoxical but often misunderstood expression of Luther's). That is, they trust that God will forgive them no matter what their actions are as long as they have faith in his mercy. Such theologians are not denying that Christians still have the obligation to do the best they know how and by no means intend to excuse sin, but only to underline their total dependence on God's mercy (Thielicke, 1964).

Traditionally, Catholic moralists dealt with the perplexed conscience by recognizing that although an action is objectively evil, a person may have subjective difficulty in forming a good conscience. For example, Jesus presents divorce as an objective evil, but people living in a culture where divorce is commonplace may have a difficult time accepting this. Jesus himself seems to have made such a distinction when he argued that the Old Law permitted divorce "because of the hardness of your hearts" (Mt 19:8). Recently, however, Charles Curran (1975, 1977a, 1985) has proposed a theory that he calls "moral compromise." Although he does not accept the extreme pessimism about human nature proposed by some Protestant theologians, he does emphasize that sin has introduced into the world a disorder that makes it impossible even for the just person always to act in a way completely consistent with the just order of things intended by God. Thus Curran (1977a) says:

> Sinfulness for the Christian always remains present in our human existence. I am not understanding sinfulness in this case as the individual single acts of a person or even the sinfulness of the person placing the act but rather the

cosmic and interpersonal aspects of sinfulness which become incarnate in the world in which we live. Sometimes the presence of sin forces us to act in a way which would not occur if there were no sin incarnated in the structures of human existence (pp. 185-186).

Curran goes on to argue that given this sinful condition, some actions that would have been objectively wrong may become objectively right. At the same time, he does not believe this situation excuses the Christian from working to overcome the sinful situations that make such compromises necessary:

> The theory of compromise recognizes that sin affects the objective order as well as the subjective order. However, compromise also recognizes that the Christian is called to attempt to overcome the reality of sin as well as acknowledging that sin will never be completely overcome this side of the eschaton. Meanwhile, the presence of sin occasionally forces us to do things which under ordinary circumstances we would not do. The word *compromise* tries to indicate the tension involved in recognizing even in the objective order the fact that sin is present, and the Christian tries to overcome it, but at times the Christian will not be able to overcome it completely (p. 186).

Curran rightly states that the sinful condition of the world affects moral decisions not only subjectively by reason of man's moral blindness or restricted freedom, but also objectively. Curran correctly points out that St. Thomas Aquinas (Summa Theologicae, I, q. 96, a. 4; II-II, q. 57, a. 3) teaches that after the fall from the state of Original Justice, war, slavery, and private property became objectively part of the natural law, although God originally intended them to be contrary to that law. The only legitimate compromise, however, consists in accepting a lesser good (e.g., achieving peace by war when the sinful condition of the world makes this necessary) rather than achieving it by dialogue. It can never be legitimate to compromise by accepting acts that are intrinsically evil (e.g., conducting a war by attacks on noncombatants). The Christian struggle against the evils of this world cannot be effectively carried out by becoming party to the injustices by which this world often achieves its goals (see 8.1-8.2).

Consequently, it is never permissible to choose the lesser evil as such. Christians must always choose appropriate means to their goals; an evil act, by definition, is an inappropriate means. Ordinarily, if there is no good means, Christians should not choose any.

Traditional moral theology, in speaking of the lesser evil, was not talking about the informed conscience, but rather about the problem of a counselor who sees that a client is determined to do something evil. In such a case, the counselor (according to most theologians) could tell the client that it would be better to do something less evil, if in this way the counselor might dissuade the client from the greater evil (e.g., to be sterilized rather than to commit an abortion). This is the principle used in the section discussing the responsibilities of counselors in *The Many Faces of AIDS*, the pastoral letter of the Catholic Bishops of the United States (USCC, 1987). This is quite different from the problem of conscientiously perplexed persons of goodwill who can always achieve moral certitude by doing what seems to them the better of two alternatives, both of which seem somehow wrong.

In view of the foregoing discussion, the *Principle of Well-Formed Conscience* can be formulated as follows.

> To attain the true goals of human life by responsible actions, in every free decision involving an ethical question, persons are morally obliged:
> 1. To inform themselves as fully as practically possible as to both the facts and the ethical norms;
> 2. To form a morally certain judgment of conscience on the basis of this information;
> 3. To act according to this well-formed conscience;
> 4. To accept responsibility for their actions.

Informed Consent

Closely related to the problem of a well-formed conscience is the notion of *informed consent* (Belmont Report, 1978; Faden and Beauchamp, 1986; John Fletcher, 1983a; Pellegrino, 1981). When one person asks another to cooperate or even to allow him or her to act on the other's person—for example, when a physician asks a patient to take a prescription, to undergo surgery, or to act as the subject of an experiment—the other's human dignity must be respected according to the Principle of Human Dignity in Community (1.5). By this principle, however, the other person, because of his or her personal responsibility for health, may not consent without an informed conscience. This implies that a healthcare professional has the duty to supply the patient with the medical information necessary for the patient to make an informed decision. When geriatric patients are concerned, this requires greater sensitivity on the part of the healthcare professional (O'Rourke, 1988b). The healthcare professional has no right to ask the patient to cooperate or submit to any medical procedure without first obtaining informed consent from the patient, or if the patient is not competent to give this consent, the informed consent of the patient's guardian (Munetz et al., 1985; President's Commission, 1982). Chapter 9 discusses in more detail some of the difficulties in making sure this ethical solution is properly satisfied in regard to research programs.

Recently, the presence of the AIDS (acquired immunodeficiency syndrome) virus has resulted in discussion concerning the need for informed consent regarding as patients in healthcare facilities (R. Bayer and Levine, 1986). The desire to protect healthcare professionals leads some to declare that patients may be tested for AIDS without obtaining informed consent. The argument is offered that testing all patients in healthcare facilities for AIDS would be the same as testing for any other blood disorder. Thus, to alert healthcare professionals to the presence of a patient with the virus, some physicians and healthcare administrators allow screening without informed consent. They argue that implicit consent is given to such testing by reason of the fact that one voluntarily enters the health facility (Welsby, 1986).

However, we believe that testing for the AIDS virus without explicit informed consent is unethical for the following reasons:

1. Testing for AIDS is not a routine medical procedure because of the harm that may result from such testing. Many persons infected with the AIDS virus are either homosexuals or intravenous drug users; thus the discrimination and opprobrium that may follow testing for AIDS infection are severe (Cassens, 1985; McCombie, 1986). Many people have lost their housing, jobs, and friends when the presence of the virus in their system has become known (Blendon and Donelan, 1988). Even people who have tested negative have been dropped as clients by insurance companies and suffer other indignities, since people surmise that someone being tested indicates that the person is in a high-risk group (Kristof, 1985; Oppenheimer and Padgug, 1986). Thus, before testing a person for the AIDS virus, the implications of the testing, whether positive or negative, must be explained clearly and thoroughly. Testing for AIDS is not the same as testing for glucose or iron deficiency.

2. Even if healthcare professionals do know which patients have AIDS, this knowledge alone does not offer any protection. Healthcare professionals may best protect against acquiring the virus only by treating all patients as though they had the virus. This advice from the Centers for Disease Control (CDC) must be implemented by healthcare facilities through provision of protective clothing and equipment (gloves, masks, etc.) (CDC, 1987). Treating everyone as though infected is the only safe course because even if the patient is tested, the tests could not be positive until antibodies have had a chance to form. Thus there is at least a few weeks' time after infection when a negative result may be inaccurate.

Clearly some testing for AIDS should be done for public health reasons, both to keep an account of the spread of the disease and to prevent its spread insofar as possible (Koop, 1986). To accomplish both goals, however, it seems voluntary and "anonymous" testing, that is, testing accompanied by informed consent and revealed only to the person tested, is more effective. Surveys show that people in high-risk groups are reluctant to submit to mandatory testing. Moreover, as long as change of behavior is the only effective way to limit the spread of the disease, voluntary testing accompanied by counseling seems to be the most effective manner of limiting the disease. Counselors should be available to help those who test positive cope with the knowledge that they have a fatal disease, but above all counselors should help infected persons realize that they will harm other people severely if they engage in behavior that spreads the virus (Michael Mills et al., 1986). Although ample justification exists for screening recruits to the armed services (the services depend on their own members for blood transfusions), we believe that mandatory screening of prisoners violates their human rights because no benefit to the public good results from such testing (Hammet, 1986). To date, there is no cure for AIDS, although it seems the fatal effects may be delayed for a time through medication. Thus the most effective way to prevent the spread of the disease is to eliminate the behavior that leads to its spread (National Academy of Science, 1988), namely, sharing infected needles for drug use, having sexual intercourse (anal or vaginal) with infected men or women, or receiving blood transfusions from donors who have not been thoroughly screened. If a cure is found for the disease, mandatory testing, without consent, would become a necessity because knowledge of the disease's presence then would lead to effective action for its elimination. This thinking underlies mandatory smallpox vaccination for children. At present, however, the main preventive measure for AIDS is to change the behavior of infected people (College of Physicians, 1986).

The Principle of Free and Informed Conscience can also be formulated as a corollary of the Principle of a Well-Formed Conscience:

> To protect the basic need of every human person for healthcare and the primary responsibility of each person for his or her own healthcare, no physical or psychological act of examination or therapy may be performed without the free and informed consent of the patient, or, if the patient is incompetent, that of his or her legitimate guardian acting for the person's benefit and, as far as possible, in accordance with his or her known reasonable wishes.

3.5 PATIENT'S RIGHTS

Choosing a Physician

Since each person has the primary obligation of caring for his or her own health, each also has the obligation to seek and choose professional people to help advise them concerning healthcare. This does not mean, however, that persons can surrender to others the responsibility of making decisions about their health. Professionals are helpers, not keepers. Frequently, healthcare professionals fail to realize how difficult it is for ordinary persons to select a physician, or how uncertain such persons are about their own rights in dealing with a healthcare institution. Healthcare professionals have an educational responsibility to help clients know how and where to seek healthcare and how to protect their own rights in doing so (Rosenberg and Towers, 1986).

No one is a good judge in his or her own case; precisely because health is so personal a value, it is something about which it is hard to be objective. People tend to delude themselves as to both how well they are and how sick they are. Even physicians need the advice of others, since most physicians do not dare diagnose themselves or their families. Psychotherapists usually undergo therapy as part of their training and return to it from time to time. Moral guides know that if they are to be of help in making sound moral decisions, they must engage in public discussion and be open to guidance themselves by responsible authority. Finally, good spiritual guides recognize their own spiritual blindness and their need for the spiritual guidance of others, above all by the Spirit. Thus, to be whole and healthy, each person must be humble enough to seek help from others more expert, or at least more objective about their problems.

Along with humility, courage and hope also are required. One out of three persons who need to see a physician fail to do so, not only because of economic and educational obstacles, but also because of fear, apathy, shame, and self-punishment (R. Blum, 1964; Llewellyn-Thomas, 1982). The most dangerous aspect of any diseased condition is that it may make the victim despair of health or afraid to seek help to obtain health. At the psychological level, neurotic and alcoholic persons notoriously deny their problems and resist therapy. Physically sick people also seem to have an almost instinctive dread of recognizing their illness and facing the pain of its cure. Even hypochondriac persons who seem only too eager to claim sickness use the illusion of one disease to hide from themselves some other sickness—perhaps at the psychological, social, or spiritual level—that would be even more painful to face. They crowd the physician's office in unconscious avoidance of the psychotherapist or some moral or spiritual counselor.

Perhaps the reason such people resist the truth about themselves is because they are organisms who tend, once an acute crisis has passed, to adapt to a chronic disease by integrating it into their way of life. Once such a distorted integration has become fixed, they sense real peril in returning to the acutely painful crisis that might be provoked by a new effort to become really well. Thus they dread physicians and avoid them as long as possible. Both psychological and physiological diseases therefore are allowed to hit bottom before these persons can submit themselves to treatment. The same principle holds at the social and spiritual levels, so that most profound moral and spiritual conversions are brought about only after a deep conviction of sin. Jesus noted that it was the publicans and prostitutes who were most likely to enter the Kingdom of God (Mt 21:31).

Even when people have the humility and courage to seek a physician, they are faced with two very serious ethical problems in choosing a good one. The first arises from their choice possibly being restricted greatly by the complex organization of modern medical care and the maldistribution of its services. Should this restriction of freedom be allowed, or is there a moral obligation to resist it? This sociopolitical issue is discussed in some detail in Chapter 6.

The second ethical issue in choosing a physician or a healthcare facility arises from today's widespread doubt about the competence and the character of healthcare professionals (Phillip Lee et al., 1988). Some authors, such as Illich (1976), have launched an attack on the whole system of healthcare in the United States. Others (D. Axelrod, 1988; Katz, 1984) without going as far as Illich, have criticized vigorously the way that American healthcare professionals live up to their professed standards. Still others seek to outline the methods that will improve medical care (Reiser and Rosen, 1984; Stillman et al., 1988). With due allowance for polemics, however, in the United States, as in most countries, the average citizen experiences difficulty in obtaining satisfactory healthcare (Aday et al., 1984).

Although Americans are convinced, and with reason, that the billions of dollars spent each year on healthcare go to support the most advanced medical technology and professional education in the world, this by no means proves that the average citizen is receiving healthcare of high quality. The life expectancy of citizens in the United States is lower than in a number of European countries and has not improved noticeably in the last 20 years. In some states the death rate is 25 percent higher than in other states.

Available studies of the quality of care (College of Healthcare Executives, 1987; R. Rubin et al., 1988) and of the actual competency of physicians in practice frequently reveal alarming percentages of physicians whose competence is substandard (Bosk, 1986; Strauss, 1984). Again, estimates show that a high percentage of surgery (50 percent in some hospitals) is unnecessary and explainable only by incompetence or greed (Margo, 1986). Finally, the studies also show that among professionals, physicians rate highest in drug addiction, alcoholism, and psychological disorders. When this is added to the growing evidence that a considerable percentage of physicians have an income well in excess of members of other professions, choosing a reliable and competent physician and a high-quality hospital is difficult (Couch et al., 1981; Steel, 1981).

Protection of Rights

The ethical issues raised by such choices are dramatized by the very titles of popular books by Arthur Levin, *Talk Back to Your Doctor* (1975); Martin Lipp, *The Bitter Pill; Doctors, Patients and Failed Expectations* (1980); William Winslade and Judith Ross, *Choosing Life or Death* (1986); and Terry Mizratti, *Getting Rid of Patients* (1986). Although we do not endorse these works, they do show the need for a careful, even aggressive attitude on the part of the patient toward the healthcare professional and the healthcare facility. This seems in strong contrast to the attitude of *trust* that has been traditionally regarded as the basis of every profession (a tradition defended in Chapter 4). These authors, however, with evidence to support their position, argue that persons who fail to take this distrustful stance toward the medical profession today are failing in their responsibility to their own health.

In every age many people certainly have been irresponsible in selecting medical guides, as well as political and religious leaders. The very fears that prevent people from seeking help also cause them often to prefer the quack (medical, psychological, social, or spiritual) to the competent guide whom they suspect may make them face a painful reality. The quack knows how to exploit these fears, this flight from real diagnosis and cure, to gain control over the patient. Not all quacks are incompetent, since very able guides can easily be tempted to use their own gifts to gain power for themselves, as the history of illicit medical experimentation evidences.

To escape enslavement to the incompetent or exploitative professional, people need to be conscious of the rights that are correlative to their responsibility to choose professional help prudently. These rights may be summed up as follows (Annas, 1973; Storch, 1982; Summers, 1985):
1. The right to the whole truth;
2. The right to privacy and personal dignity;
3. The right to refuse any test, procedure, or treatment; and
4. The right to read and copy medical records.

Also, Chapter 6 discusses the right to treatment of persons who are institutionalized, such as prisoners or those involuntarily committed to mental hospitals (Forer, 1982; Meisel, 1982).

All the rights proposed rest on the fundamental concept of informed consent. If the patient is to give free consent, the patient must also be able to refuse any test, procedure, or treatment. The right to privacy and personal dignity also amounts to the right of patients to refuse to be involved in any professional procedures that make them objects to be examined or discussed for the benefit or convenience of professionals or students rather than for the patient's own therapy. (Annas et al., 1981)

If this consent is to be not only free but also informed, the patient has the right to the whole truth, including access to read and copy medical records (Bruce, 1984; Canadian Medical Association Journal, 1985). Many professionals deny these rights on the grounds that the patient is not able to understand the technical information known to the physician and may be harmed by it. However, such difficulties do not disprove patients' right to know but only establish the professional's duty to communicate this information in ways that are helpful, not harmful, to patients so that consent may be truly informed.

Among the facts patients have the right to know is the competency and ethical integrity of the physician or healthcare facility to which they may entrust themselves. The authors already cited give much good advice on this subject. Generally, they agree that the first consideration is medical competency. In the present state of affairs, they believe such competency is most likely to be found among physicians holding assignments to a medical school–affiliated hospital, since they are most likely to be well-educated and up-to-date in knowledge and skill and subject to some form of peer review. Similarly, these authors generally recommend choosing a larger, accredited, medical school–affiliated hospital, whether a public or a nonprofit private institution, and avoiding small proprietary hospitals.

They also recommend choosing a primary service physician who is concerned with total health and who should be a family practice specialist rather than a general practitioner. Through these primary service physicians, the need for further specialized care can be ascertained and suitable specialists sought. All these authors, however, emphasize that no matter how excellent the physician, people should never hesitate to ask for consultation when doubts arise, especially when surgery is in question (Wertheimer et al., 1985; Horowitz, 1988).

Thus the underlying ethical issue of trust again emerges. Is competency the primary consideration in choosing a physician (Cousins, 1985)? Certainly it is the *specific* qualification most people seek in any professional, including their physicians. If physicians are not also trustworthy, however, in the sense that they are sincerely dedicated to helping the patient get well, then their medical competency is dangerous, as in the case of brilliantly competent surgeons eager for more bodies on which to demonstrate their skill. Thus the careful choice of a primary service physician is highly important, since it is this physician who is most concerned for the patient as a whole person. Also, persons should seek physicians who work in institutions where not only their skill, but also their professional dedication to patient welfare, is most likely to be tested and evaluated by peers.

People, therefore, should not lightly accept the idea that their personal responsibility for their own health is satisfied merely by assuming a critical attitude toward physicians and demanding their rights from them. Such a responsibility also includes willingness to trust physicians once they have been prudently chosen, to make good use of their advice, and to cooperate with their healing efforts. Although people should never be afraid to protect their rights and to insist that physicians give patients all the information they need to give informed consent to treatment, they should also give physicians a deserved respect. Trustworthy and competent healthcare professionals perform for people a precious service, for which they deserve profound gratitude, good reputation, and fair and prompt payment.

While retaining primary right and responsibility to give informed consent or refusal to any kind of professional health service, people should also remember the commendatory words of Scripture:

> Hold the physician in honor, for he is essential to you, and God it was who established his profession,

> From God the doctor has his wisdom, and the kin provides for his sustenance.

> His knowledge makes the doctor distinguished, and gives him access to those in authority.

> God makes the earth yield healing herbs, which the prudent man should not neglect;

> Was not the water sweetened by a twig [when Moses sweetened the bitter waters in the desert] that man might learn his power?

> He endows men with the knowledge to glory in his mighty works,

> Through which the doctor eases pain and the druggist prepares his medicines;

> Thus God's creative work continues without ceasing in its efficacy on the surface of the earth (Si 38:1-8).

Part 2

THE HEALING PROFESSION

Although individuals have primary responsibility to care for their own health as well as for the psychological, ethical, and spiritual aspects of their personal development, such development can be achieved only with the help of other members of the community. In advanced communities, such help is furnished by persons who have chosen and been educated for the special social roles called the professions. Part 2 considers the chief ethical issues involved in the choice of the healthcare profession as a vocation and in the educational preparation needed to fulfill the demands of so difficult a vocation.

Because the healthcare profession is only one among several professions basic to the culture of any advanced community, it is necessary first to consider the nature of the professions in general (as discussed in Chapter 4), then to define the specific role of the medical profession, and finally to identify its interrelations with other professions. The chief thesis in this section is that medical education must include the development of basic ethical attitudes. Since these attitudes are rooted in the relation of trust between professional and client, Chapter 5 deals with the specific character of this relation in the healthcare situation. Finally, since today the profession of medicine, as with that of teaching, is exercised largely in institutional settings, Chapter 6 considers the ethical issues raised by the social organization of healthcare.

The Healthcare Profession

OVERVIEW

This chapter considers first the concept of a profession in general (4.1) and then the specific task of the healthcare professional. Traditionally, this profession has been rather narrowly identified as "the medical profession" and with the role of the physician as a medical doctor (MD). The overall emphasis of this book is on the health team, but this chapter deals with the more traditional and narrower concept, considering the historical ideals of the medical profession in 4.2 and the education of physicians as it transmits these ideals today in 4.3. The concern here is not with the scientific knowledge and technical skills so essential to this profession, but rather with its ethical ideals and standards.

4.1 PROFESSIONS: DEPERSONALIZING TRENDS

As stated in the Introduction, the purpose of this book is not to pass moral judgment on the shortcomings of the healthcare profession in meeting its own standards. Rather, our purpose is to identify some of the ethical issues that are most acute for the progress of this profession today and to suggest some directions in which Catholic healthcare professionals can give witness and leadership in the resolution of these issues by the profession and by the public.

The medieval professions were divinity (theology), physic (medicine), and law. They were "person professions" (Sieghart, 1985) centered on a counselor-client relation. They did not produce goods for sale or works of art for enjoyment, but worked to heal, guide, or protect some person in a life crisis. Industrial society has greatly fostered the professions, but it has also depersonalized them. No longer are they centered on conviviality of persons (Illich, 1972), but on the productivity of an impersonal system. They no longer deal with better interpersonal communication, but with more efficient exchange of energy.

This slow depersonalizing transformation of the professions is reaching its completion today, just as industrial society itself seems about to yield to a new postindustrial society (R. Veatch, 1985). Neither progressive capitalism nor revolutionary Marxism has been able to fulfill the promises of scientific technology to produce a society of abundance and freedom. Even this promise begins to seem illusory in view of the ecological doomsday predicted by some authorities (Meadows et al., 1972; Marco, 1987).

In postindustrial society, the source of power will no longer be economic ownership (whether capitalist or socialist), but rather *knowledge and its communication.* Such power means a still greater role for the professions (Moline, 1986). This knowledge can be used to bring about greater social conformism and dependency on the professionals, or it can be used to open the system to wider and more genuine social participation by all. In either case, the professions must be radically reconstructed.

Will professionals become technocrats whose technological mastery must extend itself to behavior control? Or will they become the persons who help others to transcend the depersonalization of technological systems by "putting the good of the weaker party over one's own interests" (Moline, 1986)? If professionals choose the latter alternative, the professions must again be personalized. They must be reconstructed so as to eliminate the threefold depersonalization that the professions have suffered in the epoch of industrial society.

First, *clients* have been depersonalized by the proliferation of specialism. They are no longer thought of as organisms, but as collections of organs (Freymann, 1974). The parts are healed, not the person, such that the very meaning of *healing,* that is, "to make *whole,*" has been lost. Around each profession has grown a host of "para" or "semi" professions. However, the result is not so much integration as competition and confusion. Even the efforts of interdisciplinary healing teams never quite seem to succeed in getting it all together again.

Second, *professionals themselves* have been depersonalized by a loss of clear identity. This loss is notoriously true for the ministry (Hussey, 1988) and is now evident in law, teaching, and medicine (Freidson, 1971; Freund, 1965; Shaffer, 1987). Psychiatrists, psychoanalysts, and psychiatric social workers all perform similar tasks but are considered members of three different professions (Henry et al., 1971). Even more confusing, many ministers, lawyers, and physicians counsel clients in ways not easily distinguishable from those used by psychotherapists (H. Freeman, 1967).

Contributing to this confusion of identity today is the tension within the profession between the goals of research and the goals of practice (Lind, 1986). In addition, many areas of professional practice may soon be handed over to computers. How, then, can a professional make that type of personal commitment always regarded as a mark of a profession if it is not clear to what he or she is professed?

Third, the *validity of the professional-client relation* is being questioned. Professionalism seems to imply an elitism that is ultimately socially destructive. Illich (1972, 1978) studied the problems of underdeveloped countries and launched an all-out attack on schooling and the concept of the teaching profession and is extending the same criticism to medicine (1976). More recently,

Beriman and Navarro (1983), Navarro (1986), and Waitzhib (1983) offered similar observations. They contend that the industrial model for organizing the professions has progressively restricted access to knowledge and skill, placing them in the hands of elites on whom the public is more and more dependent, but from whom the public receives less and less adequate service (Cahn, 1986). The result is that service institutions have become "production funnels" that proliferate subordinate professions and paraprofessions. Illich wants to free people from such production funnels by giving nonspecialists easier access to the information now the prerogative of professional elites. He argues that both capitalist and Marxist politics are based on the same invalid professional ideal, and that the Third World is desperately striving to make the same mistake.

These three depersonalizations are most easily illustrated in the case of the medical profession, but they also occur in the most unlikely profession—the religious ministry, which has always claimed to be concerned for the whole person. In recent years many priests, ministers, and rabbis have deserted their calling to serve. The clergy have accepted elitist status and are neither sure of their own role nor competent to give interdisciplinary guidance to other professionals in the service of persons (John Paul II, 1984c).

Personalistic Concept of a Profession

Today the term *profession* is used for almost any prestigious occupation because it has the aura of an ideal (Moline, 1986). It is a symbol rather than a reality. The distinguished sociologist Howard Becker (1960) writes:

> The symbol systematically ignores such facts as the failure of the professions to monopolize their area of knowledge, the lack of homogeneity within professions, the frequent failure of clients to accept professional judgment, the chronic presence of unethical practitioners as an integrated segment of the professional structure, and the organizational constraints on professional autonomy. A symbol which ignores so many features of occupational life cannot provide an adequate guide for professional activity (p. 46).

Nevertheless, the sociologists have devoted much time to developing a good empirical definition of a profession. Merton (1960) explains the social value of a profession very succinctly:

> First, the value placed upon systematic knowledge and intellect: *knowing*. Second, the value placed upon technical skill and trained capacity: *doing*. And third, the value place upon putting this conjoint knowledge and skill to work in the service of others: *helping* (p. 9).

Barber (1965) proposes the following "relativistic" definition:

> Professional behavior may be defined in terms of four essential attributes: (1) a high degree of generalized and systematic knowledge; (2) primary orientation to the community interest rather than to individual self-interest; (3) a high degree of self-control of behavior through codes of ethics internalized in the process of work socialization and through voluntary

associations organized and operated by the work specialists themselves; and (4) a system of rewards (monetary and honorary) that is primarily a set of symbols of work achievement and thus ends in themselves, not means to some end of individual self-interest.

Similarly, Underwood (1972) says:

> These four concerns—concern for persons, trained skills, values and basic theory, and public responsibility—are the central themes of professional ideology always mentioned in the sociological literature on the professions and the professions' statement of purpose (p. 422).

Moore and Rosenblum (1970) use a scale to define professionalism. Professionals must rate high on the following six operational attributes:

1. Professionals practice *full-time occupations.*
2. They are committed to a *calling;* that is, they treat their occupation "as an enduring set of normative and behavioral expectations."
3. They are distinguished from the laity by various signs and symbols and identified with their peers—often in formalized *organizations.*
4. They have esoteric but useful knowledge and skills through specialized *education,* which is lengthy and difficult.
5. They are expected to have a *service orientation* so as to perceive the needs of a client relevant to their competency.
6. They have *autonomy* of judgment and authority restrained by responsibility in using their knowledge and skill (pp. 51-65, 174-186).

The problem with these definitions (which fundamentally come down to Merton's "knowing-doing-helping") is that they fail to distinguish clearly the original group of person professions from other highly developed occupations that the term has been extended to but that not deal *directly* with persons. Today engineering, architecture and the other arts, and business are considered professions because they also involve knowing, doing, and helping (Sieghart, 1985). Their immediate objective, however, is not personal but productive. This obliteration of the distinction between the person professions and productive occupations is characteristic of industrial society and its depersonalization of the professions. If they are to be repersonalized, this distinction between personal and productive professions must be drawn once more.

The need for this distinction and the importance of the counselor-client relationship in the professions has been pointed out by the sociologist William Goode (1969), who makes a fundamental suggestion:

> Specifically, I suggest that a category of occupations is set apart (as a profession) by a primary variable, upon which a considerable number of structural consequences hinge: whether the professional must symbolically or literally "get inside the client," become privy to his personal world, in order to solve the problem that is the mandate of the profession (p. 307).

According to this view, research scientists and scholars are not professionals because they are directly concerned with knowing, not doing, and with theory, not practice. The work of laboratory experimentation may appear as a doing, but its purpose is to test a theory, not to apply it practically.

To call the technologies and the arts (engineering, business, fine arts) professions is confusing and dangerous because this designation disguises that they produce *things* and do not directly help persons. Certainly the technologies should educate their practitioners to be more sensitive to the human uses to which their product will be put. This humanization of technology, however, will be hindered if industrial society continues the previous tendency of lumping the technologies and the person professions together under one name and to judge them all in terms of productivity.

A true profession, therefore, is rooted in theory but aimed at practice—a practice that does not produce things external to persons but a service directly to persons themselves (Shaffer, 1987). Furthermore, this service is not applied to persons who receive it passively but facilitates those persons' own activity. It aims at healing them, at making them whole, at freeing them to act on their own. Counselors should not act on clients, nor dominate them, but enable them to become fully, autonomously themselves. Thus a profession cannot properly be elitist. It communicates power rather than enforces dependency.

Finally, professional help in the full sense is concerned precisely with those problems that are deeply personal, that are matters of life and death. Therefore such help engages both counselor and client in a profound responsibility both to each other and to the community. This personalistic concept of a profession can reconstruct the professions and professional education for the future (Kanigel, 1988).

Physicians and Patients with AIDS

The practical results of viewing medicine as a profession, as opposed to a trade or a business, are immediately evident when considering the responsibility of physician and other healthcare workers to treat patients with acquired immunodeficiency syndrome (AIDS). Treating AIDS patients involves some risk for the healthcare worker of acquiring the human immunodeficiency virus (HIV) infection if the worker is exposed to body fluids (Marcus, 1988). Moreover, if a physician accepts AIDS patients, other patients may determine they do not wish to continue as patients. For these reasons, some physicians refuse to treat AIDS patients (Koop, 1987). If healthcare is simply another marketplace trade, and if healthcare workers are engaged merely in business, then there would be no responsibility to treat AIDS patients. Instead, physicians and other healthcare workers could refuse to treat AIDS patients either because of personal risk or because profits would be diminished.

Although some attempting to answer the question concerning treatment of AIDS patients have opted for a mitigated form of personal responsibility, most individuals and medical societies have stated that because medicine is a profession in the true sense of the word, AIDS patients must be cared for without discrimination. Thus the Texas Medical Association and the Arizona Board of Medical Examiners were willing to settle for a general responsibility on the profession as a whole, maintaining that the physician fulfilled his or her responsibility if the AIDS patients were referred to another physician who would care for the patient (Medical News, 1987; Texas Medical Association, 1987).

On the other hand, the American Medical Association (AMA, 1988a), the American College of Physicians (Scherr, 1987), and several individuals considering the topic (Pellegrino, 1987; Schwartz and Gray, 1987) declare that because medicine is a profession, individual physicians and healthcare workers have ethical and legal responsibilities to care for AIDS patients. As Emanuel states (1988): "With the understanding that medicine is a profession committed to the ideal of caring for the sick, physicians can deny emergency care, but not simply because of a person's disease, the inability to pay, or the physician's personal dislike; physicians cannot discriminate against people in accepting nonemergency patients."

If medicine is viewed as a profession, reasonable risks clearly are associated with being a healthcare worker (Emanuel, 1988). One assumes those risks on entering the profession. Such risks are associated with other occupations; for example, being a policeman and fireman exposes one to injury and death. Although the injury resulting from an HIV infection is serious, for most healthcare workers there is small danger of infection (Kelen et al., 1988; Weiss et al., 1988; Zuger and Miles, 1987). Thus, healthcare workers are not being called on to undergo undue risks when proper precautions are used in caring for AIDS patients (Centers for Disease Control, 1987). Many healthcare facilities have developed policies that state the ethical and legal responsibilities of physicians and other healthcare workers to care for AIDS patients.

Healthcare Counseling

This book is concerned with the way the personalistic concept applies to the healthcare professions because, although healthcare counseling has much in common with other types of professional counseling, it is also distinct from them.

Originally, the term *counseling* pertained to rational, moral, and ethical functioning (Pietroferg, 1983) and in particular to the legal profession, as the British use of the term *counselor* indicates. Counseling also found a place in the religious ministry, since the rabbi was a type of religious lawyer, and this role was passed on to Christian priests. As Chapter 1 argues and Chapter 14 develops more fully, however, the specific type of counseling proper to the ministerial profession is deeper than the legal and pertains to the spiritual dimension of the human person. One can also argue that the teaching profession, in arousing the creativity of the student, also reaches to this same level of intuitive life.

The medical professional often performs one or the other of these types of counseling proper to the other professions. A physician may have to discuss with a patient certain ethical and legal issues, such as those involved in an abortion decision. Sometimes a physician is involved in a patient's spiritual struggles about death and the meaning of life. Often physicians must play the role of teacher, helping patients understand their body or psyche. However, all these involvements are incidental and substitutional. A prudent physician is quick to refer the patient to experts in other professions when the issues are ethical and spiritual rather than medical.

The proper task of the medical professional is to deal with problems at the biological and psychological levels of human functioning (Pellegrino and Thomasma, 1981, 1988). At the psychological level, counseling of a certain type plays a major therapeutic role, although some deny this (see Chapters 5 and 12). At the biological level, however, it is not so obvious that the physician's role is still primarily that of a counselor. However, if the thesis argued in Chapter 3 is correct—that all persons have primary responsibility for their own health—then the physician's primary responsibility is to help patients make good health decisions, which requires a counseling process. People cannot make good decisions about how to care for their health unless they have the required information. In more complicated cases, this information can be obtained only by consulting a physician. To some extent the physician is playing the role of a teacher in giving this information. More is involved than this, however, since the information required is not abstract biological truth but a concrete assessment of personal health and the possible ways of dealing with the problems this assessment presents. This form of guidance is required of a physician, and it engages the physician in a special type of counseling.

This basic counseling relation on which the whole medical profession is built is "trusteeship" (Freymann, 1974). William F. May (1983) speaks of a "covenant" between physician and patient, as did Ramsey (1970). Technological progress in medicine has temporarily obscured the importance of trusteeship, making it appear that the physician is a scientist-technician rather than a counselor, but this same technological progress will eventually expose what it covers up. Soon not only the process of treatment, but also diagnosis itself, will become the work of technicians, while physicians will be freed once more to deal personally with patients. Moreover, physicians will be dealing not with patients so sick that they cannot think, but with responsible persons concerned to stay well. In such situations, the physician will play the role of health counselor. As Freymann states:

> The degree to which a modern patient seeks these two attributes— knower-doer and trustee—in his doctor varies. The victim of an acute catastrophe may need and want only the knower-doer. But the less clear-cut the clinical picture, the more the patient looks for both. He wants a knower-doer who can solve those problems for which there is an answer. But he wants a trustee who can comprehend *all* his problems and help him to face them, no matter what the outcome. The former calls for a scientist, but much of what the pure scientist can do now will be taken over by the technician-computer teams. The latter calls for a physician or a nurse, for no matter how man-like computers may become, I do not think trusteeship will ever be automated (p. 313).

Nursing is truly a profession because it shares in this counseling task of the physician. Today (see 6.4), the role of the nurse has become very ambiguous (Barger-Lux and Heaney, 1986; Crissman and Betz, 1987; Kluge, 1982), but Freymann (1974) was correct in saying that the medical profession has always had the double dimension of cure and care. Thus medicine always requires a distinction between the curing task of the physician and the caring task of the nurse. What is common to both cure and care is that the patient must consent to both and cooperate actively with both, so that both physician and nurse must enter into the trustee relationship with the patient.

Also, this basic relationship will not be eliminated as patients in the future relate more and more to a health team rather than one-to-one with a personal physician (Mechanic, 1985). Chapter 1 shows that personal relationships always have a social character. Group psychotherapy has proved that personalism need not be eliminated just because the one-to-one relationship with a therapist is expanded into a more complex social relationship.

The account of the professions as rooted in the counselor-client relationship, however, is very far from the reality of the professions in society today.

As cited in 2.1, Freidson stated in 1971 that the professions are no longer characterized by service to the client, nor by fidelity to a body of expert knowledge, but instead by a drive for autonomy. Thus the medical profession is often unresponsive to the health needs of the public, since the public has no way to make its needs effective in the face of this professional autonomy (AMA, 1986a).

Freidson is not alone in this opinion. Berlant (1975) denies that the medical profession in the United States and Great Britain arose to meet a social need, but rather that it developed as a "commercial class" dedicated to achieving monopoly control. He argues that historically the medical profession has gone through all the steps characteristic of any commercial class, such as (1) creation of a commodity, (2) separation of the performance of its service from any necessary satisfaction of the client's interests, (3) creation of scarcity, (4) monopolization of supply, (5) restriction of membership, (6) elimination of external competition, (7) price fixation, (8) unification of suppliers, (9) elimination of internal competition, and (10) development of group solidarity and cooperation. Of course, similar disparaging accounts can be given of the other professions, including teaching and religious ministry, which are supposed to deal with spiritual values. The following section considers these sociological criticisms of the medical profession in more detail.

4.2   TRADITIONAL IDEALS OF THE MEDICAL PROFESSION

Priest or Scientist?

To make sure that the personalistic concept of the medical profession is not a mere ideal requires a brief look at the crosscurrents of purpose that have been at work in the historical development of the profession (Galdston, 1981; Reiser and Dyck, 1977; Reiser and Rosen, 1984).

The standard histories of medicine (Garrison, 1960; Sigerist, 1951) usually divide this history into the prescientific period and the scientific period, which begins only in the seventeenth century after Vesalius and Harvey. Michael Foucault, in his fascinating book *The Birth of the Clinic* (1973), shows that the crucial step was taken as a result of the efforts of the radical wing of the French Revolution to abolish all professions, including the medical profession, as a means to establishing a classless society. The resulting chaos in healthcare then led to the reestablishment of the medical profession and its hospitals on a new basis under the domination of the scientific ideals of the Enlightenment.

Freymann (1974) has also shown that from 1700 to 1850, healthcare was fragmented and the profession at a low ebb until the Age of Pasteur, with its emphasis on the scientific education of physicians to fight acute diseases. Only now, Freymann believes, is the profession entering the Age of Darwin and Freud with the emphasis on an ecological, positive health approach. Thus medicine as an effective scientific technology is a very recent development in human history.

On closer examination, however, it becomes evident that this division into prescientific and scientific periods is somewhat misleading because it is only a manifestation of two aspects of medical tradition that have always coexisted and still do. Today, along with orthodox scientific medicine, a vast field of heretical medicine exists, ranging from naturopathy, faith healing, homeopathy, and chiropractic to osteopathy, acupuncture, and "holistic" medicine (Guttmacher, 1979), not to mention countless forms of pure quackery. These therapies evidently complement orthodox medicine because they seem to meet health needs that orthodox medicine does not (Easthope, 1986). Also, it is no secret that even within orthodox medicine the field of psychotherapy is a borderline area that many medical physicians consider unscientific.

This duality, on closer examination, reflects the mind-body or psychosomatic duality of the human being who is sick. In early times the learned professions all originated from the one rather confused profession of priest (or perhaps priest-king). Priests were looked on as custodians of sacred wisdom and power over the forces of nature, a gift from the gods, who alone possessed cosmic secrets.

In Greece (whence modern Western medicine is directly descended) the first father of medicine was Asclepius (Ackerknecht, 1982), who was so kind as the "mild god" that he was to prove a great rival of Christ as Christianity spread throughout the pagan world (Edelstein, 1967). Asclepius' priests presided over shrines (the first clinics) where the sick came to worship, sleep, and have their dreams interpreted. The symbol of the medical profession today is still a staff with entwined serpents because the serpent, symbol of wisdom and the healing power of mother earth (i.e., nature), was the cult animal at these shrines. Today in the city of Rome, the Hospital of the Benefratelli of medieval origin is built on an island in the River Tiber over remains of a shrine of Asclepius transferred from Greece in classical times. A great snake is still to be seen carved on the ancient ruins.

This myth manifests a basic truth about the medical profession: the physician to this day retains something of a priestly ministry in the service of the healing forces of nature. Something similar is true of every profession, since all professions deal with the sacred dignity of the human person and rest on the sacred covenant of trust between client and professional. This priestly ministry is especially true of the medical profession because its direct relation to life and death gives it a fundamental, primitive character. A person's trust in the physician is almost the same as trust in one's mother; it is a primordial confidence in life support.

No wonder, then, that even today the physician is a charismatic figure, surrounded by a priestly atmosphere (witness the myths of television doctor shows). Although this trust can be abused and exploited, it is valuable when it is authentic. No one can be healed without trust. Thus the most significant distinction in understanding the history of medicine is not between scientific and nonscientific medicine, but between *authentic* medicine and quackery. Authentic medicine has both priestly and scientific dimensions.

Why did it take until the seventeenth and even the nineteenth century for the rapid development of this scientific side of medicine to begin? The empirical rational method was already well understood in the time of Hippocrates, about 400 BC. Hippocrates rejected the designation of epilepsy and other ailments as sacred diseases and attempted to explain them biologically. In the next century, Aristotle (himself a son of an Asclepian doctor who was the physician of Alexander the Great), in *De Somniis,* demythologized the notion of dreams, often used to diagnose diseases, by giving such psychic phenomena a physiological explanation. This tradition of scientific medicine was further developed by Hellenistic physicians such as Galen and by medieval Arabian, Jewish, and Christian physicians. Before Harvey (d. 1657) described the circulation of blood, however, the practical fruits of this scientific approach were sparse. Why?

One explanation is that the scientific aspect of medicine was held back by its priestly aspect (White, 1896). It is not inevitable, however, that these two aspects should hinder rather than complement each other. Others have pointed out that scientific medicine could not get far until the development of chemistry and biology. But why were these sciences also so slow to develop? Perhaps the better explanation is given by some Marxist sociologists and other authorities. Greek thinkers clearly recognized the method and value of empirical science, but they were discouraged from engaging in experimentation in science and clinical practice in medicine by a social system based on the sharp division between the liberally educated freemen who despised manual work and the slaves or serfs. This barrier between theory and practice, between the spiritual realm and the realm of matter, was the major obstacle to the development of science and scientific medicine.

Elevation of the physician to the status of a learned professional increasingly separated from the suffering patient was intensified by the university education of the Middle Ages. Nevertheless, the Christian concern for the poor began to break through this Greek contempt. Glaser (1970) has shown that Christianity, particularly in its Roman Catholic form, has been the religion most concerned with organized healthcare because of its belief in personal charity and of the integral relation of the body to the human person. Despite practical efforts to realize this Christian ideal, however, the state of scientific knowledge and the level of social organization were so low that until the end of the Middle Ages, the chief efforts were directed more to caring for sick and dying persons than to healing them.

Practical and material concerns were clearly seen to have religious and ethical values only with the Renaissance and the development of Christian humanism in Catholic Europe and Calvinist emphasis on work as a vocation in Protestant Europe. Thus the groundwork for the rapid rise of empirical science and modern medical technology was finally laid. Undoubtedly the secular humanism of the Enlightenment built well on this basis, but it did not lay its foundation. The role of the French Revolution was essentially negative. It broke down the old, fixed patterns of the medical profession so that the new model might develop fully (Foucault, 1973; Vogel, 1980).

Does the previous tension between the liberal and the service aspects of medicine exist today? At first glance such a suspicion seems absurd. The modern physician is above all interested in practice, and no class of physicians has greater prestige and remuneration (Hsiao, 1988) than surgeons, who certainly get their hands dirty. A closer look, however, reveals that the emphasis on the specialist, as opposed to the general practitioner, and the building up of a pyramid of paramedical professionals in the service of the physician, who mediate between the physician and patient, is the modern version of this class distinction (GMENAC Report, 1980).

The Christian Physician

On the other hand, the rise of psychiatry and psychosomatic medicine in the twentieth century has strengthened and developed the other, priestly aspect of medicine in which the physician as counselor becomes less the scientific technologist and more the artist in direct contact with the patient (McKeown, 1980). The current debates about the humanization of medicine reflect the resurgence of this other aspect of the medical tradition, which has never died and will always be part of medicine (L. Moore, 1987). Many of the real needs of patients that nineteenth-century medicine tended to abandon to the medical heretics are now being recovered as legitimate concerns of the orthodox medical profession. These debates, however, continue. The problem of the personalization of healthcare is far from solved (Linzer, 1986), but the emphasis on patient needs speaks well for a repersonalization of medicine.

Therefore the charismatic character of the physician, which arises from the priestly side of medicine but is also enhanced by the miraculous power of scientific technology, should be respected. In all professions the charismatic atmosphere is an important element of the professional relation and is essential to the healing process. This atmosphere makes it possible for the patient, often distrustful, to place the necessary trust in professional help. It also gives medical professionals a sense of personal dignity, dedication, and responsibility that immeasurably contributes to their satisfaction and persistence in a difficult vocation.

This charismatic aspect is also a guard of other ethical values, since nothing is so likely to keep medical professionals from abusing their position for financial or other gains as this sense of self-respect. It would be disastrous if the increasing mechanization of medicine or the reduction of the medical professional to an anonymous functionary in a government bureaucracy would destroy the priestly charisma of the profession (Pellegrino, 1985b, 1987).

On the negative side, however, as with the clergyman, overemphasis on the special status of the physician is open to great abuses. The physician can become an unquestioned, dogmatic authority in medicine and in all other matters as well (Childress, 1982). The medical profession often jealously defends its authority and its prerogatives, refuses to discipline members of the profession, and claims the right to settle ethical and social questions that affect the profession on the grounds that laypersons have no right to opinions in such matters (D. Axelrod et al., 1988).

Therefore, the physician who wants to develop a sound ethical judgment must have (1) a profound respect for the medical profession as a vocation that has both scientific and priestly aspects, (2) a clear understanding of the limits of this profession, and (3) a sense of personal responsibility to develop the attitudes and skills that enable one to personalize the profession (O'Rourke, 1988a).

Christian healthcare professionals are called by their faith to understand this vocation in a special way, just as professionals of other religions or philosophies of life are called by theirs. Christians think of life as a gift of God and the body as a marvelous work of divine creation to be reverenced as a temple of God (1 Co 6:19, 2 Co 6:16). They also think of the human person not only as a living body, but also as a body living with spiritual life open to a share in the eternal life of God. Consequently, the Christian healthcare professional thinks of sickness as an evil desecrator of the temple. Even when sickness cannot be overcome, the struggle against it can be lived through as an experience that can further moral and spiritual growth. Thus the Christian physician or nurse is truly a minister of God, cooperating with him in helping human beings overcome their suffering to live more fully.

The Christian medical professional finds a model in Jesus Christ, the Healer. Although physicians do not have supernatural or miraculous powers, they do have medical skill, which is also a gift of God. They can imitate Jesus' compassion for the patient and his reaching out to the most neglected, even the lepers. This Christian attitude cannot be a matter of mere pious words; rather, it is a profound dependence on God, who gives the physician and nurse the inspiration, insight, and courage to carry out their work as professionally and as skillfully as possible.

Moreover, one should not make the mistake of thinking that the ethical aspect of medicine pertains only to its personal, priestly side. It also penetrates its scientific aspect. A scientific approach to disease is built on the devotion to objective truth and the courageous, persevering effort to advance this truth through research and criticism. The history of medicine is unfortunately replete with examples not only of outright quackery, but also of superstition and self-delusion. Eminent physicians have sometimes become so enamored of their own theories and personal reputations that they have continued to defend their theories and even to counterfeit evidence concerning them long after their fallaciousness was evident (Engler et al., 1987; Lock, 1988). Others have stubbornly refused to face new facts and new theories (Schlitz, 1987). On the whole, however, the scientific approach, with its insistence on objective evidence and critical review by peers, has a splendid record. This scientific integrity has been very effective in limiting the excessive charismatic pretensions of some physicians.

Dedication to objective truth and scientific integrity is an ethical value of the highest order. Nothing is gained if the effort to humanize or personalize medicine interjects an unhealthy sentimentalism or occultism into the practice of medicine. Sound ethical judgment can only be based on critical, scientific knowledge (Goldman, 1980).

On the negative side, however, the scientific method, as now understood and practiced, often tends to reductionism, that is, the assertion that the scientific method is the exclusive road to truth. Since the scientific method deals only with the limited aspects of reality that can be measured and experimented on, such a reductionist attitude can compel physicians to ignore and deny facts and experiences outside those rather narrow limits. When reductionism is rigidly applied, the patient is treated as a soulless machine. In the history of medicine, this mechanistic approach has been profitable to the degree that it has used the scientific method intensively, but it has ultimately limited the advance of medicine. Biologists and physicians sensitive to the holistic character of living organisms and the human person have revolted repeatedly against reductionism and opened new, broader, and more fruitful lines of research (Kass, 1985).

Thus sound ethical judgment must completely respect scientifically established medical facts, but it cannot rest on these facts alone. It must be open to all humanistic approaches to understanding and evaluating the human condition.

4.3 MEDICAL EDUCATION AND ITS BIASES

In view of the complex history of the medical tradition, medical education needs to do justice to these various aspects of the profession if it is to prepare medical professionals to make good ethical judgments. Most medical professionals tend to think all their lives in the categories learned in medical or nursing school. This outlook has become so much a part of them through the intensive experiences of their training that they are not likely to reexamine or question it; such an attitude can stifle creativity and growth (Fox, 1988; Ludmerer, 1985).

The medical profession, as well as other professions, recognizes that educational institutions often have glaring biases and defects (Ebert and Ginzberg, 1988). The medical profession in the United States has taken the lead in self-criticism in this regard (D. Bok, 1984; Eichna, 1980; Petersdorf, 1986; James Warren et al., 1985). The famous report by Abraham Flexner led the way for reform in medical education. Flexner (1910) emphasized (1) the need for professional self-criticism; (2) the unity of scientific research and medical practice; (3) the advantages of the university-associated medical school; (4) the great importance of a sound, liberal education, rich in the basic sciences as a preparation for medical school; (5) a systematic or logical, but not overburdened, ordering of the curriculum with some limited elective freedom for the student; (6) an emphasis on laboratory and clinical work; (7) the great importance of constant research in special institutes; and (8) the adequate financing and use of a full-time medical staff. On the whole, these recommendations still remain sound. Many authorities today, however, would reject Flexner's emphasis on logical ordering of the curriculum, with theoretical study of the normal body preceding clinical contact with the sick body. They would argue that from the beginning, the program theory should be balanced by clinical experience (Vivieri, 1987).

Although Flexner strongly emphasized a sound general education as the basis of scientific medical education, he did not provide equally for the personalistic aspect of the profession. He seemed to presuppose this from other sources. Thus his curriculum has little room for (1) discussion of the nature and limits of the profession itself, (2) study of the counseling skills needed by a physician, (3) study of medical ethics, and (4) sociology and ecology.

A more recent effort at renewing medical education was made under the auspices of the Association of American Medical Colleges (AAMC, 1984). The GPEP Report is too lengthy to summarize here, but the first recommendation of the report is notable. The recommendation is entitled "Shifting Emphasis" and states: "In the general professional education of the physician, medical faculties should emphasize the acquisition and development of skills, values, and attitudes by students at least to the same extent that they do their acquisition of knowledge." Because this report is recent, there is no evidence as yet whether or not it will have the far-reaching effect on medical education as did the Flexner report.

Although there has been an effort to add courses in humanities and ethics to the medical school curriculum in recent years, the success and intensity of this effort has not been uniform (Culver et al., 1985; McElhinney, 1981; Pellegrino, 1985a; Rogers and Barnard, 1979). Even when ethics or other subjects in the humanities are required, they are often on the fringe of the educational effort (Ewan, 1986; Pinkus, 1986; J. Robinson, 1985). Moreover, little effort is made to discuss goals and objectives of present and future physicians in order to design a humanistic and scientific curriculum that would fit their needs. This lack of reflection and inability to introduce progressive changes hamper the efforts of most medical schools in the United States (S. Jonas, 1978; T. McNeill et al., 1986).

The training of nurses has been forced into the same pattern, with the result that today the nursing profession is undergoing a severe identity crisis (Chaska, 1983; Crissman and Betz, 1987; Langemann, 1983; Spicker and Gadow, 1980). In the United States the physician's role has been masculine; the nurses's, feminine. The result is that the nursing profession has had to struggle to achieve the autonomy that characterizes a full-fledged profession (McCloskey and Grace, 1985). This power struggle has forced many nurses out of an expressive or caring role into an instrumental administrative or technical role. Furthermore, the relation of the registered nurse to the practical nurse and other auxiliaries is far from clear. The AMA for example, wishes to institute a new category of healthcare worker called "registered care technologist," which would require less training and education than nurses (AMA, 1988c).

The view that the nurse has a role complementary to that of the physician rather than subordinate to it (J. Ashley, 1976; L. Stanley, 1979) has not yet been generally accepted. This role cannot be accepted unless the education of nurses provides them with adequate preparation in the personalistic aspects of healthcare. Fortunately, in the last 15 years nursing education has become more and more insistent on (1) good general education, (2) emphasis on the sociological aspects of nursing, and (3) some emphasis on techniques in personal relations (American Nurses' Association, 1982; D'Amato, 1985).

Medical and nursing schools operated under Catholic auspices have an opportunity and a challenge in our pluralistic society. First, if they are faithful to their Catholic tradition, they have a set of time-tested values on which they can form an ethics of the healthcare professional. Second, they have a position in the public forum enabling them to witness to the sacredness of human life in word and action. Third, they can commit themselves to a value-centered education that will form healthcare professionals who are true Christian personalists (Drake, 1986).

To meet these challenges and opportunities, however, Catholic schools will need to be sure of their identity (Theis, 1986). If they seek only to imitate other schools or correspond to the popular trends in healthcare education, they will waste their heritage and never achieve their potential. Unfortunately, Catholic schools training healthcare professionals have a difficult time effectively stressing the development of a Christian identity because they compete in a society that often sets standards for excellence and proficiency in accord with humanistic standards.

Biases

In view of medical schools' lack of emphasis in regard to the ethical aspects of medicine, what is the ethical outlook of the medical profession at present? The empirical data of a study by Amasa Ford and associates entitled *The Doctor's Perspective: Physicians View Their Patients and Their Practice* (1967) led the authors to a series of conclusions. These conclusions have been verified by more recent studies (Colombotos and Kirchner, 1986; Ebert and Ginsberg, 1988). The quotes in the following conclusions are from Ford and associates.

1. Most physicians have a "strong sense of vocation" rooted in the original priestly character of medicine and reinforced in American culture by the Protestant Calvinist stress on vocation. However, this religious motivation has been covered over:

> The vast growth of science and technology in the four hundred years since Luther has obscured the specifically religious conception of most vocations. The physician seldom speaks of God any more when discussing his concern for the patient. Yet he still finds satisfaction in measuring up to personal standards. Vocation, thus, has come to have an ethical rather than a religious basis and to be rewarded by satisfaction rather than by salvation. To be effective, the physicians in this study have said "they must be motivated and competent and must show concern for the patient" (p. 140).

2. Another important component of this motivation is the physicians' sense of specific competence; that is, they have an important and well-defined service to offer. Much of physicians' personal satisfaction in their work depends on this sense of competence. Competent physicians are happy physicians.

3. Physicians are very convinced of the necessity of a "modern individualism," or a professional one-to-one concern. This conviction has been influenced by American economic attitudes, but it also penetrates even deeper. Most physicians believe they must "care for the whole patient," and a minority of physicians are also highly socially conscious.

4. Physicians tend to think *pragmatically,* so their basic attitude can be characterized thus:

> The physician sees himself as a professionally competent person who is in a social position to apply scientific knowledge and to exercise impartial control over the situation in order to achieve the rational goal of curing or helping a sick patient. The patient's part of the job is to trust the doctor and cooperate with him (p. 144).

This element of control implies that the physician retains a detached concern or benevolent, affective neutrality and that the patient should be cooperative and trustful. Physicians are often not very sophisticated about the question of control from a psychological point of view.

Furthermore, the study showed that physicians on the whole do not regard themselves as scientists, but rather as *applied* scientists, and that they do not clearly experience a dichotomy between the scientific and the humanistic or affective aspects of medicine. Their satisfactions are not theoretical but pragmatic.

5. Physicians take much satisfaction in their professional position as a mark of achievement. This study tended to show that this sense of achievement is more important for physicians than monetary rewards, which they do not like to think of as a primary motivation. They resent, however, (a) failure of patients to pay, or failure to receive what they consider just acknowledgment and recompense for the burdens of responsibility, or long education, and of long hours that they have to bear, and (b) limitations on their independence, since these restrictions remove important symbols of their professional position.

Moreover, although physicians gain some satisfaction from scientific interest in their work, they gain more from the therapeutic results. Physicians obtain more satisfaction from giving to the patient (in a parental, nurturing sense) than from a mutual relation. In this way, some physicians perhaps alleviate a sense of guilt over their higher social status. An important element of satisfaction or dissatisfaction is found in the sense of consistency between personal and professional ethics. The modern physician is not inclined to moralize; this factor is associated more with older general practitioners than with younger specialists.

This study, however, gives evidence that physicians do have a common sense of ethical purpose.

This well-done study by Ford and associates indicates some possible ethical biases that medical professionals need to be aware of and that medical education should strive to balance if the medical profession is to make good ethical judgments.

First, on the whole, physicians fortunately continue to exhibit the dualistic balance between the scientific and the humanistic. However, this balance is constantly imperiled by the fact that their scientific training is explicit, detailed, and specialized, whereas their humanistic and moral training is left largely to examples and symbols transmitted to them without explicit reflection or criticism (Agich, 1985; Cassell, 1984; Light, 1980; Pellegrino, 1985b; Scully, 1980). Physicians thus assume that, although science is exact, ethical discourse is vague, subjective, and a matter of opinion (Clouser, 1980). On the one hand, this assumption leads to a kind of moral skepticism, and on the other to a dogmatic rigidity, since no method of dialogue or research for critical consensus is available.

Second, physicians tend to take a pragmatic view whereby what is most valued is an immediate, practical solution (Beauchamp and McCullough, 1984). In ethical matters, this pragmatism often causes physicians to act so that (1) they will not be made to feel guilty if an action is taken against their professional or personal standards; (2) they will not seem inhumane toward the patient, yet will not become too involved in the emotional or social problems of the patient; and (3) they will not go beyond the limits of the patient to wider social problems. An example of this simplistic type of pragmatic thinking is found in the statement of the legal committee of the AMA, which declared that physicians need not be concerned about the ethics of performing an abortion as long as proper medical procedures were followed and it was not forbidden by law (AMA, 1981).

Third, because the motivation of physicians is so bound up with their sense of vocation, autonomy, and competence, they resent interference in their decisions. They believe that only physicians are in the position to make medical-ethical judgments and that they can be relied on to be decent and humane in these decisions (Brooks, 1984). This belief tends to lead physicians (as in the problem of the dying patient) to follow as their primary rule: *help the patient*, but interpret help as the duty to keep trying by every technique available to improve the patient's physiological condition. They can then rest assured and without guilt that they have done all they can do. This attitude leads to deeply felt but simplistic attitudes toward ethical questions.

Fourth, physicians are often resentful that so much is laid on their shoulders. They cannot understand why a wider sociological, religious, psychological, or interrelational view should be their responsibility. Physicians believe that such concerns are someone else's business. Moreover, when medical students select a specialty with its even more well-defined area of competency, their limits of responsibility become even narrower.

None of these attitudes is necessarily wrong. Undoubtedly they are the result of the medical professional's need to live by a clear motivation, with limited responsibilities, and to have sufficient freedom for action and personal judgment.

They often result, however, in a closed attitude that renders the physician incapable of learning from others or sharing in a team effort to improve ethical treatment of health problems on a social scale. Thus these attitudes become harmful biases that can lead to gravely mistaken ethical judgments.

The healthcare profession is noble by reason of its great heritage, its remarkable modern advances, and its great promise for the future. It deserves the type of education that will free it from its own sickness, with which it has been infected by an acquisitive society.

CHAPTER 5

Personalizing The Healthcare Profession

OVERVIEW

Chapter 4 argues that at the center of every profession there is a counseling relation between persons and that this relation takes on a special mode in the healthcare profession. Chapter 4 also points out that many healthcare professionals are untrained or not specifically skilled in how to develop and maintain such a relation. However, ethical decisions about health matters depend first on a cooperative effort of patients and professionals, without which patients lack the information they need for an informed conscience. Ethical decisions also depend on peer relations between members of the health team, who must pool their information and expertise. Such cooperation between patients and professionals and between professionals and colleagues demands trust and effective communication, which are rooted in sound personal relations. Therefore, unless such relations are established and maintained in the healthcare facility, there is little hope of ethical, humanistic healthcare.

This chapter first defines the exact nature of professional-patient relations (5.1) and then in 5.2 deals with the ethical problems of professional communication and confidentiality (5.2). Finally, one basic aspect of peer relations in the health team is discussed—the problem of peer discipline—leaving other aspects of this important question to later chapters (5.3). Again, what is said of the physician-patient relation must be understood also to apply to nurses and other members of the health team in ways appropriate to the specific role of each.

5.1   THE COUNSELING RELATIONSHIP

Models of Professional-Patient Relationships

Szasz and Hollender (1956) identified three basic models of the physician-patient relationship: (1) the model of activity-passivity; for example, the surgeon operating on an anesthetized patient; (2) the model of guidance-cooperation; for example, the physician prescribing medication and the patient taking medication regularly; and (3) the model of mutual participation; for example, the patient engaging in a program of diet and exercise with supervision by the physician. These observations have been confirmed by others (W.F. May, 1983; R. Veatch, 1981). In all three models the physician as well as the patient achieves certain satisfactions. Thus the physician derives a sense of power from the activity-passivity model and a sense of paternal superiority from the guidance-cooperation model. In a course of treatment for a particular illness, there may be progress from one model to another.

Siegler and Osmond, in a fascinating book entitled *Models of Madness, Models of Medicine* (1974), identified eight potential models of therapeutic relationships.

1. The *medical model,* whereby the physician diagnoses and treats the disease of a patient, who is relieved of blame, who is free to take time out to be treated, and whose role is to trust and cooperate with the physician.

2. The *impaired model,* whereby the physician must get the patient to accept a permanent and incurable defect and then rehabilitate him or her for a life as normal as possible.

3. The *psychoanalytical model,* whereby the therapist assists the patient to come to a greater self-knowledge, even of unconscious motivation, and to develop a more effective way of living.

4. The *psychedelic model,* whereby the patient undergoes a "trip," an unusual experience, during which he or she needs guidance to achieve personal growth.

5. The *family-interaction model,* whereby the patient is only a part of a family system that is disordered (the patient may be the member) and whereby the therapist tries to improve the quality of the system.

6. The *social model,* whereby the real problem is reform of the social order causing the problem. The therapist is a social reformer and the patient perhaps a co-revolutionary.

7. The *conspiratorial model,* whereby the patient is a victim, not merely of social disorder but of an actual effort of suppression, and the therapist becomes an advocate to expose the conspiracy.

8. The *moral model,* whereby the patient requires moral reeducation and conversion of behavior under the guidance of a moral director.

In view of the differences in professional roles, the social, conspiratorial, and moral models do not seem directly appropriate to the work of the healthcare profession. Rather, they appear to pertain to the work of the ethical counselors who deal with the level of conscious, free, responsible behavior, whether it is personal (moral model) or social as well (social and conspiratorial models). The conspiratorial model, although concerned with political behavior, also has a psychoanalytical aspect, since it involves the unmasking of hidden political forces just as psychoanalysis unmasks unconscious personal motivation. On the other hand, the medical, psychedelic, and family-interaction models clearly deal with the psychological level and are the concern of psychotherapy. The psychedelic model also raises questions for the spiritual or pastoral counselor. Similarly, the family-interaction model suggests ethical counseling because the family is the basic unit of social life. Finally, the medical and impaired models deal chiefly with the biological level of human functioning.

Psychotherapeutic Models

From an ethical perspective, issues are raised first by the medical and impaired models at the biological level and then by the psychoanalytical, psychedelic, and family-interaction models at the psychological level. Psychotherapists are well trained in the problems of counselor-client relations and are generally well aware of the ethical issues that arise. Some of the more detailed issues are discussed in Chapter 12.

What are the ethical implications, however, of the remarkable dependence of mentally and emotionally disturbed persons in relation to their therapists? The ethical significance of this relationship can be summarized by a more detailed account of the psychoanalytical model (see 12.3).

In the psychoanalytical model, the client comes to the therapist because of painful anxieties that make normal life difficult or impossible, with the goal of trying to resolve emotional conflicts whose unconscious origin is unknown to the client. The therapist's responsibility is not to diagnose the illness by labeling it, but to help the client come to an understanding of the causes of his or her problems and to cope with them more effectively. To achieve this, the therapist must gradually win the client's trust and help the client step by step to interpret the symbolism of the symptoms. The therapist must grant the client the right to have his or her behavior interpreted as symbolic rather than judged morally and to have his or her sufferings counted worthy of sympathy. The therapist must help the client not to act out symptoms, but to discover their underlying meaning and thus to come to a deep and realistic self-understanding. Finally, the therapist must help the client acquire new skills in coping with the problems of life and terminate dependence on the therapist. To do this, the therapist must personally arrive at self-understanding through the same process.

The client must come to trust the therapist, speaking more and more freely, cooperating by undertaking the task of working through symptoms, and rejecting escape from the process by suicide or even by a flight into health. The client's will to get well and become independent of the therapist must also be reinforced. This process depends on an intense one-to-one relationship in which the client withdraws from the familial and social situation in which he or she has become ill. It also demands toleration by family and society of the client's temporary withdrawal from ordinary relationships and responsibilities.

The client's dependence on the therapist is essentially a recapitulation of the parental relationship, but a healthy one rather than the unhealthy one from which the client has suffered. The therapist is a good mother in taking on the attitude of which Carl Rogers (1951), one of the foremost psychotherapists in America, called "unconditional benign acceptance." The therapist is also a good father in the increasing role of interpretation and confrontation with reality. The libidinal, erotic elements of the transference of the client to the therapist are gradually turned toward the real love objects of the client's independent life. By no means is it easy for clients to come to such total trust in their therapists, since they may have learned to distrust any mother or father. If clients are to get well, however, they have a moral obligation to try to trust, cooperate, and engage in this working-through process. Clients must accept the tasks of (1) trusting the therapist and (2) trying to recover health and normal independence.

Therapists undertake the moral burden of being faithful to this trust reposed in them by their clients. Therapists must listen, not judge, and (to a degree) must sympathize. Therapists must set limits on acting out by clients and must insist on working through. They must approve and reinforce the client's progressive achievement of insight and gradually confront him or her more and more with the demands of reality. Finally, therapists must be willing to let even favorite clients go. For therapists to be ethically true to this trust, they must be personally aware of any tendency toward *countertransference* (i.e., the development of a relationship in which the therapist begins to use the client to meet the therapist's own emotional needs) and must strive to keep this human tendency within limits (Kolb and Brodie, 1982).

Today these mutual duties, which clearly involve considerable virtue from therapists and a desire for virtue and willingness to grow through suffering from clients, are often formalized in a contract made at the beginning of therapy. In this contract, therapists make sure clients understand and accept the goals and limits of therapy and are aware that they can hold a therapist liable for the therapist's half of the contract. Thus therapists are unethical when they fail to make such a clear contract (which is an aspect of informed consent, as discussed in 3.4) or fail to adhere strictly to it. Therapists should *not* assume moral obligations beyond the limits of this contract. Thus analysts normally should not undertake any responsibility for patients who act out their symptoms outside the therapeutic setting.

Such limitations raise certain difficulties, however, the major ones being: (1) What if the patient is contemplating suicide? (2) What if the patient is contemplating some act injurious to another party, such as physical attack, theft, adultery, or divorce? (3) What if the patient proposes sexual relations with the therapist? (4) What if the patient refuses to work seriously at the therapy or needlessly delays its termination? These problems are discussed at greater length in Chapter 12. Here we need only to point out that these actions constitute a breach (perhaps not culpable) of the contract on the client's part. These actions relieve the therapist from his or her contract, but they leave the therapist obliged (not as a professional, but simply as a citizen) to prevent harm to a third party or to prevent insane persons from harming themselves (DeKraai and Sales, 1984). Consequently, the therapist can discreetly inform the family or others to guard against suicide or crime. In questions 3 and 4 the therapist can also terminate therapy. If the patient becomes worse or needs commitment, consultants should be called in or the family informed so that the commitment process can be undertaken (Belli, 1982).

Other forms of psychotherapy do not rest on such a close relationship between therapist and client, but they present essentially the same ethical issues.

Medical Model

In strong contrast to the psychotherapeutic models is the medical model, but it also has many ethical issues. Today the patient enters both models in much the same type of setting—a private office, clinic, or hospital. In the medical model, the professional goal is to treat a physical illness so as to restore normal physical functioning to the degree possible. The physician first seeks to diagnose the disease, then to prescribe a course of treatment (in which the physician is assisted by nurses and others) through medicine, surgery, nursing, or change of regimen. The physician must also make a prognosis and, if possible, offer the patient hope. The patient, on the other hand, is relieved from blame for his or her condition and from ordinary responsibilities to work and family but is expected to be cooperative with the professional staff. Families and society are expected to support the patient psychologically and to contribute to the expenses (M. Benjamin, 1985; Parsons, 1964; Pellegrino and Thomasma, 1981).

In the medical model, the patient is not expected to be as active as in the psychotherapeutic models, except in rehabilitative stages of treatment, which pertain more characteristically to the impaired model (Lebacqz, 1985). This patient passivity raises the main ethical issue characteristic of this model. If, as Chapter 3 argues, the healthcare professional is only a servant to the patient because primary responsibility for the patient's health remains the patient's, then it follows that the professional has no rights over the patient, except those given by the patient's informed consent. Thus, ethically speaking, an implicit or explicit contract must regulate all that occurs in the medical model.

What are the essential features of this medical contract (Giles, 1983; Pellegrino, 1985b). First, the contract limits the obligations assumed. In the medical model, a physician does not assume the role of a psychotherapist or of an ethical or spiritual counselor. Efforts to repersonalize medicine should not demand that the physician assume all the roles proper to a complete health team. Of course, physicians need to be aware of nonphysical factors that may be affecting the patient's health in order to seek the help of other members of the health team in dealing with such factors.

Nevertheless, the physician who provides primary care has a special relation to the patient. Studies show that 50 percent or more of patients seen by primary-care physicians are not suffering from any physical dysfunction. Some physicians regard such patients as hypochondriacs, are bored with their complaints, and get rid of them as fast as possible, or (sorry to say) keep them coming back for an easy fee. Other physicians patiently try to alleviate excessive anxiety by prescribing a placebo or tranquilizer or using a little amateur psychotherapy or a dose of fatherly advice.

The implied contract between a patient and the primary-care physician, however, obligates the physician to undertake a serious effort to help the patient discover the nature of the problem and the type of help appropriate to it, medical or otherwise. The patient who does not feel well comes to a physician as a first, obvious step in an effort to determine the source of the discomfort. If the possibility of a physical cause can be eliminated, the patient then has the information necessary to take the next step—seeing another type of counselor or other action. However, if the physician fails to listen or make an adequate examination or sends the patient away confused or with a placebo or tranquilizer, the patient still lacks the necessary information for rational decisions (Brahms, 1987; Preston, 1987). Physicians who deal in an evasive manner with patients are only reinforcing hypochondriacal tendencies.

A well-known study of hospital care (Duff and Hollingshead, 1968) showed that a high percentage of patients were incorrectly diagnosed because of the failure of physicians to listen carefully to patients' complaints and recognize nonmedical factors in their conditions. Moreover, the present system of financing healthcare has led to problems in sustaining quality of care (R. Veatch, 1986).

Second, the medical model, as with other professional relations, is based on trust. The physician, therefore, must establish trustworthiness within the limits of the contract. As it relates to this trust, the contract should have three elements.

1. *Concern.* Fundamental to the contract is the physician's concern for the patient's well-being. Trust will never exist if the patient believes that the physician is concerned only about the fee or is acting out of mere routine as a machine or a bureaucratic functionary. The physician must communicate interest in the patient as a person, not as a kidney or a heart, and a willingness to do for the patient whatever is professionally possible, not limited by mere self-interested motives (D. Cooper, 1985).

   For this reason, Ramsey (1970) has rightly emphasized that the professional contract is something more than a contract; it is a "covenant" in the theological sense. In the Old Testament, God made a covenant with his chosen people based not on their worthiness but on his generous love for them, and he confirmed this covenant by a promise not to desert them even if they did not meet all their obligations. The professional contract is analogous to such a covenant in the sense that the professional undertakes to help the client not because the client is ethically worthy of help, or even because he or she is able to pay for the service, but primarily because of human need and the essential human rights based on need rather than on merit. The professional contract also implies the promise to continue the patient's care even when the patient is no longer able to insist on its fulfillment.

   This concept of covenant, however, should not be exaggerated. God himself insists on the responsibility of his people to respond to their own obligations under the covenant. Thus the physician also has the right to demand cooperation from the patient. Moreover, the physician's contract is not universal but limited by his or her own competence. Therefore the physician is not obligated to do more than inform the patient when a problem exceeds the physician's competence and refer the patient to another specialist or another type of nonmedical counselor.

2. *Knowledge and skill in medicine.* Healthcare professionals have the fundamental responsibility, within their specialties, to be expert in both the science and the art of healthcare, up-to-date in knowledge, experienced,

of good judgment, and skilled in procedures. Personal warmth does not substitute for medical expertise. Reciprocally, however, one may say that this knowledge and skill cannot be put to their best use if the other humanistic elements are not also present (Morreim, 1986; Ozar, 1985; G. Silver, 1986). Professionals communicate such expertise to patients by evidence of their education and licensure, by reputation, and also by the care and thoroughness with which they deal with patients.

3. *Communication.* Patients retain fundamental rights over their own bodies and the fundamental knowledge of how they feel not only at this minute, but also throughout the day and in varied situations. Thus physicians cannot hope to make a proper diagnosis, carry on successful treatment, or make an accurate prognosis without adequate patient communications. Barnlund (1976) makes this observation about communication:

> When one turns to ask what is currently known about communication between medical personnel and patients, the answer is itself mystification—very little. Here is a profession founded on science, dedicated to truth, committed to inquiry, concerned with the relief of suffering, yet either oblivious or unwilling to examine its own communicative behavior. Is this simply a mote in an otherwise scientific eye? Or is it a defensive assertion of the medical mystique and the preference to do as one pleases?

Finally, in caring for the patient, the physician retains his or her own moral agency. The physician does not become the slave of the patient, especially when ethical issues are concerned (Loewy, 1986).

Healthcare Fees

To these basic ethical obligations of the physician, a fourth can be added that applies also to the psychotherapeutic models: to set or refuse an appropriate fee. In a capitalist society, one assumes that a professional should be paid as any other worker is paid according to the laws of supply and demand. One assumes that a service is just as much a commodity for exchange with a value measured in monetary terms as is any other product. Consequently, some persons argue that nothing is ethically wrong with organizing the medical profession on the basis of profit as in any other industry, and they actually speak of "the health industry" (Rafferty, 1984). They believe that the stimulus of the profit motive has been the main cause of the rapid technological development of American medicine. Rosett (1984) contends that if the free market were permitted to prevail in healthcare, the economic efficiency of the American medical system would be greatly enhanced and inflation in medical costs reduced. Logically, therefore, the courts now defend physicians' right to compete by advertising cut-rate services.

Furthermore, some argue that the fee is actually a part of therapy, since it causes the average person to refrain from asking for unnecessary services that might overload the system and deprive others in real need from obtaining proper attention. Moreover, the fee promotes a cooperative attitude from the patient and thus shortens the time of treatment.

Freud (Drucker, 1978) scandalized the Jewish physicians of Vienna (for whom the Jewish tradition of caring for charity patients was a cardinal rule) when he insisted on fees from *all* his patients. Freud stated that the subject of psychotherapy who does not have to pay a fee is very likely to waste much time before getting down to the painful task of working through resistances. Freud's practice, however, has become standard in psychoanalysis.

The question can also be raised as to whether this capitalistic assumption is a realistic and practical fact. At no time in the history of medicine has the market system operated fully in the professions because there have always been people who desperately needed professional help but could not pay for it. Either the professional had to provide free services or payment had to be made by a third party. In fact, since the rise of health insurance and Medicare, most healthcare *is* paid by a third party, the insurer or the government, who determines standard fees. Chapter 6 discusses the various ways of organizing medical systems to meet the problem of the patient who cannot pay.

If the account given in Chapter 4 of the nature of a profession is correct, it should be clear why profit cannot be the primary basis of any profession but must be considered a secondary and highly variable feature. The medical profession, as with any true profession, must rest not on bargaining but on trust; it provides a service that is concerned with life and death, matters so precious as to be priceless. No monetary value can be set on the spiritual light given by a priest, the defense of human rights provided by a lawyer, the risk of his own life provided by a soldier, or the search for truth shared by a teacher. Similarly, there is no price for the service of a physician in the battle to live.

Just because the healthcare professional performs so precious a service, it cannot be bargained for. Thus in the past the fundamental principle in all professions was that the professional must be ready to give service free to those who were in need but could not pay. Jesus said with regard to religious ministry, "The laborer is worthy of his hire" (Lk 10:7; see also 1 Tm 5:18); but he meant that his disciples should live from hand to mouth, "freely giving what you have freely received." St. Paul followed this same principle in his own way by supporting himself by manual labor, so that no one might accuse him of preaching for gain (1 Co 4:12; Acts 18:3). Thus religious professionals deserve to be supported by the public so that they can provide services purely on the basis of the client's need.

The same principle applies to all true professions because they provide services that are life-and-death necessities. Thus professional fees are not payments measured by the value of the service provided (which is truly priceless), but a *stipend* to be measured only by what professionals need to live in a manner that will free them to work without distraction. Therefore medical professionals who set their fees so high as to accumulate wealth in other businesses that distract them from their profession are not faithful to their profession (L. Eisenberg, 1986).

Official codes of medical ethics generally state that medical fees should be adjusted to the patient's ability to pay. The assumption is that richer patients will be charged enough to compensate physicians for what they lose in low or no fees charged poorer patients. The inadequacy of this as a principle becomes apparent when the fees are paid by a third party such as an insurance company or the government. Experience shows that in such a situation, physicians are tempted to charge as much as they can get, with a resulting inflation in health costs. The ability-to-pay principle is not unjust as long as it remains within the bounds of the more fundamental principle: professionals are public servants who have no right to expect in return for services anything more than a standard of living that will make it possible for them to perform those services with liberty of mind and health of body and to fulfill family and social obligations adequately.

A Christian physician, lawyer, teacher, or religious minister can only conclude that a professional living is essentially a modest one in which simplicity of lifestyle and freedom to be available to serve others is the only honorable measure of remuneration. Also, one cannot accept the argument so often put forward that since physicians spend long years of difficult study, work long hours, and assume great responsibility, they deserve to make money. The rewards of any profession are to be found not in some extraneous gain, but in the satisfactions of knowledge and of interesting and absorbing work, as well as in the joy in a baby delivered, a sick patient restored, or a dying patient made comfortable and serene. Such an ideal is not easy to realize, nor is it often realized in its purest form. Even when imperfectly realized, however, this ideal is what has given the medical profession its own vitality and health.

5.2   PRINCIPLE OF PROFESSIONAL COMMUNICATION

Listening and Truth Telling

In healthcare, as in all professional relations, adequate communication between professional and client is a fundamental ethical requirement. In the medical model, opportunities for such communication may be rather sharply restricted, but they are still crucial. Within these limits, what are the duties of physicians and nurses?

The first obligation is to listen to the patient. Often in the medical model, however, while professionals concentrate on filtering out medically significant information, patients are attempting to express their malaise in a rhapsody of symptoms, fears, fantasies, evasions, cries for attention, and so forth (Agich, 1985; Alpert, 1986). The work-pressured professional cannot afford to sit and hear a long and rambling discourse from a self-pitying patient. Even the psychotherapist, who has a special interest in all sorts of behavioral clues, must insist that patients "get to work" without evading the therapeutic process. Somehow professionals must cut through the noise and get at the real message, but they need to remember that "the medium *is* the message"; that is, the way patients are (or are not) communicating may be the most significant symptom.

Therefore, no matter how busy they may be, healthcare professionals may not ethically rush through interviews or simply rely on laboratory tests. They have the responsibility to acquire the art of medical dialogue, by which they can help patients say what needs to be said. The first rule of this art is for the professional to repeat back to the patient what the professional has heard that seems significant and to ask whether it is what the patient meant. This feedback not only reassures the patient but can also gradually train the patient in giving relevant information. A second rule is to obtain the patient's cooperation by explaining the purpose of questions, since unexpected and cryptic questions are threatening and confusing to many patients. If physicians are unable or unwilling to learn this art of dialogue, they must learn to work in a team that includes other professionals with such communication skills.

A professional must not only hear but also *believe* patients who have the basic right to be believed until they lose that right by clearly proved deception. Thus the temptation of some busy physicians and exasperated nurses to jump to the conclusion that a patient is malingering has to be resisted. Although what a patient reports may not be objectively true, it is subjectively so because it expresses what the patient really *feels* and is therefore medically significant and important (R. Baron, 1981).

Professionals also have the right to require honesty and frankness from clients (R. Gillon, 1986c). When professionals suspect deliberate deceit, they should deal with the situation explicitly and directly as a breach of the patient's contract with the professional. In most illnesses, however, psychological factors may cause communication to be distorted by unconscious elements of self-deceit, denial, confusion, or panic. Psychotherapists in particular have to deal with this perplexing inability of some patients to communicate openly, but therapists also experience in themselves something of the same ambiguity. Appleton (1972) states this opinion:

> Psychiatrists advocate honest and open communication by physicians with patients but too often do not practice what they preach. Their reasons for silence include uncertainty about the cause, treatment, and prognosis of psychiatric illnesses and unwillingness to depress, demoralize, anger, or alienate their patient (p. 743).

This observation applies to all healthcare professionals, who cannot expect truth from their patients unless they are equally truthful with them. Lack of frankness by professionals is usually excused as concern to spare the patient, but it is just as often the result of the professional's unconscious fear. Chapter 13 discusses the problem of telling the truth to the incurable or dying patient. Here it suffices to say that the fundamental principle in all such situations is that the patient has the right to the truth, however difficult it may be for the professional to communicate it (Applebaum et al., 1987; S. Bok, 1982; Speedling and Rose, 1985).

Confidentiality

Patients have the right to the truth about their health because they have the primary responsibility for their health. They also have the right to privacy about those aspects of life that do not directly affect others. Human community is based on free communication, which is impossible if confidences cannot be shared.

Thus healthcare professionals have a serious obligation to maintain such confidences that protect the patient's right of privacy (Kagle, 1984; Kotton, 1986).

How is a professional to act when questioned by others about a patient's condition? Can confidentiality be protected by lying? All Catholic moralists agree that it is always wrong to "lie," even to protect confidentiality, but not all agree on how to define *lying*. Some (C. Curran, 1975) distinguish between a *falsehood* (i.e., a false statement) and a *lie*, which is not only a false statement but also one made to someone who has the right to a true answer. Consequently, they hold that someone who has a duty to keep a secret can answer falsely to inquirers. It seems better to state, as does Knauer (1967), that the meaning of any human statement must always be determined from the context in which communication occurs. Therefore, when persons ask questions that they have no right to ask, the context renders any answer given essentially *meaningless*, so that it is ethically inconsequential whether that answer in a normal context would be true or false. Thus healthcare professionals who are questioned about confidential matters may, without lying or even giving a falsehood, reply in any way that protects confidentiality. This fact, however, cannot excuse a physician from frankly answering questions put by a patient or the patient's guardians because these persons have the right to know. Whether one has the obligation to reply to a question with unambiguous and accurate information then depends on the questioner's right to such information (S. Bok, 1982).

It is not easy to draw the line between what individuals have the right to keep private and what they may have the duty to make public. Thus the contract between professional and patient should determine this as exactly as possible. If professionals are convinced that, to follow the best course for a patient, they need to discuss the case with consultants or before other members of a team or professional staff, the professionals must obtain the patient's informed consent. Generally, this consent is implicitly contained in the contract. Thus, in most mental hospitals, it is assumed that voluntary (or even involuntary) commitment implies the right to discuss the patient's condition and progress with other members of the therapeutic staff.

Such assumptions, however, are easily open to abuse (Schmid et al., 1983; R. Schwartz, 1984). Books have been published by physicians and psychiatrists about their famous or notorious patients, living or dead (Chayet, 1966). In our opinion, much greater care must be taken to obtain explicit consent from patients with regard to matters that may be embarrassing to them, especially in the present age of medical teamwork and computerized records (Applebaum et al., 1984; R. Bayer et al., 1984; Sieghart, 1984). Most patients (or when they are incompetent, their guardians) readily permit the therapeutic use of information, but they should have the opportunity to restrict the use of this information when entering into contractual relations with the professional. It should not be too difficult for a physician or healthcare institution to work out a regular procedure by which patients are informed of their rights to privacy and asked for explicit consent for any necessary use of confidential information. One of the most difficult problems is researchers' need to have access to records, especially when doing epidemiological studies; even here, however, it should be possible to guard individuals' privacy from public knowledge (R. Gillon, 1987; Gordis and Gold, 1980).

Nevertheless, the right of privacy, sacred as it is, is limited by other persons' rights and by the individual's own limited rights of self-disposal. Patients may behave in ways that directly injure themselves and indirectly or directly injure others. For example, patients may commit suicide, seek ways to continue their chemical dependency, spread contagious diseases, or commit acts of theft or aggression against other patients or the staff (Basson et al., 1988). Some may become so seriously incompetent as to become a public danger on release from an institution, such as the epileptic bus driver who refuses to change his job. In the case of *Tarasoff v. Regents of University of California,* the court held a therapist responsible for not warning third parties that his client might be dangerous (Annas, 1976; Knapp, 1982; Mark Mills et al., 1987).

In all these cases, the family or society has an obligation to prevent harm both to the patient and to the public because all are members of a community that exists for the good of each of its members in relation to all others. Thus, in general, even when information is given in confidence, professionals have not only the right but also the duty to communicate information to those who may be able to prevent serious harm to the patient or to others (Meyers, 1982; O'Donnell, 1986).

Thus professional secrecy is not as absolute as the secrecy demanded of a Catholic priest, who may not reveal what he has learned in confession regarding a penitent's sins or defects, even to prevent harm to a third party. Professional secrecy also is not as absolute as that given by law to the confidences between accused criminals and their lawyers. With the priest, the penitent is revealing personal moral responsibility before God, which is beyond human judgment. With the lawyer, the accused is protected in his or her rights by the adversary process. In medical matters, however, patients seldom need to reveal to the professional anything that is essentially incriminating; usually the fact, at worst, might be an embarrassment. Moral fault, however, may incidentally be revealed, as when the patient voluntarily admits an intention to commit a crime and when the medical condition has moral implications (addiction, venereal disease, illegitimate pregnancy).

When what is revealed is an intention to commit a crime (including suicide), the professional has the obligation to reveal to appropriate persons whatever information is necessary to prevent such a crime. When no crime is contemplated, but there is probable danger of harm that can be prevented, the professional should discreetly do what is likely to be helpful in preventing such harm. Ordinarily this should not be done without first warning the patient of exposure if the patient refuses to desist. For example, the professional should keep the fact of addiction confidential if the patient is willing to cooperate with treatment, but the professional may be forced to make it known to the family if cooperation is refused. A professional should protect the confidence of someone illegitimately pregnant unless the intention to secure an abortion is evident. In this case, despite recent court decisions declaring the "right" of minors to free choice of abortion, professionals may be forced to inform the parents of a minor or the father of the child (Gardell, 1986). This will at least permit parents to discuss the decision with their child and attempt to protect the rights of their grandchild. In the case of venereal disease of a minor, confidentiality should be maintained unless the minor refuses treatment. In other situations, professionals should first seek to obtain the patient's cooperation and only proceed to inform the third party when this cooperation is refused and the damage feared is both serious and probable. The benefit of the doubt is in favor of confidentiality, which influences the dependence of the patient on the professional.

Certain very serious problems about confidentiality have been raised recently by the computerization of health records and also by the requirement of private and government health insurance plans that physicians report the nature of a patient's illness as a condition of receiving payment (Applebaum et al., 1984; Lako, 1986). A physician clearly does not have the right to give information of this sort without the patient's permission (Hiller and Beyda, 1981; Neville et al., 1986). This, however, leaves the larger question of how patients are to obtain the benefits to which they are entitled without giving such permission. The insurance or public agency has the right to ask proof from patients that they have used funds for a legitimate medical purpose, but the agency also has the duty to design adequate controls that do not require detailed information possibly embarrassing or injurious to the patient. Computerization of health records should always require the patient's permission, and even when permission is given, care must be taken to limit the availability of these records to a few definitely authorized persons (Murray and Pagon, 1984). Similar problems are raised in the case of peer review, a process that is becoming more and more widespread, as discussed in 5.3.

Some professionals (Szasz, 1974, 1977, 1987) argue for an extreme individualistic and libertarian position. For example, they contend that addicts should be permitted free access to alcohol and drugs, and some even believe that suicidal persons should be permitted to take their own lives if they wish. This opinion is based on such notions as: "Freedom is doing what you want with your own life," and "Immorality is only doing harm to another, nonconsenting adult." As shown in 1.2, the very nature of personhood implies involvement in a community. Self-destructive behavior is not merely of concern to the person in question, but to all with whom his or her life is intertwined. In fact, psychology seems to show that such behavior is an often unconscious cry for help (Battin, 1983; Beck et al., 1986). To let such persons destroy themselves because they claim that is what they want is actually to ignore this cry that comes from the true self. The real answer must be a social concern for persons in their real liberty, which consists in becoming more open to others, not more closed. To achieve openness, the trust of the alienated must be gained.

In recent times, the spread of acquired immunodeficiency syndrome (AIDS) (see Chapter 3, p. 68) has reminded healthcare workers of the serious responsibility of confidentiality (R. Bayer et al., 1984; Jonson et al., 1986). Mainly because of the manner in which AIDS is acquired (people infected with the HIV virus often are homosexual, bisexual, or intravenous drug users), severe discrimination is exercised against AIDS patients (President's Commission on AIDS, 1988). Thus their privacy should be protected. People seem to forget that many people with AIDS have acquired the disease through blood transfusions or were born with it. Moreover, Christian compassion demands that respect be shown for those who acquire the disease through aberrant behavior, even though the activity that brings about the disease is not valued. Jesus never asked those he healed how they became ill.

Healthcare workers therefore have a serious responsibility to maintain confidentiality in regard to AIDS patients. Those who minister to AIDS patients must be careful about gossip and casual conversation that would reveal the presence of the disease to those who have no right to this information. On the other hand, those who counsel AIDS patients should follow the same norms discussed on p. 69 concerning revealing the presence of the disease to a third party who might be injured. If possible, the AIDS patient should be persuaded to tell third parties, such as a spouse or any person sharing sexual intimacy, about the disease's presence and the danger of contagion (American Medical Association, 1988a). In some circumstances, if the patient will not reveal the disease's presence to concerned third parties, the healthcare professional might be held in charity and justice to reveal this information (Gellman, 1986).

In view of the foregoing discussion, the *Principle of Professional Communication* can be formulated as follows:

> To fulfill their obligations to serve the patient's health, healthcare professionals have the responsibility:
> 1. To strive to establish and preserve trust at both the emotional and the rational levels;
> 2. To share the information they possess with those who legitimately need it to have an informed conscience;
> 3. To refrain from lying or giving misinformation;
> 4. To keep secret information that is not legitimately needed by others but that, if revealed, might either harm the patient or others or destroy trust; and
> 5. To reveal information to those who might suffer serious harm if the information is withheld.

5.3   PEER RELATIONS AND PROFESSIONAL DISCIPLINE

Healthcare professionals need good personal relations not only with those they serve, but also with their colleagues on the health team. Problems of leadership and accountability, common decision making and cooperation in carrying out decisions, and adequate communication and mutual support have psychological importance, but they also are profoundly ethical.

Some of these issues are discussed in Chapter 6 and in the concluding Part 5 of this book. This section deals only with the especially sensitive issue of peer discipline because the problem of mutual responsibility is crucial in any group. If healthcare professionals do not care enough about each other and their common enterprise to accept the painful task of maintaining group standards in a fraternal and humane way, they cannot hope to personalize healthcare.

The recent phenomenal rise in the number of malpractice suits seems proof that the healthcare profession is currently in need of stricter discipline. The Commission of Medical Malpractice of the Secretary of the U.S. Department of Health, Education, and Welfare (Powsher and Hemmersaith, 1987; U.S. HEW, 1973) concluded (with some dissenting voices on the commission) that the main factor in this increase in litigation has been the growing number of medical injuries, real or apparent. These simply may result in part from the increasingly complex and risky procedures of modern therapy. The commission also concluded, however, that malpractice suits frequently result from (1) poor communication between physicians and patients and thus from inadequately informed consent on the patient's part; (2) patients' frustration because physicians seem unresponsive to their complaints; (3) patients' unrealistic expectations about the benefits of treatment; and (4) growing public conviction that consumers need to defend themselves against arrogant, self-serving professionals. It is noteworthy that the first three of these factors (and perhaps in large part the fourth) reduce to a failure in communication in which physicians are often not well trained. Furthermore, one is led to wonder why other members of the health team do not notice or correct such misunderstandings (D. Smith, 1984).

Two opposite remedies have been proposed for the malpractice problem. One answer is *peer review* (W. Curran, 1987). It is argued, plausibly enough, that in a field so highly technical as medicine, no one is competent to evaluate professional performance except peers in the profession or even in the same medical specialty. Professionals should judge their peers, set penalties and rewards, and, if necessary, expel serious and incorrigible offenders from the profession (A. Goldberg, 1984).

On the other hand, some authorities (American Bar Association, 1986) argue that peer discipline has never been successful in protecting the patient or even in maintaining high standards of medical competence. A profession, they contend, is too concerned with its own autonomy to be very diligent in disciplining its members. A built-in bias works in favor of protecting members of the profession rather than in the interests of patients. Consequently, these critics believe that disciplining a profession first must concern those who suffer from malpractice or neglect. Healthcare consumers must know and defend their own rights by all available economic, legal, and political means.

The first of these two positions, peer review, was adopted long ago by the American Medical Association (AMA) and the American Psychiatric Association for their membership, but it has been implemented rather perfunctorily (AMA, 1987a). As a result, many states have recently extended the authority of state licensing boards to include reevaluation of physicians' performance. Moreover, within various specialties and healthcare facilities, committees are being set up to monitor and improve professional performance (McIntyre and Popper, 1983; R. Moore, 1985). Moreover, the U.S. Supreme Court has limited the rights of peer review by physicians (*Patrick v. Burget,* 1988).

Calling to Account

The existence of a problem in regard to evaluating physician competence is clear from the title of a recent conference, "Physician Competence, Whose Problem Is It?" sponsored by the AMA, the American Hospital Association, and the Association of American Medical Schools (Medical Review Bulletin, 1988).

Since the primary responsibility for health must remain with each person, to whom the professional is only a servant, the ultimate right to call the medical profession to account must be in the hands of those the profession exists to serve. This is why the users of health services have the fundamental right to the final word in regulating the profession through public law.

In this matter it seems that the physician and the lawyer are in a somewhat different position than the minister, teacher, and scientist. These latter professions deal with objective truth as such, and the public has no right to silence the voice of truth. However, the lawyer is an officer of the court; that is, he or she is subordinated to the government's legislative and judicial officers who represent the people in determining the law. The medical professional also does not stand for truth as such, as a scientist must, but is providing a service to human physical or mental health, a service that must ultimately be judged in terms of its practical enhancement of human well-being (Siegler, 1987). Consequently, the medical profession must accept a public, practical evaluation of its services. Healthcare professionals, in their secondary role as scientists, have a right and obligation to speak out for objective truth about biological and medical matters, but this does not give them complete autonomy in the realm of medical practice.

There are many views on how to remedy the rise in malpractice suits and the great increase in insurance rates that this produces. Certainly the tendency to forget that medicine is a practical science and that unfortunate results are often not the result of incompetency must be communicated to the public (O'Rourke and Brodeur, 1986). Some blame the legal profession because the courts have too often extended vague legal rules, such as those that relate to the time allowed plaintiffs to report injuries, the application of the *res ipsa loquitur* ("the injury is sufficient evidence of fault") doctrine to medical injuries, the doctrine of informed consent, and liability based on oral guarantees of good results (Harolds and Block, 1966). Some blame the legal system also because lawyers find malpractice suits very profitable, since they receive a high percentage (usually 30 to 40 percent) of the damages awarded, according to what is called the *contingent fee system.*

Besides the poor communication just mentioned, others blame the medical profession for the unwillingness of many physicians to testify against peers. All admit, including the AMA, that physicians and other medical professionals have the duty to testify in such cases out of justice not only to the claimant, but also to the physician and the profession itself. Compassionate concern for a colleague does not excuse a professional from frank and honest testimony as to the colleague's competence or responsibility when these are in serious question, as long as due process is being observed.

The medical profession and every learned profession must have a genuine but limited autonomy. As healthcare users become more knowledgeable about what is and what is not good medical care, they will become increasingly able to detect serious incompetence or negligence in the service they receive. This awareness will only raise questions, however; it will not be sufficient in most cases to pass judgment. Res ipsa loquitur will apply in some cases of medical malpractice, but not in most. People may doubt that a procedure recommended by their surgeon is really necessary, but all they can do is either to ask the surgeon for more convincing answers to their questions or to consult another professional (Ziegenfuss, 1983).

Apparently, therefore, a satisfactory system of discipline for the medical profession must be a combination of both *peer* discipline and *consumer* discipline. A medical review board must include both professional peers with requisite technical knowledge and experience and also healthcare users (along with legal advisers) to ensure that the medical professionals are more concerned for the served than for their own self-interest as the servants. At the same time, it is essential that medical information be made more easily available to all users so that each can know and defend his or her own rights and interests (Ginsberg, 1986).

Since medical professionals now have this information, they have the responsibility to undertake the educational task of informing the public so that it can defend itself against the professionals themselves. Since professionals are inevitably biased in favor of defending their own autonomy, and since any work or public education is difficult in the face of inevitable public apathy, the prospects of such an educational program are not bright. It seems that the public does not want to assume personal responsibility for its own health, but prefers to take pills or have surgery rather than to exercise or stop eating, drinking, and smoking too much.

In the face of this dreary reality, many otherwise compassionate and humanistic healthcare professionals are inclined to lapse into paternalism. They argue that the profession will have to do what it can for the public on the basis of its own expert judgment while defending itself against annoying or even dangerous lay intrusion into health affairs.

Christian professionals cannot accept this paternalistic and defensive position. The real remedy for malpractice and unjustified malpractice litigation is a more personalized practice of medicine that will reduce misunderstanding between professional and patient and will correct human failure by professionals through mutual cooperation and discipline within the health team itself. The notion of fraternal correction is part of the Christian ethos (Mt 18:15-18). Applied to a profession, it means that the members do not simply ignore or hide the defects of colleagues out of indifference or self-interest, but are seriously concerned to help them overcome these defects and repair the consequences. Fraternal correction also implies that even those workers in subordinate positions have a right and an obligation to correct superiors and that the superiors have an obligation to listen to such corrections.

If such mutual support and discipline are to be possible in a health team, it must rest on a profound mutual trust and respect, which can be built up only by persistent effort. One of the marks of a Catholic healthcare facility, therefore, should be this striving to establish the personal relationships within the staff and administration, which will be the basis for such professional cooperation.

CHAPTER 6

Social Organization of Healthcare

OVERVIEW

Today healthcare is no longer a matter of a person-to-person relation between physician and patient, nor simply of health teams located in separate healthcare facilities, but a great network of interrelated institutions. This chapter deals with this social organization of healthcare, first explaining some of the organizational models that are under current discussion and then developing the Principle of Subsidiarity and Functionalism, which is the ethical foundation of any social organization (6.1). Section 6.2 considers the question of whether the type of medical care now dominant in the United States requires not reorganization but radical revision.

Since the hospital situation is an important factor in modern healthcare, the hospital is discussed as an institution (6.3) and as a system of interpersonal relations (6.4). Next, the special features of a hospital based on a Catholic value system are delineated (6.5). Finally, some of the resources currently available by which healthcare facilities can achieve greater humanization and personalization are discussed (6.6).

6.1   ORGANIZATIONAL MODELS AND PRINCIPLE OF SUBSIDIARITY

Models

Up to this point, this book has been developing the model of a healthcare professional as a person competent in the art and science of medicine and motivated to serve other persons, each of whom has primary responsibility for his or her own health. The Christian healthcare professional finds this model in Jesus himself who came to heal and "not to be served, but to serve" (Mt 20:28).

Since individuals are responsible for their own health and the healthcare profession has a responsibility to be of service in this pursuit of health, does society as a whole have the responsibility for the health of each of its citizens and thus for the promotion and regulation of the healthcare profession in pursuit of universal health?

American culture is paradoxical in its prevailing attitude toward this question. Long ago the principle was accepted that government should promote and regulate universal free education for all children at least through high school. For some reason, however, Americans have hesitated to accept whole-heartedly the principle that government should promote and regulate universal free basic healthcare. The medical profession itself, through what was long its principal representative, the American Medical Association (AMA), has been extremely hesitant about supporting any such principle (AMA, 1986a; Childress, 1984; Falcone and Hartwig, 1984; Mulstein, 1984). However, as Falcone and Hartwig (1984) point out, several other interest groups are now active in health affairs. For this reason, agitation and persuasion for the provision of public regulation of healthcare has increased. As Falcone and Hartwig state, "Although not happy with PSRO (peer service review organizations) or health planning legislation, AMA opposition was mild compared to the fight over Medicare and NHI (national health insurance)." Such organization as the American Association of Retired Persons (AARP) and various groups representing mentally and physically handicapped persons encourage the federal government to become more involved in providing and regulating healthcare.

Americans generally tend to compare themselves to their main competition, the communist and socialist countries (Kervasdoue et al., 1984; Kohn and White, 1976). As already pointed out (1.3), this comparison is actually a juxtaposition of two religious value systems: humanism in the First World and Marxism in the Second World. Consequently, since medical education is often woefully negligent of the social sciences, healthcare professionals tend to identify all social issues in terms of two opposing models: free enterprise versus socialism.

Realizing that various models of the social organization of healthcare are possible in the United States is helpful (Alford, 1975; deVries, 1982; C. Hill, 1986). The first of these models is the *pluralist* system, which for the most part describes the healthcare system in the United States today, but which some people regard as no system at all. Its regulatory principle is the market in which persons with health needs compete for the services of healthcare professionals, principally on a fee-for-service basis, and professionals compete to sell their services. Today, however, these professional healthcare providers no longer act merely as individuals but are organized in a whole spectrum of healthcare institutions, of which the hospital is the major one (Aiken and Mechanic, 1986; AMA, 1984).

Each of these healthcare facilities requires the cooperation of many medical specialists assisted not only by nurses but also by many different technicians and auxiliaries. Furthermore, an increasing number of physicians are organized in *group practice* of various types. In some of these, they are prepaid by patients a fixed salary or a fee based on the number of patients served (capitation). Thus, in a pluralist system, there is no single organizational structure but a plurality of health providers, some acting individually but most acting through some institutional group (R. Rubin et al., 1988).

113

The difficulties with a strictly pluralist system have become very apparent in recent years (deVries, 1982; Mitchell, 1987; Starr, 1982). It is an inefficient system because it does not provide for long-range planning and wastes resources in overlapping services and duplication of expensive plants and equipment. More serious still, this model has not provided access to adequate medical care for many socially and geographically disadvantaged groups. Also, the pluralist system has not demonstrably raised the general level of health in recent years (Eastaugh, 1981; Lee and Brown, 1981). Finally, it seems subject to ever-mounting costs, which in 1987 absorbed 11.1 percent of the gross national product (Health Care Financing Administration, 1987).

Some defenders of the pluralist system (AMA, 1987b; Doubilet et al., 1986) argue that the medical profession cannot be blamed for the unhealthy American way of life over which physicians have little control, nor for mounting costs, which have been largely produced by government intervention in the form of Medicare and Medicaid, an intervention that prevents the market system from operating effectively (Bayer and Callahan, 1985; Sapolsky, 1977). These defenders propose no remedy but the extension of private health insurance systems, with the government providing only for catastrophic illness (American Hospital Association [AHA], 1986a). To such arguments, others respond that without government intervention, the poor will be even more neglected (Lurie et al., 1986; Robbins, 1984), and that the medical profession itself has destroyed free-market controls by monopolistic practices and by creating unnecessary demands for expensive modes of treatment (Califano, 1985).

Other defenders of pluralism avoid polemics and look for ways in which free-market mechanisms can be brought into play to afford better cost control and greater effectiveness in meeting real rather than artificial needs (Sorkin, 1986). Some (Sabbatini, 1985) doubt professional monopoly is really the major factor in raising health costs. However, others assert this and call for restrictions on such monopolistic practices of medical societies as the use of ethics codes to prevent advertising and limit access to information by which consumers might be able to make competitive choices (Weikel, 1984). Other economists (Sloan, 1983) believe some degree of government regulation is inevitable but advise that it should not emphasize planning as much as provide economic motivation and encouragement for hospitals to control costs (e.g., by budgetary measures), to set limits on new hospital construction, and to shift to more outpatient care.

Centralization

Because of difficulties with the pluralist model, a centralized model was proposed (Ellwood, 1974). According to this model, the United States was to be divided into regions, each to have all healthcare organized in a unified system. Both physicians and hospitals were to be organized in three levels of care. In such a system, long-range planning would be possible, and the emphasis was to be moved from the cure of disease to preventive care. This system was partially enacted at national and regional levels (AHA, 1977). The centralized model did not succeed, however, and was gradually replaced with an emphasis on competition as a means to reduce healthcare expenditures (Myrich, 1983). Unfortunately, competition has created more problems than it has solved and does not seem to be effective as far as U.S. healthcare needs are concerned (Kinzer, 1988; Mundinger, 1985; Newhouse, 1982).

The present healthcare system is pluralist and competitive and is dominated by a desire to reduce funding, no matter what the outcome to society (AHA, 1987b). The thought is that if funding is reduced, inefficient healthcare professionals and providers will be eliminated and costs will be manageable. Thus the federal government has instituted a prospective manner of reimbursing through diagnosis-related groups (DRGs) for Medicare and Medicaid (R. Veatch, 1986). The private insurance companies also are adopting this system. Industry and businesses are seeking to contract and the physicians and hospitals seeking to provide healthcare at reduced rates. The plan to limit the federal government's expenditures and the results of this plan, as they affect the public, are indicated by the following excerpt (Sorkin, 1986):

> While the healthcare industry grew rapidly in the 1960s and 1970s, with little attempt to limit expenditures, the 1980s have brought an emphasis on cost-containment measures. Partly because of record-breaking peacetime deficits, the government has responded by cutting social programs including health activities such as Medicare, Medicaid, and veterans' health programs.

One implication of these cutbacks is that the gains that have occurred in healthcare access may be imperiled. The share of the U.S. low-income population covered by Medicaid has fallen sharply. Moreover, Medicare budget reductions will result in rising premiums and deductibles, meaning that the elderly will be expected to pay a rising proportion of their healthcare costs (Bayer and Moreno, 1986).

Employers, as well as the government, are trying to restrict healthcare spending. The percentage of employers requiring employees to pay deductibles for inpatient hospital care has increased significantly. Moreover, to limit cost increases, employers are switching from conventional health insurance for their employees to health maintenance organizations (HMOs) or preferred provider organizations (PPOs) (J. Eisenberg, 1986).

Along with the emphasis on cost containment, the healthcare industry is becoming more competitive. Walk-in clinics, ambulatory surgery centers, free-standing emergency centers, and alternative birth centers are all examples of relatively new types of healthcare organizations competing with hospitals for patients. In response, hospitals have opened their own ambulatory surgery centers, allocated space for luxurious birthing rooms, and established HMOs and satellite clinics. They have also begun to advertise extensively (Agich and Besley, 1985).

A New Model

Alford (1975) points out that it is a mistake to think of the pluralist model as free enterprise and the centralized model as socialism. Because of the monopolistic control by the medical profession, the pluralist model is in fact a free enterprise system only in a very limited degree (Reinhardt, 1988). In such a model, health consumers are seldom in a position to make intelligent choices between competitive alternatives either because they lack information or because these alternatives are very limited (Schwartz, 1987).

On the other hand, the centralized model is by no means incompatible with a free enterprise system as it now operates in the United States. The American way of life has moved toward a high degree of centralization and monopoly in industry as well as in government. Such centralization has not changed the class structure of American society in any radical way. It would be perfectly possible to set up a centralized model in such a way as to leave considerable choice to both the consumer and the provider. This model could even include voluntary health insurance and fee-for-service features. What is essential to such a system is that it be centralized on a regional basis and involve planning in acquisition and allocation of resources. Given the difficulties with the present system in regard to planning for healthcare and arranging for financing that afford adequate access for all, a new model should be considered. Such a model would be based on the view that there must be centralization and planning but also extensive participation in the planning process (Smith and Kaluzny, 1975). In a planned society, whether governed by a democratic or a Marxist bureaucratic elite, individuals receive healthcare but lose any real control over how this is done. In a market system, individuals scarcely have any more control because they lack the information or alternatives from which to choose. What is needed, therefore, according to those who seek a third model, is a system in which consumers play a real role in the planning process (Navarro, 1986).

The great problem in adopting the participatory model is the resistance of healthcare professionals. They have been educated to believe that the maintenance of high-quality healthcare demands professional autonomy and forbids interference by laypersons (AMA, 1986a). Such barriers to a participatory model can be overcome by a change in medical education to move the physician's ideal away from the exclusively scientific model toward a more humanistic model (Association of American Medical Colleges, 1984). A humanistic model is superior even scientifically because it relates the individual ecologically to the environment. Other researchers (H. Blum, 1974; Toulmin, 1986) believe that a participatory model can come about only by educating consumers to know and aggressively defend their rights. Our line of argument would lead to the conclusion that the essential steps to developing a participatory model are (1) assumption of responsibility by each person for his or her own health, (2) restoration of a sound professional-client relationship, and (3) education of medical professionals to be able to work in this relationship (Pellegrino and Thomasma, 1988).

Common Good

For Catholic healthcare professionals, the first step in seeking a better organization of healthcare in the United States and in the world must be to free themselves from the ideology that leads Americans to analyze every social issue in terms of the American free enterprise system and the tyranny of socialism and communism. Unfortunately, most American Catholics have received a kind of religious education that tried to refute accusations that Catholics are un-American by identifying Christian social teaching with the American way of life. Such identification of any human culture with the Gospel is certain to be misleading, since the Gospel stands as a prophetic criticism of every culture, approving some of its features but correcting others.

The authentic social teaching of the Catholic Church has been fully formulated since Leo XIII's great encyclical *Rights and Duties of Capital and Labor* (1891), in many papal encyclicals and documents, by the Second Vatican Council in *The Church in the Modern World* (1965c), and most recently in the encyclical *On Social Development* of Pope John Paul II (1987a). This teaching contains some strong criticisms of Marxist socialism and communism, chiefly on three grounds: (1) its atheistic materialism, (2) its denial of the right of private property, and (3) its tendency to totalitarian government. However, this teaching also contains a vigorous criticism of capitalism on three grounds: (1) its deterministic reliance on economic laws, (2) its advocacy of unregulated competition and the profit motive, and (3) its neglect of the Christian advocacy of the poor. Recent documents (e.g., John XXIII's *Christianity and Social Progress (Mater et Magistra)* [1961], Paul VI's *The Development of Peoples* [1967], and John Paul II's *On Social Development* [1987a]) have pointed out that capitalism and communism alike have become colonializing powers either politically or economically and are thus largely responsible for the wars and poverty that oppress the great majority of humankind (Curran and McCormick, 1986). Christian healthcare professionals, therefore, should base their thinking about the social organization of healthcare on the principles of the Gospel, not on the principles of the free enterprise system any more than on those of socialism.

Apart from ideological bias, no one economic system any more than one political system is simply natural, right, or Christian. Such systems are human inventions, each with some advantages and some disadvantages, to be selected according to particular historical circumstances. These merits need to be evaluated both from a theoretical point of view and from a practical, experiential point of view. In judging them ethically, both their congruity with fundamental moral and Gospel principles and their pragmatic results in a given situation must be considered. A theoretically correct system in some circumstances may result in ethical disaster, whereas it is sometimes necessary to tolerate theoretically wrong institutions because they are the best that can be hoped for at the moment. In the long run, however, bad principles will have bad consequences. Christians must constantly strive to test their understanding of principles by experience and to bring the real situation into line with these principles once they are refined.

Catholic healthcare professionals thus have the responsibility at present to study all proposals for a national plan for healthcare and attempt to judge them in terms of theoretical principles and practical experience. Such a study is beyond the scope of this book, but it may be useful to indicate the first steps in such an ethical inquiry regarding a plan for providing access to healthcare for all.

A number of plans for better access to healthcare have been proposed (Fein, 1986). The plans all include some form of universal or national health insurance (AMA, 1986a, b; Feder et al., 1980; Shareef, 1984). In accord with Catholic social teaching, the following basic concepts should be included in any plan that is finally accepted:

1. The principle of access to healthcare as a fundamental human right
2. Comprehensive coverage of all types of health problems, physical and mental
3. Emphasis on positive health, that is, on prevention of disease and promotion of optimal health
4. Emphasis on provision of quality care
5. Emphasis on the humanistic education of healthcare professionals
6. A method of financing generally in the direction of a national trust fund built up by a progressive tax based on ability to pay and without cost sharing by the actual recipient
7. Participation by both consumers and healthcare professionals in administration and planning of the system

The general shift away from efforts to develop national programs of social service through the federal government toward a more conservative strategy of decentralization, deregulation, and stress on free-market competition is now taking place in the United States. This is a result of public dissatisfaction with the apparent ineffectiveness of such programs and the mounting burden of taxation and bureaucratic intervention (Number, 1982). This shift of opinion is exemplified by a recent change in the policies of The Catholic Health Association of the United States (CHA), which represents more than 900 hospitals and long term care facilities. Formerly the association had supported national health insurance as a means of meeting the objectives just mentioned, but CHA announced in 1981 that it is rethinking this stance and is seeking ways to work toward the same objective but "in ways more compatible with the maintenance of a strong and vital private sector" (CHA, 1981).

The argument given for this shift by CHA can be summarized as follows. In an economic system based on control by the free market, as in the United States, healthcare contains no internal means of self-regulation because (1) the government encourages unlimited demand for healthcare services by guaranteeing their payment without visible cost to the customer; (2) physicians feel free to select methods of diagnosis and treatment without regard to cost; and (3) the government also stimulates supply by funding research, the training of more professionals, and capital expansion. The result is an unlimited demand and an equally unlimited rise in costs. Faced by this impossible situation, the government is forced to cut costs by increasingly burdensome regulations and ceilings that affect the quality of service. In the end, the underprivileged persons whom the government was trying to help have still heavier tax burdens and no better care (Blendon, 1986).

The conclusion seems to be that it would be better to maintain the existing pluralist system, with all its very serious faults, and seek new ways of obtaining the same major objectives that a centralized national program was supposed to achieve. The difficulty with this argument is that there is so little evidence that "deregulation of the healthcare industry" will increase competition among healthcare providers, since (as Chapter 4 shows) the American medical profession is strongly monopolistic and committed to a type of medicine based on complex, expensive technologies (Navarro, 1986). It seems more likely that healthcare costs will continue to mount, whether there is a national insurance or not (Health Care Financing Administration, 1987). The United States Catholic Conference, in its *Letter on Health and Health Care* (1981), and in its pastoral letter on *Economic Justice for All* (1986), continues to support a national system of healthcare that blends private and public providers and affords equitable access to healthcare for all. As CHA indicates in its study, the only fundamental cure for the problem would be a shift to preventive medicine, since only in this way can the demand for services find a natural limit (Engelhardt, 1980). Preventive medicine, however, demands radical changes not only in the healthcare profession, but also in the American lifestyle and even in the competitive economic system on which it is based. As Kelman (1980) has written:

> The structure of modern industrial capitalist society appears to materially and unavoidably produce a meaning of "health" intrinsically involving substantially preventable disease. Because in such a society private investment responds to cyclical and geographic fluctuations in rates of return and competitive labor markets, much of the disease structure (heart disease, stroke, kidney failure, and cancer, among others) encompasses diseases which captive citizens cannot afford to do without. To prevent those diseases through environmental and workplace cleanup, full employment, and geographic capital stability is to drive away the very private capital on which economic life is based. Consequently, those diseases which are intrinsic to modern capitalist society as the law of supply and demand are, therefore, a characteristic component of the meaning of "health," and the socially optimum level of organistic condition in this epoch (p. 143).

To face this fundamental dilemma requires radical thinking, and it is here that Catholic social thought can make an important contribution to finding new solutions. These solutions must rest on three principles that have been previously expounded in this book: (1) every human being does have a fundamental right to health, as acknowledged in the *Universal Declaration of Human Rights* (United Nations, 1948), Article 25, because human rights are based on essential human needs; (2) individual persons have the primary responsibility to promote their own health; and (3) as social beings, however, people also have the right to seek the help of others when necessary to fulfill this responsibility and reciprocally have the duty to give the same help to others as much as they are able.

Subsidiarity

The papal encyclicals and the Second Vatican Council have repeatedly proposed a universal social principle (of which this second proposition is only an application to healthcare) that is called the *Principle of Subsidiarity* or, more comprehensively, the *Principle of the Common Good and Subsidiarity*. Section 1.5

argues that the dignity of the person requires a community and is to be found in this communal sharing, or common good. Each individual, therefore, has a need and a moral obligation to contribute to the common good and a right to share in it.

Most social evils and injustices are the result of exclusion of some persons from the common good in which they have a right to share (Williams and Hauchal, 1987). The ancient evil of slavery was precisely such an unjust institution. The slaves contributed to the common good but were not permitted to share fully in it, not only in regard to economic goods, but also in regard to spiritual goods such as education, freedom, political participation, respect, and even the right to worship the "gods of the city." Thus the distribution of the common good is a fundamental demand of social justice.

Jesus, moreover, taught an ethics that clearly went beyond even this demand for distributive justice based on merit (i.e., each received in proportion as he or she contributed). Jesus proclaimed the coming of the Kingdom of God (Mk 1:15), which was not merely a heavenly kingdom but also the fulfillment of the Old Testament prophecies of the reign of God on earth (Viviano, 1988). When Jesus said to Pilate, "My kingship is not of this world" (Jn 18:36), he did not mean by "world," the earth, but the present sinful order of power struggle. He was saying to Pilate, "I am not competing with you power brokers. I am building a kingdom built on a different principle; on service, not on dominion." He taught his followers to pray, "Your Kingdom come, your will be done, on earth as it is in heaven" (Mt 6:10). The Beatitudes (Lk 6:20-22; Mt 5:3-11), in their original form, were the joyful announcement to the poor (i.e., those excluded from the common good) that at last they were to be included in that common good, not only economically, but spiritually ("the poor have the good news preached to them") (Lk 7:22). Consequently, the principle of the early Church was "from each according to his ability, to each according to his needs," a principle that Marx borrowed from the Acts of the Apostles (4:32-35). Thus the Principle of the Common Good requires love and mercy, and the distribution of the common good not according to merit, but according to need. Thus the mark of all Jesus' work was his concern for the neglected, the outcast, the leper, the prostitute, the Samaritan heretic, and the pagan unbeliever.

A Christian ethics of healthcare distribution must be based not on merit, and certainly not on the ability to pay, *but on need*, because the needy are the most neglected. (A person who can care for himself or herself does not need social help.) Moreover, social oppression is the major cause of their illness, an oppression from which the more affluent members of society profit. Thus those who are helpless by reason of poverty, disease, defect, or age (the unborn or the senile) should be the first consideration of any health plan.

However, all persons should contribute to the plan according to their *ability*. Thus the social responsibility for healthcare falls first on those who have the ability to heal, the healthcare professionals, and second on those who have the ability to pay, that is, those who have financially profited the most from society. For such affluent individuals to claim that they have made their wealth simply by their own efforts is an absurdity. They may have worked hard, but their wealth would not have been possible exclusive of the society of which they are a part. Consequently, their debt to the common good is in proportion to the wealth they have received from it.

From this notion of the common good, the idea of subsidiarity follows logically. *Subsidiarity* implies that the first responsibility in meeting human needs rests with the free and competent individual, then with the local group. Higher and higher levels of the community must assume this responsibility (1) when the lower unit cannot assume it and (2) when the lower unit refuses to assume it.

Although all persons are primarily responsible for their own health, when they cannot assume this responsibility—either because they are too young, too old, too poor, too uneducated, or possessed of any other handicap—the community at higher levels must come to their aid. If a lower level neglects to fulfill the responsibility, a higher level must correct the oversight by punishment or other remedies. The higher level should never be content merely to take over responsibility, however; it must work to return responsibility to a lower level. Thus people should be educated about personal healthcare, helped to pay for such care, and held responsible for neglecting it. *The main objection to many social reforms has been that they have not provided for this progressive decentralization.* For example, the welfare system in the Untied States has perpetuated poverty rather than helped the dependent to become independent.

The growing criticism of liberalism and the excesses of government bureaucracy, however, should not lead to identifying Catholic social thought with the conservative movement, which has grown more and more powerful in the United States since the Second World War. As Nash (1976) has shown in *The Conservative Intellectual Movement in America Since 1945*, American conservatism is of three varieties: (1) libertarianism, which advocates a laissez faire government; (2) traditionalism, which deplores the loss of Western cultural heritage through overrapid social change; and (3) nationalistic anticommunism. Catholic social doctrine has always opposed laissez faire capitalism, which the papal encyclicals label "liberalism" in the original sense the term had in the economic thought of Adam Smith and the political thought of the French Revolution. Although Catholicism defends Western cultural heritage, as Vatican II made very clear, the Gospel message is to build the Kingdom of God on earth by a radical reform of society according to the demands of peace and justice. Likewise, Catholicism opposes communism, not by a program of nationalism but of disarmament and international cooperation. Thus Catholic thinking in social matters must remain independent of both the liberal and the conservative tendencies, both of which arise from the basic assumption of humanism.

Therefore the type of healthcare program that Catholics can consistently support must aim at preventive medicine, at achieving a healthier people who can care for themselves, rather than an ever-increasing dependence on technical medical care and professional help. As Plato observed, "A society that is always going to the doctor is a sick society" (*Republic III*, 405A). To achieve this fundamental objective, society must seek the sound political and economic organization of society.

Functionalism

The popes have also stressed that one of the evils of historical capitalism and communism alike has been the tendency of both systems to concentrate all the power of decision making in the state. Before secular humanism became the dominant philosophy of modern society, Christian thinking was able to advance the notion that a society is not simply a two-level structure of government and citizenry, but an organic community containing many functions that are mutually interdependent.

This concept of the mutual interdependence of a community was enunciated by St. Paul in 1 Corinthians 12-13 and linked by him with Jesus' teaching that the greatest should become the servants of the least in the Kingdom of God. Thus the power to make social decisions ought to be kept as close as possible to those who experience those problems and are most strongly affected by the decisions concerning them. Only in this way can the dignity of the least members of a community be acknowledged and their interests effectively served by the greater. A paternalism that decides everything for those it claims to serve is really nothing but a form of domination and tends to become self-serving. Thus St. Paul, without directly attacking slavery, admonished the master that he should treat his slave not as a child, but as a "most dear brother" (Philemon 1:16), that is, as equal by reason of their mutual interdependence in Christ. The Principle of Subsidiarity therefore requires us to share decision-making power not only at various vertical levels of local, state, and federal government, but also among horizontal sectors representing various functional bodies. Thus education, as a basic function of society, forms a body of persons, some with expertise (the educators) and others (the students) who are trying to educate themselves through the services of the experts. Decisions about education pertain first not to government but to bodies of cooperating teachers and students mutually dependent on each other. The same holds true for other basic social functions—especially for the economy, with its interdependence of management, workers, and consumers—as well as for the social organization of healthcare, with its mutual interdependence of professional healers and health seekers. Each person in a society is related to as many such functional bodies as he or she has basic needs. The role of government is to coordinate and encourage the full development of these different organs of society, not to deprive them of their decision-making capacity.

This application of subsidiarity to the organization of society on the basis of social functions, rather than on the basis of a struggle between isolated individuals defending their rights and a centralized government having all the powers of social decision, is usually referred to as *corporatism* in Catholic documents. This term somewhat misleads Americans, who usually view corporations as purely economic organizations. The term has also been discredited because it has been used by fascist political parties in Europe to win Catholic support for its exact opposite, namely, totalitarianism, or total state power. The following discussion will use the term *functionalism* instead.

Functionalism is opposed on the one hand to communism and national socialism (as with that of Mussolini and Hitler) because they are totalitarian, concentrating all decision-making power in the hands of the state and the military. On the other hand, it is opposed to the competitive individualism of unregulated capitalism or free enterprise, with its hidden tendency toward monopolism, resulting in concentration of decision-making power in the hands of an interlocking power elite (Califano, 1985) or the industrial-military complex of which President Eisenhower warned. Functionalism is not a mere theory, since it has a powerful influence, through Catholic statesmen, on the formation of the European common market and of co-determination by management and labor in West Germany, Yugoslavia, Japan, and other countries. Some of its implications are also evident in Latin America in the efforts of Catholic theologians and political leaders to develop a theology of liberation that is not capitalist, fascist, or Marxist (Boff, 1986).

Politically, it might seem that functionalism would have little chance in the United States. Certain features of some institutions, however, are in fact functionalist. For example, higher education in the United States, in contrast to the statism of the lower school system, remains largely functionalist. Decisions about educational policies in our colleges and universities are made independently of government by faculties and accrediting agencies and by the right of students to choose their own schools. The student revolt of the 1960s, however, seemed to show that schools needed to allow students greater participation in policy making, and to a certain extent this has taken place, rendering the system still more functionalist (Dickstein, 1988). On the other hand, the increasing control of the government over schools by reason of their economic dependency is working strongly to destroy their functionalist character.

Similarly, after the Great Depression the growth of labor unions in the United States, to a considerable degree under the influence of Catholic social thought (Cronin, 1950), portended the eventual development of functionalism in the economic sphere. Unfortunately, the unions have largely neglected the social aspects of their original purpose and have been co-opted by the capitalist market system in which they are becoming just another monopoly. Renewed Catholic leadership in unions, including hospital unions, could remedy this neglect. Fortunately, this trend toward monopoly shows some signs of a reversal in the growth of consumerism, participatory democracy, and social ecology, as well as in the increasing dissatisfaction with resulting liberal reforms, so many of which have served only to enlarge the power of government bureaucracy. Catholics need to take advantage of this growing criticism of the so-called American way of life to propose a more personalistic and functionalist conception of society.

In healthcare, these general ethical principles of subsidiarity and functionalism have to be applied to the concrete historical situation of American medical institutions. The medical profession, as it has operated in the United States, has been influenced by three somewhat inconsistent principles: (1) the ancient ideal of a profession as service, which was formulated in the Hippocratic oath and reinforced by Christianity; (2) the philosophy of secular humanism, with its strong emphasis on human rights and the duty of man to use scientific knowledge to solve human problems; and (3) the ideology of capitalism, which has been fostered by humanism. Many liberal secularists consider this capitalist ideology to be at odds with their concern for human rights and the full application of the social sciences to the planning of economic and political life. However, conservative humanists defend this ideology as at least preferable to the philosophy of Marxism.

In view of Christian goals, a Catholic should be particularly aware of the lessons learned by the United States. The first of these is that the pluralist system did not adequately care for the poor, nor did it do much about positive health improvement (AHA, 1986a; Waitzhib, 1983). It tended to foster an exaggerated professional elitism, to place strong emphasis on monopolization and the profit motive, and it never produced a system of medical education that was personalistic. On the other hand, the pluralist system should be credited with promoting very rapid technological and scientific progress and with developing many healthcare facilities equipped to give acute care. It must be noted, however, that this progress has led to greater expenditure of resources on the sophisticated treatment of relatively rare ailments rather than to better care for the health of the majority (R.G. Evans, 1985).

A centralized system is aimed at correcting some of these defects, but not in a very radical manner. Such a system will probably greatly increase the bureaucratization, which, as evidenced by the welfare system, can cost a great deal and accomplish very little. A centralized system will provide more health-care, but there is no certainty it will promote better health. A bureaucracy also is not likely to personalize the healthcare it gives. Even if this system makes a sincere effort to humanize medicine, such effort will not be guided by a Christian concept of the person but by a humanist concept that may express itself not in concern for neglected persons, but in their extermination by abortion or euthanasia.

Therefore, although Christians should favor a national healthcare program as the only practical way available to extend care to the neglected of society, they should not have any illusions about the adequacy of such programs. To oppose national comprehensive healthcare in the reactionary way in which some Catholics fought the labor unions, the Child Labor Amendment, the United Nations, and the Equal Rights Amendment, because such reforms are favored by secular humanists of the liberal wing, only gives support to the secular humanists of the conservative wing, whose views are even less compatible with Catholic social principles. Instead, Christians should critically support the new schemes for national comprehensive healthcare, stressing the need to incorporate into these plans as many functionalist features as possible. For example:

1. Comprehensive healthcare should aim primarily at the promotion of positive health, not merely at the cure of acute disease or the prolongation of life through sophisticated techniques. Therefore, it should work for (a) removal of the environmental and social causes of ill health, including the commercial encouragement of unhealthy patterns of

living, and (b) provision of preventive health education that will give persons control over their own health.

2. Priority should be given to the problems of the most powerless, poorly informed, and least able to pay. These persons should not be cared for paternalistically, but should be admitted at once to participate in the power of decision about their own health needs.

3. Decision-making power should not be confined to a government bureaucracy, nor to autonomous professionals, but should be shared by all concerned in mutual interdependence.

4. Planning should proceed in such a way as to avoid tendencies to increase dependence on higher levels and to promote a gradually increasing decentralization in both control and funding. This decentralization, however, should not be used as an excuse for the government to neglect the monitoring of healthcare and the supplementation and correction of defects at lower levels of organization.

5. Planning must be a continuous process of decision making that adapts to experience and new needs, rather than a fixed plan based on projections that may be mistaken.

Christians may find support for various items of a functionalist program from different and opposed ideological camps. For example, ecology-minded people are convinced that environmental and social factors are the major cause of poor health conditions, but others cite this fact to defend the medical profession against the charge that it is responsible for these conditions. Again, the rights of health consumers are defended not only by civil rights and consumer advocates, but also by individuals who believe that the free market is the best method of controlling health costs. Consequently, Christians should attempt to transcend ideological biases and use a strategy of coalition to promote particular goals.

Above all, Christians should work together through various church agencies to influence the health education of consumers and the medical education of the professionals. Catholic schools, medical schools, and teaching hospitals especially should teach a personalistic approach to health and to the objectives of the medical profession. Catholic institutions must protest against the many current forces that tend to absorb them into the centralized, bureaucratic structure of society dominated by secular humanism. At the same time, Catholics should approach secular humanists with a genuinely ecumenical spirit, which seeks through dialogue to find grounds of agreement and cooperation.

The ethical principle underlying all such efforts to organize society, including its healthcare institutions, in such a way as to counteract tendencies toward totalitarian bureaucratism on the one hand, and competitive individualism on the other, can be summarily formulated in the following *Principle of the Common Good, Subsidiarity, and Functionalism:*

Human communities exist only to promote and share the common good among all their members "from each according to ability, to each according to need" in such a way that:

1. Decision making rests *vertically* first with the person, then with the lower social levels, and *horizontally* with functional social units.
2. The higher social units intervene only to supply the lower units what they cannot achieve by themselves, while at the same time working to make it easier in the future for lower units and individuals to satisfy these needs by their own efforts.

6.2   LIMITS TO HEALTHCARE

To make a sufficiently prophetic and radical critique of our American health system, special attention must be given to the question of what is popularly called "the crisis of limits." (Callahan, 1987b; Enthoven, 1980; Fuchs, 1986)

A characteristic feature of the 1970s and 1980s has been growing criticism of the ideal of unlimited technological progress and of the modern concept of specialism in the learned disciplines and the practical professions. This "crisis of limits" is occurring in both the democratic and the Marxist countries. This crisis is not easy for true believers in these value systems to endure, and they tend to react by claiming that the critics are reactionary opponents of progress. Actually, the critics are not opposed to progress, but to the myth of progress, an illusory concept of the nature of human progress (Kervasdoue et al., 1984).

Thus Illich, in his highly controversial book *Medical Nemesis* (1976), argues that Marx was correct in distinguishing between "exchange values" as a measure of welfare and "use values." Illich attempts to show that although modern industrial society has enormously increased the production of exchangeable goods (measured as the gross national product, or GNP), in some respects it has been even less effective than preindustrial society in satisfying basic human needs. Nevertheless, he does not propose that scientific technology be abandoned, but rather advocates that technologies be selected and developed that will meet needs economically, instead of increasing production of exchangeable goods at the expense of limited energy resources.

Illich chooses to study modern medicine because it is typically cited as outstanding proof of the success of technology based on the industrial type. He attempts to deflate this claim by using two arguments. First, he argues that the success of modern medicine is based on two achievements: (1) increased life expectancy and (2) improved patient comfort in the absence of cure. The first achievement, he explains, is primarily a result of relatively simple technologies that brought about the reduction of epidemics by immunization, antibiotic drugs, and improved hygiene. The whole elaborate system of hospitalization, however, has had little effect on life expectancy and is enormously and increasingly expensive. The second achievement, Illich insists, results in an "anesthetized culture" in which people do not know how to integrate suffering into personal growth, while in fact the quality of their life is not notably improved.

Second, Illich argues that modern medicine is actually producing as much poor health as it heals. These *iatrogenic* diseases take three forms:

1. *Clinical* iatrogenesis is produced by drugs, unnecessary surgery, and other harmful remedies administered by physicians and healthcare facilities.
2. *Social* iatrogenesis is produced by encouraging people to become consumers of doubtful medical remedies rather than by changing the morbid social conditions that cause their ills, especially the inequitable distribution of healthcare.
3. *Cultural* iatrogenesis takes the form of symbolic, psychological effects on the way persons perceive their bodily life as something meaningless in both its pleasures and suffering, as something to be possessed and used and manipulated, rather than as part of their person that has to live, grow, die, and be transcended.

The response to Illich's criticism usually has been to agree that his arguments are largely valid, but to claim they have already been recognized by the medical profession (Horrobin, 1980). Illich does not deny this; in fact, he has drawn heavily on certain critics within the medical establishment.

Whatever the future may be, the healthcare profession in the United States must seriously face up to the problem of *limits* (Callahan, 1987b). Healthcare problems will never be solved simply by national plans if (as in other systems of socialized medicine in Europe) they allow ever-mounting costs of healthcare, such as the 500 percent rise of per-diem hospital costs for a patient since 1970 (Sorkin, 1986). It is not surprising that similar crises exist in transportation, energy in general, or population growth, where the necessity of limits is admitted by all, even though limitation demands radical readjustments in American culture.

6.3   THE HOSPITAL AS COMMUNITY

Cure and Care

So far this chapter has noted that the social organization of healthcare in the United States is and probably will remain pluralistic, although more careful planning is needed to meet everyone's needs because resources are limited. Now consider the structure and function of the basic units from which this system is built. At present these units in which healthcare is concentrated are hospitals and medical centers dedicated primarily to the treatment of acute diseases. Long term care centers are growing in number, but their existence has little effect on the manner in which medicine is practiced and healthcare provided in the United States.

A great modern hospital is a world of its own: a strange community in which most members remain only a few days, but in which some live for months and years, and where life begins for some and ends for others. Today the trend to hospitalize patients for medical care is being reversed by developing outpatient surgery centers and other facilities designed to care for ambulatory patients. For the immediate future, however, the hospital will be the main focus for healthcare (Goldsmith, 1981). It is therefore necessary to raise some questions about the ethical goals of the hospital as a human community.

127

According to Sigerist (1960b; C. Rosenberg, 1987), the hospital evolved historically in three stages. First, the Romans established hospitals for soldiers and for work gangs of slaves for the purpose of maintaining manpower for special tasks. Second, Eastern Christians instituted *xenodochia* (guesthouses) or hospitals (hotels, inns) for the poor, a development paralleled in older religions only by the Buddhists in the second century BC under the emperor Atoka. These hospitals were copied and further developed by the Muslim conquerors of portions of the Byzantine Empire, and the Muslim hospitals in turn inspired Western Christians, at the time of the Crusades, to new efforts. These medieval institutions usually did not supply medical care in the strict sense, but only nursing and spiritual comfort. By the Renaissance, however, Christian hospitals were regularly visited by physicians and sometimes even became retirement homes for the rich. Third, in the eighteenth and nineteenth centuries the Christian hospitals were gradually replaced by modern public and private hospitals, generally under the inspiration of Enlightenment humanism with its emphasis on scientific technology and the free enterprise system. Thus, historically, the line of development has been from an emphasis on care to one on cure. A fascinating example of this development can be found in the 600-year history of the work of the Alexian Brothers studied by Kauffmann in *Tamers of Death* (1976) and *The Ministry of Healing* (1978).

Considerable sociological effort has been devoted to understanding this typical modern institution into which a good portion of national income is poured each year (Aiken and Mechanic, 1986; Donnelly and Williams, 1982). The hospital seems to be a curious mixture of several types of organization (Conrad and Kern, 1981).

1. The hospital retains something of its original character as a hotel or temporary residence, with the primary function of care and custody. This purpose is most pronounced in the impaired model, wherein the hospital becomes a permanent or long-term residence, approaching a total institution of the sort studied in Goffman's well-known work, *Asylums* (1962). As such, it is divided into the *hosts* (the administration and staff), who care for the *guests* (the patients).

2. The hospital is also a place of cure in which the medical staff provides diagnosis and treatment for the patients. Thus it consists not only of hosts and guests, but also of *healers* and *sick*.

3. Finally, the hospital is usually also a school in which there are *teachers* and *researchers* (overlapping roles, as in any modern university) with their *students* and *research staffs*. The students are engaged both in class work and in supervised clinical practice, and some are interns and residents in actual full-time practice.

Especially interesting is the fact that the nurses are at the point of intersection of all these functions (Chaska, 1983). They are often themselves students in training, but they also provide care; that is, they are the persons who actually carry out the host function of the hospital. At the same time, nurses are an essential part of the medical staff engaged in cure, since nurses execute many of the treatment procedures and cooperate closely with physicians in observing patients and monitoring treatments.

Today the organizational complexity of the hospital is further intensified by the hospital being a quasi-governmental agency for the administration of public funds for healthcare. As such, it is also staffed with social workers, who help patients return to the wider community. Thus the hospital today becomes one of the principal formative institutions of society, providing a model community that is bound to have a profound effect on the average American's understanding of social and personal interrelationships. This is evidenced by the mythical power that television dramas about hospital life seem to have over the American imagination.

A Healing Community

If the modern hospital and nursing home are to perform these varied functions effectively, they must solve several basic ethical questions. In discussing total institutions, Goffman (1962) has shown that a prison, a small village, or a monastery can never be really total because it lacks the resources to satisfy all human needs. If it is not to foster regressive behavior in its inmates, the total institution must find ways to be open to wider influences. The medieval monasteries found it necessary to develop a complex internal life enriched by the practice of hospitality, which made them centers of communication rather than mere enclosures from the world.

Thus, in the impaired model, hospitals or nursing homes in which patients remain for long periods have two special obligations. First, they must constantly seek ways for their patients to retain contact with the life of the outside world and to engage in a variety of stimulating and enriching experiences and occupations. Second, they must find ways to involve patients in some genuine participation in making the decisions that affect their lives. Obviously, senile or mentally disturbed patients may have little capacity for such participation, but too often this incapacity has been fostered by patterns of institutional life that have given them no opportunity to express their preferences or to take at least some responsibility for themselves and others.

Today, largely because of the inflation of health costs, great efforts are being made to reduce the hospital stay for surgical patients and even for acutely ill patients, so that now the average stay is less than a week. This is not only less costly, but also better therapeutically and ethically. The hospital has an ethical responsibility not to disrupt the home life of patients. Although sick persons have the right to be relieved of many ordinary social obligations (Conrad and Kern, 1981), they need to be helped to experience sickness as a part of life, not as an interruption in living.

Consequently, despite inconveniences to the staff, better hospitals and nursing homes no longer discourage visitors, not even small children, but find ways to facilitate continued family contact and opportunities for the family to share in the therapeutic process. Similarly, when their condition or convalescence permits, patients should be encouraged to assist their fellow patients. The sense of isolation, abandonment, and helplessness is perhaps the most traumatic aspect of being sick, but sickness can also be an important occasion to draw people together in a shared effort of healing. Whenever possible, patients should be given an opportunity to exercise freedom of choice.

Today, within necessary limits, hospitals and nursing homes provide such freedom, but there must also be a constant, imaginative effort to enlarge the scope of patients' activities. This should be measured not by the convenience of the hospital staff, but by therapeutic and human values.

Moreover, the public should also share in making the policies by which healthcare facilities are governed as public institutions. Most members of the public will have to use a hospital or nursing home at some time, and all have an interest in the type of institution their taxes and gifts support.

The communal orientation of a hospital or nursing home as described here is primarily patient centered. Patients will not be treated as persons, however, if the professionals who care for them are themselves alienated by feelings that their own needs are neglected or their rights infringed. These healthcare professionals invest much of their lives and energy in the life of the healthcare facility and are rightly convinced that they have special rights based on their dedication, expert knowledge, and experienced judgment.

Perhaps the most important of these professional rights is the *autonomy of professional judgment*. Physicians need to be free to examine their patients and to order the treatment they think best. Nurses need to believe that their responsibility for their patients is just as professional as that of physicians. How can this necessary autonomy be reconciled with the communal character of the hospital as an institution? Can the hospital administration permit physicians to use their facilities or require cooperation of nursing personnel for purposes that, in the administration's judgment, are either unprofessional or unethical, such as abortion or sterilization? Chapter 9 discusses some of the concrete ethical questions that may arise.

Generally speaking, however, professional freedom in healthcare institutions, as with academic freedom in universities, must be vigilantly protected (Loewy, 1986). The trustees and administrators not only have such disciplinary responsibilities, but also a positive duty to unify the institution's multiple functions in a manner that permits both the patients and the staff to form a truly human community and not merely a "health factory." Faulty communications between physicians, nurses, auxiliaries, and administration, and within these subgroups produce an atmosphere of tension deleterious to the services that can directly affect the psychosomatic health of the patients, especially in mental hospitals. Modern administrative and communications theory affords important resources for improving such situations, provided they are used as tools to achieve ethically acceptable goals and not merely to oil an impersonal machine.

Finally, as the inflation of healthcare costs continues, many ethical questions arise from the economic policies of hospitals, reflecting the severe pressures from which they suffer. Here two important patient rights come into question: the right to emergency care and the right to treatment once the patient is admitted. Rankin and Duffy (1983) show that the courts have generally upheld the legal obligation of hospitals with emergency wards (and even of those not so equipped to the extent of their resources) to care promptly for all persons who come to them in serious need of medical attention and to continue to care for them until they are ambulatory or can safely be transferred to another hospital willing to receive them. The courts are beginning to develop a doctrine on the rights of patients in so-called custodial institutions to treatment as well as to care (Kindred, 1984). In some states there are laws against "dumping" (sending endangered patients to other hospitals), and all healthcare commentators declare dumping to be an unethical practice (Friedman, 1982; Schiff et al., 1986). Christian and humanist ethics both have accepted the teaching of the Parable of the Good Samaritan (Lk 10:25-37), but in public institutions this concern for one's neighbor must be legally enforced.

All these ethical and legal questions, which arise from the ideal of the hospital as a community of care and cure, faced with the realities of modern depersonalized and competitive society, can be solved only at the price of an unremitting effort to give priority to *persons* over institutions and properties. Every hospital suffers from the proliferation of bureaucratic rules intended to protect the institution from exploitation by the crazy or the crafty. This red tape is destructive to patients and staff. The chief remedy against this ever-present danger is training the staff to deal with borderline situations in a flexible and prudent manner and to provide a variety of methods by which self-criticism can be promoted and outside criticism can be heard. To achieve this interplay, it is necessary to develop the staff not merely as a hierarchical structure of command responsibility, but as an interacting *health team*.

6.4 THE HEALTH TEAM

Physicians and Co-Workers

Because of the highly specialized character of modern medicine, health seekers must entrust themselves not to a single physician within the hospital, but to a *health team* (Brower, 1985). The medical staff of such a team may include physicians, nurses, and psychologists, and perhaps paramedics or medical assistants. The nursing staff will include registered nurses, practical nurses, and aides, and perhaps nursing unit managers and nursing clerks. The medical departments will include physicians who are pathologists, along with many medical technologists (e.g., specialists in hematology, chemistry, microbiology, serology, histology, and cytology), other physicians who are radiologists and radiation therapists with their assistants, technicians in encephalography and electrocardiography, and finally therapists skilled in occupational and physical therapy. They will be supplemented also by a social services department (staffed by medical social work professionals), a pharmacy, a dietary department, and a health science library. (It is noteworthy that because of the ever-increasing number of drugs, physicians are beginning to give pharmacists a greater role in determining the precise drugs to use and the mode of administration according to the physician's diagnosis and general plan of treatment.) In addition, persons will be in charge of patient services such as admissions, hospital records, environmental services (housekeeping), laundry, and purchasing. The business services department involves admissions, accounting, budgeting, and credit and collection, and the buildings are cared for by a plant department.

Personnel and public relations departments are essential to secure and care for this complex body of skilled people, and the whole institution requires an elaborate administration, with its governing board and administrative staff. Finally, a healthcare facility makes use of the services of such outside professionals as architects, accountants, attorneys, special consultants, and sales representatives.

This (incomplete) list of the various diversified professional and subprofessional roles required in a modern healthcare facility emphasizes that any patient entering a hospital or nursing home is confronted with a small army of persons. These people are supposed to serve the patient, but the patient must deal with them and perhaps must protect himself or herself from them.

This section discusses only the health team in the somewhat narrower sense of those members the patient must deal with very directly—the physician, the nurse, and the social worker—in order to determine what reciprocal ethical obligations exist between the patient and these three types of professionals. Then the issue of protection of the patient's rights by some type of advocate is discussed.

Traditionally, the chief decision maker in any health team is the licensed physician, the medical doctor (MD). Supposedly, licensure guarantees that physicians have the basic, integral knowledge of the human body and its essential life processes to be reasonably certain about a patient's condition and therefore able to decide (1) what emergency care is necessary and (2) what should not be done to the patient without further examination. Consequently, no serious step toward treating the patient can be taken without a physician's permission. Of course, much emergency care is provided by first-aid persons who may have very limited training, but it is generally conceded that any patient has the right to be seen by a physician as quickly as possible (Sanders, 1984).

Today the concept of the licensed medical doctor as a general practitioner has been vastly altered by the growth of medical specialization. In 1950, only about 36 percent of physicians in private practice were specialists, whereas today about 70 percent are specialists (Ginsberg et al., 1984). This growth is not clearly related to patient needs. There are too many surgeons and only about 30 percent of the required number of radiologists and psychiatrists, 40 percent of anesthetists, and 50 percent of pathologists. This imbalance is largely the result of decisions by the physicians themselves, who prefer a particular type of work because it is interesting, convenient, prestigious, or profitable. The possibility of a free choice of specialties is one of the features of free enterprise medicine most valued by the profession.

This rapid decline of the general practitioner as the primary-care professional has deprived patients of the advantages of having their health problems evaluated by someone who knows the patient in his or her family context over a long period and who thinks of the patient as a whole person with a continuous biography. Recently, there was a trend among medical students to specialize in family medicine as a way to reconcile specialization with an interest in primary care, but this trend has not continued (AMA, 1988d). Otherwise, primary care is usually given by a specialist in internal medicine for adults and by a pediatrician for children. Another approach to this problem is the diagnostic clinic in which a patient is examined in an orderly manner by a whole crew of specialists, who then attempt to synthesize their findings so as to obtain a total understanding of the patient. Again, patients have been encouraged to have an annual checkup, which can be done in a clinic and may even be largely computerized, so that the patient's health is continuously monitored and problem areas identified for further study and treatment.

None of these developments seems as yet to provide a completely satisfactory answer to the problem of how to provide the kind of primary healthcare that will keep the total person in clear focus while making use of all the advantages of specialized knowledge and skill (Strauss, 1984).

Nurses, Social Workers, and Patient Advocates

Perhaps the key to this difficulty is to be found in a better understanding of the nurse's proper role, which today has become ambiguous (McCloskey and Grace, 1985). Originally, the nurse was the person most concerned with caring for and having continuous contact with the patient. Therefore, the patient-centered type of healthcare this book is advocating would dictate that the nurse is the *central* professional figure, not the physician. Primary care is the nurse's task, not that of a general practitioner, family specialist, or others.

Nurses, however, have been burdened with other tasks. For too long they spent much of their energy in housekeeping chores--making beds, carrying trays, and so forth. Today they have been largely relieved of these tasks by auxiliaries, but they are still much occupied with such technical tasks as temperature taking, injections, medications, and intravenous feeding. Moreover, they are oppressed by the sexism implicit in the notion that caring is a maternal role suitable only for women (J. Ashley, 1976). This sexism is reflected in the fact that until recently, female physicians were a small minority, whereas in the Soviet Union and other countries their number more than equals male physicians. Fortunately, this trend is now reversing, and within the next generation as many as 30 percent of physicians in the United States will be women. This freeing of medicine from sexism would also be furthered if men were encouraged to enter the nursing profession in larger numbers.

Under present circumstances, however, as nursing education has advanced, able female nurses have sought administrative and teaching posts as the only way of advancement open to them. They would find nursing itself much more interesting, however, if it became the real focus of healthcare, so that the role of the nurse, female or male, in direct contact with the patient is seen as primary care and the real source of unity in the health team. Then the nurse assigned to a given patient would become the authority having responsibility for the patient as a person and assisting the patient in making use of all the resources furnished by the health team.

This personalistic, mediating function today is often performed by the medical or psychiatric social worker. Sociological study of the medical profession has led to acknowledging the great importance of the social dimension in treating disease. Thus persons trained in social process have been added to healing teams. The social worker interviews patients to discover possible social factors of ethnic culture, economic status, and family structure that may have caused the disease, may hinder treatment, or may prevent rehabilitation. Such workers typically help patients regarding their legal rights, their opportunities for public financial assistance, and other matters connected with illness. They also act as liaison with the patient's family and help find ways to ensure family stability in the absence of the patient from the home. Finally, social workers undertake the patient's reentry into society. In the case of psychiatric patients, this involvement is of major importance, since reentry into normal life is difficult for mental patients and may lead to recommittal.

In comparing the role of the social worker with that of the nurse, the social worker is chiefly concerned with patients in their normal life patterns, and the nurse with patients undergoing the actual experience of sickness and healing. Consequently, these two roles are very closely connected and together constitute primary care in the strict sense of direct concern with the patient as a person. The physician's role, on the other hand, is more specialized because it is focused precisely on the diagnosis and treatment of a pathological condition or its future prevention. If this analysis is correct, the physician cannot be the sole decision maker on the health team. Rather, the patient has the ultimate decision and is helped in this decision first by the nurse and social worker, who are acquainted with patients in their total personalities and life situation; second by the primary-care physician; and third by various specialist physicians.

Recently, some hospitals have begun to recognize the need for pastoral care, not as an occasional intervention of religious ministry from outside the institution by a visiting member of the clergy, nor as a convenience for patients who wish religious ministration by a resident chaplain. Rather, pastoral care is being seen as a regular part of patient care, since all patients, religious or secular, have problems of ultimate concern that affect the success of the healing process (Marty and Vaux, 1982). This issue is discussed at length in Chapter 14. Here we only say that pastoral care has to be closely linked to the role of the nurse and the social worker, since it adds depth to their firsthand concern for the patient as a person.

For reasons Chapters 4 and 5 discuss, physicians will not find it easy to reconcile their proper professional autonomy with the requirements of teamwork or to relinquish the idea that they have sole decision-making power in healthcare and all others are merely their executive assistants. The readjustment necessary in their education and self-identity might be compared to what Catholic priests are being forced to undergo since the Second Vatican Council. If the health team concept is to have real significance, physicians, along with priests, must come to acknowledge that they need the help of others not only in carrying out decisions, but also in making them, if the people entrusted to their care are to be well-served.

Often, when continuing education programs on ethical policies are offered to a hospital's professional staff, the nurses take advantage of these, but the physicians are notable by their absence. The most propitious method for introducing ethics into the medical school and speciality training programs seems to be by discussing ethical dimensions of medical problems at conferences and grand rounds. However, after specialty training is over, many physicians no longer have the opportunity to attend conferences and grand rounds. Because physicians occupy a leadership role on a healthcare team, they must be as well-acquainted with the ethical policies of the institution as are other members of the staff; yet they often excuse themselves because of their heavy workload, as if the nurses had it easy. It would be entirely reasonable for Catholic institutions to specify as a condition of granting hospital privileges to physicians, or for medical staff and residents, attendance at a certain number of hours of continuing education on the institution's ethical policies. A hospital administration that puts this issue on a professional, rather than an informal, level will find that physicians will accept this responsibility as they do many others. Further, physicians will soon come to view it as a reasonable and necessary part of the continuing education demanded of all healthcare professionals today.

The new profession of paramedic or physician assistant is being developed. This new role can be defined in two ways. For some, a paramedic is merely a substitute for a physician justified by the so-called doctor shortage, and a medical assistant is merely a technician. Others, however, see that the physician's work can be subdivided into several roles of a professional character, but not all demanding the full competency of a physician. In this last model, medical assistants may share in decision-making processes and not only in technical execution, and they are not mere emergency substitutes (Schneller, 1978).

Another aspect of the health team concept is the question of the defense of patients' rights. Recently, there has been much argument that patients need an *ombudsman* or "patient's advocate" to support patients in their efforts to insist on adequate care (Marks, 1986; Storch, 1982). Ravich (1986) sees the patients' representative as one who helps "personalize the patient's hospital experience." Citing state laws concerning patients' rights, she presents different models for this task. In summary, we believe that the advocate should have the following powers: (1) full access to medical records, (2) ability to call in consultants, (3) ex officio participation in hospital quality-of-healthcare communities, (4) power to lodge complaints directly with the hospital executive committee, and (5) access to all patient support services.

It seems a mistake to confuse the notion of patients' advocate or ombudsman, which pertains to the strictly legal or ethical dimension and is most properly a task for a lawyer, with the notion of patients' representative. The latter role seems proper to the work of the nurse, the social worker, and the pastoral care person, who provide primary care and who mediate between the patient and the rest of the health team. They would inform patients of the availability of the advocate and call the advocate in to help all patients who believe their rights may be imperiled.

6.5   THE CATHOLIC HOSPITAL AND LONG TERM CARE FACILITY

Catholic Identity

Catholic hospitals and long term care facilities were founded principally by religious orders of sisters and brothers to give healthcare to the neglected and, especially in areas where Catholicism was not the chief religion, as a means to witness to the ethical and spiritual aspects of healthcare in accordance with Catholic values. Healthcare has always been considered an apostolate of the Church, whether offered in the home or in a more formal institution. Today in the United States, the dominance of secular humanism as a philosophy of life has so influenced and pressured the operation of such Catholic institutions that many wonder whether these institutions are any longer Catholic and are able to be conducted as an apostolic endeavor (Commission for Catholic Health Care Ministry, 1988).

What characterizes a Catholic hospital or nursing home? In the United States such a facility has several obvious characteristics.

1. This institution has a Christian and Catholic ministry and therefore receives apostolic direction from the bishop of the diocese. Under his guidance and interpretation, it follows the *Ethical and Religious Directives for Catholic Health Facilities* approved by the United States Catholic Conference (USCC, 1971), which outline the spiritual care patients should receive, the duties of the facility as a representative of the Catholic Church, and the medical procedures prohibited in Catholic healthcare facilities. The fact that a medical-ethical rule (e.g., concerning abortion and sterilization) is contained in the *Directives* does not give it any greater doctrinal validity than it had before being included in the *Directives*. Many of the ethical problems presented in this book are treated in the *Directives,* but some of the more recent issues, such as transsexual surgery, in vitro fertilization, and behavior control are not considered. The *Directives* were revised slightly in 1975, and the need for a more extensive revision has been agreed on by the NCCB (1988).

2. A Catholic hospital or nursing home is usually sponsored by a religious community or a diocese; that is the community or diocese usually owns the facility and has responsibility for determining policy. A few Catholic hospitals and nursing homes in the United States are sponsored by laypeople (Modde, 1985).

3. The facility has at least a priest chaplain (resident or nonresident) who regularly conducts mass and is responsible for sacramental administration to, and even pastoral counseling of, the patients and staff.

4. Such institutions usually are marked by various Catholic symbols, statues, pictures, crucifixes in the rooms, evidence of some sisters or brothers and the chaplain in religious clothing, and so forth.

All these characteristics (even the last) are more than superficial. They express the character of the facility as a ministry of the Catholic Church, based on the interrelations of the whole person in all the biological, psychological, social, and spiritual dimensions dealt with in this book.

There is something deeper, however. Catholics essentially conceive of the healing ministry as an extension of the ministry of Christ (O'Meara, 1983). Jesus was prophet or teacher, king or shepherd, priest or sanctifier. The Second Vatican Council has taught that this threefold ministry should be reflected in all the works of the Church and in every member. Healing is part of the shepherding function of the Christian community, since building this community entails concern for each weak member who needs restoration to vital life and participation.

Jesus healed people *radically* by penetrating to the spiritual core of the human personality and liberating the person from original or social sin and also from individual, personal sin, with the more superficial but real effect of healing them also psychologically and physically. A Christian healthcare facility, therefore, is also concerned with the radical healing of those for whom it cares. The experience of sickness and healing in such a hospital should also be an experience of personal spiritual growth through suffering and redemption.

What should make a Catholic healthcare facility a special kind of community and a model for other healing communities is that its members, both professionals and patients, are clearly aware of the presence of Christ the Healer in the midst of the community making use of his ministers—physicians, nurses, technicians, administrators, and patients in relation to each other—in his work of healing. This presence of Christ should also be celebrated ritually through the sacraments and proclaimed through the words of Scripture and of preaching, with Christ's promise of renewed life more powerful than death. In an effort to help Catholic hospitals understand and achieve their identity, the Catholic Health Association has instituted several studies and designed several programs over the past 15 years. Among the more recent studies and programs are *Evaluative Criteria for Catholic Health Care Facilities* (1980), *Health Care Ministry Assessment* (1983), and *No Room in the Marketplace: The Health Care of the Poor* (1986). A special group, the Commission for Catholic Health Care Ministry (CCHCM), sponsored by the USCC, the Leadership Conference of Women Religious (LCWR), the Conference of Major Superiors of Men (CMSM), and CHA, analyzed the present healthcare situation and projected a vision to ensure the continuance of healthcare as a ministry of the Church. This study is called *A New Vision for a New Century* (CCHCM, 1988). In addition, many Catholic healthcare corporations sponsor numerous educational programs to help their healthcare professionals understand and internalize the mission and meaning of Catholic healthcare. The need for education and formation of healthcare professionals is recognized as a vital need if Catholic healthcare facilities are to continue in existence (CCHCM, 1988).

Such a religious conception of a healthcare institution should not weaken but rather enhance its competence in all the arts and sciences of modern medicine. In a secular humanist hospital, which is usually considered nonreligious, the vital principle is the value system of secular humanism described in 1.3, with its dedication to scientific progress, its concern for human rights, and its faith in the power of human reason and human cooperative effort to overcome sickness. Without that commitment to humanist ideals, a secular hospital becomes a depersonalized machine that hurts as much as it heals. In the same way, unless a Catholic hospital receives its vitality from its own religious faith and system of values, it will become more hurtful than healing, a scandal rather than a witness of Christ's presence in a suffering world.

A significant development in Catholic healthcare is the recent development of healthcare systems or corporations in which several hospitals under the sponsorship of the same religious congregations, or of different congregations, are united in a single corporation. This corporation is able to provide the individual hospitals with much needed research and education and a more effective public voice in influencing public healthcare policy (Connors, 1986; Donnelly et al., 1978). It is essential that such large corporations give as much attention to the Christian values to which they are dedicated as to economic and administrative problems.

An especially difficult problem for Catholic hospitals is the problem of unionization. Following the teaching of the papal encyclicals, the U.S. bishops have always favored the right to unionize. However, the formation of a union in a Catholic hospital is often resented and resisted by the administration, not so much because of wage policy, but because of a feared loss of administrative control in an already very complex operation. The attention this ethical issue deserves cannot be given here, but note that the solution to the presence of unions in Catholic healthcare facilities should not be doctrinaire or one-sided (O'Rourke, 1978). The goal of a Catholic institution should be to recognize the right of employees not merely to have fair wages and good working conditions, but a real voice in decisions that affect them. Both administration and employees, however, must put patient care before their private benefit (Maida, 1982; Texas Catholic Conference, 1983).

One of the reasons Catholic healthcare facilities sometimes fail to understand all the aspects of social justice questions that must be considered in making ethically sound decisions is because their boards are made up largely of professional and business people and do not include representatives of labor or the underprivileged. This is understandable in view of the need for the advice and support of experienced business and professional experts. Nevertheless, Catholic healthcare facilities also serve the working class and those who require public assistance. A serious effort should be made to see that these consumers of services are adequately represented on any board.

6.6 ETHICS COMMITTEES AND MISSION EFFECTIVENESS COMMITTEES

Many hospitals today are trying to meet the growing number of bioethical problems by establishing ethics committees that include representatives of administration, medical staff, and ethicists or clergy (Brodeur, 1984). Although long term care facilities do not encounter the variety of ethical issues that surface in acute care hospitals, these facilities should institute ethics committees as well. In addition to the ethics committee, Catholic hospitals and nursing homes should consider creating a committee whose concern is to foster mission effectiveness, that is, to ensure that the institution's apostolic objectives are clearly understood and that programs are instituted to help achieve these objectives. After discussing the purpose and function of the ethics committee, we consider the mission effectiveness committee. While these two committees have different matters of concern, in Catholic healthcare facilities it is not unfitting that one committee consider both matters of concern (O'Rourke, 1989). However, if one committee considers matters pertaining to both medical and institutional ethics, this fact should be made clear in the committee's statement of purpose.

Purpose

Recently, one of the first empirical evaluations of ethics committees in hospitals was published (Lo, 1987). According to the study, ethics committees are used for everything from "acting as a public relations tool for justifying unpopular decisions resulting from discontinuing unprofitable services" to "serving as an alternative to the courts." Although most ethics committees have a more limited purview, the study showed that some committees believe they should be involved at some time in particular medical decisions concerning patient care. Basing considerations on the nature of the physician-patient relationship, it seems that the responsibility of ethics committees should be more limited. The ethics committee helps both physicians and patients (or proxies), since both have something to contribute to the medical care decision. Primarily, the patient or proxy expresses the desires and values of the person seeking medical help. Primarily, the physician makes a diagnosis and designs a medical care program in accord with the patient's expressed wishes. Ethicists are able to help physicians prepare for medical decision making according to the accepted ethical norms, but ethicists may never replace physicians. If we are to preserve the integrity of the physician-patient relationship, the ethics committee should be envisioned as a group of people fulfilling the role of the medical ethicist. Thus they offer to healthcare professionals and their patients only education and consultation, and they formulate policies that have the administration's approval.

With this somewhat more specified function assigned to medical ethics and ethics committees, several observations are in order:

1. Ethics committees should devote intense activity to self-education. If the committee is to sponsor education and consultation in accord with accepted ethical principles, it must be knowledgeable about the principles in question. Common sense does not suffice for sound ethical decisions. The President's Commission on Ethical Issues in Medicine and Research (1983d) has developed some principles for our pluralistic society. The Catholic Church, in accord with its notion of human dignity, has also developed ethical norms for medical care. Depending on the character of the healthcare facility, the ethics committee should school itself in one or both sets of these principles.

2. The membership of the ethics committee need not include people "from all walks of life." When stating regulations for ethics committees, there is a tendency to require membership of people who are "nonscientific," who "represent the community," or who are "consumers of healthcare." Clearly, when membership of "outsiders" on ethics committees is

recommended, it is assumed that ethical decisions on medical care will be based on public opinion rather than on accepted ethical principles and the knowledge of medical practice. People from all walks of life may serve effectively on ethics committees in healthcare facilities if they are knowledgeable about ethics. They do not qualify as ethical experts, however, simply because they are "outside" the profession of healthcare. Rather, people qualify for ethics committees through their ability to analyze issues from a well-reasoned ethical perspective.

3. The ethics committee should sponsor education programs for all people associated with the healthcare facility. The formulation of policy in regard to ethical issues, such as policies for do-not-resuscitate (DNR) orders or transplantation of organs, is simply more specific educational programs. If consultation on an ethical issue is requested by a physician or patient (or proxy), the purpose should be to help the physician and patient (or proxy) sort our their thinking (LaPuma et al., 1988). The ethics committee does not replace the physician or the patient. The concept that the ethics committee becomes some sort of jury before whom evidence is presented is a travesty of medical decision making.

4. The size of the ethics committee would depend on the size and nature of the health facility. It should include a balanced representation of the administrative and medical staffs, including physicians, nurses, and representatives from the pastoral care and social work departments. Although it is important that the pastoral care department be represented, the ethics committee should not be identified with that department; the implementation of ethical norms is a responsibility of all associated with the facility, not merely of those in pastoral care. One member of the committee should be a theologian, whose function is to help inform the whole committee about the teaching of the Catholic Church and theological developments in understanding this teaching (Kelly and McCarthy, 1984).

5. The medical ethics committee is a committee of administration, not a committee of the medical staff. Hence, it is responsible to the board of trustees, through the CEO.

Mission Effectiveness Committees

Mission effectiveness committees have a different purpose than ethics committees (Fitzpatrick and Gaylor, 1987; Vaughan, 1987). Their purview is broader because they are concerned with the effectiveness of the institution as an apostolate of the Church. This type of committee evaluates whether or not the healthcare facility truly carries on the healing ministry of Jesus.

Some of the questions every Catholic hospital needs to ask itself through a mission effectiveness committee are the following (CHA, 1980):

1. Jesus taught us in the Parable of the Good Samaritan that God's call to ministry usually comes through the presence of a neighbor in need. Who in our community needs our help to attain healing?

2. How does this institution witness to the presence of Christ in this city, county, or state by its special concern for the most neglected, the poor, and the sinful, and for the dignity of life and person? Do we obscure that presence by red tape, excessive financial worry, Pharisaism, or conformism to secularist values?

3. Are the patients involved as much as possible in their own care? Is a patients' advocate available who can assist patients to secure their rights?

4. How are employees treated in the institution? Are the principles of social justice and subsidiarity respected in their case? Is there any attempt to form a Christian community? Do employees realize their importance in establishing Christian identity? Is there a routine way to achieve reconciliation when communication breaks down? Are there ways and procedures to protect the rights of all employees in regard to employment, assignment, working conditions, salaries, and wages?

5. Is there a department of pastoral care with trained personnel who are recognized as a part of the regular staff and who provide both patients and staff with adequate counseling and sacramental services? Are these liturgical and sacramental services celebrated in ways that meet the needs of patients involved in the healing process?

6. How does the healthcare facility deal with controversial medical-moral issues? Does it have procedures to deal with difficult cases and to remain faithful to the *Ethical and Religious Directives* in a way that is pastoral rather than merely legalistic? Is there an effort to provide Christian alternatives to such forbidden practices as contraception, sterilization, abortion, and in vitro fertilization? Are there provisions for ethical genetic counseling and sex instruction and therapy?

7. Does the hospital conduct adequate educational programs to inform all members of the hospital community of the objectives, Christian value system, and areas for dialogue and exploration in such matters? Does it try to elicit the experiences and views of all in developing and refining these values and objectives?

8. Does the hospital maintain a vital relation with the local church and other Catholic healthcare facilities? Does it consult local pastors whose parishioners are subject to its care for their cooperation? Does it relate ecumenically to the healthcare facilities of other Christian churches and other local faith communities? In institutions where many of the staff or patients are not Catholics (a typical situation today), the ecumenical aspect of the ethics committee is of great importance. Specific Catholic identity and ecumenism are by no means opposite goals, but great charity and an understanding of ecumenical method are essential in harmonizing them (O'Rourke, 1983).

9. Does the institution play a civic role in promoting better health legislation and planning?

10. Does the hospital manage its financial affairs responsibly in view of its primary responsibility to the poor, as well as to others? In seeking

funding from either private or public sources, does the hospital ensure that it will remain free to pursue its Christian purposes without compromises that would defeat these purposes?

Where there is more than one Catholic hospital in a diocese, the local bishop may find it impossible to coordinate the work of all directly. It may be useful in such dioceses to establish a diocesan healthcare committee to assist the local Catholic hospitals to collaborate with one another. Collaboration among Catholic healthcare facilities was not vitally required when funding was more generous. At present, Catholic hospitals are often forced into competition with one another, to the detriment of the overall apostolate (Commission on Catholic Health Care, 1988).

6.7   HEALTHCARE, ETHICS, AND PUBLIC POLICY

The federal government has made some attempt to give ethical guidelines for social policy in regard to healthcare. In the late 1960s and early 1970s, Congress became uneasy, in fact disturbed, about the implications of scientific research. Revolutionary advances in science and technology were predicted, such as genetic engineering and DNA splicing, and it was feared that these advances might have damaging effects on individuals and society. At the same time, public outrage arose over some scientific research projects that had violated the human rights of some individuals. For example, a study was made public in which aborted fetuses were decapitated in order to perform pharmaceutical tests. Also, the Tuskegee Syphilis Study, in which the cure for syphilis was withheld from some poor black men afflicted with this disease, was exposed in the press (Jones, 1982). Because of general apprehension about revolutionary scientific developments and the sharp public reaction to specific abuses in the area of research, Congress established the Commission for the Protection of Human Subjects of Biomedical and Behavioral Research (CPHS) in July 1974 (PL 93-348). As its name indicates, the mandate for this commission was to set ethical guidelines for research projects involving human beings, especially those whose rights might be violated. When the life of this commission expired, the Secretary of the Department of Health, Education, and Welfare appointed an Ethics Advisory Board (EAB) in the spring of 1977 to continue the study of ethical issues and public policy. The advisory board was superseded a few months later (November 1978) by another group created by Congress, called the President's Commission for the Study of Ethical Problems in Medicine and Biomedical and Behavioral Research (PCEMR). This commission, having declared its work complete, disbanded on March 31, 1983. In 1985, Congress instituted the Congressional Biomedical Ethics Board (PL 99-158), composed of representatives and senators, who will be assisted in their work by a 14-member advisory committee of scientists, ethicists, and lawyers. The board will remain in existence until further legislative action is taken. Whether this study group will be as productive as the former ones remains to be seen. However, because of the nature of the board, it seems its deliberations will become politicized. Selection of the advisory board has been delayed for this very reason, and to date no studies have been undertaken.

The productivity of the first three federal commissions has been impressive. The CPHS published more than 10 studies in its four-year life on subjects such as research on fetuses, children, prisoners, and mentally infirm patients. It also studied psychosurgery, put forth ethical guidelines for delivery of healthcare by government agencies, and set standards for institutional review boards. In the Belmont Report (1978), the CPHS sought to synthesize the ethical principles it had used in its studies. The EAB, because of its short existence, studied only one ethical problem at length, that of in vitro fertilization. The PCEMR was commissioned by Congress to consider many ethical issues, such as brain death, access to health services, withdrawal of life-support systems, and testing in regard to genetic disease. During its existence, the PCEMR published 10 studies on these and other topics.

Evaluation

Although we do not attempt to evaluate the documents emanating from these federal commissions (CPHS, EAB, PCEMR), we offer the following general comments.

1. The very fact that Congress recognizes the need for ethical norms in the field of research and therapy is a step forward. For the most part, the norms set forth by the commissions are useful and protect the rights of scientists and physicians as well as subjects and patients.

2. The norms formulated by the commissions are designed with our pluralistic society in mind. Thus these norms seek to enunciate what most scientists, politicians, and religious thinkers will agree on. Although the norms do not state it explicitly, it is clear that they avoid controversy, so some of the more difficult and important ethical issues are not considered, such as the value of fetal life, the time when human life begins, the purpose of healthcare, and the difficult decisions that limited public funds will require in the future.

3. Although some of the more important norms concerning physician-patient relationships are considered, such as informed consent and justice in selection of research subjects, there is insufficient consideration of the pressing ethical questions arising from the society-physician-patient relationship, such as: Is there a right to equal healthcare for all? Should all feasible care be financed publicly? and, What are the goals for U.S. national health programs?

4. The basis on which these ethical statements are formulated is not the nature of the human person, the covenant between physician and patient, the just society, or religious teaching. Rather, the basis is what is culturally acceptable, that is, what norms seem acceptable to the American public. As a result, the conclusions are pragmatic and usually balance rights rather than defend them. Deciding ethical responsibilities in this manner is dangerous because it justifies whatever is popular. The ethicist should continually question and evaluate what is culturally acceptable, judging it on more fundamental values.

143

5. Motivation for observing the norms of the federal commissions is mainly monetary. If a person or institution does not observe these norms, the person or institution will not receive federal funding and might be subject to malpractice litigation. Thus, in a certain sense, these "ethical statements" emanating from the federal commissions are legal norms as far as the motivation for observing them is concerned. Although ethicists may differ in detail as to the proper motivation for ethical activity, no ethicist considers avoiding legal sanctions to be the ultimate justification for ethical action.

In sum, the deliberations of the federal commissions have been worthwhile in that they have brought to our attention the need for ethical norms in the field of research and therapy. However, because the commissions avoid some of the more important questions and concentrate on expressing consensus, and because the norms are based on a weak foundation, it is clear that more rigorous thinking must be applied to the modern ethical issues in medicine, research, and healthcare.

At the private level, there is also an extensive interest in bioethics and in the effort to develop and publicize ethical norms as widely as possible. At present, more than 20 private centers are sponsored by universities or corporations that seek to educate people in one way or another concerning ethical issues. Although most of these centers serve a local or regional constituency, some seek to serve a national audience.

The Pope John XXIII Medical-Moral Research and Education Center in Braintree, MA, considers the ethical issues in medicine, healthcare, and research from a Catholic perspective. During recent years, the center has published several books on seminars held to probe contemporary ethical issues.

The Hastings Center Institute of Society, Ethics, and the Life Sciences at Hastings-on-Hudson, NY, studies ethical issues affecting all facets of society. Although the ethical issues arising from medicine and research have been considered by members of the institute's study commissions, such issues as ethics in business, in government, and in the military have also been the subject of their study. The Hastings Institute proceeds from a humanistic perspective.

The Kennedy Institute of Bioethics at Georgetown University, Washington, DC, has published the important *Encyclopedia of Bioethics*, sponsors the National Reference Center for Bioethics Literature, and produces *The Bioethics Line*, a computer-assisted method of searching for literature on questions of ethics and public policy. The Kennedy Institute proceeds from an ecumenical perspective, with a special concern for ethics and values in the Judeo-Christian tradition.

In addition to the publications and services offered by these institutes, more than a score of periodicals publish articles concerning ethical issues in medical healthcare and human research.

Part 3

BIOETHICAL DECISION MAKING

Part 1 deals with the ethical responsibilities of persons for their own health, and Part 2 with the ethical responsibilities of professionals. Part 3 outlines the process for resolving ethical controversies and arriving at sound ethical decisions espeically from the Christian perspective. In these chapters we use the term "bioethics" rather than "medical" or "healthcare" ethics in order to signify the whole range of interrelated problems that are discussed in current ethical literature.

CHAPTER 7

The Logic of Bioethical Decisions

OVERVIEW

Chapter 7 discusses the logical *form* of ethical reasoning, and Chapter 8 its *content*. An understanding of the different logical forms of ethical reasoning is important, since sometimes groups with very similar values (the content of ethical reasoning) can still violently disagree on how to solve concrete problems because the forms or methods of their reasoning differ. In order to understand the Christian approach to ethics, special attention should be devoted to the scriptural basis for the various principles, and the manner in which a principle differs from a rule.

7.1   THE LOGIC OF BIOETHICAL DEBATE

Ethical Pluralism

Piaget (1929) and Kohlberg (1973, 1981) have shown that groups of adults include persons at different levels of ethical development, corresponding to the three main phases a child must pass to full ethical maturity.

1. In the *preconventional* phase, decisions are made on the basis of the immediate consequence of an action, its rewards and punishments.

2. In the *conventional* phase, decisions are made on the basis of social approval. Conformity to group norms becomes paramount, and satisfactions can be delayed and suffering incurred to achieve the praise of others.

3. In the *postconventional* phase, maturity increases through the internalization of moral judgments. Decisions are made on personal standards, whereas the standards of society become subject to criticism.

Most public ethical controversies are carried on at the second level. Only when people begin to think critically for themselves do they begin to question society's assumptions about what values are important. Even before individuals can do this, however, they must ask themselves, "What method am I following or should I follow in trying to solve my ethical problems?" In seeking a good method of ethical reasoning, people must keep in mind that no method of *practical* reasoning can be expected to give the same clarity or even the same certainty that sometimes is achieved in purely theoretical reasoning. Moreover, not only is ethical reasoning practical rather than theoretical, but it deals with ultimate problems of life and death, of self-fulfillment and self-destruction. Consequently, ethical reasoning is often obscured by people's conflicting emotions, their own sinfulness, and the sin of the world around them. Therefore, to think about ethical problems with the measure of clarity and certainty that is possible in so difficult a field requires a good method, and today bioethicists struggle to find one (Engelhardt, 1986b; Pellegrino and Thomasma, 1988; R. Veatch, 1981).

To present the main ethical methodologies developed in our civilization, a single example will be used: the problem of abortion. The purpose here is not actually to debate that issue, which is dealt with in Chapter 9, but to show how different modes of thinking could be applied to a single problem.

Deontological Versus Teleological Ethical Methodologies

Current bioethical writers divide ethical methodologies into those that are *deontological* (from the Greek for "reasoning about duty") and those that are *teleological* (from the Greek for "reasoning about a goal"; i.e., the means to be taken to achieve some end) (H. Brody, 1981; B. Brody, 1983a; T. Shannon, 1987.)

Deontologists think of ethics according to the model of our duty to pay our debts. For them, the question of moral right and wrong always reduces to obedience to some code of laws, customs, or norms that obliges us because of the authority of someone who has made these laws, or who at least approved these customs or norms. Deontologists thus reduce moral right and wrong to the *will of some authority*, and thus they are *voluntarists* who believe that ultimately something is right or wrong because "the boss says so" (Bourke, 1970). This does not necessarily mean that the boss is somebody else, since people can be their own bosses.

Teleologists, on the other hand, think of ethics according to the model of the reasoning craftsman who begins with an idea of something he wants to create and then tries to figure out how to achieve that goal. Therefore teleologists trace back the norms of right and wrong not to the will of an authority, but to some *intelligence* (their own or that of someone wiser than they whom they can trust) that is able to see the alternative means to the end and to select the most effective. They are *intellectualists* rather than voluntarists.

So defined, these two methods of ethical reasoning are not necessarily exclusive. Deontologists need not hold that the authority they obey is *arbitrary*. They may be convinced that the boss has good reasons for his or her rules, although it is not necessary to know those reasons, just to obey them. Teleologists, on the other hand, can admit that laws, customs, and norms are an important and sometimes necessary guide to good decisions about which means to use to achieve an end, provided that the authority who made these rules was an expert who can be trusted. Nevertheless, it is important to clear thinking to decide which of these methodologies is primary and which secondary and instrumental.

Unfortunately, this clear-cut distinction between teleological ethics and deontological ethics, as these terms were historically understood, has recently become confused. In reading current bioethical literature, it is important to steer clear of these confusions, which come from three main sources. The first mistake is to identify teleological reasoning with *consequentialism* and to say that all teleologists determine whether an action is right or wrong only by its consequences, whereas deontologists maintain it can be right or wrong no matter what its consequences. The second is to identify the acceptance of *exceptionless norms* with deontological reasoning, that is, rules whose violation no circumstances can justify, and teleological reasoning with the view that under certain circumstances any norm can be broken. The third is to speak of *mixed systems* that are in some respects deontological and in others teleological.

The first of these confusions arises from a failure to notice that not all types of teleological ethics need be consequentialist (B. Brody, 1983b), and deontological ethics does not necessarily ignore the moral significance of the consequences of human actions. The second confusion arises from the failure to notice that exceptionless norms can sometimes be derived in both teleological and deontological systems, and in both systems circumstances can modify the morality of an action. The third results from the failure to see that although these two methodologies are not necessarily exclusive, one must decide which is primary and which is secondary and instrumental, not merely "mix" them in an eclectic manner, which can only lead to paradoxes (McCullough, 1986).

The importance of this distinction has been evidenced in the abortion debate. Some have attempted to resolve the abortion issue deontologically by referring to the law, the courts, or majority opinion. Others appeal against the law, the courts, and majority opinion to "natural law" arguments, that is, to teleological reasons drawn from the relation of the act of abortion to the goals of human life in the community. Is an act right or wrong because an authority wills that it be so judged? Or must that authority, if it is to be legitimate, will that it be so judged because it seems an effective or destructive means to the true goals of human living? To answer these questions is to choose either a deontological or a teleological method of deciding about the morality of abortion, but it is only the first step and may conceivably lead in either direction. Until that first step is taken, however, any debate on the question will be at cross purposes.

The following description of the main varieties of deontological and teleological ethics points out their strengths and weaknesses. Figure 1 assists the reader in following this discussion.

Figure 1. Types of Teleological and Deontological Ethics

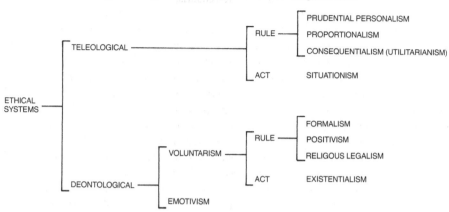

7.2   DEONTOLOGICAL (DUTY) METHODOLOGIES

Emotivism

At the beginning of most discussions of an ethical issue, people express felt attitudes. For example, I am horrified at the idea of abortion and especially at the way so many people are now ready to approve what they previously regarded as a shameful crime. You, on the other hand, are indignant at the presumption of anyone who would force a woman to bear a child that she does not want, especially when that child will be defective and live a miserable life; you are pleased that more liberal, humane views are beginning to prevail. From the outset it appears that this discussion will get nowhere. How can we discuss the obviously sincere but purely subjective, feelings of another person?

However, we cannot rest content with this initial impasse. Feeling cannot be an ethical criterion that is beyond criticism, no matter how sincere it may be. People are often led by their feeling to do things that turn out to be very destructive not only to others, but also to themselves. You may "feel" it is all right to destroy a fetus, but what if you also feel it is all right to kill blacks or Jews? I may "feel" it is wrong to permit a woman to have an abortion, but what if I feel it is wrong to permit my child to be given a necessary blood transfusion?

Some modern ethicists hold that an emotivist ethics of this type is the only one possible, since any discussion of values is a discussion about subjective, emotional attitudes (Ayer, 1936). Some ethicists modified this position of Ayer by asserting that "ought" statements are not mere expressions or descriptions of emotion, but are prescriptions stating what people "feel" should be done, although the grounds for such prescriptions still are subjective feelings, not the knowledge of some special fact (MacIntyre, 1981).

This reduction of moral statements to mere subjective attitudes does not seem very convincing. However, a more plausible form of emotivism can be defended as follows: certainly not all feelings can be trusted, but can't we trust our better nature, our humane feelings? The great philosopher Rousseau (1753) argued that if people would free themselves from the prejudices acquired by bad education and the influence of a corrupt civilization and return to their natural human feelings, they would make much better ethical judgments. Such is the basis of our American confidence in the common sense of the people. We believe that the "common" person is closer to nature and reality than is the sophisticated intellectual. We take opinion polls on many bioethical problems because we assume that what most people "feel" is right probably *is* right.

There is much truth in this view because natural human feelings of family love, loyalty to one's group, sympathy for the underdog, opposition to arrogance and tyranny, and fairness and compassion are better guides to morality than current fads or the fanatical ideologies of armchair philosophers out of touch with basic human realities (R. Baron, 1981). In discussing abortion, the fact cannot be overlooked or denied that most women are very reluctant to have an abortion, even when they think it right to do so. On the other hand, who could be insensitive to the anguish of a woman faced with bringing a deformed child into the world?

If people attempted to live only by natural feelings, however, the progress of civilization would be impossible. Freud, in *Civilization and Its Discontents* (1930), added to Rousseau's analysis the bitter truth that civilization is an absolute necessity if people are not to be destroyed by the contradictions of their own instinctive drives. Without such civilization and the discipline it makes possible, there could be no modern medical science.

Consequently, it seems necessary to accept the view of Aristotle in *The Nicomachean Ethics* (H. Veatch, 1971), who taught that emotion is to be trusted only when it has been refined, educated, and disciplined by virtue. Recently, ethicists have again been insisting that good decisions are not possible merely by following rules. People need *character* if they are consistently to meet the crisis of decision making (Hauerwas, 1981; Palmour, 1988). Decisions made by people who have a respect for persons, reverence for life, and compassion for the suffering are likely to be good decisions, whereas decisions made by persons who are insensitive and lacking in sympathy are likely to be morally bad. Thus what people *do* is the outcome of what they *are* (McCabe, 1969). This is why persons often make the statement, "I would rather trust physicians or nurses of good character to make ethical decisions than all the experts in bioethics in the world."

This point is well taken. Ultimately, all ethical decisions do involve a degree of moral sensitivity, fairness, and compassion that is only found in psychologically healthy and mature people, in civilized, decent human beings. Character is all important. But what is decency? What are the standards or principles by which good characters are formed? The German physicians who carried out Hitler's evil medical experiments were men who thought themselves (and were considered by others) decent, ethical professionals. However, they probably were not in the habit of reflecting about the ethical standards of their profession (Alexander, 1949; Lifton, 1986).

In view of the foregoing description of emotivism, should it be classified as deontological, teleological, or perhaps some third type of ethics? Since emotivism is *noncognitive* (i.e., it does not rest on what people know but what they "feel"), it cannot be teleological, since the teleological method requires the agent to understand the relation between means and ends. Emotivism also is not obviously deontological, since deontology implies obedience to the *will* of the lawmaker rather than to one's own feelings. Nevertheless, emotivism is best classified as deontological because emotions resemble the will; both are noncognitive, affective faculties that differ only in that emotions relate more directly to imagination, and will to reason. Thus emotivism is the type of deontologism that teaches each person has the duty to follow the law of his or her own natural and psychologically healthy instincts or feelings as the best authority as to what is right or wrong.

Religious Legalism

Many theists ground ethics in a direct appeal to the will of God, who is the ultimate authority and who alone determines what is right and wrong. As St. Paul said, "We ought to obey God rather than men" (Ac 5:29). The Jewish, Christian, and Muslim conviction is that God has revealed his will through prophets as recorded in the Bible or Koran. This *Divine Command Morality* (Idziak, 1986) is simply defined as "obedience to the commands of God," such as the Ten Commandments (Ex 20:7-17) or the great commandment of love (Mk 12:28-34).

Among Christians this type of deontologism has been common, and among Protestants it has predominated (Gustafson, 1978, 1983; Mehl, 1971). Although a great variety of Protestant ethical systems exists, most of them teach that since the fall persons have been unable to distinguish correctly between right and wrong because they have deluded themselves with Pharisaic self-righteousness and self-justification. People can be freed from this blindness only when confronted by the righteousness of God as revealed in the Word of God, especially in Jesus Christ the Incarnate Word. Even with this biblical revelation, the will of God remains essentially mysterious to people, so they can never hope to understand why God makes such demands, but can only obey him in absolute trust.

Although Catholic theologians have also developed similar systems, Catholics generally have not favored this approach because the emphasis on blind submission to God's will does not seem to do justice to the biblical doctrine that humankind is created in the image and likeness of God. True, this image has been profoundly distorted by human sin, so that without God's revelation, we could never arrive at a correct idea of our true nature or divine destiny and be raised to friendship with God; without the grace given us in Christ, we would never be able to achieve this goal. It is true, however, that the gifts of human intelligence and freedom given us by God at creation, in which this image and likeness primarily consist because they open us to God's call to friendship, remain a part of our human nature even in the fallen state (Haring, 1968).

After we are reborn through grace, these gifts are again freed to enable us not only to obey God blindly, but to obey him intelligently and freely. God's will remains in many ways mysterious; however, it is not an arbitrary will, but rather God's wisdom, which he shares with us so that by his grace we can cooperate with his plans for our lives. Thus Catholic moral theology strives to go beyond deontologism to an ethics that insists that God wants us to understand his wise purposes and to use our own intelligence and experience in executing them (Finnis, 1983; Grisez, 1983). Thus Jesus' Parable of the Talents (Mt 25:14-23) might be read as indicating that when God commands us as his servants to carry out a task, he also demands some creativity from us in obeying these commands. Legalism does not seem to take this creativity into account.

Positivism

Probably most Americans tend to think of morality in terms of a code—the Ten Commandments or federal or state laws. The secular form of deontologism identifies morality with what is *legal*. This is what is called *legalism*, or *positivism* (from the term *positive;* i.e., law "posited" by the will of the sovereign). For many, the Supreme Court decision settled the question of whether abortion is right or wrong. Its opponents, on the other hand, betray the same way of thinking when they label abortion a crime, that is, a breach of law. Sociologists and anthropologists believe that morality is determined not so much by written laws (which are easily changed) as by unwritten law or custom. For them, morality simply means conformity to the accepted social standards of a particular culture (Varga, 1978). They point out that in some cultures abortion is considered immoral and that in others, at least in some situations, a moral duty. This view—that there is no such concept as a universal, transcultural standard of right and wrong—is *moral relativism* (Sumner, 1986).

The case for positivism is strong because it is true that people form moral standards only in a social context with the help and guidance of their community. No individual is capable of working out a personal system of values merely on the basis of his or her own limited experience and insights. Also, people could not live with others if each one lived by merely personal ethics. Thus some type of law or at least a custom is necessary concerning abortion to protect the rights of both mother and child and to educate and give direction to the ethical thinking and attitudes of all the adults involved.

Man-made laws or accepted customs, however, are not ultimate criteria of morality for two reasons:

1. Legal morality is always broad, crude, and unrefined. In personal living, the law must be supplemented by more refined, sensitive personal standards.
2. Man-made laws and customs may be destructive and, even when originally just, often become obsolete in changed circumstances. Therefore it is necessary to criticize them, refuse to obey them, or work to have them changed.

Thus those who believe the anti-abortion laws are unjust, work for their liberalization, whereas those who favor these laws work for a constitutional amendment to make it possible to reinstate them.

Formalism

The inability of Catholics and Protestants to resolve problems about the conflict of religious and theological issues led ethical thinkers of the Enlightenment in the eighteenth century to present a purely rational ethics not based on revelation, which would be more consistent with their new religion of secular humanism. Rousseau's emotivism was one such system, but there was also a new form of deontologism proposed by Immanuel Kant (Auxter, 1982; Shell, 1979). Kant was deontologist in the sense that he accepted the idea, derived from his pietist Protestant background, that morality is a matter of legislation, but he also believed human beings must legislate for themselves. Morality cannot be heteronomous (a law from outside) from society, nor can it be theonomous (from a God beyond understanding), but must be *autonomous,* with each person legislating for himself or herself. We must be confident that if we each legislate for ourselves reasonably, God will ratify and sanction our decisions.

It might seem that this self-legislation would lead to the crudest form of emotivism. However, Kant insisted that people must legislate not emotionally but rationally; thus his system is sometimes called *ethical rationalism.* Kant argued that this type of legislation required that moral norms be completely free of any mere self-serving or self-interest; thus his system is also called *moral purism* or *altruism.* All moral norms or maxims must take the form of the categorical imperative: *act so that the rule of your action can be the norm for all persons equally.*

This rule offers no actual ethical content, but it does contain the *form* of pure disinterestedness or universalizability that any moral rule must have to be truly moral (Frankena, 1980); thus the name *formalism.* For Kant, the content of such rules has to be supplied from a consideration of the consequences, as judged by feelings (so thought Rousseau, whom Kant admired) and experience. Thus Kant argued, "It is our duty never to lie, no matter what the consequences" because if everyone lied, the mutual trust on which society is founded would become impossible. I cannot expect you to tell the truth to me unless I tell the truth to you.

Kant's theory in its original form is usually rejected today as unrealistic. It is doubtful that psychologically speaking, this pure disinterestedness is even possible as a normal human attitude; nor is it clear that this method can produce concrete yet exceptionless rules. Numerous modern ethicists, however, have tried to revise Kant's duty ethics in a more acceptable form. A popular version is that of Rawls (1971, 1981), which attempts to found morality on an implied contract by which human persons agree to protect each others' rights. Another version is that of Frankena (1980), who proposes two principles, *beneficence* and *justice,* that all other moral rules can be reduced to and that, in case of conflict, must be reconciled with each other as well as possible. Frankena justifies these rules much as Kant would by arguing that only if such norms are legislated will a human, social life be possible. Ramsey (d. 1988) (1973), a distinguished bioethicist, used this approach effectively in opposing abortion, basing his ethics on the great commandment of love of God and neighbor; this, however, requires a considerable deductive process, since the Bible contains no explicit command concerning direct abortion.

Existentialism

The foregoing forms of cognitive deontology are all characterized by the fact that they are *rule* deontologism (i.e., obedience to general laws). Existentialist atheist philosophers such as Jean Paul Sartre, however, have developed an *act* deontology. This denies the existence of divine laws, revolts against the injustice of positive laws, and denies the power of human reason to legislate for itself in advance of the unique situations that every individual must confront (Jeanson, 1980). Existentialists believe that it is up to the individual confronted by the absurdity of the world and its injustices to create his or her own values. Morality consists in being *responsible,* that is, in responding to life situations in one's own way and then accepting the consequences without blaming anyone else. Some Christian theologians, notably Bultmann (1958), have given this type of ethics a Christian interpretation. They emphasize the notion of a radical obedience to the surprising, unpredictable call of God, such as his command to Abraham to sacrifice his son Isaac, in seeming contravention of the moral law (Gn 22).

The strength of this moral theory is that it seems to account for the fact that many greatly admired heroes and saints have not been content merely to keep some rule, but rather have been innovative, meeting new problems in new ways. This type of thinking is manifest in the abortion debate when someone says, "I think that abortion is tragic, but when a woman is faced with a crisis in her life because of pregnancy, she should have the courage to decide for herself, no matter what others think or what the law or the Church says." The weakness of existentialism, however, is that (1) it gives the puzzled individual no help in making a decision; and (2) it destroys communal decision making, without which society is impossible. No doubt each of us is responsible for applying general norms to unique situations, and this requires not mere conformity, but intelligent creativity. Without general norms, however, people cannot act together for the common good.

7.3   TELEOLOGICAL (MEANS-ENDS) METHODOLOGIES

Teleology and Natural Law

Teleologists insist that an ethics of law, whether that be the law of God, the state, or the individual, cannot be the ultimate source of morality because laws, to be reasonable and binding, cannot be arbitrary but must be based on human nature and its needs. If God created men and women, he must will that they act in accordance with the nature he gave them. If the state makes laws, these must take into account the needs of its citizens. If I make laws for my own conduct, I must take into account who and what I am by nature. Consequently, teleological ethics, broadly understood, is a *natural law ethics* (Finnis, 1983).

At first it seems paradoxical that natural law should characterize teleology, which does not make law the ultimate basis of morality, rather than characterize deontology, which does. In fact, the term *natural law* came into common philosophical usage through the Stoics, whose ethics were the most deontological of all the forms of Greek philosophical ethics, but it probably originated with the great Jewish thinker Philo (Koester, 1968). In such a deontological system, the notion of natural law served the purpose of explaining why there is a higher and more universal law that seems to bind all humanity and that therefore is not the positive law of a particular society or the religious law of a particular religion. The natural law, the Stoics believed, is *instinctive* to the whole human race. The Roman Stoic and jurist Ulpian even believed natural law was common not only to all human beings but also to animals as well (e.g., the laws of self-preservation and procreation).

In the Middle Ages, however, the scholastic theologians, influenced by the strongly teleological ethics of Aristotle, interpreted "natural law" differently. For them it no longer meant some type of instinct for what is right and wrong, but a type of reasoning that leads beyond all verbally expressed laws to the nature of the human person created in God's image. Human beings act morally when they live in such a way as to satisfy those needs basic to human life and common to all human beings in a consistent and harmonious way (Aquinas' *Summa Theologiae*, I-II, q. 94, a. 2).

Although some influential ethicists such as G.E. Moore (1903) maintained that the values natural to us as human beings are known directly and intuitively (*intuitionist ethics*), most versions of natural-law ethics do not contend that the natural law is self-evident. It is not self-evident that abortion is always wrong or sometimes right. Rather, it is known by generalization from human experience, along with whatever can be learned about human nature from the behavioral and life sciences (Finnis, 1980; Macquarrie, 1970). Also, this does not mean, as it is sometimes asserted, that natural-law ethics is necessarily conservative because it is based on past experience. Human reason is creative and experimental, so the norms of natural law are open to continuing development as people seek to know more about themselves and to improve ways of meeting basic needs.

Thus teleological ethics appeals to natural law not precisely because it is the will of some authority, but because it expresses human nature and its needs as these can be discovered by human reason and satisfied by appropriate means freely but wisely chosen.

Utilitarianism

In some forms of teleological ethics, the needs of a human person are considered to be purely *individual*. This is called egoism, or what Ayn Rand (1964) calls "the new selfishness" and others call "libertarianism." At first, this view is shocking and the very opposite of Kant's ethics, which was based on the idea that any self-interested action is immoral by definition. Kant's puristic duty ethics, however, is less credible than egoism. Certainly each person has the responsibility (section 3.4) to care for his or her own needs and interests. A person cannot demand that others do everything for him or her, nor is he or she justified in criticizing others because they take care of themselves. Even Jesus Christ, in giving us the great commandment that sounds so altruistic—"Love God and your neighbor as yourself"—indicated that people must also love themselves. The efforts of some theologians who defend duty ethics to explain away that "as yourself" have not been very successful (Frankena, 1985; Outka, 1972).

Section 1.2 shows that self-love is not necessarily selfishness. Genuine self-love not only is consistent with the love of others, but also demands that a person love others, because the deepest human need is for those spiritual goods that can be best enjoyed in community. To seek personal good is not to remain selfishly individualistic, but to learn to share in communal life. Such sharing is what makes persons images of God, since God himself is a communal trinity of Father, Son, and Holy Spirit who share one being and life and who generously share this being and life with us through creation and redemption.

Thus egoism is inadequate, not because it approves self-love, but because it proposes an incomplete view of human needs. Therefore, the abortion issue cannot be argued merely in terms of the woman's *private* convenience. Her need as a member of society should be considered to protect the rights of all human beings (of course, this accounting does not settle the question of whether the fetus *is* a human being). Catholic theology has never rejected the notion that self-love is legitimate. In fact, it condemned as heretical the theory of pure love that some quietists proposed, according to which true saints should become indifferent to their own happiness (Knox, 1950).

Few ethicists have accepted egoism; rather, they have opposed Kantian duty ethics by a utilitarianism based on the notion of the greatest good for the greatest number (Singer, 1980). In its current forms, utilitarianism is often called *consequentialism* and is probably the most favored ethics in modern U.S. society, where humanism dominates (Kurtz, 1988). Any teleological ethics is based on evaluating the effects of an action as a means to an end, but there are different ways of estimating these effects. Utilitarian consequentialism makes this estimate by a calculation of positive gains and negative losses *quantitatively*, enumerating these gains and losses as comparable items. Its model is that of an economic exchange in which gains and losses can be calculated in terms of a uniform monetary measure. No wonder such an ethics, with its cost-and-benefit analysis, is very understandable and acceptable in American society, which is used to thinking in this kind of computerizable logic. Some people identify this type of logic with reason itself.

Situationism

One form of utilitarianism is *act utilitarianism*, exemplified by the situationism developed by Joseph Fletcher, one of the pioneers of bioethics (1954, 1988). Fletcher's approach is intelligible because he is reacting to the duty ethics prominent in the Protestant tradition, to which many Catholic conservatives also seem to have committed themselves. For Fletcher there is only one absolute moral rule, that of love (*agape* in New Testament Greek). People must always do what is loving. Fletcher settles abortion cases, not by saying that abortion is always wrong or always permissible, but by judging the consequences of having or not having an abortion for this particular woman in this particular situation in view of "loving action."

But what is loving action? It has generally been pointed out by Fletcher's critics (Cox, 1968; King, 1970; McCormick, 1981; Outka, 1968; Ramsey, 1965) that in his actual solution of cases, Fletcher has been forced gradually to develop various generalizations and rules. Furthermore, he asserts without proving (1) that the rule of love is a universal rule (egoists do not admit this) and (2) that no other rules are universal. Fletcher's only argument for this second assumption is that, with sufficient ingenuity, a hardship case can always be imagined in which it seems difficult to apply the usual rule. However, this argument only proves that ethical decisions can be difficult. The same objection can be brought against the rule of love, which is certainly very difficult to apply in many cases.

Consequently, most utilitarians reject pure situationism (Engelhardt, 1986b) and advocate some form of *rule utilitarianism* (as Fletcher seems to do in practice) whereby cost-and-benefit calculations must be made on the basis of experience formulated in normative generalizations, that is, moral rules.

Whether any rule admits an exception cannot be decided a *priori*. In dealing with scientific facts, the formulation of any natural physical law is only approximate and must be refined (e.g., Einstein's refinement of Newton's gravitational laws). Moreover, a prediction based on natural physical law is always merely probable because in the concrete instance another law may modify the outcome (e.g., the law of gravitation is offset by the law of electromagnetic attraction when a magnet is used to lift a piece of metal). Why is it surprising, then, that moral natural laws, which have a basis in natural facts, need to be reformulated as knowledge of human needs and situations increases, or that there may be a conflict of laws in concrete cases? Many rule utilitarians make this point by saying that moral rules have only a prima facie obligation (Beauchamp and Childress, 1983; Ross, 1930); that is, they are assumed to be binding unless sufficient reason is found to make an exception. Thus many ethicists today would consider mothers to be bound first by the rule that in general abortion is wrong, but that in some cases special circumstances shift the cost-and-benefit balance in favor of an abortion.

Ethical debate based on utilitarianism, however, also tends to end in an impasse. To many it seems based on a very superficial, overly economic view of the needs of human persons and human communities. It calculates cost-and-benifit consequences by treating human values as quantitatively comparable *items*, without taking adequate account of the unified, hierarchical, interdependent structure of the human person or the person's relation to a community sharing higher values, as discussed in Chapter 1. Some utilitarians, such as John Stuart Mill (1863), have tried to introduce a *qualitative* element into their system, but to do so consistently demands an essentially different type of ethics, which is described next.

157

Proportionalism

David Kelly (1979), in a study of the development of Catholic thinking on medical ethics, contrasts what he calls a "classicist mentality" and a "historical mentality." Kelly sees a tendency among Catholic moralists to abandon the former static world view based on the concept of an unchanging human nature and to adopt the later dynamic, evolutionary, historical, and cultural world view that takes full account of scientific progress, the variety and variability of human culture, the pluralism of value systems, the differences between unique persons, and the novel situations of contemporary life.

As a result of this shift, a system of teleological ethics has been developed that is typically called *proportionalism*. It originated with an important essay by the German Jesuit, Peter Knauer (1967), and was further explicated by the distinguished moralist of the Gregorian University in Rome, Josef Fuchs, SJ (1971, 1980, 1984), and by Bruno Schuller, SJ (1973). In the United States, proportionalism has been vigorously defended by Richard A. McCormick, SJ (McCormick and Ramsey, 1978; McCormick, 1981, 1984b) and Charles E. Curran (Curran and McCormick, 1979) has become the center of considerable controversy (Hoose, 1987).

Proportionalism is sometimes accused of being merely utilitarianism or consequentialism, but this is not the intent of its proponents (Cahill, 1981). According to McCormick (1973a, 1981, 1984b; McCormick and Ramsey, 1978); proportionalism accepts the classical thesis of Aquinas that the morality of a human act is determined by its object, its circumstances, and the intention of the agent. Proportionalism, however, departs from the classical interpretation of this thesis, according to which an act can be rendered immoral by reason of the moral object alone, if this object, apart from the circumstances and the agent's intention, is *intrinsically evil*. For proportionalists, the object of a human act, apart from its circumstances and the agent's intention, is only a *premoral* object that involves certain human values and disvalues. It becomes a moral object, which is morally good or bad, only when consideration is given to the proportion of values to disvalues involved in the concrete act taken in its circumstances and in view of the agent's intention.

The practical importance of this rather subtle technical distinction was brought out in an important article by Fuchs (1971). He defended proportionalism on the grounds that it was more "objective" than the classical methodology because it based moral judgment on the concrete act rather than on some abstract "nature" of the act. Fuchs also admitted, however, that proportionalism eliminated, at least in theory if not always in practice, the possibility of "absolute" or exceptionless moral norms. Theoretically it is always possible, according to proportionalism, to imagine circumstances in which any human act might be morally good, even those acts, such as torture of innocent persons, generally considered evil. Fuchs is also much influenced by the *intuitivism* of Scheler (Deeken, 1974), according to which absolute moral values are never realized in human existence except in a merely relative manner (O'Connell, 1974). McCormick, however, in his revision of this theory, seems now to admit some absolute norms, while still rejecting the concept of intrinsically evil moral objects (Cahill, 1981; McCormick and Ramsey, 1978).

An important implication of this theory is that the distinction between the *direct* intention of an intrinsically good act from the *indirect* intention of its possible foreseen bad side effects is no longer necessary. For example, classical moralists justified the abortion of a child resulting from a necessary hysterectomy for uterine cancer on the grounds that what the surgeon *directly* intended was not the abortion but the removal of the cancer. They forbade, however, the direct abortion of a child to save the life of a woman suffering from kidney disease on the grounds that this required the surgeon to directly intend the child's death as an evil means to a good end. For proportionalism, however, the two cases are not significantly different in regard to intention. Considered premorally, the value of the child's and the mother's lives and the disvalue of their deaths are only premoral or "ontic" values (to use the term proposed by Janssens, 1972). These values take on moral value only when the agent, who, if he or she observes the principle of proportion (i.e., if he or she chooses only acts in which the ontic values equal or exceed the disvalues), intends a morally good act.

The strength of this methodology, according to the proportionalists, is that while preserving the traditional norms of Christian morality, it provides a simple, honest, and direct way to solve conflict situations where rigid adherence to the norm would seem to violate the overriding Christian principle of love for persons. Those who reject proportionalism, however (among whom are the authors of this book), point out that it is difficult to reconcile this theory with the firmly established view in Christian tradition (which continues to be followed by recent popes in their moral teaching) that some acts (e.g., direct abortion) are *always* morally evil no matter what the circumstances or the agent's intention (John Paul II, 1984a). To this, proportionalists reply that their view is a legitimate development of traditional teaching that will make it more adaptable and less legalistic without radically undermining it. Whether this reply can really be justified is discussed after we first present what we consider a sounder revision of classical moral thinking, which we call *prudential personalism*.

7.4   PRUDENTIAL PERSONALISM

Criteria of Morality

Much current ethical debate, especially that on medical-moral and human sexuality topics, polarizes into what seems an irreconcilable dichotomy between a deontological ethics with absolute moral norms and a consequentialism with a cost-and-benefit calculus. If Catholic moral theology is to respect its own tradition, it must avoid both extremes.

As Haring (1966) has shown, the basic reason Catholic moral theology finds itself in this quandary is that after the Council of Trent, the textbooks used in seminaries replaced the means-ends ethics of the medieval theologians, which emphasized the development of the virtues coordinated by Christian love and prudence, with a duty ethics emphasizing the Commandments. Protestant theologians during this period also generally taught a duty ethics, to which Kant finally gave a philosophical systematization. This widespread theological trend reflected the attitudes of secular society that, in the Age of Reason, stressed the need for centralized sovereign authority acting through codified laws and clear lines of command.

At the end of the nineteenth century, however, the Thomistic revival in Catholic theology and the antirationalistic reaction in Protestant theology began a trend back to a means-ends ethics, which is clearly evident in the documents of the Second Vatican Council (1965c). These taught that the "objective criteria" of moral right and wrong are based on "the nature of the human person and human action" (*Pastoral Constitution on the Church in the Modern World*, n. 51).

Charles Curran (1977a) has argued that such an ethics is a "mixed form" rather than a pure duty ethics or a means-ends ethics. Such a mixed form of ethics would agree with duty ethics that objective criteria of morality cannot be reduced exclusively to the consequences of an action, but it would also agree with a means-ends ethics that these criteria must include such consequences. Curran calls this third model "an ethics of relationality and responsibility" (Curran, 1988; Jonsen, 1968; H. Niebuhr, 1963). People cannot claim complete control over their lives (as means-ends ethics seems to assume), nor can they reduce their responsiblities to obedience to general norms (as duty ethics assumes). Rather, they have to respond to the persons and events that confront them in life in ways that maximize human values, making creative use of the resources available. Curran believes that such an ethics is more in keeping with a Christian understanding of dependence on the grace of God and encounters with other persons than is a duty ethics, with its danger of legalism, or a means-ends ethics, with its danger of illusions about a person's rational control over his or her life.

It seems that Curran's ethics of relationality and responsibility should be classified not as a mixed form, but rather as a personalist form of means-ends ethics. We also would insist that any modern Christian ethics must stress that the "ends" of human action are always *persons* and the community of interrelated persons responding to each other. At the center of this community is a tri-personal God with whom the initiative always belongs and on whose grace we completely depend to make any fully human response (Kiesling, 1986). However, to respond to persons is to direct action to the good of persons, and this always is a matter of free choice of means to ends, of acts that relate persons to persons or alienate them from each other.

As already argued, a deontological ethics is inadequate because it only traces the criteria of morality back to the will of some lawmaker, whether that lawmaker is God, the government, or the autonomous individual. But the question must still be asked, Why is the will of the lawmaker itself righteous? The ultimate answer to this query must be given in terms of the practical wisdom or *prudence* by which the legislator makes wise rules for the benefit of those who are to obey. As soon as "benefit for someone" is considered, one is constructing a means-ends type of ethics, which measures the rightness or wrongness of human action by its helpful or harmful consequences, that is, as an effective means to the goals of human life (the satisfaction of human needs).

We accept this means-end type of ethics wholeheartedly, and we use the term *prudential* because it indicates the practical, goal-seeking character and even the situational or contextual character of this ethics. For a prudential ethics, morality ultimately is not a matter of obeying rules, but of intelligently seeking appropriate, concrete behavior by which to achieve human personal and communal goals. This is not to deny the value of laws, rules, or principles (see 8.1), but only to contend that what makes such laws obligatory is their helpfulness in guiding prudential decisions to successful goal achievement.

This still leaves the following question unanswered: what goals are morally right for a human being? As noted, the Second Vatican Council answered this by saying that these goals are determined by "the nature of the human person and human action." Theologically, this can only mean that the ultimate measure of morality is the pattern of Jesus Christ, in whom alone has been revealed what it is to be fully human, undistorted by sin (Ep 5:1-20).

Jesus as Model

The United States' bishops, in their joint pastoral letter *To Live in Christ Jesus* (United States Catholic Conference, 1976), have written:

> All of us seek happiness: life, peace, joy, a wholeness and wholesomeness of being. The happiness we seek and for which we are fashioned is given to us in Jesus, God's supreme gift of love....God reveals to us in Jesus who we are and how we are to live. Yet he has made us free, able, and obliged to decide how we shall respond to our calling. We must make concrete in the particular circumstances of our lives what the call to holiness and the commandment of love require. This is not easy. We know, too, that decisions may not be arbitrary, for "good" and "bad," "right" and "wrong" are not simply what we choose to make them. And so God gives us his guidance in manifold forms (p. 8).

Thus a teleological ethics that goes no further than consequentialism, utilitarianism, or situationism is inadequate not because it judges actions in terms of their consequences, but because it fails to evaluate these consequences in the light of a correct understanding of authentic human goals. Rather than being determined by a particular culture's customs or by individual preference, these goals are determined by "the nature of the human person." Thus we speak of the ethics we advocate as "personalism" because it evaluates human goals and the means to these goals in terms of the self-actualization or fulfillment of the human person in community.

Historians of ethics usually characterize this approach to morality as an ethics of self-realization and cite Plato, Aristotle, Hegel, Royce, and even Dewey as typical proponents (MacIntyre, 1967, 1981). We accept this classification provided that two points are kept clear:

1. The ethics we propose is not based on intuitionism or idealism of any sort, since its principles are derived from human, historical experience, especially the experience of perfect human actualization in the historical Jesus and (less perfectly) in his true disciples throughout the history of the Christian community.

161

2. This ethics of self-realization should not be understood as individualism or egoism, but as essentially *communitarian,* in accordance with the notion of personhood developed in Chapter 1.

A prudential personalism, therefore, proposes that the rightness or wrongness of human actions be judged by asking, "How does this action in its context contribute to the growth of persons in community?" Thus the effects of any human act must be evaluated not in terms of immediate pains and pleasures, or even in terms of other immediate qualitative values, but must all be referred to the actualization of the human person in relation to other persons. Because consequentialists and utilitarians fail to provide such a conception of full human personhood as the goal of every human action, but content themselves with more superficial values, they create an ethics of expediency in which the end justifies the means, that is, *any* means. Following consequentialism or utilitarianism risks wasting our lives in the pursuit of unsatisfying and often inconsistent goals, which ultimately leave our deepest human needs frustrated.

Constructing a prudential personalism raises questions about the inherent needs of the human person and of the subordinate needs of all those functions that integrate the human person as a complex whole. These inherent needs are not themselves something that can be chosen, since we cannot choose to be human. By God's gift we *are* human. We can only choose how to realize the humanity in its fullness by morally good action or frustrate its fulfillment by bad action. Moreover, growth and fulfillment as human persons has a twofold aspect: on the one hand, our growth is a response to the vocation that God gives to each of us in our unique existence; on the other hand, it is our response to the common essential humanity that unites us to others in the human community (Rahner, 1975).

Basic Common Needs

It is at this point that the philosophers and theologians who have influenced the development of utilitarianism on the one hand and proportionalism on the other raise a difficulty about how to come to an understanding of the human person or of the nature that makes the person human. Utilitarianism was developed by English philosophers in the sceptical tradition of David Hume, who had denied that we know anything about the human self except our own stream of consciousness. Such philosophers left the study of human nature to the biological and psychological sciences, which *ex professo* refuse to deal with questions of value. Utilitarian ethics was developed as a method of dealing with ethical problems in terms of observable consequences without reference to any human self or any human nature. As shown, proportionalism was developed by German ethicists in the continental tradition of idealism and phenomenology, who leave to science the study of human nature as an object to be observed and measured, and who reserve for philosophy the study of the *subject* in his or her cultural world of human-created values.

It is not necessary here, however, to refute these competing philosophies nor to work out a better metaphysics of the human person before constructing a personalist ethics. As Adler (1970) has argued well, it is sufficient to begin ethics with a common sense notion of what it is to be human. Of course, the more this understanding can be enriched and deepened, both through the behavioral sciences and through theological reflection on the life of Christ, the more adequate and refined moral judgments will be. What can be learned in particular from the proportionalist trend is that an understanding of the human person must not be merely abstract but must take into account human historicity.

Human beings never exist simply as human, but as members of a particular community with its particular culture at a given time in history. Moreover, each individual is unique in his or her constitution and experience. Consequently, what it is to be human varies and can be deepened and enriched or distorted and trivialized by culture. Again, human nature itself is not absolutely unified, as is evidenced by genetic differences between members of the human race; nor is it absolutely stable, since it is subject at least to some extent to the continuing evolutionary process of natural selection. Some of these changes also result not from natural causes but from cultural ones, and with increasing knowledge may fall under human control. This means that at any given moment of history for any given group of people, their moral understanding will be profoundly conditioned by their history. One needs only to read the Old Testament to become aware of how differently the ancient Jews interpreted the Ten Commandments than people do today.

Nevertheless, historicity itself implies continuity, identity, and community. There would be no biographies if people were mere streams of consciousness. It is only because we each remain essentially ourselves from cradle to grave that we have personal histories. Similarly, unless the human race shared a common nature that was at least relatively stable for vast periods of time, there would be no human history and today there would be no global human community. Therefore human persons all have some basic common needs that characterize them as human and make possible cooperation as a human family. Prudential personalism rests on the conviction that such needs can be known and can be, with some success, separated from cultural variations. Thus it becomes possible to make these basic needs the goals of authentic human life, which guide people in their choice of appropriate means to those goals and in terms of which it is possible to criticize culture. What these goals are has already been mentioned in the description of the human person (1.1) and is further discussed in the next chapter.

Thus a prudential personalism provides a logic of moral decision that takes the following form:

1. People need to be very clear about the goal of human life set by the Creator for human beings in common and for a particular human being in his or her uniqueness. This self-understanding has to be achieved by making use of all the types of information of the conscience described in 3.4.

2. This effort at self-understanding does not result in a single principle (e.g., Jos. Fletcher's "act lovingly"), but in an indefinite number of principles reflecting the complex, multidimensional constitution of the

human person (1.4). Therefore the Principle of Totality and Integrity (2.4) comes into play as persons attempt to assign priorities among these various basic goals and realize their independence. Out of this reflection comes a system of values needed to formulate the moral rules that help persons to make prudent choices.

3. In terms of this value system expressed in moral rules (which are open to development as self-understanding grows), people strive to inform their consciences concerning particular moral choices (3.4) in a prudent manner, that is, by keeping in mind both goals with their relative priorities and the concrete circumstances, risks, and foreseen special consequences of a particular act. Such a moral logic is therefore "prudential" in its practical, intelligent effort to reach goals, and it is "personalist" in that it works not for superficial goals but for the total realization of the inherent needs of the human person in community.

7.5   AN EVALUATION OF ETHICAL METHODOLOGIES

Prudential Personalism Versus Proportionalism

At present the chief rival methodologies in Catholic bioethical literature are undoubtedly the so-called classical methodology, of which prudential personalism is a revision, and proportionalism, which, although it was first put forward as a revision of Thomism (Dedek, 1979), has been shown by several scholars (Carney, 1978; Connery, 1973, 1981; W. E. May, 1977a) to be a radical departure from Aquinas (Patrick Lee, 1981; W. E. May, 1984). To compare and evaluate these two methods more precisely, the way in which prudential personalism arrives at ethical decisions is first explained in greater detail.

As one type of teleological ethics, prudential personalism begins its analysis of a moral act from the ultimate goal of human life, that is, the self-actualization of the person in relation to God, other persons, and the world. People are not free *not* to want to be happy, but are free to commit themselves to different concrete realizations of happiness (e.g., pleasure, fame, God). To choose unreasonably as an ultimate goal (or "fundamental option"; McInerny, 1987) what people know will not satisfy all their basic needs is to "build our house on sand" (Mt 7:26). The Gospel says that nothing can satisfy all human needs except life with God and with his friends in the Kingdom of God, a kingdom that is eternal but into which people enter even here on earth.

Ethics, however, deals not only with the goals of life but with free choice of appropriate means to these goals. People especially need ethical reasoning when they are faced with decisions that demand actions they foresee will have not only good consequences but bad ones as well. Jesus himself said sadly, "I have not come to bring peace, but division" (Lk 12:51), meaning that his very work of peacemaking would also result in quarrels.

The word "consequences," however, is somewhat ambiguous. Most properly, it refers to those effects that follow on the act itself, but one must remember that a free act, in its very performance, has an effect first on the agent. One of the great insights of Christian ethics is that morality originates not in the outward deed but in the inward motive (Mt 15:18-20). In acting, persons may not actually accomplish the good they intend or suffer the harm anticipated, but the primary effect of the free act is in themselves and follows inevitably (McCabe, 1969). The first question must always be, "Will this act make me more truly human as Jesus was, or less so?"

To judge among alternative means, people rationally (but also with the sensitivity of attention that healthy, disciplined feelings promote) measure each means by the goal toward which it is supposed to lead. To act in this reasonable way in view of basic needs, all of which must be met to attain self-actualization, is to act in accordance with our God-given nature, and this is the same as obeying the natural law. The law of Christ that is the Gospel (Ga 6:2) confirms a correct understanding of human nature and, furthermore, calls us to that higher happiness of intimate friendship in the Trinity, which is beyond human powers and attainable only by grace (Kiesling, 1986).

Chapter 1 lists some of these basic needs that must be met if the ultimate goal of living is to be reached. Aquinas (Aquinas' *Summa Theologiae* I-II, q. 94, a. 2) conveniently reduces these basic needs to four: to preserve life, to preserve the human race through procreation, to advance in knowledge of the truth, and to live in community with other persons. Unless people preserve their lives, self-actualization is not possible. If the human race is not propagated, there can be no human society. If there is no human society, persons cannot progress in the knowledge of truth, especially that highest truth, which is to know God and other persons in intimate friendship.

In making an actual moral decision, therefore, three things are necessary:

1. I must first ask myself whether I am acting for the right end.
2. I must then ask whether the act I am considering is an effective means to that end. I may discover that the act is intrinsically evil, that is, directly contradictory to one of my basic goals (e.g., killing innocent people is directly contradictory to my need for society), in which case such an act is morally evil.
3. If, however, the act in itself appears to be an appropriate means, I must consider whether in my circumstances, here and now, its normal effectiveness is destroyed, in which case an otherwise morally good act becomes evil.

Proportionalists, however, deny that human acts taken in themselves apart from circumstances can be said to be intrinisically and determinately *morally* good or evil, but only premorally (ontically) to have certain values and disvalues (Keane, 1977). For example, the act of killing certainly has serious disvalues since it terminates precious human life. It can be judged morally, however, only when one takes into account the circumstances and the agent's intention, which may make killing in self-defense or in capital punishment a morally good act, since in these circumstances the values of self-defense and of justice outweigh the disvalues of the death of an aggressor or a criminal. Thus a proportionalist might consistently consider that killing a child by abortion might be a morally good act in certain circumstances.

We believe that this theory has serious and indeed fatal difficulties. We first mention three objections that have been raised by others (Connery, 1981; Grisez, 1983; W. E. May, 1984) and then offer another objection we consider more fundamental. The first objection is that proportionalism advocates "doing evil that good may come from it." Proportionalists deny this because they hold that when the ontic values outweigh the disvalues, the act as a whole is *morally* good and only premorally bad in some respects. However, we must ask, How can we can measure or weigh the relative values or disvalues in an objective manner? Can happiness of one individual be compared to the life of another? The second objection is that proportionalism is merely consequentialism or utilitarianism. Proportionalists deny this because for them the values and disvalues of an act include not only its consequences but its intrinsic effect on the agent. But does not consideration of the intrinsic act lead us to put forth some values that should never be violated? The third objection is that to apply the principle of proportion in practice is impossible, since the values and disvalues of human acts are not commensurate—cannot be reduced to some common denominator—and thus cannot be weighed together. Proportionalists reply that moralists have always admitted that a "proportionate reason" is one of the determinants of morality, and this implies that somehow the values and disvalues of human acts can be weighed.

Ontic Values and Disvalues

In our opinion, the essential error of proportionalism is in the notion of the ontic "values" and "disvalues" of the act premorally considered. Janssens (1972) defines ontic evil as "any lack of perfection at which we aim, any lack of fulfillment which frustrates our natural urges and makes us suffer." But how are these disvalues and values to be weighed so as to find their proportion? If we consider the ontic aspects of a human act and judge them to be values or disvalues of a certain weight, we must either do so in relation to the true end of human life or not. If we consider them as a means to this end, however, we are already considering them *morally*, since morality consists precisely in this relation of means to end.

On the other hand, if we consider these values simply in themselves apart from this relation (and this is what the proportionalists claim to do), they have no *morally relevant* value or disvalue. For example, the act of killing a human being viewed in relation to such goals of life as self-preservation and the preservation of society can be said to have value or disvalue, but apart from such goals it has no determinant value. To say that killing has ontic disvalue because it is the destruction of a living body is meaningless, unless we first grant that preserving the human body is a *moral* good. Thus proportionalists use the terms *ontic* or *premoral* contradictorily; the only way we can connote value or disvalue is by relating an act to an end, which thereby constitutes a moral or ontological, not merely a premoral or ontic, value or disvalue. In the proportionalist methodology (as in the philosophy of Martin Heidegger and Max Scheler, in which it seems to have originated) we are imprisoned in a cultural relativism that determines our judgment of values; thus human historicity swallows up any transcultural human nature on which ethics might be based.

Prudential personalism does not fall into this trap because it holds that the act *premorally* considered, (i.e., antecedent to the agent intending it as a means to the true end of life) already possesses a natural teleology that a free human act, if it is reasonable, must respect. Thus the so-called premoral or ontic character of the act is the primary determinant of the act's morality, much as the nature of an instrument determines the uses to which it can reasonably be put. Given the end, some tools are excluded as counterproductive, but usually some freedom of choice among other tools remains. Thus a knife is not a fork and cannot be used as such. Poison cannot be chosen as food, but there is considerable freedom of choice for food among nonpoisonous substances. Discovering this teleology requires increasing one's understanding of the human body-person and its relations to other persons, in its transcultural nature as well as in its historical development.

Notice that the difference between the systems is not that the proportionalists require that an act's values outweigh its disvalues, whereas the prudential personalists ignore this proportion. For any teleologist the means to the end must be proportionate to it. The difference is that prudential personalism judges this proportion to the end first by (1) whether the character of the act renders it an appropriate means or not and (2) whether the circumstances of the act might destroy this intrinsic appropriateness. The proportionalist, on the other hand, claims that circumstances or good intention can sometimes make an inappropriate means appropriate, if the values achieved outweigh the disvalues incurred. How, then, can the proportionalist determine what counts for a value or disvalue in ethical decisions?

Knauer (1967), faced with the objection that the many types of values of an act are difficult to reduce to a common denominator, argues that the way to tell whether an act's disvalues exceed the values is by the test of whether "in the long run and for the most part" the means is "counterproductive" in achieving the end. This seems to be circular reasoning, however, because this proportion was supposed to determine if the means was counterproductive. Prudential personalism does not get into this vicious circle. By its method, if the act in its intrinsic character is not proportioned as a means to the true end of human life, then "in the long run and for the most part" the act obviously must be "counterproductive," even if in the short run, because of accidental circumstances, its values seem to outweigh its disvalues. For example, lying may seem to do more good than harm in the short run; but it is essentially counterproductive because it makes the speaker a liar and destroys fundamental human trust, thus eventually leading to evil results greater than the good accomplished.

Connery (1981), in his detailed refutation of the claims of proportionalism, points out that in practice proportional methodology makes moral decisions extremely onerous, if not impossible, since it requires us to make an exhaustive analysis of every foreseeable consequence. The classical method, on the contrary, provides a way of first eliminating those means clearly unsuitable to the true end of life and then clarifying the nature of a licit direct intention. Then, provided that the foreseen evil consequences are not evidently disproportionate, so that they could not be intended only *indirectly,* the act is judged licit. Proportionalism, however, suffers the severe practical disadvantage that, on the one hand, it is open to arbitrary balancing of values in favor of laxity and, on the other, to a scrupulous rigorism because it furnishes no objective way to determine the proportion of the alleged ontic values and disvalues. Peter Singer (1980) has argued that moralists of this school use the classical method to make a prima facie determination of an act's morality. Then, if this seems to result in an unfavorable conclusion, these moralists strive to make a case for a more convenient conclusion by finding values and disvalues that will tip the balance in favor of an exception to the general norm.

Physicalism

Proportionalists, with their rigid distinction between the premoral and the moral act, have a special dislike for what Charles Curran (1968, 1977b, 1979, 1985, 1988) calls "physicalism" or "biologism," for which they criticize classical moral theology. Thus Curran admits that ontically considered, a homosexual act has disvalues; that is, it is abnormal (a conclusion that has raised protests from some homosexuals). Curran judges that such acts are objectively moral, however, if this disvalue is outweighed by the values to homosexuals of expressing a genuine human love and meeting their sexual needs. It seems to him "physicalist" to suppose that the abnormal physical character of the act could outweigh these high personal, even spiritual, values. Similarly, in the contraception controversy, moralists of the proportionalist school could not see that the slight alteration in the physical act of intercourse by artificial methods had any great moral significance that could outweigh the spiritual good of the marriage it was supposed to promote. Thus, proportionalist thinking tends to be a form of dualism in which the physical character of acts is dismissed as only of ontic significance, which leads us back to the central problem of proportionalism: how are the values and disvalues of the act ontically considered values at all? And how can they be weighed?

In calling our revision of the classical method *personalism* and defining the human person as "embodied intelligent freedom," we retain the classical methodology and stress even more strongly than was traditional the unity of the human person as a body-person. All human acts, however spiritual, are also acts of the body, as the Jewish tradition has always taught (Novak, 1985; Ratner, 1977). Consequently, for an act to be true human, it must respect the inherent teleology or normal biological functions of the body and its organs, not because these are superior to other dimensions of the person, but because their functions are not merely animal but truly human and absolutely necessary to think, love, and act as human beings (Sacred Congregation for the Doctrine of the Faith, 1987).

For these reasons, we believe that the classical methodology of moral judgment, which we include in prudential personalism (but to which we add more attention to human historicity in our understanding of human needs and the means available to satisfy them), is superior to that of proportionalism. Thus it is understandable why the popes and bishops continue to use the classical methodology and deplore the erosion of traditional norms. This erosion has resulted from the ingenuity of some proportionalists in finding exceptions to these norms by weighing supposed values and disvalues without showing how these are related to the universal structure of the human person—the basic needs and innate biological and psychological structure of the human person that classical methodology endeavors to respect.

Application of Methodologies

To complete this evaluation of these moral systems, we now return to the example of abortion to see how in practice these systems work out. A deontologist faced with an abortion decision will ask if there are rules requiring or forbidding abortion. If no rule is discovered, the deontologist feels free to do what seems convenient. If there is a conflict of rules, the deontologist will seek another rule to resolve the conflict or fall back on the rule to do the lesser evil.

A utilitarian or consequentialist faced with the same situation will consider the probable consequences of having or not having the abortion and will attempt to judge whether it will be of greater or lesser benefit to the persons concerned. The utilitarian will evaluate "benefit" either in terms of subjective satisfaction or in terms of what appears desirable or undesirable, but without seeking to ground such evaluations in any teleology *intrinsic* to the persons concerned. Abortion will thus be judged in terms of the subjective sufferings or relief of the mother, the possible sufferings of an unwanted or defective child, the various advantages to society, and so forth.

A proportionalist also will look at the proportion of values and disvalues that he or she can foresee as included in the act of abortion and all of its foreseeable consequences. The proportionalist then will judge if, in this case, the values of the abortion outweigh the prima facie disvalues that are traditionally attributed to it.

A prudential personalist will try to take into account all the consequences mentioned but will evaluate them in terms of the self-realization of the persons involved and of the community of persons of which they are a part. Thus he or she first must determine whether the fetus is a person. Then the various consequences of abortion or of bearing a child must be evaluated in terms of the needs inherent in the mother and the child, both as unique individuals and as part of the total human community.

When we speak of inherent needs in the human person, we are brought back to the modern ethicists' puzzlement about how to get from facts to values, from the *is* to the *ought*. As Henry Veatch (1971) has shown, this problem had its origin in the mechanistic view of the world favored by many modern scientists. If a human being is a machine produced by the blind forces of evolution, what is the sense in speaking about inherent goals and purposes in the human person?

169

In such a view, human goals or purposes are simply a matter of individual choice, or they are imposed on people by the laws and customs of the culture in which they have been raised.

The discoveries of modern science can be accepted, however, including our evolutionary origin, without accepting the mechanistic interpretation of these facts. One also can accept scientific discoveries without denying either the common sense of Christian conviction that human persons have been created for a purpose and that this purpose is manifest in their genetically determined physical and psychological constitution as individuals and as part of the human species. This dynamic structure of human nature with its innate needs is a part of the order of facts that one can determine empirically by the life sciences, if one avoids the sociobiologist's deterministic exaggerations (Barlow and Silverberg, 1980; Callahan, 1980) and interprets philosophically to provide a unified view of what it is to be human. Such an empirically grounded view furnished the basis for an ethics that goes beyond cultural relativism (Rachels, 1986). Thus, whenever this book refers to basic human needs or to human nature, it implies a philosophical account of the human person that considers fully the findings of modern biology and psychology and that is in keeping with what healthcare professionals know about the human body and psyche.

When human needs are viewed not merely as static facts, but as goals to be achieved, they become values, that is, goods to be desired and sought. Thus it is a biological fact that people need to eat in order to live. However, when we perceive this necessity and begin to make free choices about how we can best fulfill this need in various circumstances, human intelligence, freedom, and creativity enter into the biological process of nutrition and it takes on a truly human, ethical meaning. Considered in their totality as a system of needs, these genetically inherent requirements of life become genuinely obligatory *oughts* because we need to be ourselves and to use our freedom to achieve self-realization.

This need for self-realization is itself a fact of human biology and psychology. Indeed, self-realization is the central unifying feature of a human person, an embodied intelligent freedom. We act morally when we perceive this fact and freely respond to its practical challenge; we act immorally when we refuse to respond realistically to this challenge and yield to disorganized and inconsistent impulses. As McDonagh (1979) has argued, moral living is an openness to a call and a stewardship of a gift. The gift is our human personhood, and the call is the purpose inherent in that personhood.

Thus, when we discuss such an issue as abortion, an adequate logic of ethics forces us to go beyond mere utilitarianism and to ask such questions as, For what purpose are we gifted with sexuality? Is the unborn child a gift of God, and for what purpose has he created it? For what purpose are we created social beings who are inclined to care for the helpless and also for women in the crisis of pregnancy? For what purpose are we gifted with the intelligence and the skill of medical art: to further life or to destroy it?

Healthcare professionals cannot shrug off such questions as philosophical or theological problems outside their field. They have received a predominantly scientific education that may have led them to be suspicious of any philosophical effort to read values into facts. When philosophers speak about the human person, a scientifically educated person may prefer to talk about the human organism, reducing everything directly to observable facts systematized by some mathematical or quasi-mathematical theory. No matter how foreign to their regular way of thinking it may be for scientists to reflect on the value implications of biological or psychological facts, however, such reflection is inescapable if there is to be harmony between medical-ethical decisions and medical science.

On the other hand, some philosophers and theologians are intensely uncomfortable with any effort to root ethics in biological or psychological structures. They are afraid that this will result in a fixed and static conception of human nature, and they would prefer to relate ethics to history and the humanities rather than to the sciences. To this view we would respond that the evolutionary view of humankind, at both the biological and the anthropological levels, is in no way contrary to the prudential personalism we have outlined here. We do not have in mind some type of timeless human nature, but simply the historically existing human species made up of unique individuals. All have their own biographies or "stories" but nevertheless form a community based on certain common needs that are not the product of culture but its source. For the Christian this historical community is centered in Jesus of Nazareth, God's Word revealed in perfect humanity.

SUMMARY

Ethical decisions are always made within some value system, and American society has a plurality of such systems. Therefore Christians need to be fully conscious of their own value system and to enter into dialogue with others to reduce conflict and to find some area of consensus. Thus bioethical matters require a logic that will help people make decisions consistent with the Christian system of values, but a logic that will also enable them to recognize analogies between their system of values and those of others.

The logic of emotivism solves ethical questions by references to emotional preferences. This can serve as the basis of dialogue if one can distinguish between sincere, humane, decent feelings and the opposite of these. Another logic, deontologism or duty ethics, solves ethical questions by reference to the will of God, to recognized laws or customs, or to personal principles of behavior. This also can serve as a basis of dialogue if the parties can find authorities in common or moral principles with which they can agree, perhaps for their own reasons. The line of reasoning in consequentialism, utilitarianism, or situationism attempts to find a solution that seems to bring the most satisfaction and the least hurt to all in the concrete situation. This type of thinking is practical and realistic and must certainly form an important element in every public discussion in a pluralistic society. Utilitarianism may result, however, in proposals that some members of the community will reject as unprincipled, merely expedient, shortsighted, and immoral.

To resolve this impasse that arises between those in a community who take their stand on absolute principles or authoritative laws and those who argue for pragmatic solutions, Catholic moral theology has attempted to find a middle course, which we have formulated as a teleological prudential personalism. Such an approach attempts to think in terms of any action's effects for the good of the persons and the community involved. Prudential personalism evaluates these effects, however, according to needs and purposes that have been established not by subjective preference, nor merely by abstract laws, but by the constitution of the human person in its individual and communal dynamism.

CHAPTER 8

Norms Of Christian Decision Making In Bioethics

OVERVIEW

In this chapter we are concerned with the *content* of Christian ethical reasoning concerning issues in bioethics. Beginning with a discussion of the relationship between Christianity and ethics (8.1), we describe ethical principles and relate them to human need. Our human needs are satisfied through the practice of faith, hope, and charity, so we discuss the principles of bioethics under these three headings. As an expression of faith (8.2) (a form of knowing), we present five principles, some of which have been discussed previously, that pertain to the formation of a prudent conscience. Under the title of Christian love (charity) (8.3), we consider four norms that are concerned with affective needs, whether this affection is for ourselves or others. Next we consider the three norms directed to the future or concerned with the eschatological aspects of ethics, gathering these norms under the heading of Christian hope (8.4). Finally, we seek to coordinate the principles presented by aligning them with the four basic human needs (8.5).

8.1 IS THERE A CHRISTIAN ETHICS?

Today the question is debated whether there is a distinctly Christian ethics (Curran and McCormick, 1980; Gustafson, 1975; Langan, 1988; Macquarrie, 1970; MacNamara, 1986). The moral values of the New Testament are also found in other religions and philosophies of life. Section 1.3 illustrates this fact by referring to the list of such values in the *Universal Declaration of Human Rights* (United Nations, 1948), to which all the nations of the world, whatever their ideologies, have subscribed. As 1.3 argues, however, two value systems may agree on a list of important values but differ greatly in their *hierarchy* of values. Thus we would expect that a Christian ethics would be characterized primarily by the priority it gives to certain values and the reasons for these priorities. Christian reflection on the human values listed in the *Universal Declaration* will prompt certain emphases and meanings in the light of the Gospel of Jesus Christ.

The great disciple of Jesus, St. Paul, summarized these Christian priorities as *faith, hope,* and *charity* (1 Co 13:13). Moreover, Paul emphasized that for him all these primary values take their full meaning from the conviction that the full life of the human person will be achieved only through a personal union with God in eternal life through incorporation in the risen Christ. A secular humanist, a Marxist, a Muslim, and a Buddhist would all agree that faith, hope, and love are important human values, but they would differ in the emphases they would give these among all values, and they would not understand them in this Christological way. Thus faith, hope, and love are common to many value systems, but only in an analogical, not in a univocal, sense.

To stress this analogy of common ethical terms, however, is not to deny that these same terms may mean different things to different persons. Analogical terms may refer to quite diverse experiences, or they may refer to one and the same experience understood in somewhat different ways. For example, the term *love* may be used by one person to refer to an experience of sexual love and by another to refer to an experience of love for the poor. The experiences are quite different; the term is the same, but it is used analogically. On the other hand, when *love* is used by a Christian, a Buddhist, and a humanist to refer to sexual love, the experience for all may be very much the same; however, the term is still used analogically because of the very different ways in which each of these three interpret that experience in the context of their different views of life and different value systems.

Consequently, although Christians may be aware when they use such terms as *faith, hope,* and *love* that they use them with a special meaning that is only analogical to the way these terms are used by non-Christians, this need not entail that the Christian believes that non-Christians do not *experience the realities* to which these terms refer just as the Christian does. Some Christians think that non-Christians have no experience of grace nor of the true God who reveals himself by grace. However, Catholic theology has always admitted that non-Christians may be living by grace in a sense as real as Christians do; that is, they experience the same realities as Christians, but they do not name them in the same way, or even when they do name them similarly, non-Christians do not understand them in the same way (O'Meara, 1973). Moreover, since the Second Vatican Council (1965a), many Catholic theologians admit that grace may act not only on those of other religions, but also *through* these religions in different symbols and languages. Christians do not claim a monopoly on the true God or his grace, but only that the gracious God has made himself most fully, explicitly, and intimately known to humanity in Jesus Christ (Vatican II, 1964a).

By love, the Christian understands first the charity, or *agape,* God has for persons and that by grace he gives them as a power to love him more than themselves and their neighbor as themselves. Jesus taught that the great commandment of love, understood in this sense, sums up all other ethical rules (Mk 12:28-34; Mt 22:34-40; Furnish, 1972; Spicq, 1963). This Christian love, however, is not a mere feeling, as an emotivist might think, but is based on faith in the Incarnate Word, Jesus Christ, who tells us who God is and what our relation to him and to our neighbor must be. Thus Christian faith moves people from an emotivist to a cognitivist level of ethical understanding, since besides being a blind trust, faith is also a genuine understanding of God's purpose for people, an imperfect but real share in God's wisdom. Christian faith, therefore, moves beyond a duty ethics of mere obedience to God's will to a means-ends level of intelligent, creative purpose and free choice.

Furthermore, a person's relation to God and neighbor is not something simply fixed; it is teleological, in a process of actualization that will not be complete until ultimate intimacy with the Triune God is reached beyond this present life. Until persons reach this goal, they also need Christian hope—by which they do not trust in their own powers, but in the promises and grace of God manifested in Christ's death and resurrection—in order to achieve individual and communal goals. Thus a "theology of hope" (Moltmann, 1967) or of "liberation" (Boff, 1986; Gutierrez, 1977) gives to Christian ethics an open, creative outlook analogous to but very different from the progressivism of pragmatism or the revolutionary hope of Marxism.

These three Pauline terms—*faith, hope,* and *love*—can serve as a way of classifying and developing a set of ethical principles specifically Christian that can be applied to bioethical questions. These principles are expressed in terms that are common to most ethical systems in the analogical way just explained.

Some would call these principles philosophical as contrasted to those of a theological ethics (moral theology, Christian ethics). The terms *philosophical* and *theological*, however, are themselves distinguishable only in function of some world view, so that this distinction has to be made in different ways in different world views. Thus it is preferable to consider these principles and the terms in which they are expressed simply as analogically common to most ethical systems, whether these systems are characterized as philosophical or theological. We then give them a specifically Christian interpretation in this chapter, leaving others to interpret them analogically according to their own thought systems. A Christian theologian of a particular school, such as a Thomist or a Barthian, can also give them a philosophical interpretation in terms of the way the relation of philosophy to theology and of natural reason to revelation are understood in that theology (Bourke, 1951; Finnis, 1983).

What Is an Ethical Principle?

In speaking of principles, we are by no means opting for what McCormick (1977) has called a "deductive ethics" or what David Kelly (1979) calls a "static classical ethics" in contrast to a historical, existential ethics. On the contrary, we do not accept the notion of deontological or institutionist ethics that we can establish a priori principles from which practical, ethical rules can be deduced in the manner of an axiomatic system. Ethical principles are not predetermined laws nor predetermined conclusions.

By *principles* we mean general statements concerning human behavior derived from human experience and constantly tested and refined in experience. Moral decisions cannot be deduced from them, but they can be used to guide intelligent analysis of concrete ethical situations. Actual ethical decision (see 3.4) depends not merely on abstract reasoning, but on *prudence*, in which several other factors are also involved. At the same time, we would not agree with consequentialists that these principles are merely statistical generalizations or prima facie rules (Ross, 1930). On the contrary, they are grounded in an understanding of what it is to be a human person and what it is to be a human person redeemed by Christ.

As Chapters 1 and 7 show, humanity is defined by human *needs*, the actualization of which constitutes authentic happiness, the true goal of life. Faith, hope, and charity work toward the satisfaction of the deepest human need, namely, to live in the society of persons centered in God (the Kingdom of God of which Jesus preached). This need for a God-centered society is "embodied, intelligent freedom" (see 1.1), but it has been marvelously deepened by grace so as to become an effective need not only for society with God and neighbor but an intimate and everlasting union in the community of the Trinity. This union with God and neighbor through Christ is Christian love. As a dynamic movement toward the perfect realization of God's Kingdom, even here on earth, it is Christian hope. As the conviction that God has called men to this Kingdom and is willing to give them the power to attain it, it is Christian faith. Christian prudence is this faith in its practical aspect as it enables us to be open to the guidance of Christ's Spirit, who alone knows the way to God and who alone can overcome those barriers of alienation that divide one person from another. Thus faith, hope, and love, as they fulfill the deepest needs of our being, are the ultimate principles of Christian ethics, and Christian prudence guides us in actually realizing these values in concrete historical situations.

By reason and faith we have some understanding of our natural needs and the still deeper needs awakened in us by God's grace, but this understanding is not complete. It can be deepened and refined by historical experience, study, prayer, and dialogue with other world views. That this insight has universal (although analogous) validity for Christians and non-Christians is evident from the *Universal Declaration of Human Rights* (1.3).

When bioethical debate is shallow and fruitless, it is usually because such simple basic insights are ignored or minimized, with no effort to understand them as they appear, at least analogically, in the opponent's value system. By using these insights, ethical decisions can be made more sensitive to deep human needs, just as some of the impasses that today divide persons of different world views can be ecumenically transcended.

8.2 NORMS OF CHRISTIAN FAITH

The first five principles or norms (some of which have been discussed previously) pertain to the formation of a prudent conscience (see 3.4). Since conscience is key to intelligent decision making, it is directly cognitive, a type of *knowing*, a strengthening and deepening of human insight and reason. Christians are acutely aware that sin and the sinful structures of the world have blinded human self-understanding (Rm 1:18-32). God has not only called Christians to be freed from this blindness, however, but has also invited them to share in his own glory and transcendent wisdom (Rm 5:1-3; 11:33-36). This enlightenment of human conscience is the work of Christ's Holy Spirit through the gift of faith. Thus the Christian understanding of these principles, analogically common to many different ethical systems, interprets them in view of the Christian model of what it is to be human, a model found perfectly realized only in Jesus Christ. Only to the degree that this model of Christ is used is it possible for us to discriminate adequately between moral good and evil (Grisez, 1983; Gustafson, 1976; Schnackenburg, 1965).

Principle of Well-Formed Conscience

The distinguished French biologist Jacques Monod, in his book *Chance and Necessity* (1971), argues that there really is only one moral value—scientific truth—since any ethics not based on realism and "facing the facts" is an immoral form of self-delusion. Monod's notion of truth is narrow and reductionistic, since the scientific method is only one way of arriving at truth, but he is correct in saying that the need to know the truth is the deepest need of human nature on which all morality depends. If a person's real needs are not known to him or her, this person cannot develop a means-ends ethics. This does not mean that the only value of truth is its practical use as a guide to living; truth is also something enjoyable in itself, as even the pragmatic Dewey (1920) admitted.

This value of truth, both as practical and as something enjoyable in itself, has been emphasized in the *Universal Declaration of Human Rights* (United Nations, 1948):

> Article 18: Everyone has the right to freedom of thought, conscience, and religion; this right includes freedom to change his religion or belief, and freedom, either alone or in community with others and in public or private, to manifest his religion or belief in teaching, practice, worship, and observance.

Christian moral theology also has insisted on the fundamental character of truth for all other values. The deepest and most profound truth is the truth of faith found in Jesus Christ and in his teaching and life, which alone can give true freedom (1 Jn 5:1-12). Catholic Christianity, however, has always believed that this faith by no means exempts the Christian from also seeking truth through human reason and science. Critics are inclined to say, "You Catholics talk a lot about reason and natural law in ethical matters, but when it comes right down to it, you really rely only on the dogmas of the Church. Your use of reason is merely a rationalization of what you believe by blind faith." The only answer Catholics can give to this is to acknowledge responsibility as Christians to be honest and faithful *both* to the light of faith and to the light of reason and to make the intellectual effort to bring these two sources of knowledge into an authentic harmony with each other. To sacrifice one to the other is itself unethical because it betrays the truth, whatever its source.

Christians, however, are not really in a different situation in this matter than are adherents of other religions, including Marxism and humanism. As 1.3

shows, all human beings have some form of religion or equivalent philosophy of life, a world view and a system of values that rests ultimately on certain basic convictions not accepted by adherents to a different system. Thus Monod, as a humanist, has a basic conviction in the power of science that many others would not accept without qualification (Polyani, 1964). This conviction is the foundation of Monod's philosophy of life. Christian faith rests on other basic convictions. A pluralistic world ought to respect these fundamental differences and be willing to work through ecumenical dialogue to achieve a greater consensus. Everyone ought to be willing to argue for his or her basic convictions, and Christians surely have no need to be ashamed of theirs, since the Christian world view is unquestionably one of the major ethical systems of human history and has earned a right to be heard in any ethical discussion.

This commitment to truth is expressed in the *Principle of Well-Formed Conscience*, which is developed at length in 3.4. The formulation is repeated here:

To attain the true goals of human life by responsible actions, in every free decision involving an ethical question, people are morally obliged to:

1. *inform themselves as fully as practically possible about both the facts and the ethical norms.*
2. *Form a morally certain judgment of conscience on the basis of this information.*
3. *Act according to this well-formed conscience.*
4. *Accept responsibility for their actions.*

Note that this principle is founded on a basic human need, namely, the need for truth as one of the necessary goals of human life. This need is both for truth for its own sake (ultimately the knowledge of God and created persons) and for practical truth, a guide to that goal. Practical truth includes the arts and applied sciences, of which medicine is both a science and an art; however, technological truths only guide persons to goals freely chosen, and these goals must be harmonized with ultimate or life goals. For example, medicine guides the physician in treating a patient; however, whether to treat a dying patient with the latest, complex technology becomes an ethical question, a question of conscience, and conscience must be guided by this principle of prudence.

The specifically Christian understanding of the Principle of Well-Formed Conscience derives from the information required to act as a Christian (Delhaye, 1968). Christians need whatever human information is available from personal and social experience and from the sciences; in view of the Christian goal of life, however, they must also turn to the Word of God in Christ for the model. Christ is known both in his historical reality and in his actual presence in the world today only in the Christian community, its Scriptures, its tradition, its official pastors in their teaching role, and its sacraments as they are experienced in the actual life and prayer of individual Christians. Consequently, all these sources of information must be sought and listened to if this principle is to have a full Christian application.

Principle of Free and Informed Consent

The *Principle of Free and Informed Consent* plays a primary role in bioethical discussions today. It can be stated as follows:

To protect the basic need of every human person for healthcare and the primary responsibility of each person for his or her own healthcare, no physical or psychological therapy may be administered without the free and informed consent of the patient or, if the patient is incompetent, of his or her legitimate guardian acting for the patient's benefit and, as far as possible, in accordance with his or her known and reasonable wishes.

This principle is simply a corollary of the Principle of Well-Formed Conscience. If, as a physician or nurse, I must act according to my own informed conscience, it is unethical for me to ask *other* persons to cooperate with me or to permit me to act on them unless I share with them the relevant information required for both of us to decide, each according to our own consciences, whether such an act is ethical. Thus I cannot ask for the consent of another unless I have helped that person to have an informed conscience and unless I believe him or her to be free to act on it. If, however, the person is incompetent, I must decide for this person if I am his or her legitimate guardian or, if I am not, I must obtain the free and informed consent of that guardian before I attempt therapy. The theological basis for this principle, therefore, is the same as for the Principle of Well-Formed Conscience.

The Principle of Free and Informed Consent is not always easy to apply, and its meaning is developed in more detail in the next chapter (see 9.5) in connection with research involving human subjects.

Principle of Moral Discrimination

Moral beings thoughtfully and freely choose what to do or not to do in view of the life goal to which they are committed and its subordinate goals determined by basic human needs. Most people have a rather vague understanding of what the central purpose in their lives may be, and they often act impulsively and inconsistently, obscuring the plan and unity of their lives. Jesus spoke of people as "wandering sheep" (Mk 6:34; Lk 15:4-7) whose lives seem without purpose or plan. In every person's life, however, a fundamental commitment is evident, shaping every important decision. Thus it is often said of a physician or nurse, "There is someone who really cares about people, and it shows in everything he or she does in both private and professional life," or "That one may be an expert professional but is a selfish person who is always acting for personal advancement or money." This fundamental commitment (or "fundamental option" as many moralists call it today) (E. Cooper, 1972; Hart, 1970; McInerny, 1987) is the foundation of all morality. Jesus said, "Seek first the Kingdom of God" (Mt 6:33). Morality is thus first a matter of fundamental commitment or *intention of the ultimate end*, that is, the general intention that gives unity and pattern to one's whole life.

The Bible indicates in many places (e.g., Ps 1; Dt 30:15-20; Pr 1-9; Rm 8:1-3) that ultimately there are only two life commitments: "wisdom" and "folly." McDonagh (1979) has characterized these as the "open way" and the "closed way." People committed to the open way accept the truth whenever it confronts them and seek to understand themselves and all of reality, and then they act in accordance with truth, constantly widening and deepening their love of all persons and things. Whoever honestly pursues this open way is moving toward the light, since it is God who is drawing that person to himself.

The closed way is what the Scriptures frequently refer to as "idolatry," commitment to a false god of darkness and hatred who turns out to be simply a symbol of the false self as it contracts on itself and feeds on itself, locked up in the prison of its own prejudices, illusions, and hatreds. This false self seeks to dominate and use all other persons and things for itself. Although this evil way is focused on the idol of the self, this is not the true human self made in God's image, but a corrupted self. Those who seek the open way seem to lose themselves, but they find their true selves made by God for himself (Mk 8:35).

Thus physicians and nurses committed to the open way of life are always growing as persons and professionals, always widening their interests and concerns, and always fulfilling themselves by giving to others and receiving from others with humility and gratitude. Physicians and nurses committed to a closed way of life, however, are always contracting more and more into a selfish world, preoccupied with status and power, hedged in by prejudice, pride, and fear of competition, and deadened by pessimism, cynicism, and apathy.

The term *mortal sin* so familiar to Catholics really refers to this commitment to a closed, selfish, idolatrous life. The choice of such a life is not usually made, without a long preceding process of alienation from God and neighbor. Little by little, through a thousand acts of petty selfishness, indifference to others, superficial thinking, vanity, and deception, persons finally come to the breaking point at which they decide to serve themselves rather than to serve God and neighbor. Jesus said, "No one can serve two masters. He will either hate the first and love the second, or treat the first with respect and the second with scorn. You cannot be the slave both of God and of money" (Mt 6:24). "Money" here means any idol, that is, the closed self.

Actions that do not do serious harm to oneself or others but that still are harmful and, if they are not remedied, may soon turn into a pattern of behavior leading to mortal sin, are called *venial sins*. Morally speaking, they are totally different from mortal sin because they do not change the fundamental orientation of a person's life as does mortal sin, but they confuse and weaken movement toward one's true goals and can finally end in a mortally sinful break with that commitment. They might be compared to the many little quarrels, insensitivities, and neglects that are part of the married lives of most people. If a couple admit these faults and try to remedy them by positive acts of love, such acts and omissions may not harm the marriage greatly. If they are passed over, however, these small problems gradually cool love, widening the distance and lack of communication between the couple, until at last the marriage is broken by rejection and the death of love.

Thus falling into mortal sin is a process, but it is also a crucial event. The breaking point comes when a person breaks off the commitment to openness toward God and withdraws into the closed self. Such an act of mortal sin can take place either *explicitly* by a deliberate turning away from a true goal in life, from God or at least from that search for the Ultimate Good, or it can take place *implicitly* when a person chooses to do something that he or she knows to be seriously contradictory to that commitment. "If any one says: 'My love is fixed on God,' and hates his brother, he is a liar" (1 Jn 4:20). One cannot be open to God, to light, to love, to truth, and at the same time do serious harm either to a neighbor or to one's true self. Thus mortal sins are acts that explicitly turn people from their true end, from the open way of life, or acts that do so implicitly by contradicting that way of life and what it implies. The healthcare professional who claims to be religious or respectable, but who knowingly and deliberately seriously neglects or misuses professional skill or status so that others are harmed or the professional's own development as a person is impaired, commits mortal sin and makes a commitment to idolatrous goals in life.

Because people often act unthinkingly or are too often influenced by emotion or lack of needed information, they may act with good intention and yet do much harm. Although the very root of morality is *subjective* intention or goodwill, this is not sufficient to attain a person's goals unless it includes the effort to make one's actions *objectively* effective (Aquinas' *Summa Theologiae*, I-II, 20). A physician who wants to heal a patient, but who keeps making mistakes in diagnosis and treatment, deserves credit for goodwill, but the patient will not be any the better for it. Moreover, unless physicians make an effort to correct their mistakes, they cannot really claim to have goodwill at all. Thus morally good actions are first to be judged on good *intention*, but they must also be judged objectively. All the good intentions in the world do not save people from the bad consequences of objectively wrong actions, nor from the responsibility of repairing these wrongs, which stand in the way of achieving true human goals. Thus moral rightness or wrongness is constituted by the *relation* between a particular action and this true goal of human living, as this relation is perceived and freely intended by a human person.

Relation of Act to Goal

This relation between action and goal, however, is not simple; it is conditioned in several ways, as mentioned in Chapter 7, but these are illustrated here in more detail as they apply to medical-moral decisions. First, goals cannot be reached simply by a general intention but only by taking definite steps. As the saying goes, "If you will the end, you must also will the means." It is not enough to intend to love God, unless as St. James says, this love expresses itself in concrete acts of care for a neighbor (Jm 2:14-17). Thus each particular act specifies the remote and general intention by a proximate and specific intention called the act's *moral object* or *purpose*. Note that this proximate intention is not different from the general intention, but rather a further, concrete determination of it: I love God by bandaging this patient's wound.

181

Second, a moral object has both a form and a content. The moral form of the act of bandaging wounds is the intention to help patients regain health through a particular healing procedure; the content of the act, however, is the therapeutic procedure itself, considered as a process of cleansing, medicating, bandaging, and so forth that has an intrinsic teleology, that is, determined effects. At this point, medical facts and moral values come together to form a single act, which is at the same time a physical, biological, and psychological process and also a moral act invested with human meaning. It is a medical act, but it is also a moral act expressed by the term *care*, which implies not merely technical skill, but also human personal concern for the patient.

How can facts and values meet in this way? It is because the act of healthcare, taken in its biological and psychological aspects, already has values, or actions that are harmful or beneficial to the human organism. The bandaging process is helpful to the human organism because it furthers the natural processes within the organism itself toward health and optimal functioning. There may also be negative values (disvalues), since the bandage may impede circulation and so forth. However, if the bandaging is essentially helpful to nature, a professional faced with the decision of whether to bandage or not to bandage can ethically decide to do so. When this decision is made in view of the patient's good and the professional's commitment to caring for the patient, then this merely biological and technical act, simple as it is, becomes a moral act with a moral object. Thus, in any moral object, one can distinguish the content of the act (technically referred to as the *physical* or *nonmoral* object) and the specific moral purpose that makes the physical act into a moral act (*finis operis*) (Pellegrino and Thomasma, 1988).

Third, specific moral acts are always performed in a context or situation; for example, the act of bandaging is frequently performed by a nurse in a hospital or clinic during daytime hours. As long as the situation is an ordinary or normal one, the moral character of an action is not modified. Sometimes, however, unusual features of the situation may be morally significant; for example, if the nurse bandages the wound of a fugitive criminal without reporting him, she may find herself an accomplice to his crime. Thus, in determining the morality of an action, once the specific moral object is known (finis operis), any special circumstances that might modify the action's moral significance must also be determined. These circumstances can be of place, time, or person (as in the example just cited). They can also be a matter of *intention* when, in addition to the specific intention of the act (finis operis), the agent has some additional and special motive. For example, the nurse may bandage the patient not only to help the patient, but also to teach an aide how to perform the procedure. Such an intention is a *circumstantial* intention (*finis operantis*).

Note that the term *intention* has now been used in three different senses: (1) the general intention of a person's life goal (fundamental option), including the harmonious satisfaction of basic human needs; (2) a person's specific intention manifested in this particular moral act as a means to that goal (finis operis); and (3) possible additional motives extrinsic to the action performed (finis operantis).

The special circumstance of an action that is of itself morally wrong can make it worse; for example, it is usually more irresponsible for a nurse to neglect a child patient than to neglect an adult. If the action is good, circumstances can make it better; for example, a nurse deserves more credit for attention to a difficult patient. But can circumstances make a bad act good? Catholic moral theology has traditionally held that if a moral object in its own specific intention is morally wrong (intrinsically evil), it cannot then be made morally good by any special circumstance (John Paul II, 1984a). For example, killing a suffering patient, because the act kills an innocent person, can never be morally justified, no matter what the special circumstances of the patient (age, member of one's family, degree of suffering, etc.) or the good intention of the agent (e.g., intention to end the patient's pain). Recently, proportionalists have wondered whether this traditional teaching requires revision. Chapter 7, however, proposed prudential personalism, rather than proportionalism, as the type of revision that better advances moral sensitivity without abandoning the past achievements of classical moral theology.

Moral Discernment

How, then, following the methodology of prudential personalism, does one discriminate between moral and immoral actions? Two basic questions must be asked of oneself and others:

1. Does it *directly* alienate me from my authentic life goal of loving God above all and my neighbor as myself?
2. Does it *indirectly* alienate me from that goal by neglecting or rejecting some intermediate goal necessary to attain that ultimate goal?

If either is the case, the action is a *mortal* sin. If it is evil but falls short of such radical rejection either (1) because the action is not serious in the injury it does or (2) because a person does not consent to it fully and deliberately, the action is a *venial* sin; that is, it hinders full movement toward the goal but is not contradictory to it.

Determining whether any given human act is essentially contradictory to the true ends of human living so as to be intrinsically evil is not a simple process. One should never be quick to conclude that any act is mortally evil or to generalize judgment in the form of absolute norms. The possibility that such a norm prevails is real, however, and in some cases it is obviously realized. Furthermore, when such absolute norms have become an accepted part of the standards of culture or of the Church's ordinary teaching, Christians ought to consider them prima facie binding in conscience unless careful study shows they need modification or clarification.

This is the same caution that is observed by the sanely conservative physician who knows that professional responsibility to the patient requires the use of well-tested treatments and not merely experimental ones. Those who are willing to base their lives or to counsel others to base their lives on some "new morality" must justify such modification of traditional norms with strong, critically tested arguments. At the same time, persons also fail in their obligation to inform their consciences when they close their eyes to new suggestions about how to improve their previous moral understanding. Being blind to new thought may be a sin against the light and the Spirit, a deadly sin indeed.

The Principle of Well-Formed Conscience is admitted, although with varying interpretations, by all the ethical methodologies discussed in Chapter 7. These different interpretations must be made explicit if the principle is to serve as a practical guide in decision making. This can be done for prudential personalism by the following formulation of the *Principle of Moral Discernment*. Proportionalists have to substitute for this the Principle of Proportion, utilitarians their Principle of Maximum Utility, and so on.

> *To make a conscientious ethical decision, one must do the following:*
> 1. *Proceed on the basis of a fundamental commitment to God and the authentic dignity of human persons, including onself.*
> 2. *Among possible actions that might seem to be means of fulfilling that commitment, exclude any that are intrinsically contradictory to that commitment.*
> 3. *Also consider how one's own motives and other circumstances may contribute to or nullify the effectiveness of the other possible actions as means to fulfill one's fundamental commitment.*
> 4. *Among the possible means not excluded or nullified, select one most likely to fulfill that commitment, and act on it.*

The specifically Christian understanding of this principle derives from the revelation in Christ that the goal of human life is to share in the life of the Father, Son, and Holy Spirit (Mt 11:25-30; Lk 10:22; 1 Jn 1:3). Every moral choice must be guided by a longing to reach this goal, which absolutely excludes mortal sin, that is, acts against God or neighbor that would turn a person away from that goal directly. All intelligent freedom must be used to facilitate this journey to God for ourselves and others. In this pursuit, we must use our own creativity to the fullest, but we must also respect the creative wisdom of God, which has made us what we are and which guides us providentially in the concrete circumstances of our lives. In this we imitate Jesus, who remained faithful in all his actions to the call his Father gave him, even in the historical situation of his times and under the shadow of the cross.

Principle of Double Effect

As already noted, a good moral act may involve not only values, but also disvalues. Persons are often puzzled by the undesirable side effects of actions they feel morally obliged to do. The moralists of the proportionalist school discussed in Chapter 7 use this principle to handle all such cases that offer moral conflict. For them an action is morally good when the agent acts so as to maximize values and minimize disvalues (C. Curran, 1975; Knauer, 1967; McCormick, 1981). Thus proportionalists reduce many moral decisions to "choosing the lesser evil" (which classical moral theology never approved but merely tolerated, while still condemning "the lesser evil" as sinful) in the many moral dilemmas that arise in lives today. They claim, however, they are not proposing that persons do moral evil, but rather that persons are morally obliged to choose the alternative that involves the lesser disvalues (premoral evils).

As already explained, such considerations, although not invalid, are insufficient moral guides. A person must not only avoid causing more harm than benefit by an action, but also must refuse to do something that is intrinsically immoral, even if in some circumstances it seems that this action may lead to greater benefit than harm, or that refusing to do it may lead to greater harm than benefit. Ultimately, intrinisically immoral actions, because they give a wrong basic orientation to one's course of action, in the long run will lead to greater evil than good, no matter how attractive and beneficial they may appear in the short run. For example, a lie undermines the trust on which a good relation between human beings rests and thus corrupts the whole relation, with at least the risk of harmful long-range consequences.

It might seem, therefore, that one should never perform any action for which one foresees harmful results but should insist on performing only those actions that have only good consequences. Otherwise, one would seem to be responsible for the harm and to have at least partially done evil as a means to a good end. This position of *moral purism* or *rigorism* (or *tutorism*; i.e., doing only what is morally safe), however, is no sounder than proportionalism because it makes action almost impossible in a world where even the best actions have some harmful results. Since refusal to act is itself often a neglect of duty, this kind of purism actually leads to sins of omission or withdrawal from one's responsibilities.

Consequently, moralists in the nineteenth century (Connery, 1981), relying on the formulation of the Principle of Moral Discrimination explained before, also formulated the *Principle of Double Effect* as a more precise way of applying the former principle to conflict cases (R. Gillon, 1986a; Mangan, 1949). It is usually stated in such terms as follow (F. Connell, 1968):

> *To form a good conscience when an act is foreseen to have both beneficial and harmful consequences, the following conditions should be met:*
> 1. *The* directly *intended object of the act must not be intrinsically contradictory to one's fundamental commitment to God and neighbor (including onself).*
> 2. *The intention of the agent must be to achieve the beneficial effects and to avoid the harmful as far as possible (i.e., must only* indirectly *intend the harm).*
> 3. *The foreseen beneficial effects must be equal to or greater than the foreseen harmful effects.*
> 4. *The beneficial effects must follow from the action at least as immediately as do the harmful effects.*

The first of these conditions follows directly from the Principle of Moral Discrimination, as formulated by prudential personalism, but is rejected by consequentialists, situationists, utilitarians, and proportionalists. Proportionalists contend that the third condition, which is their Principle of Proportion, is the only necessary condition. For prudential personalism, however, the first condition is essential and the second condition is also needed to avoid moral purism, since these recognize that, to do good directly, people are sometimes indirectly responsible for some harmful effects. Connery (1981) points out that the purpose of both the third and fourth conditions is to guarantee the first two, since unless one refuses to perform an action foreseen as doing more harm than good (third condition) or judged to be the use of an immoral means to a moral end (fourth condition), one cannot honestly claim to be intending the harmful side effects only indirectly. Moreover, Connery shows that the third condition does not require that difficult and perhaps impossible detailed weighing of values and disvalues demanded by proportionalism, but only the assurance that we are not obviously doing more harm than is justified by the good we directly intend.

For example, when a physician decides to remove a cancerous but gravid uterus, he or she must directly intend to save the mother's life and may only indirectly intend to abort the child. The physician is not called on to weigh the value of one life against another in terms of every possible consequence, but only to decide if he or she is directly intending a good that is comparable to the harm the physician knows will also result. Unless this rough proportion exsits, the physician cannot honestly say that he or she only indirectly intends the harm to the child; and if the physician does intend harm directly, he or she is violating both the first and the second conditions.

The purpose of the fourth condition is to exclude the use of an evil means to achieve a good end, since such action would also violate the first requirement. This final condition is not always easy to verify. Because of these difficulties, there have been several recent attempts to reformulate it. The suggestion that seems the most persuasive is made by Grisez (1970b) who points out:

> ...The ambiguity of ambiguous actions can be of two kinds. In one type the destructive aspect of the action is the means by which the positive aspect is realized. In the second the two aspects are really inseparably linked in one action; the positive aspect does not produce the destructive, nor does the destructive produce the positive; the act embraces both results directly (p. 140).

Grisez cites as an example of the first condition the traditional practice of castrating boy sopranos for the purpose of producing beautiful music. In this case the act of mutilation is one act (a means) intended for the sake of another distinct act (making music). This is doing evil for a good purpose, because the intention of the first act is to mutilate (an evil), although the intention of the second act is to make music (a good). On the other hand, the second type of ambiguous action is illustrated by castration of a boy to prevent the spread of cancer. In this case only one indivisible act is intended, namely, an act of healing (good) which, however, contains two effects (one good, one bad) inseparably connected. The essential ethical difference between the two cases is that in the second the *evil* need not be intended but only permitted (indirectly intended), whereas in the first case the agent *must* directly intend the evil (otherwise the act would never be performed), although the agent intends it only as a means and not an end.

It might seem that Grisez's suggestion is itself ambiguous in application, since it requires deciding when an act is really indivisible. Grisez shows, however, that although in given cases the answer is not always obvious, it can be worked out objectively by analyzing the actual free choices open to an agent. The advantage of this new formulation is that it no longer forces consideration only of the order of physical causality in an act (i.e., whether in a procedure the mutilation of the body or the healing follows directly from the surgical incision), but takes this physical order along with the moral intention that gives unity to all the act's physical elements.

Charles Curran (1975) has also reviewed the various new views on double effect and grants that Grisez's formulation has much to commend it. He prefers, however, the route taken by the Principle of Proportion theorists, who have reduced the Principle of Double Effect, first to "commensurate reason" (Knauer, 1967) and then to the Principle of Proportion. We, on the contrary, believe the Principle of Double Effect should be retained, but its importance should not be exaggerated. It is only a corollary of the more fundamental Principle of Moral Discrimination. Usually double effect comes into play as a way of discovering whether an act that is clearly good in intention is in fact an excuse for the use of a morally evil means. When a prudent examination of a course of action does not reveal this lack of integrity, one has every right to take the benefit of the doubt and judge on the basis of the good practical intention. Thus medical ethics would begin with the assumption that, if the professional intends the patient's good and undertakes the most effective therapy known medically to achieve this good, the procedure is ethical *unless* clear reasons show this involves *demonstrably* evil means. The Principle of Double Effect, either in its previous form or in its reformulation by Grisez, suggests some tests that can be applied; ultimately, however, the discrimination remains prudential, a prudence that ordinarily requires reinforcement by professional and community consensus or legitimate moral authority. Thus the Principle of Double Effect is not a legalistic formula, but rather is helpful in discerning when an action is morally acceptable, even though the action may involve an effect that would be immoral if the effect were directly intended.

The essential point to grasp in understanding double effect is that one must always intend to do only what is *morally* good; the evil side effects must be *physical*, not moral, evils (not intended and would be avoided if possible), or they must be evil acts of *other agents* that one cannot prevent.

The specifically Christian understanding of this Principle of Double Effect arises from the biblical understanding of the origin of evil in the world, which differs greatly from the Buddhist idea that evil is an illusion, or the secular humanist idea that evil is an inevitable part of evolutionary progress (Bowker, 1970). Christians believe that they, as the community of the human race and in some measure as individuals, have rebelled against God's loving will for them and chosen to "know good and evil" (Gn 3:4), that is, to live in an ambiguous world where good and evil are mixed confusedly. To find a straight path through such a world is impossible without the guidance of Christ and the Holy Spirit he has sent. This also requires people to use their intelligence to the fullest, however, to separate what is essentially good and accidentally evil from what is essentially evil and accidentally good. Jesus calls on Christians to be "cunning as serpents, yet harmless as doves" (Mt 10:16) and rebukes the witless imprudence of some of his followers (Lk 16:8).

Principle of Legitimate Cooperation

From what has been said, it follows that people must be careful not to cooperate in or promote the actions of others when these acts are immoral (G. Kelly, 1958). Obviously, it is immoral to cooperate with an evil action by suicide because one wishes to be rid of the burden of a relative, although one would never actually murder the relative directly. To actually intend the evil purpose is *formal cooperation*, no matter how small one's share in the actual physical execution. Advising, counseling, promoting, or condoning an evil action, even when sometimes done merely by being silent when one has a duty to speak up or express an opinion, is formal cooperation because such actions signify agreement with evil.

Material cooperation, on the other hand, is any type of cooperation in which one does *not intend* the evil effects, but only the good. When such material cooperation is *immediate* (e.g., nurses who assist physicians to perform an abortion, which they personally disapprove), it amounts to the same as formal cooperation because it is a direct contribution to an evil act in which the cooperator shares the responsibility for the act (Burtchaell, 1988; Merkelbach, 1959). On the other hand, *mediate* material cooperation, which can be proximate or remote, under certain conditions is sometimes justified and even necessary. These conditions are as follows (McFadden, 1967).

First, the more remote the cooperation, the easier it is to justify. For example, the manufacture of morphine is remote from drug abuse because morphine also has important and legitimate medical uses. However, the sale of morphine is closer to actual abuse and must be carefully regulated to ensure that it is put only to legitimate uses.

Second, the good achieved by the cooperation must outweigh the contribution of the cooperator to the evil and the degree of evil. Thus persons whose livelihoods depend on a job (because it is impossible or difficult to get another similar job) are justified in working for certain institutions where abortion is performed, provided they disapprove and do not immediately cooperate with an abortion.

In such institutions there are many different degrees of cooperative proximity, ranging from the nurses whose cooperation is very proximate to the janitor of the building whose cooperation is very remote. All have the moral responsibility of deciding, however, if sufficient reason exsits to justify their material cooperation with the destruction of innocent persons, just as the same responsibility rests on participants in a war effort in which obliteration bombing of noncombatants is regularly employed.

When this justification exists, it is only because (1) the cooperation is not formal (the person does not want the abortion and would try to prevent it if possible), (2) the material cooperation is mediate because most of the person's work does not contribute to the abortion (except if the institution is an abortion clinic where all or most of the work is abortion related), and (3) the loss of a job is a serious matter.

Third, the evil effects of scandal, that is, the bad example that can be set, must be weighed. Even the appearance of cooperation with evil helps this evil to continue. The Christian has a serious duty to take a stand against destructive actions and to share in them as little as possible. Thus Christians should take as active a part as is practically possible in protesting against injustices at institutions in which they work or from which they benefit. Catholic hospitals in particular have the responsibility to consider the type of example they set in a community even by appearing to condone injustices (see Chapter 9 for more specific norms of cooperation in regard to abortion).

If persons refused even remote material cooperation in the affairs of a community, they would also sin by *omission*, since doing good also would become impossible. A Christian purist would be unable to act as a citizen or to share in any institution because every government, human institution, and even or-ganized religion commit some evil and unjust acts. By belonging to such an organization, a person somewhat cooperates with these evils. People have a moral obligation to belong to social institutions, however, since only through them can legitimate human needs be served.

Charles Curran (1975) has shown how the Second Vatican Council, in the *Declaration on Religious Liberty* (1965b), advanced Catholic moral thinking by permitting a degree of cooperation by Catholics with non-Catholics in their religious activities that moralists had previously considered unjustifiable. In part the Second Vatican Council grounded this on a more benign view of the religious truth found in such practices, but also on the respect due to the consciences of others, even when these others may be in error. Thus a person may sometimes cooperate with other *persons* out of respect for their right to act according to their conscience, even when one cannot in good conscience cooperate with their *acts as such*. Curran points out that if this type of cooperation is permitted in so sacred a matter as religious worship, it must also be permissible in lesser matters, such as many of those that medical ethics treats. We would agree with this important observation but emphasize that it would not justify immediate cooperation in intrinsically wrong acts (e.g., suicide), especially when they involve the rights of a third party (e.g., abortion), no more than such cooperation would be permitted in religious matters that involve intrinsically wrong acts (e.g., polygamy, ritual murder).

Thus the *Principle of Legitimate Cooperation* is nothing more than an application of the Principle of Double Effect to the situation where an act is performed by more than one person with different purposes. It can be formulated as follows:

To achieve a well-formed conscience, one should always judge it unethical to cooperate formally with an immoral act (i.e., directly to intend the evil act itself), but one may sometimes judge it to be an ethical duty to cooperate materially with an immoral act (i.e., only indirectly intending its harmful consequences) when only in this way can a greater harm be prevented, provided (1) that the cooperation is not immediate and (2) that the degree of cooperation and the danger of scandal are taken into account.

Note that in this case, as in the Principle of Double Effect, the reason that a proportion between benefit and harm is required is to ensure that the evil effect is not directly intended, since that would render one's own act of cooperation morally evil. The moral acceptability of the action does not result from weighing good and evil, but rather from judging one's intention in regard to the evil effect and how intimately one participates in the action that brings about the evil effect.

Principle of Professional Communication

Truth cannot be arrived at simply by individual effort. No single person has all the information needed for good decisions, nor can one arrive at truth except by a social effort. Every human institution, particularly every modern healthcare institution, is an enormously complex system of *information*. The moment a patient enters, a process of history taking, of performing tests, of filling out records, of keeping charts, and so forth begins. Furthermore, an endless amount of research contained in the medical library and in the brains of a network of technologists and specialists begins to be applied to the process of diagnosis and prescription for the patient's treatment. Moreover, because the institution is an administrative network of cooperating personnel, problems of interpersonal relations arise among the staff and the patients themselves.

This whole network essentially depends on good *communication*, which is impossible without (1) trust, (2) contact among the people who have information, (3) clear articulation and expression of information, and (4) continuous feedback by which failures in communication can be corrected. Modern communication theory has shown that this work of communication depends first on good emotional relations among the communicators, since emotional conflict is a powerful barrier to communication and brings into play all sorts of uncontrollable, unconscious factors. It thus becomes a serious moral duty in every institution to promote an emotional openness among both the staff and the patients.

Since the application of the *Principle of Professional Communication* is discussed in detail in 5.2, the principle need only be repeated here:

To fulfill their obligations to serve patients, healthcare professionals have the responsibility:
  1. *To strive to establish and preserve trust at both the emotional and rational levels.*
  2. *To share the information they possess that is legitimately needed by others in order to have an informed conscience.*
  3. *To refrain from lying or giving misinformation.*
  4. *To keep secret information that is not legitimately needed by others, but that if revealed might either harm the patient or others or destroy trust.*

190

Note that this principle is also founded in the basic human need for truth. If human beings cannot trust one another for the information they must use to guide their lives, this need cannot be satisfied. Since the Principle of Informed Conscience requires that persons obtain from others, especially from expert professionals, whatever needed knowledge cannot be achieved by themselves, persons have a right to true and relevant professional advice.

The Christian specification of this principle arises from the Christian understanding of trust and forgiveness. Jesus, in the case of Nicodemus (Jn 3:1-21), the Samaritan woman (Jn 4:1-42), the adulterous woman (Jn 8:1-11), and elsewhere, is represented as dealing with individuals in a way that won their trust and their confidence in his full acceptance of them even in their sinfulness. The Church, in its sacrament of reconciliation, has established the confessional seal of total confidentiality so that people might feel free to unburden themselves not merely of physical and psychological problems but of their real guilt. For the Christian, therefore, professional confidentiality is not only professional; it expresses respect for the dignity of the human being, whom only God has a right to judge (Mt 7:1-5).

8.3   NORMS OF CHRISTIAN LOVE

Motivation

The norms just listed that relate directly to the knowing, reasoning, and judging process in decision making are all rooted in one of the basic human needs, the need for truth. Next come the norms that relate more to affective *motivation*, since motivation powerfully influences judgment for good or ill. Such motivation has both a structural, or relational, aspect and a dynamic, or processive, aspect. The structural aspect involves the interpersonal relations that bind persons together in community, and the ethical norms that govern these relations can rightly be called norms of love, as distinguished from the norms of conscience just discussed.

Love means not only a feeling, but also the practical *will* that leads one person to be concerned about another person and that person's true needs. Furthermore, love motivates people to help others fulfill these needs by sharing with another the values they themselves enjoy.

In any Christian ethics, the fundamental truth is that there is a Triune God and that "God is love" (1 Jn 4:8). God loves us not because he has first needed our love, but because his love for us has made us lovable:

> In this way God's love was revealed to us: God sent his only Son into the world that we might have life through him. This is love: not that we have loved God, but that he loved us and sent his Son as an expiation for our sins....If we love one another, God remains in us and his love is brought to perfection in us (1 Jn 4:9-10, 12).

The great theologians have all taught that the essence of the Christian life is the sharing by grace in this love of God, by which we love him and one another through the very same love by which he has created and redeemed us (Gilleman,

191

1961). God's love is thus a life-giving and healing activity, and the healthcare ministry is a work of love by which persons cooperate with God in giving life and healing sickness. Love of God can never be merely sentimental because it is built on faith and on all the truths derived from human reason and science. Therefore the healthcare professional's love must be a love informed by the best available medical knowledge and skill.

Christian professionals know that God loves them and that whatever love professionals have is a share in this divine love. This must be shared in turn with others, not by a minimal performance of duties, but as a generous concern and realistic care for those in need. Under the pressures of daily work with its frustrations, however, this vision and realization of God's personal love as the source and motivation of that work can become very dim and can fade into a deadly routine. Jesus, the great physician, found the pressure of the sick so great that he, too, had to retire into a desert place to pray and to regain hope and strength.

> The whole town was gathered at the door, and he cured many who were sick with various diseases....Rising very early before dawn, he went off to a deserted place where he prayed (Mk 1:33-35).

Three particular norms help to define the content of Christian love: (1) every person must be valued as a unique, irreplaceable member of the human community (Principle of Human Dignity in Community); (2) every person must be encouraged to play a role in the common life and fully share its fruits (Principle of Common Good, Subsidiarity, and Functionalism); and (3) all persons must be helped to realize their full potential (Principle of Totality and Integrity). Previous chapters have developed these three principles. Here they are restated with some reflections on their specifically Christian understanding.

Principle of Human Dignity in Community

Although today the unique value of every human being is affirmed by all religions and philosophies of life and the inalienable rights of the person are guaranteed by the constitutions of most governments, these rights are silently contradicted by three trends that seem to characterize contemporary life:

1. Persons are swallowed up in totalitarian, bureaucratic institutions.
2. Persons who are unnecessary for the efficient operations of these institutions—women, the very young, the very old, uneducated and defective persons—are treated as nonpersons.
3. Even successful persons find their happiness not in sharing their lives with others but in private, individualistic satisfactions.

Section 1.5 shows how the right understanding of human personhood and mankind's essentially social nature can help overcome this contradiction. That section concludes with the following formulation of the *Principle of Human Dignity in Community*:

All ethical decisions (including those involved in healthcare) must aim at human dignity, that is, the maximal, integrated satisfaction of the innate and cultural needs of every human person, including his or her biological, psychological, ethical, and spiritual needs as a member of the world community and national communities.

This principle rests on a basic human need that must be satisfied to attain true happiness, namely, the need of every person for society, since it is only in community that this dignity is recognized and supported. Moreover, this principle not only states one basic need but includes all other basic needs whose satisfaction is required by a person's dignity. In short, human dignity in community sums up the true goal of human life: self-actualization in relation to God and neighbor.

The Christian specification of this principle comes from what Jesus Christ added to our understanding of ourselves as created by God in his own image to share his eternal Triune life in total personhood as bodily and resurrected beings. The community in question, therefore, is not only this temporal human community, but also the Kingdom of God into which even the least and most unworthy human beings are called.

Principle of the Common Good, Subsidiarity, and Functionalism

The Principle of Human Dignity in Community requires that various levels of responsibility be established within the community. Chapter 3 argues that the primary responsibility for health rests with the individual concerned and that the whole work of healthcare professionals must be conceived as a cooperative service to individuals in their personal search for health. At the same time, individuals are not self-sufficient in this search for health, and they can achieve health only with the help of the community. Consequently, it is also essential to give attention to the *Principle of the Common Good, Subsidiarity, and Functionalism*, which is discussed and formulated in 6.1 and repeated here:

Human communities exist only to promote and share the common good among all their members "from each according to ability, to each according to need" in such a way that:
  1. *Decision making rests* vertically *first with the person, then with the lower social levels, and* horizontally *with functional social units.*
  2. *The higher social units intervene only to supply the lower units what they cannot achieve by themselves, while at the same time working to make it easier in the future for lower units and individuals to satisfy these needs by their own efforts.*

This principle is only a way of spelling out the implications of the Principle of Human Dignity in Community by showing the respective roles of the individual, subgroups, and the total community, so that by this division of labor the dignity of every member of a community will be fully recognized and actively promoted. It has its source in our basic need to preserve life.

The Christian specification of this principle is given by St. Paul in 1 Corinthians (12-13), where he shows that the Christian understanding of the person based on Jesus' concern for "the little ones," "the least brethren" (Mk 9:33-37), must be the principle that governs the Church, conceived as the Body of Christ, ensouled by the Holy Spirit, which is the model for the coming Kingdom of God. The conception of social authority as service rather than domination (Mk 10:41-45) is at the heart of the Gospel.

Principle of Totality and Integrity

The *Principle of Totality and Integrity* is discussed in detail in 2.4 and is repeated here:

> *To promote human dignity in community, every person must develop, use, care for, and preserve all of his or her natural physical and psychic functions in such a way that:*
> 1. *Lower functions are never sacrificed except for the better functioning of the whole person and even then with an effort to compensate for this sacrifice.*
> 2. *The basic capacities that define human personhood are never sacrificed unless this is necessary to preserve life.*

This principle makes explicit another aspect of the Principle of Human Dignity in Community by requiring *self-respect* as well as respect for each other. Unless a person respects his or her own personal integrity, which includes one's natural bodily and psychic integrity, and seeks to preserve and perfect one's own gifts, that person cannot expect the community's respect. One of the effects to be feared from the current drive of some medical professionals to use technology to remake the human body by sterilizing it, making human beings into robots, or using them as guinea pigs, is a gradual erosion of respect for human life by society.

A certain analogy exists between this principle and the Principle of Subsidiarity, but only an analogy. Both reflect that the community and the person are complex systems of mutual interdependence of the whole and its parts. They differ radically, however, because the human person is a natural, primary unit in which the parts depend completely on the whole and exist for its sake. On the contrary, the community is a system made up of primary units, that is, human persons, and exists for their sake, not merely as isolated individuals but as sharers in a common, profoundly interrelated life. Fallaciously to turn this analogy into an univocal concept falls into the error of totalitarianism, which sacrifices the person to the communal state.

Human wholeness consists in the interdependence of higher and lower spiritual and bodily functions. Consequently, the lower functions cannot, without qualification, be sacrificed to the higher functions. This sacrifice might be to the advantage of the higher function but will not be to the good of the whole person, since that good is essentially complex, irreducible to the good of one part, even if that part is the highest.

To be a complete human being, therefore, is not merely to have the higher level of functions but to have the basic human functions in harmonious order. This order requires the subordination of the lower functions to the higher but also forbids their total sacrifice. This dependence also cannot be supplied simply by some means external to the person. For example, the ability to produce babies in test tubes does not justify the elimination of the reproductive power of human beings, nor does the possibility of intravenous feeding justify the elimination of the human alimentary system. Human perfection requires that people reproduce and eat in a human manner. Substitutions of external means of life may be justified temporarily out of necessity, but they do not improve on human nature.

Human body functions contribute to higher functions by supplying what is needed for physiological brain functions, but they also supply part of the human experience that is essential to human intelligence and freedom. Bodily feelings (movement, eating, sexuality, manipulation of the environment) develop one's self-awareness and relation to the community. Thus, if a child were conceived in a test tube, gestated in an artificial womb, and then raised in a laboratory, it is doubtful that he or she would have essential human experiences. The following norms pertain to human integrity:

1. Primarily, human health is not merely a matter of organs but of capacities to function humanly.
2. Generally speaking, any particular human functional capacity can be diminished when necessary for the good of the whole person, that is, so that the person can better exercise all other human functions.
3. Secondary functions can always be sacrificed to more basic ones. For example, a finger can be removed to the save the use of the hand because the capacity of action given by one finger is secondary in relation to the capacity given by the hand as a whole.
4. Primary or basic functional capacities, however, cannot be destroyed to promote even more important capacities, except when it is necessary to preserve the life of the whole person. For example, the capacity for emotional feeling must not be sacrificed to the power of scientific thinking. The capacity to think humanly cannot be sacrificed to think more technically.

Why, then, is it sometimes permissible to sacrifice one of these basic human capacities to preserve life? The reason is because, in this case, it is not a question of sacrificing one basic capacity for another, or for the better functioning of all other human capacities; it is a question of sacrificing one function so that the whole person can continue to function. Only in such extreme necessity does basic integrity yield to the good of the totality.

The great importance of the Principle of Totality and Integrity for medical ethics is that it establishes a norm for setting priorities when one human value must be subordinated to another. Chapter 2 works out this hierarchy of values in terms of the biological, psychological, social, and spiritual dimensions of human personality. The spiritual and social values have higher priority than the psychological and biological values, but such priority must not be understood *dualistically* as if the lower can simply be sacrificed to the higher values. Rather, in the human person there is a mutual interdependence of the body and the soul, the lower and the higher, as expressed in this Principle of Totality and Integrity.

This principle is rightly classified as one of the norms of love because it expresses the sense in which each person must have a proper love of *self*, without which the love of others is impossible and is a mere sentimental altruism. Its specific Christian character arises from the Incarnation, in which the Word of God became flesh, lived a bodily life, died, and was resurrected in the body transformed in glory. Consequently, Christian anthropology admits both a certain polarity in the human person because of a commonality with the animal and earthly world and a spiritual intelligence, freedom, and openness to God, but it opposes any form of dualism that would deny the dignity of Christ's human body, our resurrection, and persons are "temples of the Holy Spirit" (1 Co 3:16). This principle is well expressed by the writer of Ephesians (5:21-33) when he makes the analogy between Christ's love for humankind, a man's love for his wife, and one's love for one's own body.

8.4   NORMS OF CHRISTIAN HOPE

Having discussed the norms of faith and love, we now consider what theologians call the *eschatological* (looking to the final coming of Jesus Christ in the fully realized Kingdom of God) aspect of ethics. The human person and the human community are not structures of static relations but are dynamic—living, growing, developing, and evolving. This is why we have opted for a teleological, goal-directed, means-ends ethics. Furthermore, human goals are not always clearly envisioned in advance. As persons progress toward goals, these goals themselves take on a new look. They open out ahead of us as does the horizon of a landscape. Dewey (1920) made an important contribution to ethics by stressing this dynamic character of human goals, which is vividly experienced in American culture. Sometimes Christian thinkers have not taken this dynamism of life fully into account in their ethical discussions, yet Jesus centered his teaching on the theme of the Kingdom of God, a goal so mysterious that Jesus could express it only in terms of parables.

Recently, Christian theologians such as Jürgen Moltmann, Johannes Metz, and Wolfhart Pannenburg (Capps, 1970) have begun the construction of "theologies of hope" to bring out the many ways in which the Gospel is not merely a message about the superiority of heaven to earth, but a call to transform the earth as we journey heavenward. In this way they are finding areas of agreement between humanism and Marxism that also emphasize that to be human is to work for the future. Christian faith sees in every earthly event (even if that event is a crucifixion) a promise, an opportunity to be used, an invitation by a God of the future to share in building the future. In healthcare this sense of hope is the source of all healing, so that to be a healthcare professional is constantly to affirm the possibility of turning suffering into a victory over disease and death.

The question, What is the relation of hope to basic human needs? might receive the reply that it is founded on one's natural need to preserve one's life and to transmit that life to future generations. This is true because life cannot be preserved except through growth and creative activity, as well as our need for eternal life, a need awakened by Christ's resurrection.

Three ethical norms relate in a particular way to Christian hope. Our hope enables us not only to endure the sufferings of life courageously, but to grow as persons through this experience *(Principle of Growth through Suffering)*. Hope also enables Christians to entrust themselves to another in the lifelong commitment of marriage and to look forward to sharing this gift of life and love with a family and the future *(Principle of Personalized Sexuality)*. Moreover, not only do we have hopes for our families but for the whole of human society and the good earth, which is its home *(Principle of Stewardship and Creativity)*.

Principle of Growth through Suffering

In any teleological ethics, the ultimate criterion of morality is *happiness*. An action is morally good because it leads to happiness for persons. People sometimes fail to take into account, however, that in the actual conditions of human existence, not all that appears to be happiness is really so. The only authentic happiness is one that satisfies the whole person in his or her deepest and most ultimate needs and does so permanently. Thus it is possible for persons to think they are happy because they have achieved goals that are partial, superficial, and unstable. On television we witness the extravagant joy of winners in giveaway contests, knowing that such happiness will quickly fade and prove to have been utterly fake. It is also possible for persons to have really achieved goals that are encompassing, profound, and lasting and yet to be in a state of great suffering because circumstances do not yet permit the full experience of satisfaction. A great writer who has completed a masterpiece, a scientist who has achieved the discovery of a lifetime, or a statesman who has successfully carried through a great reform may feel exhausted, torn by inner conflict, and depressed. Such persons are to be envied, however, because ultimately they know they have reached the goal of their whole lives.

Thus, from an ethical point of view, it is essential to realize that true human happiness cannot be measured merely by pleasure, comfort, or freedom from anxiety, tension, and guilt. Normally, pleasure, comfort, and peace are the *consequences* and the *signs* of the achievement of authentic human goals and the fulfillment of true human needs, and thus they are good and desirable. They are *secondary* signs, however, not the proof or measure of real human achievement.

This is the reason why a hedonistic ethics is unrealistic. The person who judges a marriage, for example, by the satisfactory orgasms he or she has or by the lack of discomfort or tension in the marriage is making a serious mistake (Masters, Johnson, and Kolodny, 1986). These are normal signs of a satisfactory marriage relation and can be ethically desired and enjoyed, but they do not constitute the true core of a successful marriage, whose goal, as the Principle of Personalized Sexuality (discussed next) shows, requires the integration of pleasure with love and family living. Sometimes complete hedonistic satisfaction can exist in a marriage that is profoundly inadequate. Sometimes such satisfaction is defective, at least temporarily, in a truly sound marriage.

Medical professionals should recognize the truth of this principle. They know that pain is typically a sign of something wrong in the body and comfort a sign of health, but they also know that these are not fundamental. Pain is often an accompaniment of a healing process or even of necessary exercise. Pleasure and comfort may mask a serious disease. Thus physicians use pain and comfort as preliminary *signs* that lead to further investigation, but they know that such signs are not themselves healthy functioning nor proof of it. The psychiatrist knows the same concept. Patients may claim to be happy and comfortable, but unconsciously they may have deep psychological ills. On the other hand, anxiety and crisis may be a part of a healing or growth process. Psychological comfort and freedom from anxiety, however, can be *signs* of increasing health and as such are to be respected.

Relevant to ethical questions, therefore, people need to look at the *deeper* and more *total* needs and not to measure good and bad merely in terms of pleasure and pain. Short-range goals, that is, immediate satisfactions, have to yield ethically to long-range goals. Since the 1960s this concept has been criticized by some on the grounds that an ethics that is always delaying human satisfaction to the future while requiring sacrifices in the present is a pie-in-the-sky ethics and that emphasis also has to be given to the "now," to the need for pleasure and satisfaction in life.

In reply, we must admit, "Man cannot live without bodily pleasure," as Aquinas said (C. Williams, 1974). Pleasure is necessary for physical and mental health, for self-understanding (Marmer, 1988; Milhaven, 1977), and for the maintenance of determination and courage for long-run goals. Short-range pleasures and comforts must be present to a moderate degree, and strains and pains cannot be endured too long. Thus *leisure recreation* (the restoration of human powers through rest and satisfaction) is an essential need of human life, and *contemplation* ought to become a predominate quality of life (Pieper, 1964). A work ethic by which life is simply striving for a far-off, never-attained goal is a bad ethic (Adler, 1970). Authentic fulfillment, however, is not to be found by the maximization of sensual pleasure (as hedonism insists), but rather by intensifying deeper spiritual pleasures along with moderate sensual pleasures. Thus a good marriage depends not so much on increasing concern for the techniques of successful orgasm as it does on a shift from a relation based on sensual satisfaction to one based on deeper and more lasting satisfactions, real community of interests, and friendship. The effort to make sensual pleasure infinite is misplaced because it aims at an impossible goal and is bound to be frustrated. The only infinite goods are of the spiritual order. Sensual pleasure at best is a recreation that prepares us for continued effort to gain these spiritual goods, or it is simply a spontaneous, effortless, and unsought consequence of the achievement of higher goals.

It is also untrue that even spiritual goods have to be left to the next life. Christians have experienced that interior peace, and spiritual joy can be achieved, perhaps not perfectly, yet really and substantially here and now.

The healthcare profession, therefore, although its task is to relieve pain and restore health, should not regard pain and suffering as the greatest of evils. Rather, healthcare must help the patient use times of suffering as means of total personal growth. However, this requires people to face the mystery of suffering and death honestly.

People suffer in many ways. In a certain sense, there are as many ways of suffering as there are specialties within the field of healthcare. The types can be limited by categorizing suffering as physical or psychic. Although every physical or psychic suffering does not lead to death, suffering and death are connected intimately. Suffering, whether physical or psychic, is a violation or subversion of a person's bodily integrity or psychic stability. Death is the ultimate and complete violation or subversion of the human person (E. Becker, 1973; Bloom, 1987; Gatch, 1969; A. Mack, 1973).

The Christian faith, therefore, looks on suffering and death in two distinct ways. On the one hand, death is evil because it is the result of sin; on the other hand, it is a liberating and grace-filled experience if the proper motivation is present. These two ways are not contradictory; rather, they are complementary. Suffering and death, joined to the suffering and death of Jesus, represent not dissolution but growth, not punishment but fulfillment, not sadness but joy. God allows suffering and death to enable persons to live with Christ now and forever.

This mystery, because it is a mystery, can never be adequately formulated in words. For purposes of ethical discussion, however, the *Principle of Growth through Suffering* can be expressed as follows:

> *Just as bodily pleasure should be sought only as the fruit of the satisfaction of some basic need of the total human person, so suffering and even bodily death, when endured with courage, can and should be used to promote personal growth in both private and communal living.*

This principle, supremely exemplified in the cross of Christ, is rooted in the basic human need to preserve life, since people suffer only to achieve a renewed, purified, and enriched life.

Principle of Personalized Sexuality

> *The gift of sexuality must be used in keeping with its intrinsic, indivisible, specifically human teleology. It must be a loving, bodily, pleasurable expression of the complementary, permanent self-giving of a man and woman to each other which is open to fruition in the perpetuation and expansion of this personal communion through the family they responsibly beget and educate.*

This *Principle of Personalized Sexuality* is based on an understanding of sexuality as one of a person's basic aspects that must be developed (personalized) in ways consistent with an enhancing of human dignity (Sacred Congregation for the Doctrine of the Faith, 1975a). Because human sexual life is not merely a matter of animal instinct but requires free decisions, it sometimes raises serious ethical dilemmas. These problems might be considered under norms of love, but more properly they belong to the norms of hope because sexual love in a very special way looks toward the future. The survival of the human community, as well as the maturation and fulfillment of the individual, notably depends on the right use of the gift of sex.

Sexuality is a complex of many values that are generally recognized in every ethical theory, but whose interrelation and priority are the subject of much disagreement. These generally recognized values can be summarized in four major categories:

1. Sex is a search for sensual pleasure and satisfaction, releasing physical and psychic tensions.
2. More profoundly and personally, sex is a search for the completion of the human person through an intimate personal union of love expressed by bodily union. Ordinarily, it is also conceived as the complementarity of the male and female by one another so that each achieves a more complete humanity.
3. More broadly, sex is a social necessity for the procreation of children and their education in the family so as to expand the human community and guarantee its future beyond the death of individual members.
4. Ultimately, sex is a symbolic (sacramental) mystery, somehow revealing the cosmic order.

These values are usually recognized in all the great religions and philosophies of life and are protected and developed in every viable human culture.

In our modern culture, dominated by secular humanism, these values are generally thought to be combined in sexuality by sheer accident through the purposeless process of biological evolution (Harris, 1985). Consequently, many today argue that we are free to combine or separate these different values according to our own purposes and preferences. Thus, for secular humanists, it seems entirely reasonable sometimes to use sex purely for the sake of pleasure apart from any relation to love or family; sometimes to use it to reproduce (making babies in a test tube) without any reference to pleasure or love; and sometimes as an expression of unselfish love but without any relation to marriage or family (Kurtz, 1988).

Moreover, for secular humanists, if sex is a symbolic mystery, it is because love and sexual ecstasy are often considered the highest happiness in life, without which no one can be complete as a person. Consequently, many secular humanists believe sexual morality can be reduced to two fundamental norms: (1) laws or social attitudes that hinder human freedom to achieve these sexual values in ways the individual desires are unjust and oppressive, and (2) sexual behavior, at least among consenting adults, is entirely a private matter to be determined by personal choice, free from any moral guilt (Kurtz, 1983).

The Christian attitude toward sex agrees with that of secular humanism in recognizing these same four values of sexuality. Christians differ in their conviction, however, that sexuality is a gift of the Creator, who in his wisdom and love for humanity created us in his image and has so intertwined these values that we cannot separate them without injury to that same image. The Catholic

Church has often been accused of a negative attitude toward sexuality. In the course of the Church's long history, the expression of its teaching on sexuality has sometimes been colored by the secular culture in which the Church has lived. Consequently, the pagan philosophies of Plato, who taught that sex is a result of the fall of the human soul into the tomb of the body, and of the Stoics, who rejected physical pleasure and erotic love as unworthy of a philosopher and saw no value in sex except procreation, as well as current secular humanists, have sometimes distorted the ways Christians have thought and spoken about sex (Noonan, 1965).

Nevertheless, genuine Christian teaching on sexuality is clear enough in the Scripture and was given a rich and accurate expression by the Second Vatican Council, Paul VI's encyclical *Humanae Vitae* (1968), and John Paul II's *Familiaris Consortio* (1981b) based on the Council. Genesis 1-3 teaches that God created persons as male and female and blessed their sexuality as a great and good gift. Jesus confirmed this teaching and perfected it by affirming that men must be as faithful in marriage as women (Mk 10:2-12; 1 Co 7:10). Nevertheless, Jesus also taught that although sexuality is a great gift, its use in marriage is only a relative value, which can be freely sacrificed for the sake of higher values. Thus, for the Christian, the celibate or single life, with its freedom from domestic cares to be of service to others, can be even more personally maturing and fulfilling than married life. St. Paul (1 Co 7:25-35) also emphasizes the value of the single life but teaches that marriage is a sacrament in that love of husband and wife is a symbol showing us the love of Christ for his people (Ep 5:22-23).

From biblical teaching it is clear why the Second Vatican Council and the papal encyclicals teach that sexuality was given to us to help us love one another, whether we freely choose to marry or to live the single life of service to society. Any use of sex outside marriage is ethically wrong because (1) it is a selfish pursuit of pleasure apart from love, as in masturbation, prostitution, or casual or promiscuous relations; (2) it expresses love but not a committed love involving true self-giving, as in adultery or premarital sex; or (3) it is committed but practiced in a way contradictory to its natural fulfillment in the family, as in contraception or the relations of committed homosexuals. The reason such actions are ethically wrong is not some repressive rule of the Church, but because they are contradictory to the intrinsic value and meaning of sexuality as designed by the Creator and blessed by him. Human culture and customs have undergone many revolutions, but such changes cannot alter the basic structure of human nature without destroying humanity itself.

Principle of Stewardship and Creativity

The hope that leads human beings to endure the inevitable pain of human existence and to overcome the sentence to death by the perpetuation of the human community also leads us to struggle with the environment. The author of Genesis 3 profoundly symbolizes the evil of death by the expulsion from the Garden, the burden of sexism by the curse on Eve, and the burden of struggle with the environment by the curse on Adam. These are the fundamental realities of the human situation, but Scripture says they are not what God wanted for humanity. He has given persons the power of intelligence, restored by grace in Christ, the new Adam, by which they deal with these problems. Although persons may deal with these evils well or poorly, however, they cannot escape the struggle and still remain human (Gn 3:16-19).

Section 3.3 deals at length with the *Principle of Stewardship and Creativity*, which has become even more important in modern times as a guide to the use of modern medical technology:

> *The gifts of multidimensional human nature and its natural environment should be used with profound respect for their intrinsic teleology. The gift of human creativity especially should be used to cultivate nature and environment with a care set by the limits of actual knowledge and the risks of destroying these gifts.*

This principle requires us to appreciate the two great gifts that a wise and loving God has given: the earth, with all its natural resources, and our own human nature ("embodied intelligent freedom"), with its biological, psychological, ethical, and spiritual capacities. Recently, we have come to recognize that our earthly environment is a marvelously balanced ecological system without which human life could never have evolved. Although we certainly have a need and a right to cultivate and perfect our earthly home, to till and irrigate its soil, to build cities, and to use its raw materials for the wonderful devices of modern technology, we should not do this ruthlessly. We must take the utmost care to conserve our ecological system unpolluted and unravished and to recycle its raw materials and its energy supplies. We have already discovered how much damage thoughtless exploitation of natural resources can do to our own lives.

Similarly, our own human nature, our bodies, and our minds are wonderfully constructed. We have the need and right to improve our bodies and to develop medical technologies that prevent and remedy the defects to which they are liable. We must do so, however, with the greatest respect for what we already are as human beings. Our bodily and mental functions have natural teleologies that cannot be eliminated or misdirected without injury to our humanness.

Consequently, a technology based on the false principle, "If it can be done, it should be done," is a misuse of our creative intelligence. Rather, we should ask ourselves, "Should it be done?" and only if the answer is "Yes" develop and use the technology to do it. Thus the God-given gifts of our environment and our humanity are ours in stewardship, but because the greatest of our gifts are intelligence and freedom, the stewardship should be creative. Our creativity should be used as co-creativity with the Creator, not as reckless wasting of his gifts.

This principle is rooted in the basic need for truth, since it is God-given human intelligence, the capacity for truth, that makes persons co-creators with God. Its specifically Christian character derives from the risen Christ being the pledge that the Kingdom of God will eventually be built. The coming of his Holy

Spirit gives persons the power to share in this building of the Kingdom, the house built not on the sand of pride but on the rock of faith (Mt 7:24-29). The Gospel does not encourage Christians simply to wait until the Lord returns, indifferent to the world's fate, as Marxists and humanists accuse. Rather, Christians are called to play a historical role in the liberation of the human race from poverty, disease, and oppression with the assistance of God's power.

8.5 COORDINATION OF THE PRINCIPLES

A study by Beauchamp and Childress (1983), *Principles of Biomedical Ethics*, proposes five principles: (1) autonomy, the right of persons to care for themselves; (2) nonmaleficence, that is, "do no harm"; (3) beneficence, or seeking the patient's benefit; (4) justice to all concerned; and (5) the trust required by the professional-patient relationship. Of these principles, autonomy serves much the same purpose as our Principle of Informed Consent; trust as our Principle of Professional Communication; whereas those of nonmaleficence, beneficence, and justice are similar to our Principle of Human Dignity in Community, Principle of the Common Good, and so on.

Why have we chosen to list 12 principles rather than a few broad ones? The main reason is that in the actual process of bioethical decision making, each of these 12 plays an important role. In fact, these could be still further multiplied by additional corollaries. Our list, however, can be coordinated and simplified by showing how it flows from the four basic needs of human persons:

1. *To preserve life:* the Principles of Totality and of Growth through Suffering
2. *To procreate:* the Principle of Personalized Sexuality
3. *To know the truth:* the Principle of Well-Formed Conscience with its methodological specification by the Principle of Moral Discrimination, along with rules for resolving conflict cases (Principles of Double Effect and of Legitimate Cooperation), and finally the Principles of Free and Informed Consent and of Professional Communication, which provide the conditions for a prudent conscience
4. *To live in society:* the Principles of Human Dignity in Community and of the Common Good, Subsidiarity, and Functionalism; along with the Principle of Stewardship and Creativity, which relates human society to the environment and to the use of all gifts for the common good

Note that this coordination does not imply that each principle has only one source in human needs; for example, although the Principle of Personalized Sexuality rises primitively from the human need to procreate, it is also closely related to the Principles of Human Dignity in Community, of the Common Good, and of Stewardship and Creativity. Of these principles, that of the Common Good is the most inclusive, since it is only in the common good (for the Christian, the Kingdom of God) that human dignity can be fully realized, stewardship and creativity exercised, and growth through suffering supported. The principles related to the need to know the truth (for the Christian, both truths of faith and of reason) precede the Principle of the Common Good in the sense that they help persons judge how to apply the other principles. However, these principles are also ultimate in the sense that the common good concretely consists in the union of each person with God and neighbor in loving and trusting truth.

To sum up this discussion of the principles that govern bioethical decisions from a Christian point of view:

1. Faith requires persons to act with an informed conscience, which requires the intellectual effort of moral discrimination between right and wrong, even in complex cases in which moral actions involve evil side effects or material cooperation. Faith also requires a relation of trust between persons, especially between professional and client, in which there is an honest exchange of the information necessary for an informed conscience.

2. Hope requires persons to accept growth through suffering, to continue the human community through the institution of the family, and to fulfill in a creative manner their stewardship of their own nature and the world God has given them.

3. Love requires a profound respect for human dignity, no matter what the condition of the person. Love also requires a proper love of oneself and a responsibility for one's own health. Finally, love requires persons to work for and share in the common good. One must accept the social responsibility of promoting the distribution of healthcare for all.

DIFFICULT BIOETHICAL DECISIONS

Part 4 considers specific problems which frequently arise in medical ethics. These more prominent ethical problems might be aligned in any number of ways. We have chosen to make the following divisions.

First are questions that concern the limits of medical care; that is, Who is the patient to be treated? and What procedures may be performed upon a person? Hence, Chapter 9 considers the ethical issues concerned with abortion, triage, and research upon human subjects. Because sexuality is such an important dimension of the human personality, all the ethical issues concerning sexuality and reproduction are gathered in Chapter 10. The human person may be altered through surgery or by means of genetic engineering. The surgical methods of changing human persons are already a part of medical practice; genetic engineering is a future possibility but ethical foresight is needed in order to avoid human tragedies. Various methods of changing the human body, phenotype and genotype are considered in Chapter 11, "Reconstructing Human Beings."

Psychotherapy in its various forms and methods is another area of ethical concern. The problems arising from this discipline are considered in Chapter 12. The last chapter in this section, Chapter 13, considers the many ethical issues concerned with death and care for the dying.

CHAPTER 9

Medical Limits: Abortion, Triage, and Research Involving Human Subjects

OVERVIEW

Chapters 3 and 4 show that a profession has limits that are set not merely by professional expertise but by the fundamental *purpose* of the profession. To act outside these limits in a way extraneous or contradictory to this basic purpose is to act unprofessionally and unethically. The purpose of the healthcare profession is to serve human persons (who are more agents than patients) to achieve physical and psychological health as dimensions of human wholeness.

Thus two basic ethical decisions must be made before a healthcare professional performs any medical procedure: (1) Who is the human person (or persons) being served? (2) What can be done to benefit this person's (or these persons') health? This chapter explores some of the ethical difficulties involved in answering these apparently simple questions.

In response to the first question, we discuss the process by which we recognize human identity and the meaning of the term *personhood* (9.1). In response to the second question, we discuss some medical actions that are questionable concerning the benefit to human persons. Specifically, this chapter considers abortion (9.2) and whether the civil law resulting from Supreme Court decisions recognizes the biological facts associated with personhood (9.3). Triage (9.4), and research involving human subjects (9.5) are then considered. Abortion involves both the aforementioned questions; triage and research are more concerned with the second question: how to ensure that medical therapy benefits the persons who are in need of help.

9.1 DECIDING WHO IS THE HUMAN SUBJECT OF MEDICAL THERAPY

Ordinarily, the professional can easily recognize the patient. But just who is the woman who is pregnant, or the body whose heart is beating but whose brain exhibits only a flat electroencephalogram, or a criminal who is in excellent health but who has agreed to be the subject of a medical experiment that may make him very ill? Is the pregnant woman one person or two? Is the body a person or not? Is the experimental subject someone who has health needs (Mackie, 1985; Rush, 1984)?

Some would question whether the medical profession deals only with human persons. What of veterinary medicine? What of "the rights of animals" urged by antivivisectionists, or even of the total biosphere urged by ecologists? Serious ethical questions arise about cruelty to animals and depredation of the environment. Undoubtedly, a lack of reverence for life or its sanctity opens the way to ruthlessness toward human persons (Rodd, 1985; Mulvanney, 1986). It is also true, however, that if the distinction between respect for human rights and respect for subhuman nature is blurred, the value of both may be minimized. Some argue that, after all, experimentation on animal subjects and on human subjects is only a difference of degree (Singer, 1986). For reasons elaborated in Chapters 1 and 2, this book assumes that the healthcare profession deals with human persons whose rights are valued differently from the respect due to other forms of life, although that respect is of genuine ethical importance.

Today also, some argue that the terms *human being* and *human person* are not identical nor coextensive (Engelhardt, 1977, 1986b). *Human being* seems to be a biological term equivalent to "member of the human species," for which definite empirical criteria exist, just as for *elephant* or *pigeon*. The term *human person*, however, seems to be a legal, philosophical, or theological term whose value is relative to a particular culture or social system. How is the healthcare profession going to deal with this issue honestly without at the same time getting bogged down in philosophical debates beyond its competence?

The medical profession should work toward consensus on this issue first on the basis of what it knows best, namely, biology and psychology, plus its own professional *self-understanding* (Burtchaell, 1980). Such considerations may need to be tempered by legal, philosophical, or theological reflections, which in turn must take into full account and be consistent with direct professional experience. It would be a gross evasion of responsibility to follow the example of the Nazi physicians and leave it to others to determine which human beings are persons and which nonpersons (Lifton, 1986).

If healthcare professionals proceed in this manner, the issue is not as obscure as some pretend. First, in deciding who a human person is, healthcare professionals should begin with the basic certitude that they—physicians, nurses, and medical researchers—are not only human beings but human persons. Understanding what it is to be a person must begin from such self-understanding. It cannot be merely external and behavioristic, nor can it rest simply on cultural or semantic conventions.

The long controversy over behaviorism in psychology has established that although scientific research should always strive to make definitions operational to maximize objectivity, the element of *empathy* can never be completely eliminated from psychology. To understand psychological phenomena, the observers must first study themselves to be objective about their own observations and interpretations. This is only another application of the basic epistemological principle (familiarized by the theory of relativity), according to which observers can never stand completely outside what they observe. Their observations are part of the processes that they are observing.

Consequently, medical professionals must always try to understand the patients in relation to themselves. They must recall their own experience of what it is to be sick or well (Natanson, 1981). This also is essential for sound ethical decision making, as is clear from almost all great ethical teachers having agreed that the Golden Rule, *Do unto others as you would have them do unto you*, is basic to any humanistic ethics.

How does the physician, nurse, or medical researcher know he or she is a human person and not a computer, a piece of medical apparatus, a corpse, a bit of tissue, or even an experimental animal? The basic reasons, argued in Chapters 1 and 3, are that the professional experiences himself or herself (1) as an intelligent person capable of abstract reason and free decision and (2) as a member of a human community, with which he or she shares a common life of thought, feeling, and moral action. Section 4.3 also suggests that modern medical education sometimes tends to obscure rather than to develop this human self-awareness in the medical student (T. McNeill et al., 1986). Perhaps this accounts in part for the current confusion about this issue of personhood.

Healthcare professionals have to integrate this fundamental self-awareness of personality with their biological and psychological knowledge, beginning with their own bodies. Why is *my* body a human body that gives me membership in the human species? To ask this question is to become aware at once that a definition of human personhood must necessarily define a type of being who is not static and fixed but essentially a being in *process*, a being *becoming*. A person cannot define himself or herself as a fixed, timeless object, but must include the notion of *biography*, or life history, in the definition.

It is no accident that the usual first step in all medical practice (and it has been since the time of Greek medicine) is taking the patient's history. A body cannot be called a human person without taking into account its past and also the future open to it. A corpse is no longer a person because it has no capacity for a human future. An unfertilized ovum, a sperm, or any isolated body cell also is not a person, since of itself it has no inherent capacity to become an organism with a human future.

Thus philosophers who insist that a definition of a human person cannot be merely "substantialist" are correct (Goldenring, 1985). It must be processive. It is an error to conclude from this, however, that in a process universe all processes are merely gradual changes, such as a rise in temperature or an increase in size or velocity. Such a conclusion is a radical distortion of process philosophy as developed by Hegel, Marx, Bergson, Whitehead, Dewey, and Teilhard de Chardin. As Whitehead (1929) so vigorously emphasized, the essence of any process view of reality must allow for genuine *novelty* in the world. In the complex processes of becoming new, entities emerge that are continuous with the past *materially* but discontinuous with it in actuality and activity. Process is not always a mere reshuffling of what was already there or its intensification or adulteration, but the emergence of new realities radically distinct from those that previously existed.

Therefore an appeal to the process way of looking at reality, so congenial to the scientific mind, does not eliminate the problem of identifying novelty and origination. We still need to ask exactly when in the long process of biological reproduction is the critical point at which a new organism, which did not exist before, comes into existence so that where there was one organism, there are now two, or where there were two, there is now a unique third. Anyone who has studied under the microscope the complex way in which one-celled organisms reproduce by fission knows that long and elaborate processes precede and follow the moment of separation, but no observer can doubt there is a critical point.

Biography

Thus a definition of the human person must not merely be synchronic but diachronic. It must be biographical. Unless the same identical human person enters the hospital and leaves somewhat healthier, unless sickness and healing are processes that take place as episodes in the life of a person with a continuous identity, and unless coming alive and dying are not merely arbitrary divisions, the whole work of healthcare becomes meaningless.

Now the biography of any human person also includes remarkable morphological and functional changes. The difference in morphology and behavior of the newborn infant, the preadolescent, the mature adult, and the senile elderly person are not as startling as the differences between a caterpillar and a butterfly, but they are remarkable indeed. The practicing physician does not doubt, however, that he is the same person as the medical student whose trials and learning experiences he so well remembers, as the young boy who first dreamed of being a doctor, and as the infant whom he cannot recollect but whose scars and immunities he still bears in his adult body and understands as part of his own medical history. Also, this physician does not doubt that the child whose prenatal existence he first confirmed, whom he helped deliver, and whose health he has assisted to adulthood and beyond is the same person. Perhaps the growth of specialization in healthcare somewhat obscures this view of the patient as a man or woman with a long life history, but it certainly does not put it in doubt.

Thus a medical definition of human personhood begins with the notion of the person as a conscious, intelligent, free adult, but it must include the entire biography of the unique organism, whose personhood is fully self-conscious and fully evident in morphology and behavior only at certain periods of that biography. This means that even if personhood is defined behavioristically, not only *actual*, here-and-now performance must be taken into account but the capacity or potentiality for behavior.

The term *potentiality* has many senses in current usage. It is necessary, even at the cost of pedantry, to distinguish some of them, since confused uses of the term are at the bottom of many current arguments about the origin of the human person (Holbrook, 1985). First, any stuff or material has the potentiality for being made or formed into an unlimited number of very different types of things. In this sense, the subatomic particles are potentially all the things that make up the universe, and the gaseous nebula from which the earth's galaxy originally came was potentially the human race. Potentiality, in this sense of mere "stuff," is something *passive*, as clay in the hand of the sculptor.

There are other senses, however, in which potentiality is conceived *actively* as the power to mold and develop passively potential material. Thus the sculptor has the active potentiality (i.e., capability) to form clay into a variety of figures. It is this active sense of potentiality that is especially useful in understanding living organisms. At any given moment of its biography, an organism has both a structure and a variety of functions. These functions are active potentialities that depend on the existence of the structure as an actuality; for example, a bird has the power to fly only when its wing structures have been actually developed. What is more important, however, is that basic to all the functions of an organism is the potentiality for *self-development*, that is, to elaborate its own structures and thus to acquire more diversified functions. This capacity for self-development is the function that gives unity to all the others and guarantees the biographical identity of the organism.

This potentiality for self-development, as with any function, presupposes some kind of organic structure, but it is necessarily a minimal structure, since on its relatively simple basis the organism is able to elaborate itself into its adult complexity. Modern embryology has shown clearly that this minimal or initial structure must be understood in an *epigenetic*, not in a preformist, way (I. Kaiser, 1986). This means that the original, simplest structure is not a miniature model of the completed, elaborated structure, but it does contain the information necessary to develop this total structure. It is entirely inadequate to think of the genetic endowment of an organism as a small mock-up of the adult. Even to call it a blueprint is misleading because no blueprint can even reproduce itself, let alone produce a building. Rather, a developing organism contains the *potentiality for active self-development*, a potentiality based on a minimal actual structure, yet containing all the information necessary to produce a maximal actual structure.

Thus the zygote, or fertilized ovum of a sexually reproducing species, is not a "blob of protoplasm"; it is a complete, unified structure, although that structure is very simple compared to that of the adult into which it will develop itself. This simple structure somehow contains all the information and all the active potentiality of self-development necessary to live its whole biography of interaction with its environment. It is this minimal structure that makes it actually a member of a definite species. The zygote of a cat, biologically speaking, is not potentially a cat; it is actually a member of the cat species with the potentiality of becoming a perfectly self-developed cat. Of course, only the adult cat can carry out all the various functions of cat life because only at maturity is the cat structure elaborated and diversified to the point that it has all the active potentialities of cat life. From the beginning, however, the cat zygote had the basic active potentiality to develop all these structures and the functions following on them.

When these distinctions are applied to the origin of the human person, it is obvious at once that it is a mistake to argue that if the fetus is a human being "potentially," then so are the ovum and sperm. Biologically, the ovum and sperm are not complete organisms, nor does either possess the genetic information necessary for self-development into a human being because they are haploid (i.e., they have only half the requisite set of chromosomes and genes).

In the past 15 years, the evidence supporting the declaration that human life begins at fertilization is more and more conclusive. All do not agree, however, that personhood begins at fertilization (Engelhardt, 1986a). However, as we understand this issue, personhood is not a quality bestowed by society, but rather a characteristic that proceeds from nature (O'Donovan, 1984). Some philosophers who equate the beginning of human life and even personhood with fertilization defend elective abortions because they maintain that the rights of the mother, a reflective conscious person, take precedence over the rights of the fetus, a nonreflective, nonconscious person (Scarlett, 1984). This latter opinion is based on a consequentialist morality that does not recognize inalienable rights but rather balances rights. There is also a tendency to limit abortion by reason of medical advances, which is an admission that the Supreme Court decision in the *Roe v. Wade* case does not make as much sense in light of contemporary medical knowledge (Callahan, 1986; Pollner, 1985).

Thus it seems difficult for a scientifically educated healthcare professional to doubt that he or she has been the same person with a continuous biography since that unique zygote began to develop itself into this adult who can look back over this personal history and acknowledge it as his or her own. Nevertheless, in the past some objections have been raised against these biologically well-established conclusions. Two recent works (Lotstra, 1985; McCartney, 1987) offer a summary of these objections. For the most part, these opinions are no longer as prominent as they were 10 years ago, mainly because of the growing biological evidence that a fetus is human from its earliest stage of development.

Puzzles

However, some still offer specious objections against this well-established biological conclusion. First is the claim (Häring, 1976) that perhaps 50 percent of all zygotes perish at an early stage of development, although a recent study indicates this may be closer to 30 percent, as determined from the earliest stages of fertilization (Wilcox et al., 1988). Does this mean that so many members of the human race came into existence and perished so soon? In answer to this difficulty, two points should be made:

1. Through most of human history, at least 50 percent of all infants perished in infancy. Therefore, if this argument proves anything, it proves that infants are no more persons than fetuses.
2. Evidence suggests that the complex process of fertilization frequently fails to be successfully completed (J. Diamond, 1975; Wilcox et al., 1988). Probably many of these zygotes are only apparently such and would not be complete organisms or human persons according to our definition.

A second objection, which has greatly influenced certain Catholic theologians (C. Curran, 1975; Dedek, 1972; Häring, 1976; see also B. Brody, 1975), rests on the notion that after fertilization is completed, there remains a period (perhaps as long as two or three weeks) when the unique identity of the organism still is indeterminate. The evidence offered for this is that during this time the zygote sometimes divides to produce twins or even multiple offspring.

How is this phenomenon of monozygotic twinning to be interpreted biologically? Although no clean conclusions are presented, it seems that monozygotic multiple births result partly from genetic factors (K. Moore, 1988; Thompson and Thompson, 1980). It makes no biological sense to say that up to the time of monozygotic twinning, there was simply a mass of cells rather than a single human organism. If that were the case, how does one account for the normal development of the zygote up to the point of twinning? And how would the event of twinning produce two or more organisms out of what is not an organism? A much more probable explanation would be the following (B. Ashley, 1976).

Every diploid cell of the body apparently has the basic potentiality to develop into a complete individual. Thus in the future it may be possible to clone or reproduce human beings asexually, not from germ cells but from any body cell (Hyde and Hyde, 1984). This potentiality is inhibited in embryological development by the process of somatic cell differentiation into various fixed types and remains actualizable only in germ cells. It is not strange, therefore, that at a very early stage of development some cells of an embryo may become detached and develop independently into a twin, or that the embryo may divide into two equal parts, each of which may develop as two new organisms of the same genetic composition. Such events do not prove that previously no human being existed, but only that this existing human being has given rise to a clone *asexually* or has ceased to exist and given rise to new twins by asexual fission. This occurrence, as with any process of multiple birth in the human species, is an accident of development that results from some genetic defect or environmental accident.

In the recent past, some argued that the fetus is only a part of the mother's body (Wahlberg, 1971) or that the fetus is similar to a tumor. Thus the embryo is not a distinct organism until implantation in the uterine wall or until the fetus is viable independently of the uterus prematurely or by normal delivery (Wasserstrom, 1975). As we have noted, no biological evidence exists for this opinion, and it is no longer proposed seriously. Such arguments ignore two basic biological facts:

1. The zygote has a new genetic composition different from any part of the mother's body. This difference is not merely caused by some mutational defect (as perhaps is the case in some tumors) but results from a unique combination of genes that gives the zygote the potentiality of development into a complete adult.

2. The embryo does not depend on the mother for further genetic information or guidance in development, merely for nourishment and shelter. The newborn infant still depends on the mother for nourishment and protection. Finally, every organism, even the adult human person, always remains dependent on an appropriate environment. In this respect, the adult and the embryo differ only in degree.

A final biological argument is that of the Aristotelian theory of *delayed hominization*, which has greatly influenced Catholic thought because of its adoption by the medieval theologians Albert the Great and Aquinas, and which has been recently revived by Pastrana (1977) and Donceel (1970, 1985, 1986).

Aristotle argued that until an organism has developed to the point that it has a central organ with the minimal structure required for psychological functions, it should be considered a vegetative, rather than an animal, being. For Aristotle, this "primary organ" is the heart. Donceel and Pastrana argue that in modern biology the "primary organ" is the central nervous system, especially the cerebrum. Since the cerebrum is observable in the fetus only toward the end of the third month, this would mean that before this stage the embryo or fetus is not even an animal organism and *a fortiori* not human.

The weakness of this argument is that it defines incorrectly the minimal structure necessary for the organism to be a human person in the sense already explained, that is, an organism that actually has the active potentiality to develop itself into a human adult capable of intelligent and free activity. We now know, as Aristotle and Aquinas did not, that before the appearance of the brain as the primary organ of the fetus, a sequence of primordial centers of development in the embryo goes back continuously to the nucleus of the zygote. This nucleus has contained from the beginning all the information and active potentiality necessary to eventually develop the brain and bring it to the stage of adult functioning. Thus, although it is true that the developing fetus first exhibits vegetative (physiological) and animal (psychological and motor) functions and finally (long after birth) specifically human functions, it possesses from conception the active potentiality to develop all these functional abilities. The minimal structure necessary for this active potentiality of self-development (even on the basis of Aristotle's and Aquinas' philosophical principles) is required for an organism to be actually a human person, not the brain structures necessary for adult psychological activities (Australian Research Commission, 1985).

Thus a healthcare professional, beginning with a self-understanding of personal identity and attempting to trace this back to its origins by the light of biological science, can scarcely doubt that the critical point is at completed conception. Nevertheless, this conviction will be attacked by some on legal, philosophical, or theological grounds. Western legal tradition (for reasons 9.2 explores) has always been ambiguous on this question (Horan et al., 1987; Shaw and Dondera, 1983).

Advocacy of Personhood

These legal doubts have led some recent philosophers to argue that personhood as the subject of rights cannot be determined merely by biological criteria, but must be defined by social consensus (see discussion of these views by Atkinson, 1979). They contend that although such consensus should not rest on merely arbitrary criteria such as those proposed by racists, it can never be absolute, since only adults capable of actually functioning as free citizens are unequivocally persons. The advocates of such views generally argue for a dividing line late in fetal development at the beginning of sensation (L. Sumner, 1981), brain activity (Goldenring, 1985), viability, birth, or even one or two months of infancy. They propose also excluding seriously defective children from personhood (Engelhardt, 1986a; Tooley, 1983).

213

This book is not the place to answer these types of arguments in detail. It suffices to point out the dubious assumptions on which they are based (Cannon, 1985). The legal arguments assume a legal positivism, according to which human rights are the result of law rather than the basis against which the justice of the laws is to be measured. Even those who appeal to the venerable tradition of Jewish religious law must ask whether the tradition on this point is the final word or whether, in light of modern science and modern views of human dignity and equality, a stricter view on the origin of human personhood conforms more to the fundamental ethical principles of Judaism (L. Meier, 1986; Rosner, 1986).

The philosophical arguments seem to rest on the assumption stemming from idealism that ethical values are simply human constructs relative to a particular culture. If our definition of the human person and thus of human rights is merely man-made, how is it possible to criticize the laws as unjust or a culture as inhumane? There must be an appeal to criteria that transcend man-made laws and values. This is why many persons in the United States have always appealed to the "inalienable rights of man," as does the *Universal Declaration of Human Rights* of the United Nations (1948). This need of a prophetic criticism of man-made laws and customs has always been the basis of the Christian theological insistence that the definition of personhood should be broad and should extend to the unborn (Dougherty, 1985; Noonan, 1985).

Thus healthcare professionals apparently should begin with the attitude of giving the benefit of the doubt, or what Kass (1985) calls "knowing the truth about nature, and our own nature." As a group of professionals who have the clearest notion of the biological criteria of human personhood, healthcare professionals have a responsibility to defend these rights socially and politically against possible doubts on the part of other professions less biologically knowledgeable. They also must explain these rights clearly to the laity, who are likely to judge more by appearances and popular impressions than by scientific fact. Healthcare professionals should be just as ready to protest a lack of respect for the unborn as they should be to oppose the biological fallacies of racism or antifeminism.

9.2   ABORTION

Traditional Views

Abortion is the termination of a pregnancy with resulting death of the human fetus. Abortion may occur spontaneously, in which case it is usually called a *miscarriage*, or it may be caused deliberately, which is called an *induced* or *procured abortion*. Catholic theologians also distinguish between those procured abortions that are direct and indirect. A *direct abortion* is one in which the direct, immediate purpose of the procedure is to destroy the human fetus at any stage after conception or to expel it when it is not viable. Most procured abortions are direct in nature. An *indirect abortion* is one in which the direct, immediate purpose of the procedure is to treat the mother to radify threatening pathology, but in which the death of the fetus is an inevitable result that would have been avoided had it been possible. Two examples of indirect abortion are surgery for ectopic pregnancy and surgery for a cancerous uterus when the woman is pregnant (*Ethical and Religious Directives for Catholic Health Facilities*, 1971, nn. 13, 16).

Today it is generally conceded by Catholic theologians that such indirect abortion may be justified by the principle of double effect (Connery, 1977) because:

1. The act itself is directly for the purpose of treating the mother and is thus ethical.
2. The mother and physician do not have any evil circumstantial intention; that is, they would save the child if they could.
3. The death of the child is not the *means* by which the mother is treated, but only a result of the treatment; that is, it is not a cause but an effect of the act.
4. There is a proportionate reason if the treatment is necessary to save the life of the mother, especially since the child is doomed anyway.

The real area of difficulty, therefore, concerns *direct* abortion, of which many millions are now performed each year in the world. On this subject there is an age-old controversy. Although in all human cultures people have valued, loved, and protected their children, and this care has been recognized as one of the most basic of ethical responsibilities, direct abortion has also been widely practiced. A study of primitive cultures (Devereux, 1955) shows that the motivation for abortion in these cultures is highly varied, including not only pragmatic reasons, but also religious and symbolic reasons arising from unconscious urges, such as hostility to male domination. This was also true of the ancient civilizations, although here economic and demographic factors came more and more to prevail. Thus, in the Greco-Roman world in which Christianity arose, abortion and infanticide in some places produced rates of reproduction below the zero-growth level (Noonan, 1967). For these cultures, it can be generally said that abortion and infanticide were not strictly distinguished (Carrick, 1985). In Roman culture, for example, an infant did not have legal status until accepted by the *paterfamilias*. This gave rise to the tradition that illegitimate persons are, in effect, nonpersons.

In contrast to these views is the attitude in the Jewish Scriptures. For the Jews, all human life has as its author the One God, whose creative power produces the child in the mother's womb and brings it step-by-step to full life. The parents play only an instrumental role in this creative process, so that from the beginning a direct, personal I-Thou relation exists between the Creator and the human being whom he is creating, just as truly as he created Adam. Several of the prophets of Israel express the profound religious conviction that it was God who formed them in their mother's womb for a special purpose. These texts led to later theological speculations among the more mystical or philosophical Jewish thinkers on the time of the "infusion of the human soul." These speculations joined with Greek philosophical tendencies that enhanced the respect for the dignity of the unborn. In any case, Orthodox Jews are convinced that when the child of a Jewish mother becomes a "living soul," it is destined for the Kingdom of God, although this membership in the Chosen People requires that it be sealed after birth by circumcision for the male. Thus death in the womb does not exclude salvation (Feldman, 1986b).

Jewish thought in practical ethics, however, has been dominated by the legislation of the Torah, which in time was elaborated by the system of rabbinical interpretation that became normative for post-biblical Judaism. The Torah inculcates a high respect for human life, and the rabbis insisted that since the principle of justice is "an eye for an eye, a tooth for a tooth, a life for a life" (Ex 21:23-25; Rosner, 1986), one cannot sacrifice one human life for another unless that other is an aggressor or criminal in some way. Consequently, Judaism has resolutely opposed any form of infanticide and has required Jews to accept martyrdom rather than to kill innocent persons.

In conflict situations where the life of the mother is endangered, however, the rabbis believed that the child could be considered an "unjust aggressor" or "pursuer" against whom the woman could defend herself. In such cases, therefore, induced abortion was permitted, and the child was not considered to have a full right to life until birth, or "when the head emerges." This reasoning was confirmed by the fact that the law in Exodus 21:22 does not set capital punishment but only a monetary fine for one who causes an abortion by striking a pregnant woman. Rabbinical casuistry led some to stricter views, which drew the line at the stage when the fetus was of human form (as evidenced by the Hellenistic Septuagint translation of Exodus 21:22), whereas others wished to draw the line 30 days *after* birth if the delivery was premature. There were also wide differences on what degree of danger to the mother justified induced abortion, with some even accepting psychological reasons as sufficient justification when they threatened the married life of the couple. Underlying all these debates, however, is the basic Jewish conviction of the high value of marriage and of children in view of the preservation of the Chosen People (L. Meier, 1986).

Jesus did not repudiate the Jewish Scriptures, nor even their rabbinical application, but he gave them his own characteristic interpretation by stressing that God's care extends to every human being, no matter how sinful, ignorant, or ritually unclean. Jesus preached the good news of God's love for the "little ones," the outcasts rejected by secular and religious authorities, including powerless little children, whom he declared should be given special respect as privileged members in his Father's Kingdom (Mk 9:33-37). Far from being un-Jewish, Jesus' attitude represents the deepest prophetic spirituality of Israel.

The Christian Church, confronted with the widespread Greek and Roman practices of infanticide and abortion, evaluated such customs in the light of this teaching of Jesus on the dignity of children. Luke, in his infancy narratives based on Judeo-Christian sources, takes up the Old Testament theme of the prophetic vocation and pictures John the Baptist as called to his mission by the Holy Spirit in Elizabeth's womb. In striking parallel to this, Jesus as the new Adam is created by the overshadowing Spirit in the virgin earth of Mary's womb, where he is already Lord, the Holy One, the Son of God. Thus the Old Testament conviction that God is the creator of human life from the moment it begins, so that the human person is defined primarily by this unique I-Thou relation to its Creator rather than the legal provisions of Exodus, came to be the guiding theme of Christian thinking about the unborn child.

In the practical moral exhortations of the New Testament Epistles, abortion is never explicitly mentioned. In the *Didache*, however, a manual of Church discipline written in the same period probably in Jewish-Christian circles, it is explicitly forbidden. This opposition to direct abortion has remained what Noonan (1970a; 1985) calls "an almost absolute value" throughout the history of the Christian Church.

The consistency of this position has been only partially obscured by the theological controversies that, as with most of the teachings of Christianity, it has occasionally engendered. These controversies will be examined here only briefly; readers may refer to the detailed studies of Connery (1977), Lotstra (1985), McCartney (1987), Noonan (1970b); and Ramsey (1973).

One difficulty arose from contact with Greek thought and took the form of the question, When is the human soul infused into the body? Platonists believed that this human animation was at conception. The Aristotelians, however, more concerned with biological processes, thought that it could not be at conception, when the embryo is (as they believed) simply unformed menstrual blood, but must be at about 40 to 60 days of pregnancy, when the fetus has definite organic form. Those influenced by Stoic philosophy even believed it was only at birth that the child breathed in the "vital spirit."

Christian thinkers respected all these views of ancient biology, but the great authority of St. Thomas Aquinas (who was a convinced Aristotelian) led to the general acceptance of the theory that ensoulment takes place when the fetus has a definitely human form between one and two months of gestation, which (as 9.1 notes) still has its defenders. Nevertheless, for Aquinas, abortion was a grave crime because it interrupted the creative work of God in nature, although it was not murder in the technical sense if it took place before ensoulment. Thus Catholic teaching traditionally regarded early abortion as a crime equivalent to murder, but not identical with it.

A second difficulty arose from the question of whether the gravity of the crime of abortion was aggravated because it prevents the child from receiving the baptism Christ required for salvation (Jn 3:5). Today the Catholic Church still insists on the importance of infant baptism, even in emergency situations such as spontaneous abortion, but theologians generally no longer conclude that this practice implies that unbaptized children cannot be saved. Chapter 14 discusses the reasons for this theological change and also the pastoral administration of baptism in emergency situations.

Other controversies have arisen over the correct way to deal with conflict situations where the life of the mother seems threatened. As already noted, the Jewish rabbis permitted therapeutic abortion, and as Connery (1977) has shown, some Catholic theologians in the past also favored this view, as do some Protestant and Eastern Orthodox churches, even at present (J. Davis, 1984). Recently, some Catholic theologians are also attempting to revive this opinion (C. Curran, 1979; D. Maguire, 1986). Since as far back as 1679, however, the popes have repeatedly repudiated the notion that the killing of one person could ever be a means of therapy for another because such a practice seems utterly inconsistent with the equal dignity of human persons. Nevertheless, this disagreement on how to deal with conflict cases does not negate the basic agreement among all the Christian churches (1) that abortion is contrary to the will of God, who creates each human person, and (2) that if abortion is ever permissible in a conflict situation (and this is denied by some), it can be justified only by the most serious reasons.

As to why the Roman Catholic Church has taken the most strict view on direct abortion, the most authoritative recent statements on this subject are the *Declaration on Procured Abortion* (Sacred Congregation for the Doctrine of the Faith, 1974) and the *Instruction on Respect for Human Life in Its Origin and on the Dignity of Procreation* (Sacred Congregation for the Doctrine of the Faith, 1987). These documents are elaborations of the condemnation of abortion by the Second Vatican Council, which linked it with infanticide (*Pastoral Constitution on the Church in the Modern World*, 1965c). The *Declaration on Procured Abortion* argues as follows:

> The first right of the human person is his or her life. A person has other goods and some are more precious, but this one is fundamental—the condition of all the others. Hence it must be protected above all others. A society or public authority may not in any form recognize this right for some and not for others: all discrimination is evil whether it be founded on race, sex, color or religion. It is not recognition by another that constitutes this right. This right is antecedent to its recognition; it demands recognition and it is strictly unjust to refuse it. Any discrimination based on the various states of life is no more justified than any other discrimination. The right to life remains complete in an old person, even one greatly weakened. It is not lost by one who is incurably sick. The right to life is not less to be respected in the small infant just born than in the mature person. In reality, respect for human life is called for from the time the process of generation begins. From the time that the ovum is fertilized, a life is begun which is neither that of the father nor the mother. It is rather the life of a new human being with his or her own growth. It would never be made human if it were not human already (nn. 11-12).

Note that this authoritative Catholic position does *not* depend on the view argued in 9.1 that human personhood begins at conception, but rather on the following proposition:

> From a moral point of view it is certain that even if a doubt existed whether the fruit of conception is already a human person it is an objectively grave sin to dare to risk murder. "The one who will be a human being is already one" (Tertullian; n. 12).

The reason underlying this statement is given in note 19 of the *Declaration*:

> This declaration expressly leaves aside the question of the moment when the spiritual soul is infused. There is not a unanimous tradition on this point and authors are as yet in disagreement. For some it dates from the first instance, for others it could at least precede implantation. It is not within the competence of science to decide between these views. It is a philosophical

problem from which our moral affirmation remains independent for two reasons: (1) supposing a belated animation, there is still nothing less than a *human* life preparing for and calling for a soul in which the nature received from the parents is completed; (2) on the other hand it suffices that this presence of the soul be probable in order that the taking of life involves accepting the risk of killing a human being, who is not only waiting for, but already in possession of his or her soul.

Although the statements quoted are not solemn definitions, the most recent statement of the Holy See on this matter calls the teaching in regard to procured abortion "unchangeable." As Connery's study (1977) shows, the issues involved have been very well debated over a long period, and the advance of medical knowledge, far from weakening the Church's position, has tended to reinforce and sharpen it.

Why, then, have controversies arisen among Christians as to the question of therapeutic abortion and other questions that came out of conflict situations? Some of these disagreements stem from situations in which there are severe conflicts between the rights of the mother and the rights of the fetus. The traditional Catholic teaching is that the right to life must be preserved in "conflict situations"; thus direct abortion is immoral. Some theologians maintain, however, that the rights of the mother might predominate in conflict situations, and therefore the theory of *probabilism* enables people to follow this opinion. Daniel Maguire (1986), for example, after agreeing with Charles Curran (1979) that abortion may be performed for "grave but real threats to the psychological health of the woman or for other values of a socio-economic nature in extreme situations," states that this opinion is acceptable because of probabilism. Maguire declares: "Probabilism taught that in health and moral matters one might follow a solidly probable opinion even though other opinions were entertained by experts and Church officers and sustained by plausible reasonings." Maguire is referring to the rule of probabilism that "a doubt as to the fact" (in this case whether the embryo is human in the sense of having human rights) makes it probable that there is no obligation to defer to the rights of another in seeking one's own goals (in this case the mother's life and well-being).

In the use of probabilism and probable reasoning in general, however, it is essential first to determine carefully on which side the presumption of right lies. Generally, the presumption is in favor of freedom from an obligation, but this must yield in situations where very serious rights such as the right to life are in question, in which cases the *more* probable course must be followed (Prümmer, 1960).

Neither Maguire nor anyone else has established that it is *more* probable that the fetus is not human; rather, as 9.1 shows, the arguments for the personhood of the fetus, even from conception, are much the more probable biologically, philosophically, and theologically than the contrary. It is more certain that an adult woman is a human person than that her unborn child is a human person. Nevertheless, when it is certain that this woman is pregnant, it is then also certain that a living child already exists who is much more probably human than not, and whose basic and very serious rights may not be ignored. Furthermore, these rights require particular advocacy precisely because the child is helpless in his or her own defense. Thus the moral theory of probabilism while legitimate in some circumstances, may not be used in conflict situations arising from pregnancy (McCormick, 1984b).

Significantly, Charles Curran (1973) and other Catholic theologians tend to solve such conflict cases not by probabilism in the classical mode, but by a theory of moral compromise or by the new proportionalist methodology, which we discuss in 7.5 and find inadequate. Many Protestant theologians follow much the same type of reasoning, trying to balance the good and evil consequences of abortion in concrete circumstances. However, even if this manner is used, it is not at all clear that abortion can ever be judged the right solution.

Woman's Right to Decide

Frequently, a pregnant woman may in good faith believe that not to have an abortion will do more harm (not only to herself but to others) than to have one. Denes (1976), Francke (1978), and Reardon (1987) have documented this in a very sensitive way from interviews with women. Some of the considerations frequently cited in favor of a woman's right to make this decision for herself are as follows:

1. A woman has to bear the risk and burden of pregnancy, delivery, and child care, which she will hardly be able to sustain unless to do so is her own choice.
2. Sometimes in the case of very young, inexperienced, or retarded women and in the case of incest or rape, a woman has little or no responsibility for the pregnancy, yet she must bear the consequences.
3. Even when she has shared in the responsibility for the pregnancy, the woman nevertheless has the right to a normal sex life, on which her marriage and care of other children also depends; however, contraception does not give her complete control over pregnancy. Therefore she has the right to use abortion as a last resort.
4. For a woman to bear an unwanted child is a disaster for the child as well as for herself, because no matter how the woman may try, she may not be able to provide the child with the necessary psychological atmosphere. As a result of her own psychological tensions, this may be led to child neglect or abuse.
5. A woman who discovers she has a defective child, especially a genetically defective child who may perpetuate the defect, has an obligation not to bring a child into the world whose life will be one of suffering and a burden to society (Fletcher and Berg, 1985).
6. A woman cannot depend on help from society to care for her unwanted child, nor to provide for the child's adoption. Such help is often insufficient and given on degrading conditions.
7. A woman should not be forced to obtain an abortion from an illegal and probably dangerous abortionist, perhaps at the risk of death and perhaps of future sterility.

8. Modern women should be free to fulfill their duty of contributing to the solution of the very serious modern problem of population control by using abortion as a backup when contraception fails or is unavailable.

9. Women should not be inhibited in their use of this right of choice by suffering interference from others who attempt to impose their own religious value systems on others or to arouse neurotic guilt feelings in those who choose abortion (B. Harrison, 1984).

The advantages for the woman and for society are very tangible. In a concrete situation, many may concur that the opposite disadvantages of pregnancy seem so overwhelming, especially if the woman is poor, already heavily burdened with children, and physically or psychologically ill, that the woman may believe that there is no other way out. As Wahlberg (1973) puts it, "Those who are not involved personally with an unwanted pregnancy tend to discuss the philosophical, medical, or moral questions. Those who face nine months of pregnancy and 15 to 20 years of child raising are more concerned with the immediate crisis."

Faced with a woman in such a dilemma, any compassionate healthcare professional may also believe that it would be utterly cruel and inhumane to refuse the medical cooperation she requests. Physicians (and also pastoral counselors) dread this situation and find it extremely difficult to refuse the requested help. This is especially difficult when they are convinced that the woman may have the abortion anyway from an illegal abortionist or by self-inflicted methods, or may even commit suicide, so that their refusal will not save the child. Therefore it is contrary to the command of Jesus, "Do not judge, and you will not be judged" (Mt 7:1), for Christians to condemn as murderers such women and the physicians who assist them out of conscientious conviction. Instead of judgment, Christians must seek ways to assist women to escape such anguishing dilemmas, while at the same time show an equal compassion for the helpless child.

The right of the mother to compassion, however, is based on the same grounds as the child's right to life, so that human sympathy and justice must be given to both. Thus some of the effects of permitting abortion must also be considered.

1. By choosing to abort the child, the mother seeks to defend her own rights by destroying another human being, an action that is radically unjust to another and contrary to her own moral dignity as a person. It is true that the continued existence of the child places a woman in a unique relation to another person existing within her own body, yet the harm she suffers from this is (except in the most extreme case) only a relative harm for which other remedies may be sought. However, the fetus suffers the absolute loss of the right to live, for which no remedy is possible (Krason, 1983).

2. Abortion of children in difficult cases encourages the widespread practice of abortion in much less justifiable cases because it becomes the easy way out. Thus the preponderance of evidence is that the social approval of abortion will imperil many more lives of children than social

disapproval, even taking into account the prevalence of illegal abortions. Furthermore, children raised in a society where it is known that abortion is permitted, or that their mothers have had an abortion, lack the important psychological assurance of unqualified parental acceptance if the child, once born, is found defective.

3. Women are encouraged and even forced by society to act in a way contradictory to their love and care for their own and others' children. It is risky to suppose that apparent social approval of abortion will do more than cover up the deep conflicts that this introduces in a woman's self-regard or in society's appreciation of the dignity of women as persons. Furthermore, the physical risks of abortion (including sterility) are not negligible, nor is the argument significant that the risks are less than those of childbirth, since maternal mortality with proper medical care today is very low.

4. Abortion policies tend to exclude the father from his proper responsibility for pregnancy and for the child and from his role of supporting his wife and sharing her burdens. Thus he, too, is degraded as a person and burdened with deep conflicts.

5. Unmarried women, mentally retarded women, and victims of rape and incest deserve the protection and care of society, which is too likely to dispense itself from this obligation simply by providing abortion as a solution. The same is true of poor women, whose rights to raise a family are ignored by the encouragement of abortion to keep down welfare expenses.

6. The family institution, which is basic to society, is further weakened when the values of parenthood and of the child as a gift of God are undermined by the spreading practice of abortion; today more than one million abortions a year are performed in the United States. Little evidence suggests that such practices encourage an attitude of responsible parenthood; rather, they promote irresponsibility by providing an easy way to escape its consequences. Thus, although very effective in population control, abortion is not a sound long-term solution for a long-term global problem.

7. Easy abortion encourages in society and in individuals an attitude of low regard for the human person, as such, and favors a merely functional evaluation of persons in terms of their actual, present contribution to economic productivity and subjective well-being. This is contrary to the advance of the concept of the dignity of the person and of inalienable rights, on which modern democracy is based.

How, then, are so many positive and negative consequences of abortion to be balanced one against another so as to apply the principle of proportion without falling into mere utilitarianism? As McCormick (himself a strong proponent of the proportionalist method) has concluded (1973a, 1984b), it is difficult to see what collection of values favoring putting to death an innocent human being could be proportionate to the one basic value of that person's right to live. How can even the rights of the mother or of society outbalance this, since the mother's rights have the same foundation as those of the child, that is, the human personhood that mother and child are equal in and that the prime purpose of society is to protect? It should be emphasized that however tangible and certain are the rights of the mother, the evil consequences to the child are still more tangible, certain, and immediate. A woman who threatens to kill herself or who may die in childbirth is still faced only with a possibility of death, which may never occur and which may be prevented. Abortion, however, dooms the child irretrievably.

Thus, in the abortion question at least, even the Principle of Proportion goes right back to the intrinsic and absolute right of the child to live, just as does the more traditional position based on the rule that direct killing of innocent persons is intrinsically evil and therefore exceptionless. Some defenders of the proportionalist method believe that sometimes the balance of advantages to the mother may outweigh the value of the life of the child, but they never explain how this evaluation can be made. It seems that what really lies behind their position is the view that precisely because the problem is so complex and incapable of an objective solution, it must be left to the mother herself to decide because she is the one most affected. This is to forget the child, however, who is affected even more directly. Also, this abdicates society's responsibility to protect the child, even against the mother, a responsibility generally accepted without question when it concerns child abuse or infanticide, although infanticide has its current defenders (Tooley, 1983). No one would argue today and defend that a slave master should be left free to do with his slave what he thinks best because the slave is *his* property.

Thus, authoritative Catholic documents consistently support the moral rule that direct killing of innocent human beings can never be ethically justifiable. This does not necessarily exclude capital punishment, since a criminal is by definition not an innocent, although Catholic theologians today generally oppose capital punishment. This also does not exclude killing an aggressor in self-defense or in war, provided that the moral object intended is to stop the aggressive act rather than the direct killing of the aggressor. One obvious exception to the rule, however, has been proposed by some critics of the authoritative Catholic teaching against direct abortion, which they believe reduces the position to absurdity, that is, the case where a physician can only save the mother by killing the child, but seems required by this rule to let both die.

This criticism can be answered in several ways. O'Donnell (1976) provides a detailed analysis of the so-called medical indications for therapeutic abortion. He shows that today the medical profession has solved this dilemma by providing the physician with the means to save both mother and child, or at least to deal with the problems of both when both are at risk, without attempting to choose the life of the mother against that of the child. Grisez (1970a) and Joseph Boyle (1980) answer it by a more careful formulation of the Principle of Double Effect, which they believe permits the physician in extreme situations to kill the child *indirectly* in saving the mother. These authors agree that the rule against direct killing of innocent persons is without exception, and that in practice the physician may not sacrifice the child's life for the mother's but must do whatever he or she can for both. They do not demand, as would the Theory of Proportionality, that the impossible task be attempted of trying to weigh the many incommensurable advantages and disadvantages involved, instead of facing the clear fact that direct abortion deprives one human being of its most fundamental right for the sake of another's less fundamental rights.

J.J. Thomson (1971, 1983), in a widely quoted article, argued that a woman has an abortion not to deprive the child of the right to life but only to defend her right, in some circumstances at least, to refuse her body for the child's support. The most plausible case is that of the rape victim who is forced to care for a child for whom she has never willingly taken responsibility. This argument fails (M. Davis, 1983; Grisez and Boyle, 1979), however, because when only one person can save the life of another, the former is obliged to make considerable sacrifices to do so, even if the latter is a stranger. In pregnancy, even one that has resulted from rape, the mother is the only one who can save the child's life. (Although perhaps in the future, if it became possible with only proportionate risk to remove the child and sustain it in a surrogate mother or an artificial womb, this might no longer be true.) This argument is similar to the theory of rabbinic origin, already referred to, that the child is an unjust aggressor. It is questionable to consider the child as attacking the mother, even when, because of her physical condition, it is accidentally harmful to the mother, since the defect is on the part of the mother, not of the child. Also, even if one accepts this description of the child, it remains true that in fending off any aggressor one can only *indirectly* (according to the Principle of Double Effect) intend the aggressor's death, which is not the case in direct abortion.

Conclusions

What practical conclusions for healthcare professionals can be drawn from this discussion? The following norms are drawn from a pastoral document issued by the National Conference of Catholic Bishops (1974) and are helpful in determining what to do in particular situations.

1. Catholic hospitals cannot comply with laws requiring them to provide abortion services, even on the ground of material cooperation (*Ethical and Religious Directives for Catholic Health Facilities*, 1971, n. 12).

2. Catholic physicians, nurses, and healthcare workers who work in facilities that provide abortion services may not take part in such procedures in good conscience. Their rights of conscience in this regard are recognized by federal law (E. Rubin, 1987).

3. Physicians, nurses, and healthcare workers should give public witness to their belief in the sanctity of life, the integrity of every person, and the value of human life at every stage of its existence by their compassion and care for their patients.

4. Physicians, nurses, and healthcare workers who work in facilities that provide abortion services should notify the institution in writing of their conscientious refusal to participate in such actions.

5. Abortion is a serious and immoral action. Catholics who perform or obtain an abortion, or persuade others to do so, are doing grave harm to

another human being against the Christian commandment of love of neighbor. All who willingly and deliberately assist in abortion procedures share the sinfulness of this destructive act. This is particularly true of the attending surgeon and the healthcare personnel who administer abortifacient drugs or other abortion procedures.

6. Cooperation in the sinful act of abortion would not ordinarily extend to preparing patients for the procedure or providing aftercare. Christian witness, however, may well require Catholic nurses to avoid even those actions, which (although not necessarily evil in themselves) may be interpreted as a compromise of Christian values.

7. Under Church law, those who perform or obtain an abortion or deliberately persuade others to do so incur an automatic excommunication (C.I.C., c. 1398). The purpose of these severe penalties is to reinforce the Christian tradition that the Second Vatican Council (1965c) repeated when it declared, "Abortion and infanticide are unspeakable crimes." Of course, it must be understood that this automatic excommunication applies only to those who know that they are incurring it, yet freely chose to do so, understanding that they are committing a serious sin. This excommunication, as with all others, can be removed by sincere repentance and confession, with the purpose of trying to make amends to others for the harm done, insofar as this is possible. The tragedy of at least a million lives a year destroyed in the United States by the medical profession through abortion can only be contemplated with profound sorrow and the determination to work to educate people about its great injustice in the same way as to work against racism and war.

9.3 THE LAW AND PERSONHOOD

In 9.1 we discussed the biological facts concerning human personhood and the ethical norms that follow from these facts. Worthwhile laws are built on relevant facts and are based on ethical norms. Have the legislators and courts in the United States who have made statements about human personhood and the rights deriving from it been consistent with biological fact and ethical reasoning? This is the consideration of the following discussion.

Since the very nature of a profession involves a certain autonomy, as recognized by the Principle of the Common Good, Subsidiarity, and Functionalism (see 6.1 and 8.2), it is understandable that healthcare professionals are very reluctant to permit laypersons, including legislators, to prescribe limits for professional activities. The autonomy of the profession, however, is relative to its purpose of serving the health not only of individual patients, but also of the community. Laws have to be made to restrain lawyers, and even the clergy have had to submit to some government regulation of their activities (e.g., the clergy may not perform marriages between parties who do not have a license). The medical profession has generally accepted such regulations as those relating to dispensing narcotic drugs and to issuing death certificates.

Far more important is the question of the legal definition of the human person, which necessarily determines who are the subjects whose rights must be respected in every medical decision. Defining the human person affects the question of abortion and also concerns many of the problems concerning death, discussed in Chapters 11 and 13. It would seem obvious that laws should supply such a definition, yet historically it has been assumed that the matter is so obvious as to require no definition (St. John-Stevas, 1961, 1971). That this assumption is unfounded is evident from the history of slavery and racial discrimination in the United States, where there has been a long struggle to have members of the racial minorities recognized as full persons with rights equal to those of the majority.

Medieval and British common law regarded abortion as a serious crime, although the courts were not always clear as to whether or at what stage of pregnancy abortion was to be punished as homicide. In 1803, the first statute law in the United States on the subject declared abortion to be a crime punishable by death if the child had "quickened" and by lesser but serious penalties if the child had not. Throughout the nineteenth century in England and in the United States, increasingly strict laws were passed against abortion, but with exceptions for therapeutic abortion to save the mother's life. Such legislation was strongly supported by the American medical profession, partly because the medical risks for the mother in abortion were still high, but also because the advance in embryology had convinced physicians of the humanity of the fetus (Mohr, 1978).

A number of factors, however, were at work in the opposite direction. First, in Europe and the United States, the value systems of humanism and Marxism, with their emphasis on human technological control over life, came to dominate the professions; thus, as abortion became medically safer, it seemed to many just another effective method of controlling human destiny. Second, the antiabortion laws proved increasingly difficult to enforce equitably, since women of means could obtain an abortion on therapeutic pretexts, whereas poorer women could not. This reason seems to have greatly influenced many clergymen and physicians who worked with the poor, as has Dr. Bernard Nathanson (1983; Nathanson and Ostling, 1979). Nathanson recounts his change of mind to an antiabortion position after seeing the enormous increase in abortions, which he and his associates had not anticipated when they worked for permissive legalization. Third, the increasing concern over the population explosion and the growing tax burden for social welfare suggested that abortion was a very effective method of reducing the birth rate, at least as a backup to contraception. Fourth, the feminist movement, which originally opposed abortion, began to favor it as giving women more control over their own lives and greater equality with men. Fifth, the emphasis on the right of privacy in sexual matters increased with the spread of new contraceptive methods.

The Supreme Court Decision

New York, Colorado, and California adopted very permissive laws with regard to abortion in the 1960s. Finally, on Jan. 22, 1973, the U.S. Supreme Court, in *Roe v. Wade* and *Doe v. Bolton*, came to the decision that it is unconstitutional for any law to infringe on the right of privacy, by which a woman has the sole power of decision as to whether to have an abortion, just as couples have the same right to the practice of contraception (Krason, 1983). Although some laws regulating medical procedures, especially after the first trimester of pregnancy and even more restrictively after the second trimester, were not automatically excluded by the court as having possible constitutional validity, the right of the woman to decide was stated unequivocally. Also, the court reinforced this in later cases by declaring that a woman did not need the consent of the child's father to have an abortion, nor did a minor need the consent of her parents. Surprisingly, in *Maher v. Roe* (1977), the Supreme Court ruled that this right of the woman to have an abortion does not imply that she has the right to have assistance for such an abortion from state or federal funds, since the government as a matter of public policy can favor childbirth over abortion provided that it does not infringe the woman's freedom. Several states have sought to limit the practice of elective abortions by specifying requirements in regard to informed consent or parental permission, but for the most part the courts have declared this legislation unconstitutional (E. Rubin, 1987). Critics point out that this decision again introduces the factor of inequity, which had been one of the strongest arguments for liberalization; that is under previous laws poor women could not have an abortion, but well-to-do women could.

The main criticism, however, that can be brought against the present stance of the Supreme Court is not that it has moved to protect the woman's rights, which is entirely in accord with its main historical effort to strengthen and extend human rights. Rather, the primary criticism is that the court has simply evaded the question of the child's rights on the very flimsy pretext that it is a speculative question on which there is no general agreement (Dellapenna, 1987; Noonan, 1979). One may well ask, When *has* there been general agreement on the issue of rights for racial minorities or for women? It is just because such issues are highly controversial and, if you prefer, "speculative," that the Supreme Court has the duty to face them squarely. In fact, the court has decided that the unborn child is not a human being with human rights, but it has not done so honestly, nor persuasively, as will be evident to anyone who checks the unscholarly history of the controversy with which it documented its decision (Ely, 1973). As Callahan (1973a) has said:

> It is often thought that when the State withdraws from resolving "speculative" questions (by definition those which command no consensus) then freedom is somehow served; that was the gist of all those arguments which would leave abortion decisions up to individual choice and conscience. I have always found that an odd kind of contention, one which, if followed rigorously, would leave all decisions bearing on concepts of "justice," "equality," "the general welfare," and the like up to individual consciences as well. For what notions could be more speculative in their final meaning and implications, to judge from all the disagreement they provoke (p. 7).

Some who favor the Supreme Court's stand have tried to blunt this issue by arguing that the court has not only considered the mother's rights, but has in effect also protected the right of the unborn child not to be born into a world where the child is unwanted and may suffer from physical or psychological disabilities. If a child does have such a paradoxical right, however, then the child has the right to choose to live or not live, just as the mother has the right to choose to abort or not. This right of the child to choose to live is denied when the mother exercises her right to abort. Thus the question of conflict of rights cannot be evaded (Garfield and Hennessey, 1984). Either the rights in question are not truly rights, or some way to balance them must be found. The Supreme Court has simply confused this question.

The result of the Supreme Court's evading the fundamental issue of whether the child as well as the mother is the subject of human rights has led to a vigorous pro-life movement. This movement favors a constitutional amendment that either would define the human person as beginning with conception or would permit the states to deal with the question individually. Some urge the adoption of this amendment by the Congress and its ratification by the states; others urge a special constitutional convention to debate it. Others believe Congress could constitutionally define legal personality as beginning with conception. The Catholic bishops have expressed support for some type of amendment, leaving the choice of its exact form to public discussion, and have launched a campaign of education on the "respect life" question. The pro-life movement is by no means a Catholic movement but includes a large membership of other faiths (J. Davis, 1985; McClendon, 1986). As for public opinion in the United States, it would seem that the majority would permit abortion in hardship cases but would probably not support "abortion on demand" (*New York Times*, Dec. 1, 1987).

The pro-life movement, however, is severely criticized by some groups in the United States who have been the strongest supporters of human rights and social justice. These proponents of civil liberties point out that the pro-life members seem to focus all their concern for human rights on the unborn, while showing little concern for the social injustices suffered by those already born (Jackson, 1988). One might ask if social justice and civil rights enthusiasts are not equally inconsistent when they hail *Roe v. Wade* as a triumph for civil liberty and connect abortion with the cause of women's rights. Both sides need to realize that human rights can only be furthered by a broad and consistent effort to extend legal protection for every human being regardless of race, sex, religion, and age, from conception to death. Moreover, the debate about how best to protect human rights must not be clouded by accusing this or that party to the debate with imposing their religious values on others, when in all such debates every side, religious or secularist, is necessarily advocating a particular value system with which others will differ.

Pluralism

American pluralism demands that minority groups have a right to advocate their own values and to attempt to assign these values an influential role in public decisions (Reichley, 1985). Catholics begin to wonder what will happen to their values if the courts, in the name of women's rights, begin to require Catholic hospitals and Catholic healthcare professionals to cooperate in abortion. So far, the law and the courts have been rather careful to protect the consciences of healthcare professionals in such matters, but this protection may break down as Catholics become integrated into a national comprehensive healthcare program.

Consequently, despite the bishops' advocacy of pro-life, some Catholics are hesitant. They argue that Catholics should work to educate the public to the evils of abortion but should not favor laws against it, since in a pluralistic society this can only be divisive and ineffectual (Cuomo, 1985; Donceel, 1985). But what, then, of the rights of the powerless unborn?

Charles Curran (1975, 1984), in a theological analysis of the problem, shows that the authoritative Church documents, including the *Declaration on Procured Abortion* of the Sacred Congregation for the Doctrine of the Faith (1974), waver somewhat between the traditional conception of the relations of Church and state and the clearer position adopted by the Second Vatican Council in its *Declaration on Religious Liberty* (1965b). The newer position recognizes that the state, although it has the duty to protect and foster human rights, must also take into consideration that these rights include the freedom of conscience of all groups in the community to make personal decisions about what is right and wrong to the degree that this is compatible with public order and the rights of others. Curran concludes:

> ...three criteria—as much freedom as possible for the individual, the criterion of public order to justify state intervention by law, and the recognition of pragmatic, prudential, and feasible aspects in the law—constitute the framework for the proper understanding of the relationship between law and private morality. Note that in this understanding of law there is what some have called an idealistic function of law insofar as it must support peace, justice, and an order of morality, but there is also the recognition of the rights of freedom of individuals and at the same time the recognition of prudential and pragmatic judgments about the effectiveness and function of law itself. In this way the danger of an idealistic approach, which does not give enough importance to freedom and considerations of feasibility, is avoided as is the danger of a purely pragmatic approach, which sees law as totally distinct from considerations of justice and peace and merely accepting the mores of a particular society at any given time (p. 134).

Curran concludes by favoring "a moderately restrictive law such as that proposed by the American Law Institute which would allow abortion in certain particular situations." The argument for this is that it would be useless to pass a strict antiabortion law that could not be enforced with a success comparable to that of other criminal laws, since ineffective laws can harm public authority and their own moral cause. Considerable weight must also be given, as Curran himself says in the preceding quotation, to the "idealistic" aspect of law by which it proposes clear standards of right. If this were not the case, then the whole history of the United States with regard to civil rights legislation, which has always proved very difficult to enforce consistently, would be meaningless.

Catholics, therefore, if they are to be true to their belief in the advocacy of helpless and neglected persons, need to work vigorously for practical legislation—first a constitutional amendment, and if that proves impossible, then the type of restrictive laws Curran proposes that will do as much as possible for the protection of the unborn. At the same time Catholics must work also for the rights of women and other oppressed groups. Curran has wisely urged practicality, rather than fanaticism, in this campaign for human rights. Political pragmatism does not mean fear to take risks, however, nor does it imply a moral purism that refuses to work with people of different motivations and ideologies.

Some fear the pro-life movement because some of its members are too narrow in their social concerns or indulge in distasteful rhetoric. To demand that all persons working for a particular goal agree on all issues or always have good manners is idealistic indeed. What is rather to be feared is the kind of polarization over an issue that leads people to believe favoring one set of human rights is opposing another. This occurs when feminists believe that to support women's rights, they must forget the rights of children, or when pro-life members believe that to support the rights of children, they must oppose the feminist movement. Such polarization has led us in the past into believing that to be against Communism is to favor Fascism, or to favor Israel is to neglect the Palestinians, or to favor peace is to oppose all revolutionary social movements.

Reading the materials prepared by the American bishops on the respect-life issue will show that Church leadership in the United States is making a great effort to propose a consistent program of social justice in accordance with papal teaching, of which the defense of the unborn is only one part (Bernadine, 1986; National Conference of Catholic Bishops, 1984, 1986). The problem is that this consistent peace-and-justice stand is little noticed in the public media, nor well communicated from the pulpit, nor emphasized in Catholic religious education.

Undoubtedly, the task of Catholics as a community should first and last be educational rather than merely political. Jesus has taught trust in the power of truth, love, and forgiveness rather than in the power of law or law enforcement. Political action cannot be neglected, but it must be informed by a still deeper educational effort. In this effort to promote respect for life and the rights of the human person, the struggle over abortion is only one element, although a type of bedrock issue (Hitchcock, 1984). What confronts Catholics is the religion of humanism with its own value system supported by the economic, cultural, and political power of the elites who dominate modern life (Hitchcock, 1982; C. Rice, 1979).

The healthcare professional and Catholic healthcare institutions have crucial roles to play in this educational effort regarding all medical-ethical issues and their social impact. They have the biological and medical information necessary to understand such issues, and they have the professional prestige and influence to be heard. Above all, they deal with the concrete situations in which a respect for life can be most clearly witnessed. In using this legitimate power, they need not think that they are imposing their religious views on others, provided they seek to listen to and respect the conscientious convictions of others in the debate, without un-Christian attitudes of judgment and labeling.

Undoubtedly, the outcome of all the struggles over laws that affect the medical profession will be various forms of compromise that shift and change in each generation. Nothing is wrong with compromise when required to achieve common action in a society. It is wrong, however, when the form this compromise takes is determined by the cowardice of those who should have spoken up for persons who cannot speak for themselves.

9.4   TRIAGE AND THE LIMIT TO EXTENDING CARE

After discussing how to determine who is the human subject of healthcare, now the following question must be addressed: What should healthcare professionals do when they are unable to give full healthcare to all those who have a right to it? The issue here is not what to do in the long range, since that issue can be settled only by finding ways to provide more healthcare personnel and more equipment, a problem treated in Chapter 6. Rather, the issue is what to do in the *short* range when resources are fixed.

This is the problem of *triage*, a French word meaning "to pick or sort according to quality." The term came into medical usage as a result of wartime experiences and was first explained by Jean Larrey, chief surgeon of Napoleon in his *Memoirs* (Hinds, 1975), as follows:

> ...those who are dangerously wounded must be tended first, entirely without regard to rank or distinction. Those less severely injured must wait until the gravely wounded have been operated upon and dressed. The slightly wounded may go to the hospital in the first or second line; especially the officers, since they have horses and therefore have transport (p. 9).

Recently, however, triage has come to have a wider significance, applying to any situation where patients must be selected for treatment because limited resources dictate that not all can be given equal care (Kesset, 1985).

Ethicists generally agree that triage is just procedure in face of emergency or scarce resources, although the type of justice involved is not one of strict (commutative) equality, but of distributive equality (Winslow, 1982). In applying triage, two questions must be asked: Who is in greatest need of treatment? and Who will benefit most from treatment? In the classical cases of wartime or disaster emergencies, these two questions yield a threefold division of victims: (1) the dying, whose need is great, but who will benefit least from treatment and who should be made comfortable and left to die; (2) the wounded who will survive without treatment because their need is little and who can be left to care for themselves; and (3) the wounded who will die unless treated, but who will probably survive if treated. Since these last persons have both the greatest need and can benefit most, they deserve the chief attention.

Today triage problems arise not only in emergency situations, but also in situations where no real emergency exists (Kesset, 1985). For example, it is necessary to select which patients are to be given the drugs to alleviate the effects of the acquired immunodeficiency syndrome (AIDS) virus (Eckholm, 1986) or a drug when a sufficient supply for all is not yet available. Again, in supportive health facilities where patients require almost unlimited attention for chronic, debilitating diseases, similar selective problems are common.

To apply triage, it may be necessary to use some random principle of selection not based on need or benefit, such as lottery or the rule of *first come, first served* (Beauchamp and Childress, 1983). Such approaches are not unfair if the need and benefit are approximately the same for all, or if there is no way of discriminating on a need-and-benefit basis.

The Principle of Subsidiarity (6.1) provides that charity begins at home; that is, those closest to us and whose need is best known to us should be cared for first. Thus it is not unjust for a family to seek the best obtainable care for family members, or for physicians to give special attention to their regular patients with whom a special relation of trust has been built. The same principle, however, requires that those who have responsibility for a large group should attempt to distribute resources to protect the basic rights of all, but to give the greatest care to those who have most need and will benefit most (Margolis, 1985).

One of the most difficult problems in applying this kind of justice arises when a choice has to be made between supplying a few patients with expensive and lengthy treatment that may only keep them living for a while in very restricted activity (e.g., liver or heart transplantation) and supplying a larger number of persons with simple treatments (e.g., a vaccine or dietary supplement) that may keep them normally active for many years. On the one hand, benefit for the many is great. On the other hand, for each of the few who have transplantations, the need is great indeed and the benefit (from their point of view) very real. But does benefiting the few represent the just use of public resources? It seems that in the social distribution of healthcare, priority ought to be given to that form of preventive medicine or treatment of acute disease that will raise the general standards of health for the many, especially for the young, over elaborate modes of treatment for the aged or seriously handicapped persons (Callahan, 1987b).

The compensation for the individual who is aged or handicapped is to be found not so much in prolongation of life or expensive treatment as in the personal attention that will make what remains of life as meaningful as possible. In this sense, the need of such persons is great and the benefit they will receive also great, but what is required is not sophisticated medicine but wise and loving concern from the community. Sometimes such concern is better shown in cultures where medical technology is underdeveloped than it is in a modern culture.

Even more difficult questions arise when the triage principle is extended to problems of healthcare distribution on a global scale. The brief discussion of this topic here may exceed the scope of this book, but we believe that American healthcare professionals must think about health in global terms. This problem of social triage was dramatized by Hardin (1974, 1980) in his proposal of a "lifeboat ethics." He explains that because of the crisis of the population explosion and world hunger, the developed countries are faced with a hard choice. To continue to send medical aid and food to underdeveloped countries will only increase their overpopulation, with the result that even more people will starve than are starving now. Consequently, Hardin advocates either food be given only with the condition that these countries institute very stringent (even compulsory) population controls, or all foreign aid be terminated.

Hardin further argues that the developed countries would be foolish to lower their own standards of living and health for the sake of poorer countries, since they need all they have to raise healthy, well-educated children, who are the only hope of the human race for the future. No matter how much is given to poorer countries, they can never produce such children.

Joseph Fletcher (1975) points out that Hardin is not advocating mere selfishness but is using the utilitarian principle, *the greatest good for the greatest number*, with which Fletcher himself agrees. Fletcher is not sure that the emergency is yet as great as Hardin supposes, but he praises Hardin for his realism. We, too, believe that ethics should be hardheaded and realistic, but we do not believe that Hardin is so much hardheaded as hardhearted (Clements, 1985). A realistic effort at distributive justice must take a broader point of view (Reich, 1985).

If Hardin is right in believing that the crisis is so close that only short-range solutions are possible, it is doubtful that anything at all can be done about the situation because social policy seldom can move so rapidly. Moreover, most experts believe that, in the long term, various possibilities still exist for bringing world population and food resources into balance. The present situation has come about because the developed countries have introduced modern medical technology into the underdeveloped countries, not merely for humanitarian reasons, but to further their policies of political and economic colonialism. Unwittingly, by introducing modern medicine, the advanced countries also upset the ecological balance and produced a rapid population growth, without at the same time producing the standard of living that motivates and facilitates responsible parenthood in developed countries. Thus justice demands that the developed countries help restore the balance that they themselves destroyed (G. Johnson, 1986).

The United States and other wealthy countries need to undertake such a restoration of justice not only for its own sake, but also for the sake of self-preservation. It is unrealistic for the wealthy nations to suppose, as Hardin does, that they can sail away in their lifeboat and leave the rest of the world to sink. There is no place to sail to and no ocean to absorb the millions who look enviously to the wealth we hoard. Also, it is not true that these countries are without power, since the ultimate weapon may turn out to be not the atom bomb, but sheer numbers.

The popes, in their recent social encyclicals (John XXIII, 1961; Paul VI, 1967; John Paul II, 1987a), have repeatedly declared that the only solution to this crisis of population and resources is distributive justice, with the distribution made not by the superpowers but by international agreement and cooperation. Implicit in the argument of Hardin and other similar positions is the assumption that quality of life and hope for the future depend on an elite group of scientific technologists. Since it is the misapplication of scientific technology that has produced the present crisis, it is not so evident that this elite is really the hope of the future.

Thus, in the social triage situation, as Rawls (1971) has argued, the fundamental principle must be equal justice for all members of the world community, even the least privileged. If resources are scarce, these resources must first be assigned to those members of the community who can use them best and most justly for the good of all. Whoever makes this selection, however, must avoid the danger of being judges in their own case. Even according to Hardin's argument, would it not be wiser to attempt to select from *all* countries those citizens on whom the future of the race can most securely depend, rather than waste these resources on so many in the United States who consume much and contribute little?

Healthcare professionals have a responsibility to employ sound social triage principles in developing healthcare policies, taking care that all members of the national and the world communities play a role in determining priorities and criteria of selection. When faced with situations in which they find no practical way to achieve this broad justice, healthcare professionals must do what they can to give the best care to those who need it and can most benefit from it. In general, these patients are the poor and neglected whose need is greatest and whose opportunities in life will be most enhanced. The privileged have ways to take care of themselves.

9.5   EXPERIMENTATION OR RESEARCH ON HUMAN SUBJECTS

After healthcare professionals have determined who is the subject of medical care endowed with human rights (9.1 and 9.2), they must respect those rights, especially the person's right to health, that is, optimal physical and psychological functioning (2.1) insofar as resources are available (9.4). Let us now consider procedures that are or appear to be genuinely medical, but where there is real question as to the true purpose of the professional. Is the purpose to benefit the patient, or is it actually to manipulate or use a human subject, not for his or her own benefit, but for the researcher's benefit and perhaps of others who may profit from the researcher's discoveries (Annas, 1985b; Caplan, 1985; Levy, 1983)? The procedures under study in this section are called research, or experimentation, on human subjects. Research or experimentation on human subjects may be defined as seeking generalizable knowledge concerning human function or behavior through empirical studies (Belmont Report, 1978).

Potential Difficulties

When science takes man as its subject, tensions arise between two values basic to Western Society: freedom of scientific inquiry and protection of individual inviolability (p. 1).

These words introduce a major study by Katz et al. (1972) concerning the legal and ethical issues of human experimentation. That research on human beings is often useful and often necessary for the common good is undeniable. Many beneficial vaccines and other therapies, such as smallpox and poliomyelitis vaccines, open heart surgery, and successful treatment of certain birth defects, have required research with human subjects, and the whole world attests to its value. At the same time, human experimentation undoubtedly has also been abused. The world should never forget the horrors of the human experimentation carried out on innocent human beings in the name of scientific progress in Nazi concentration camps (Lifton, 1982; Mendelsohn, 1982). Aside from such atrocities, other egregious violations of human rights have occurred in the United States, such as the withholding of newly discovered penicillin from patients in the Tuskegee syphilis study (Jones, 1982); the Willowbrook experiments, in which retarded children were used as experimental subjects (Krugman, 1986); and the injection of live cancer cells in unknowing subjects in the Jewish Chronic Disease Hospital case (Faden and Beauchamp, 1986). Psychological experimentation has also given rise to serious debate about behavior control (Macklin, 1982). Such abuses often are not the product of demented or perverted minds; rather, they result from lack of care and ethical sensitivity on the part of well-motivated researchers who overlook the rights of human beings in an effort to ensure scientific progress or academic advancement (Shapiro and Charron, 1984). Today, in an effort to obviate excesses and facilitate progress, the federal government requires that every institution that carries on research projects with public funds establish an institutional review board (IRB) (President's Commission for the Study of Ethical Problems, 1983e). The federal government will not fund research projects unless they have been first approved by an IRB.

In their account of research on human subjects, Katz et al. (1972) state:

> Human experimentation in the practice of medicine is as old as the practice of medicine itself only during the last hundred years, since the age of Pasteur, has medicine become aware of the need for deliberate and well-planned experimentation (p. 1).

The heightened concern in regard to human experimentation on the part of ethically serious people results in part from the growing number of research projects involving human subjects. Since 1947, approximately one-quarter million projects involving human subjects have been carried out, about one third of which have been supported by the government (Chalkley, 1975; C. McCarthy, 1983). Another source of concern is the fact that the frontiers of science are being rolled back further every day. Thus human experimentation not only affects the rights of human persons in the future, but may also condition and change the very core of human nature itself (L. Shapiro et al., 1986).

Several categories of human subjects may be involved in research programs: (1) normal healthy adults, including the investigator, and elderly persons; (2) sick adults, usually referred to as "patients," including the acutely and terminally ill; (3) prisoners, soldiers, and students living in highly controlled situations; (4) children, both healthy and ill; (5) mentally incompetent adults and children; (6) unborn children or still-living aborted fetuses; and (7) the aging. Each of these categories presents special problems (see various studies of the National Commission for the Protection of Human Subjects of Biomedical and Behavioral Research, U.S. DHEW, 1975).

Experimental research on human subjects should be sharply distinguished from therapy, since the primary purpose of research is not to heal but to learn (Applebaum et al., 1987). It has become customary to classify research as either

235

therapeutic or nontherapeutic. *Therapeutic research* studies the effects of using diagnostic, prophylactic, or therapeutic methods that depart from standard medical practice but hold out a reasonable expectation of success. Thus the research may give greater benefit to the human subject than standard treatment. Clearly, what begins as human research may later become standard medical practice. *Nontherapeutic research*, on the other hand, is not designed to improve the health of the research subject; rather, it seeks to gain knowledge or develop techniques that may benefit people other than the subject (Belmont Report, 1978).

The proper manner of conducting these types of research on the various categories of human subjects has become one of the most discussed bioethical questions of recent years (R. Levine, 1981, 1983; President's Commission for the Study of Ethical Problems, 1983b). Through seminars, studies, and the work of the various federal commissions, some ethical principles have been developed to serve as a guide for researchers and for those who support research. As a result of such studies by legal, medical, and ethical groups throughout the world, especially in the generation after World War II, these principles have become widely accepted, even though there may be disagreement concerning their applications in particular cases. Interestingly, the norms produced by medical and legal experts of the World Health Organization (WHO), such as the Nuremberg Code (1946) and Helsinki statements (1964), are largely in harmony with the teaching of the Catholic Church on human dignity and research in that they admit to exceptionless ethical norms. However, later statements of research groups, such as the Warnock Committee, are not in accord with Church teaching because they follow a consequentialist method of reasoning (O'Rourke, 1988d).

Principles of Research on Human Subjects

These norms of research on human subjects that are summarized and discussed here relate chiefly to three ethical principles: the Principle of Totality and Integrity (2.4), which is especially relevant to therapeutic experimentation; the Principle of Human Dignity in Community (1.5), which relates to the limits of nontherapeutic experimentation; and the Principle of Informed Consent, a corollary of the Principle of Well-Formed Conscience (3.4; 8.1), which relates to the capacity of the various categories of human subjects to participate freely in research programs. Thus the following norms:

1. The knowledge sought through research must be important and obtainable by no other means, and the research must be carried on by qualified people.
2. Appropriate experimentation on animals and cadavers must precede human experimentation.
3. The risk of suffering or injury must be proportionate to the good to be gained.

Because the Principle of Double Effect (8.1) is used to justify the possible ill effects of human experimentation, the relation between risk and potential benefit is most important (R. Gillon, 1986a). Of course, predicting the degree of risk with certitude is seldom possible. Moreover, sometimes, as in the case of poliomyelitis inoculation in 1954 when the use of some poorly prepared live vaccine resulted in the death of children, or in the 1980 swine flu inoculation disaster, some risks are far greater than predicted. Thus absolute certainty in regard to the nature and degree of the risk cannot be required. To demand such certitude would paralyze all scientific research and would very often be detrimental to the patient. Care must be taken, however, to predict as accurately as possible the nature and magnitude of risk from any particular human experiment, and the bias of enthusiastic researchers in favor of the promise of some new procedure must be subject to review by an institutional review board (IRB) (R. Levine, 1985).

When determining the degree of risk that a person might undergo, one must bear in mind the difference between therapeutic and nontherapeutic research. If research is therapeutic, persons may undergo greater risk, and possibly even death form the illness or malady that the researcher is trying to cure. The Principle of Totality and Integrity (2.4) is involved in therapeutic experimentation.

The same Principle of Totality cannot be invoked in the case of non-therapeutic experimentation because one person is not related to another person or to a group of persons (the state) as part of the whole. Although a relationship of extrinsic finality exists between and among different people, a relationship of intrinsic finality or form does not. Thus one person does not exist for the other, nor is one person ordered to the other in total finality. Each individual person is an end, or being in himself or herself, and cannot be sacrificed for another. This is the basic reason why the public authority has no right to sacrifice individuals for "the interest of the state or for scientific progress" (Pius XII, 1952; John Paul II, 1986). Experiments carried out for the good of the state or for scientific progress may provide new knowledge or medical techniques and thus seem beneficial, but they do so and are so at the expense of human rights and human dignity and therefore are immoral.

Although it is sometimes fitting that researchers themselves participate in experiments, they are bound by the same restrictions as other subjects (Altman, 1987). The Nuremberg Code (1946) is rather unclear about this stipulation, implying that researchers may take greater risks than others (n. 5). Pope Pius XII (1954) expresses a more accurate view:

> He (the doctor or researcher) is subject to the same broad moral and juridical principles as govern other men. He has no right, consequently, to permit scientific or practical experiments which entail serious injury or which threaten to impair his health to be performed on his person, and even to a lesser extent is he authorized to attempt an operation of experimental nature which, according to authoritative opinion, could conceivably result in mutilation or even suicide (p. 315).

A special ethical issue arises in double-blind research (Koppleman, 1986; Marquis, 1986). The objectivity of scientific research depends largely on the use of controlled experimentation in which a group of subjects is divided into two subgroups, one of which receives the experimental therapy while the other, the control group, receives the standard therapy or a placebo. Sometimes three groups are used, one group receiving the experimental therapy, one receiving a placebo, and one receiving standard therapy or no treatment at all. This sometimes is called a *randomized* clinical trial. To ensure even greater objectivity, *double-blind* control may be used: not only are subjects not informed as to which form of treatment they are receiving, but even those researchers who evaluate the effects of the treatments do not know which subjects have received which therapy. Only the double-blind technique can eliminate the *placebo effect*, that is, the improvement frequently experienced by patients who expect it and the effect of bias on the part of scientists. This raises ethical questions, however, since it seems (1) that those patients who do not receive the new therapy are at a therapeutic disadvantage and (2) that none of the patients in the double-blind experiment could have given informed consent to a specific treatment (Louis and Shapiro, 1983; Marquis, 1986).

Thus in double-blind experiments the subjects should be informed that, if they consent to the experiment, some will receive the new treatment and others will not, but that none of the subjects will know. The potential subjects will then be free to consent to these experimental conditions or to refuse to participate. If the clinical trial involves a placebo for the control group and the project aims at finding an agent that will mitigate or cure a lethal or disabling disease, a special ethical issue arises, because the control group may not be receiving adequate therapy for their illness or disease (Koppleman, 1986). This is especially true if there is some justification for thinking that the new therapy might be much more effective than previous ones. Thus the same protocol may be therapeutic for some and nontherapeutic for others. IRBs and researchers then must be doubly cautious when a double-blind placebo protocol is being designed or reviewed. If the new therapy proves to be effective, the protocol must be modified and the new therapy made available to all. Of course, a rush to judgment concerning the efficacy of a new therapy must be avoided.

4. Subjects should be selected so that risks and benefits will not fall unequally on one group in society.

Justice demands that the burdens associated with human progress be shared equitably. In recent years, the poor of the world, especially in the United States, have borne an unequal burden in relation to medical research (Belmont Report, 1978). The causes of this situation are psychological as well as economic. Research protocols must be designed to offset this imbalance and ensure that when the poor take part in an experiment, their human rights are respected and they are given the freedom that their human dignity demands. Given the nature of the situation, it may not be possible to guarantee that the poor will not be numerically dominant in human experimentation, but it is possible to protect their rights. The same consideration holds for those categories of subjects who are chosen because they live in restricted and controlled circumstances where the researcher has easy access to them, such as prisoners, soldiers, or those confined to rest homes or mental institutions (Davis and Mahon, 1984; Denham, 1984). Such persons are in need of advocacy lest they be too easily persuaded to join in experiments by group pressure or by rewards that their situation makes excessively attractive. Prisoners, offered parole in return for participation in a dangerous experiment, may find this one hope of freedom too compelling to resist (*Scott v. Casey*, 1983).

> 5. To protect the integrity of the human person, free and informed (voluntary) consent must be obtained.

This is perhaps the most important and the most debated of the principles involved in human research and is a form of the Principle of Well-Formed Conscience (3.4), which is the very basis of all ethical decision. According to one of the more recent statements on the subject (Applebaum et al., 1987), free and informed consent means the following:

> The idea of informed consent is the notion that decisions about medical care a person will receive, if any, are to be made in a collaborative manner between patient and physician. The concept also implies that the physician must be prepared to engage in—indeed to initiate—a discussion with the patient about the available therapeutic options and to provide relevant information on them (p. 12).

The Belmont Report (1978) states that the elements of informed consent on the part of the patient are knowledge, understanding, and freedom. Despite extensive descriptions of informed consent published in ethical literature, serious discussions and disputes still arise concerning the concept of informed consent and its application. Many question, for example, whether prisoners can ever give *free* consent because of their situation (Lidz, 1983). Others question whether double-blind procedures, an integral part of some experiments, can ever be employed. We believe, however, that both experimentation on prisoners and double-blind procedures can be performed if extra care is taken in obtaining consent (Katz et al., 1972; Pellegrino, 1981).

Proxy or Vicarious Consent

The most puzzling problems, however, occur in situations in which one person gives consent for another for whom the first is morally responsible. The need for such consent occurs when unconscious people are dying, as well as in research programs (Reed and Olson, 1985). Such consent is usually called *proxy consent*, an unfortunate term because properly speaking a legal proxy is an agent acting on behalf of another by the other's consent, which is precisely what is lacking in the case under consideration. It would be better to call it *vicarious consent* because a vicar fulfills a duty for another irrespective of whether the other has authorized it. It should be distinguished also from *implicit* consent and *presumed* consent. Persons consent implicitly when they actually consent to some general line of action, which implies more detailed permissions, as when a patient consents to surgery without specifying what anesthetic is to be used. Consent is presumed when it is highly probable that someone who is not able to give consent because he or she is absent or unconscious would have given it if present or conscious, as when a surgeon presumes a patient would expect the physician to remove a diseased appendix that the patient was unaware of but that the surgeon notes in the course of other abdominal surgery. Proxy or vicarious consent, according to some, is a form of presumed consent, but other explanations are possible. As such, it simply means that one person who represents the interests of another by some legitimate title gives consent for the experiment in place of the subject because that subject is incompetent (John Paul II, 1980b; M. Shannon, 1985).

Children and retarded, infirm, and dying persons are often considered as subjects for human research (Davis and Mahon, 1984; Stanley and Stanley, 1981; J.W. Warren et al., 1986). It is sometimes argued that this gives them an opportunity that they might not otherwise have of contributing to the common good. Since they are not competent, or at least not fully competent, to give free and informed consent, consent can be given in their case only by the proxy or vicarious consent of a parent or guardian. Decisions of proxy consent must be made in view of the good of the individual person, not for a higher good, for a class good, or for the good of another person, which would amount to manipulation of the person as a mere means. Thus, if the experiment is therapeutic, there would be reason for the proxy to allow risk in proportion to the person's best interest. If nontherapeutic experimentation is involved, however, the decision is more difficult.

In recent years, the responsibility of a proxy in regard to children has been discussed rather intensely. Some authors (W.E. May, 1976; Ramsey, 1970) maintain that the person issuing proxy consent has no right to expose a ward to *any* risk. The justification for this position is that a proxy should make a decision in accord with the best interests of the subject. In nontherapeutic experimentation the interests of the subject are not clearly evident, however, and since the subject does not have the capacity to make a free choice about the matter, the proxy (guardian) has no right to presume or say anything on behalf of the ward.

Other authors (Ackerman, 1979; McCormick, 1974a, 1976; B. Miller, 1982) allow for exposing children and others who cannot consent for themselves to "minimal risk." Thus proxy consent is interpreted as a form of presumed consent. The justification for their position is that there are some things a child as a human being *ought* to do for others, for example, to take part in research when hope exists of "general benefit" and only minimal risk. The U.S. Commission for the Protection of Human Subjects, when determining the norms for fetal experimentation, followed the minimal risk theory (O'Rourke, 1975).

We follow the more protective opinion, maintaining that proxy consent is not licit in nontherapeutic experimentation, even when the risk is minimal. Our main reason for this opinion follows.

Guardians have responsibility for wards who cannot care for themselves because of the Principle of Human Dignity in Community, which affirms that no person can achieve fulfillment without sharing in the common good and contributing to it. Thus, when a guardian or proxy consents to subjecting a ward to experimentation, the proxy has the right to do so not on the basis of the presumed consent of the ward, which is merely hypothetical, but on the basis of an actuality, namely, the need of the ward for care. Therefore theories of presumed consent based on what the ward *ought* to do if the ward *could* consent are weak.

However, it may be granted that if a guardian in a concrete case is sure that the ward will suffer less than minimal risk and therefore gives proxy consent, the guardian does not fail in his or her responsibility to care for the ward, since "little counts for nothing," as the saying of the moralist goes. In other words, a guardian should be an advocate, jealous of the rights of the ward, not ready to yield these rights for the sake of others who cannot act for themselves, nor for the hypothetical rights of future generations of other children.

Another group of human subjects who have been subject to research protocols are living human embryos (C. Baron, 1985; Fletcher and Schulman, 1985; Lejeune et al., 1984). Some study groups have approved of this type of research (DHEW, 1978; Warnock Report, 1985). Other commissions have disapproved such research (Australian Research Commission, 1985; Council of Europe, 1985; Dickson, 1988). Committees and ethicists who approve of embryo research often assume a pragmatic, short-range view of the situation and usually proceed from consequentialist theories (Mendelhoff, 1985).

The Catholic Church recently issued a strong statement rejecting any form of research on human embryos that is nontherapeutic. Therapeutic research, still in beginning stages (Hendren and Lillehi, 1988), was approved; nontherapeutic research was rejected. The reasoning put forth in the statement of the Church is as follows (SCDF, 1987):

> The fruit of human generation from the first movement of its existence, that is to say, from the moment the zygote has formed, demands the unconditional respect that is morally due to the human being in his bodily and spiritual totality. The human being is to be respected and treated as a person from the moment of conception; and therefore from the same moment his rights as a person must be recognized, among which in the first place is the inviolable right of every innocent human being to life (p. 699).

6. At any time during the course of research, the subject (or the guardian who has given proxy consent) must be free to terminate the subject's participation in the experiment.

The reason for this guideline is that the consenting subject or proxy may not have been able to anticipate correctly the subjective factors involved, the amount of suffering, or the anxiety or depression until these begin to be actually experienced. Also, the subject or proxy may even discover the information given was inadequate or deceptive or imperfectly communicated; or the subject or proxy may have second thoughts about his or her own understanding or freedom when the consent was given. The subject or guardian cannot consent to give away the primary responsibility for defending the subject's own health and integrity, since this is an inherent right and obligation. Consequently, if during the course of the experimentation the subject or proxy begins to see that serious risks to the subject's well-being may be involved, the subject or proxy is ethically obliged to stop participation.

Psychological Experimentation

Special problems are involved in psychological research (Macklin, 1983; Szasz, 1982). To discuss these problems more fully, we defer the topic to Chapter 12, after the nature of psychotherapy and its distinctions from medical therapy are more thoroughly explained. At this point, however, we can state that in such research all the precautions necessary in medical experiments must be preserved, especially informed consent, careful calculation of risks and benefits, and precautions against the bias of researchers in favor of their own freedom. We must also add the following special rules.

7. In psychological research, which shades imperceptibly into social research, the researcher should work *with* rather than *on* the human subject (Morrison et al., 1982; Sider, 1983). That is, the researcher must gain the cooperation of the subject in the experiment so that the subject will participate with the purpose of gaining greater insight into himself or herself as a person in order to become freer and more realistic in coping with life's problems and also with the purpose of sharing this knowledge and freedom with others.

This principle is based on the fact that psychological experiments with a human subject are also psychological *experiences* for the subject that can be healthy and psychologically therapeutic or traumatizing reinforcement of bad behavior patterns. In very few cases can such experiences be merely neutral. Even the experience of filling out a questionnaire can be educational or terrifying. Any experience in which the patient is treated as a passive object rather than as a person cannot be a beneficial experience. It is questionable whether such treatment can even be experimentally useful, since in such a situation the human person is no longer acting humanly, but subhumanly. Thus persons should not permit themselves to be treated in this way because those who seek to reduce them to objects are violating their human rights. Psychological experimentation must involve the human, active cooperation of the subject and produce some learning and growth benefits.

8. The researcher must avoid breaking down human trust by lying or manipulation, although subjects can give free and informed consent to experiments in which they have to learn to interpret ambiguous communications or meet puzzling situations.

In many psychological experiments, the experimentalist does not seem to have any qualms about lying to subjects. Not only is lying (in our opinion) intrinsically wrong and contrary to professional ethics (5.2), it is also psychologically harmful to the subject because it breaks down the social trust on which human relations are built. Common-sense proof of this is that those who have been subjected to such manipulation often react indignantly when they discover the deception and believe they have been treated unfairly (Cupples and Cochnauer, 1985; C. Smith, 1981).

This is especially true when dealing with mentally disturbed patients, since elements of distrust, withdrawal, and paranoia present in most forms of emotional disturbance can only be reinforced by deception from professionals who claim to be especially trustworthy and authoritative (Davis and Mahon, 1984).

This rule against lying, however, does not prohibit experiments in which previous warning is given that the experiment may involve games with ambiguous clues and the subject's possible embarrassment and defeat. These are risks of the experiment to which the subject must have a chance to give free and informed consent or refusal. Deception in such a case is not what moral theologians define as a "lie," because traditional moral theology has always insisted that it is permissible to use ambiguous clues or language in situations where others are forewarned either explicitly or by the very nature of the situation.

Such games do not usually break down trust if the experimenter sticks to the rules. Moreover, they may be highly educational for the participant, since through them the subject gains insight as to how important it is to base one's interpretation of reality on solid evidence, rather than on ambiguous evidence or subjective feelings.

9. Researchers must not take serious risks of reducing the subjects' ability to perceive reality as it is or to make free choices except as a temporary experience through which the subjects can learn to cope with distortions of truth and attacks on their freedom.

This rule states more exactly the special risks involved in psychological experimentation. It excludes permission for any more than temporary damage to patients' ability to remain or become free in managing their own lives. Thus an experiment would be forbidden if it might cause organic brain damage or induce drug addiction. This also applies to experiments that might make the subject unduly liable to hypnotic control or to compulsive patterns of behavior or that might create recurrent hallucinations. A special case of psychological research that may involve risks to freedom is research in dealing with human sexuality. This issue is discussed in Chapter 12 in connection with therapy for inadequate or perverted sexual behavior.

CONCLUSION

These nine norms for ethical research are founded in the Christian concept of respect for persons and in the concept of responsibility that individuals have toward human community.

CHAPTER 10

Sexuality and Reproduction

OVERVIEW

In Chapter 8 we discuss the various principles or norms for virtuous human action, describing how these principles are related to the fundamental virtues of faith, hope, and charity. As one norm relating to the virtue of hope, we discuss briefly in Chapter 8 the Principle of Personalized Sexuality. Because human sexuality gives rise to many ethical issues in medical therapy and surgery, we believe that the matter of human sexuality should be considered more thoroughly. Thus, before considering the main ethical issues that arise in medicine from human sexuality—contraception (10.2), family planning (10.3), sterilization (10.4), artificial insemination (10.5), and treatment of rape victims (10.6)—we consider the norms for optimal function of sexuality from a Christian perspective (10.1). We conclude this chapter with a discussion of the pastoral approach to problems of conscience that arise from an effort to live effectively as sexual human beings (10.7).

10.1 PRINCIPLE OF PERSONALIZED SEXUALITY

Modern ethics insists that sexuality as much as any other basic human function must be understood as specifically human and personal (Lawler et al., 1985). It is often asserted that ancient ethics treated human sexuality simply as an animal function requiring restraint, lest it turn human beings into brutes. Although such assertions are caricatures of the past, a sound ethics certainly must guide human beings to love humanly, just as much as to work or to think humanly.

Human sexuality is not merely one item in human personality, but a dimension affecting every aspect of human living (Sacred Congregation for the Doctrine of the Faith, 1975a). In this regard the Church teaches "the human person...is so profoundly affected by sexuality that it must be considered one of the principal formative influences in the life of a man or woman. In fact, sex is the source of the biological, physiological, and spiritual characteristics which make a person male or female and which considerably influence each individual's progress toward maturity as members of society."

Thus human sexuality is a complex of many values that are generally recognized in every ethical theory, but whose interrelation and priority are the subject of much disagreement. These generally recognized values can be summarized in four chief categories. First, obviously sex is a search for sensual *pleasure* and satisfaction, releasing physical and psychic tensions. Second, more profoundly, sex is a search for the completion of the human person through an intimate personal union of *love* expressed by bodily union. Ordinarily, it is also conceived as complementing the male and female by one another so that each achieve a more complete humanity. Third, more broadly, sex is a social necessity for the *procreation* of children and their education in family values so as to expand the human community and guarantee its future beyond the death of individual members. Fourth, ultimately, sex is a *religious* mystery, somehow revealing the cosmic order. These values are recognized in all the great religions and philosophies of life and are protected and developed in every viable human culture.

In modern culture dominated by humanism, these values are generally thought to be combined in sexuality simply by accident through the purposeless process of biological evolution (Harris, 1985). Many today argue that human beings are free to combine or separate these different values according to their own purposes. Thus, for humanists, it seems entirely reasonable sometimes to use sex purely for the sake of pleasure apart from any relation to love or family or sometimes to use it to reproduce (e.g., by artificial insemination) without any reference to love or pleasure (Kurtz, 1988). For humanists, moreover, if sex can be said to have a religious value, it is because romantic love and sexual ecstasy are often considered the highest happiness in life, without which human experience is incomplete. Consequently, for many humanists, sexual morality can be reduced to two fundamental norms: (1) laws or social attitudes that hinder human freedom to achieve these sexual values in ways that the individual desires (as long as no other person is harmed) are unjust; and (2) sexual behavior (at least among consenting adults) is entirely a private matter to be determined by personal choice (Marcuse, 1972; Menninger, 1942).

The traditional Christian value system differs from humanism not, as some humanists suppose, in denying any of the four values of sexuality, but chiefly on two positive points. First, these values of sexuality are ethically *inseparable* by human choice because their combination is not the result of mere evolution, but of God's wise provision for human good. Second, the religious value of sex is that it provides an experience of love that teaches people the meaning of other kinds of love, especially the love between God and the human community (John Paul II, 1984b). Fully allowing for Sacred Scripture presents many themes concerning sexuality rather than a concise systematic teaching (Schnackenburg, 1965) and also for the historical developments within the Scripture, the Bible always treats the four values of *pleasure, love, family,* and *sacramentality* as intrinsically related and inseparable, and it has always disapproved of sexual behavior that separates them (B. Ashley, 1981).

245

Inseparable Values

These four values are inseparable because sexual pleasure without love is a type of lie in which the best possible expression of love in the natural language of bodies says what is not really meant. Such a lie destroys the fundamental trust on which human society rests; thus a society in which prostitution, promiscuity, and infidelity are common becomes a cynical, disillusioned, paranoid, and alienated society. The honey of hedonism becomes the bitter gall of distrust. On the other hand, love without pleasure makes intimacy a burden that becomes too heavy for most men and women to bear.

Moreover, sexual love that does not lead to procreation because of direct human intervention is not a complete expression of the love between man and woman. Sexual union may be all that they immediately seek, and it may seem for the moment to be the ultimate fulfillment of their love because sex is a natural mystery not fully understood by young lovers. The full meaning of sex, however, only gradually unveils itself as the couple live out their lives together. In this living they discover a deep need to express their love through children, who will enrich their lives and perpetuate their love beyond their own aging and death (John Paul II, 1981b).

In becoming a mother or a father, moreover, hidden aspects of the personality of a woman and a man emerge that neither previously had guessed, actualizing each as a person and further deepening their love. Thus the perfect expression of sexual love is not simply a series of orgasms, but a shared life expressed in many ways, of which intercourse may be the most intense, but family life the most rich and enduring.

Finally, for the Christian, this delightful and fruitful love of man and woman cannot be separated from its sacramentality. Such love seeks to perpetuate life beyond death; not merely a life of the delight that comes from bodily functions and transmits bodily life, but an eternal resurrected life in which the body will share the eternal delight of the soul, in which the intimacy of communication will know no barriers of time or place or limits of energy, and in which all generations will be contemporaneously young.

In view of this dignity of sexual love as a fulfillment of a basic human need, it would seem that the celibate life exemplified by Jesus falls short of complete human self-actualization. Indeed, if the world had never been distorted by sin, no doubt every Adam would have his Eve, and every Eve her Adam. In the sinful world, however, sex and the family are no longer an unmixed joy but in some ways a burden. To carry this and other burdens, society needs a division of labor. Those who choose marriage have its joys and its sorrows while sufficiently perpetuating the race, whereas those who choose the single life are freed for other secular and religious services to society while paying the price of a degree of loneliness and asceticism. Although this second choice is harder for human beings to appreciate, Jesus, Paul, and countless Christians in vowed religious life or in single lay life have freely chosen to devote their undivided energies to prayer, study, and social service.

The Church's teaching on marriage and celibacy are the two fundamental themes affirmed by Jesus in the texts forbidding divorce, in which Jesus appeals to the order of creation (Mk 10:2-12; Mt 19:3-9, 5:31-32; Lk 16:18; 1 Co 7:10) and calls on his disciples to leave all things to follow him (Mt 19:29 and parallels) in the celibate life he lives (1 Co 7). The religious or sacramental meaning of sexuality is most clearly expressed in Ephesians (5:22-23), where the writer takes up the Old Testament symbol of Yahweh as the husband of the chosen people and, building on Jesus' own references to himself as the bridegroom (Mk 2:1-20), transforms this into a symbol of the love between Christ and his community. Thus married love becomes an analogue through which is learned how God loves humanity and what its response to him through love of neighbor should be.

Often it is said that the Christian attitude toward sexuality, compared to that of the Jews (e.g., as expressed in the frank sensuousness of *The Song of Songs*) has always been negative. This is to be blamed, it is said, on the influence of the Greek and Roman Stoics, who rejected sex except for procreation, or of the Neoplatonists, the Gnostics, or the Manicheans, for whom the body was a prison of the soul. Again this supposed negative attitude of the Church to sex is attributed to a celibate clergy envious of those who were free to enter into sexual experience. Finally, particular blame is laid on St. Augustine for influencing Christian thought in this dualistic direction, supposedly as a result of his personal struggles with lust and his previous adherence to Manicheism (Kosnik et al., 1977). These historical assertions, although cited today by many authors (Keane, 1977; D. Maguire, 1986), are in fact half-truths that fail to take into account that the Catholic Church, as Noonan (1965) has shown, has consistently striven through the centuries to strike a positive balance between the dualistic rejection of sex on the one hand and its exaltation to a mystique on the other. As for St. Augustine, he was the first to present a complete theology of marriage that acknowledged sexual intercourse would exist even if Adam and Eve had never sinned. In striking this positive but realistic balance, the Church was influenced not so much by pagan authors as by the Bible, which contains a corrective for pagan exaggerations. By affirming both that the God-given purpose of sexuality is permanent fidelity in a fruitful marriage and that, nevertheless, human fulfillment can also be achieved in the single or celibate life, the Church glorifies both sexuality and its value for human happiness.

Reasons for Christian View

Undoubtedly, the Christian view of what human sexual behavior should be, which in the past won the admiration of so many pagans, today seems to many persons very unrealistic and even pernicious. The arguments of these critics will first be presented and then evaluated.

In the last 40 years, empirical studies on human sexual behavior (Kinsey et al., 1948, 1953; Masters and Johnson, 1966; Hite, 1976, 1981) have given extensive evidence (if anybody doubted it) that most human beings fall far short of the Christian norms for sexual integration. Before marriage, most Americans apparently engage in masturbation and casual sexual encounters, frequently homosexual ones. It is estimated that about five percent of the population of women are exclusively homosexual in orientation (Becker and Kavoussi, 1988; Gebhard, 1972). A high percentage of marriages end in divorce, and extramarital sex is often concurrent with marriage. Furthermore, many children are unwanted or abused, and even more suffer serious psychological damage from conflicts between parents. At the same time, contraceptive practice seems to predominate in American sexual life and is backed up with the widespread practice of abortion, so that the United States birthrate has achieved the zero-growth level (Kolata, 1988).

The pressure of this sexual revolution and the worldwide concern about the population explosion press especially hard on the Catholic couple who are deeply committed to the Christian life and are loyal to the Church (Finnis, 1985). At one time, it is claimed, a large family was an economic asset because the children contributed to the family's living. Today in the United States, the large family seems a heavy debit, particularly since modern healthcare ensures the survival of most children, and modern education requires long and expensive years of dependency on the parents. At the same time, the mother of the family has been educated to expect a life as an autonomous person to whom constant pregnancy and child care may be a continual frustration. With the mobility of American life, the breakup of the extended family, and the difficulty of obtaining inexpensive help, the mother of today may feel oppressed by a continual burden of child care. The father, on the other hand, forced by economic conditions to be away from home a large part of the day, is under growing pressure to provide for his family. The result, as evidenced by the divorce rate, is greatly weakened family stability and great psychological strain on the parents.

Moreover, to these critics the Church seems completely inconsistent (1) when it teaches that sexual love is personalized, yet also insists that it be confined to the legally enforced institution of marriage, and (2) when it teaches that parents must be responsible about parenthood, yet forbids them to use contraception. Has not the first inconsistency led to loveless marriages? And has not the second led many Catholic couples to disobey Church teaching rather than to imperil their marriage (and thus imperil proper care for their children) through prolonged or periodic abstinence from the fostering of their love by intercourse? Is it not a further inconsistency that a church which forbids contraception and abortion also frowns on new ways of helping infertile couples to have children by artificial insemination and in vitro fertilization?

Critics also stress that Catholic couples have hanging over them the fear of mortal sin, that is, separation from God and denial of the right to receive the sacraments, if they resort to forbidden sexual practices. Even if in their own consciences they believe themselves justified, they still have the burden of feeling guilt resulting from the conflict between their own consciences and the authoritative teaching of the Church. Granted that heroism is sometimes required of the Christian, is it reasonable to expect such heroism of the average person through many years of daily family living? And if these pressures are heroic for the normal man and woman, what about those who suffer from various forms of physical or psychological weakness or abnormality?

The Catholic Church is not the only one accused of lack of realism. Although the Protestant churches may be more permissive about contraceptive practices, they also generally propose to their people a rigorous ideal that excludes extramarital sex. Is it any wonder, then, that the traditional Christian understanding of sexuality seems antiquated and unrealistic, not only to humanists but also to many Christians?

Realism, however, depends on one's total vision of reality—one's world view and value system. Humanism has dominated the growth of modern society in the last 200 years and, naturally enough, has used scientific research and technology to promote its own perception of reality and to implement its own values. The stable family has not been a major objective of this society, as it would be for a social order shaped by a Christian vision (Kurtz, 1983, 1988). It is not surprising, therefore, that the Christian understanding and living of sexuality as essentially *family living* today appears increasingly outmoded and impracticable. The theology of liberation, however (Boff, 1986), is beginning to make us aware that minority groups (and active Christians are a minority in the modern world) must no longer allow the powerful to define reality for the weak. Consequently, rather than simply conforming to dominant views of what practical, realistic sexual life should be, Christians must work for changes in social structures that will make it practical and realistic to live the biblical understanding of family life.

Moreover, for the future the Christian view of marriage and family may prove more realistic than the present sexual revolution. Promiscuity seems to lead to fear of intimacy rather than to sexual fulfillment (Gabriel, 1987). The data of anthropological and behavioral science (Leslie and Korman, 1985) reveal that amidst the vast variety of sexual customs in the human race, two features stand out as universal:

1. Every human culture that has endured regulates sexual behavior by social norms that are diverse in some respects.
2. The primary social function of these norms is to protect the basic family unit as the chief means of educating the children, on whom the future of the community depends.

Technology and Values

Of course, many believe that because today's technological capabilities extend far beyond those possessed by former cultures, these technologies must be used to promote a humanist system of values, particularly a humanist view of sexuality (D. Maguire, 1986). Technology, however, can be used to promote Christian values just as well as humanist values.

The real question is *what* values should be promoted in sexual behavior. The answer must depend not only on what technology can accomplish, but on the human persons in community whom this technology ought to serve. This book argues throughout that the human person has basic needs that cannot be morally ignored because these needs define what it is to be human. Satisfaction of these needs constitutes this self-actualization, which is the supreme principle of ethics, the goal that measures every means as moral or immoral.

Realistic inquiry, in the light of the behavioral sciences as to what sexual needs of human beings have been manifested in all viable societies throughout history, reveals first that the basic pattern is monogamous marriage. This fact is intelligible in view of human biology, which is unique in two important respects:

1. The time of gestation and child care is remarkably long because of the time required to develop the complex human brain and to teach basic behavioral patterns to a child who, because of his or her excellent brain, is highly teachable.

2. Sexual intercourse is not confined, as in most mammals, to a mating season but ties the man and woman together in a lasting bond. This guarantees the woman and her child the concern of the male, who is no longer merely an impregnator but a father who shares in the burden of prolonged child care. The need for this continuous companionship of the father with his wife and children has necessitated the social institution of the family, which varies from culture to culture. (The chief variant has been polygyny, one father with many wives—a variant that is impractical for most men and consequently a status symbol for the elite.)

Some theologians today argue that since the function of sex for the human species is not only procreation but also the bonding of man to woman (in contrast to the male bonds of working and fighting groups, which also characterize the human species), sex therefore has two *separable* functions, of which the bonding function is more human than the procreative one (Kosnik et al., 1977). This obtuse argument ignores that this bonding is rooted in the need of the child, not in the necessary condition of the adults, since evolution might have produced human beings all of one sex, in which case male-female bonding would have been pointless. Thus human biology as such gives priority to procreation and has adapted human beings to family living precisely to care for the needs of large-brained human children.

This does not mean, however, that procreation is morally superior to the love that bonds man and woman, but only that the love that bonds them is truly human in itself and even more human in its extension to the children, who are the superabundance of that love. Just as Christians believe that they must love God and neighbor by a single love, likewise in the natural order the love that bonds man and woman is the same love that leads them to beget and care for their children. Thus procreation in the human species is unique because it is not the fulfillment of blind instinct nor a compulsive drive for pleasure, but a free act of commitment—the commitment to love another through bodies that will die, but not before they have transmitted human life.

Recent studies have revealed more information about intimate bonds between the child and the mother and father. Research has demonstrated that for days or weeks after childbirth the mother is in a special psychohormonal state that facilitates a maternal-infant bonding of lasting significance (John Fletcher, 1983b). The formerly typical practice in hospitals of separating the mother from the infant has been shown to be harmful to this bonding, which is essential so that certain basic emotional attitudes of trust may be "imprinted" in the child. Breast-feeding, which today is again urged by many pediatricians who have discovered its important physiological and psychological functions, helps to intensify this bonding.

The human father is himself unique in the animal kingdom; even more characteristic of the human species is the mother, whose role is the most highly developed in all mammalian species (Wilson, 1978). The fact that polygyny is the chief variant of marriages, and that in most societies a considerable degree of male promiscuousness and infidelity is tolerated, only underlines the uniquely human fact that, for the most part, human males settle down to one wife and take enormous pride in their children, making great personal sacrifices for both wife and offspring. Just as the mother plays an essential role in the child's initial emotional development, as the child grows, the father also plays an increasingly important role in that prolonged social education necessary for human living. This need of the human community to transmit and to develop its traditions results in culture. Modern psychology, of whatever school, has discovered how very deep in the unconscious are the roots of culture—that is, the basic relations of man and woman, parents and child—as well as the vast importance for a human person to live in a normal family.

In view of these simple facts that modern research more and more enforces, it is difficult to understand why so many (but not all) humanists believe that the current lack of social support for stable families is a healthy or inevitable consequence of technological advance, a "wave of the future." Some predict the demise of the family, or at least a sharp separation of sex from procreation. They believe that children in the future will be produced in the laboratory so that women can be totally liberated from pregnancy and child care, that children will be raised by experts and without parents, that sex will become an entertainment having no necessary connection with love, and that romantic love will be freed from every restriction as to the sexual partner. Such fantasies are as old as Plato, and they have always turned out to be a joke.

In particular, the present conviction that even those who have families should have only one or two children overlooks such views as that of the distinguished psychologist Eric Erikson (1968), who says that the Victorian suppression of sex has now given way to the suppression of a natural desire for children. For the child, too, there are great advantages of being raised with at least two or three brothers and sisters so as to learn social ways in the small unit before venturing into larger ones. It seems almost ridiculous to emphasize these points except that modern culture either overlooks them or minimizes them with the argument that they pertain to past cultures rather than acknowledging that these facts are evident in all cultures, precisely because they are rooted in fundamental human anthropology.

Most sociologists today do not see any evidence that the family is disappearing or will disappear in the immediate future (Glick, 1985; Leslie and Korman, 1985). They believe that its present weakness is caused by a cultural transition in which some of the family functions, particularly its economic and educational ones, have been partially taken over by other institutions. If this transaction leads to a new stability that respects basic human needs, the outcome may be a superior type of family life, promoting a greater sense of equality between the man and woman and a less repressive and exploitative education for the children. There is good reason to hope this will be the case, since the progress of the behavioral sciences will expose the fallacy of many current notions. If the culture destroys the family, however, it will destroy itself. The old adage must be remembered: "God forgives always, man sometimes, nature never."

Personalized Sexuality

As a result of the advance of the behavioral sciences and of the bitter controversies over sexual morality that have characterized this century, theologians have been struggling to develop a richer and more positive theology of sexuality and marriage.

Beginning with the work of Herbert Doms (1939) and Dietrich and Alice Von Hildebrand (1965, 1984) and culminating in the Second Vatican Council (1965c), Paul VI's encyclical *Humanae Vitae* (1968), and most recently John Paul II's *Familiaris Consortia* (1981b), a new formulation of the theology of marriage has taken on authoritative status in the Catholic Church. The former language that spoke of the value of procreation as the *primary end* of marriage has been abandoned, and the meaning of marriage is not said to be *love*, but love of a special kind—love that leads to a covenant (C.I.C., c. 1055). The characteristics of this *covenanted* love are that it is *human, total, faithful, exclusive,* and *fruitful.* The terms *human* and *total* indicate that it involves the whole human personality and thus includes the values of bodily pleasure along with the other aspects of male-female love. The terms *faithful* and *exclusive* indicate that this love is permanent and monogamous, and the term *fruitful* indicates that it is normally completed by children. This conception of sexuality, therefore, describes *human* sexuality in its specific character as human and not merely animal, although it includes human animality. The Council, Paul VI, and John Paul II emphasize this by indication that procreation is not irresponsible or fatalistic, but "responsible parenthood." That is, a couple should beget children precisely to express their love for each other and their concern for society. Thus procreation should be limited to those children for whom the couple can care and educate with the proper community assistance, although generosity in deciding on the number of children is a Christian responsibility.

Such a conception of sexuality is personalized because it attempts to use sex for truly interpersonal purposes (SCDF, 1987). Thus it excludes bestiality and autoeroticism as truly human uses of sex because these are efforts to achieve sexual satisfaction separated from the expression of love for another. This separation of pleasure from a truly human purpose (as 8.3 explains) leads to an addictive or compulsive pattern of behavior that restricts human freedom and makes it more difficult to form interpersonal relations (Carnes, 1983). Personalized sexuality also excludes sexual relations outside the permanent commitment of marriage because these are contrary to its character of the person's total giving. Finally, it questions homosexual unions because the love so expressed lacks the complementarity of male and female related to the fruitfulness of marriage. In all these forms of sexual relations, the full meaning of sexuality is essentially frustrated and its integrated values separated.

Of course, it can be argued that if for some reason persons cannot achieve all the values of sexuality, why may they not at least achieve those possible to them? For example, why cannot lonely old people satisfy themselves by masturbation or homosexuals by a loving relation with another member of their own sex? Certainly it is sometimes justifiable for married people to realize some of the values of marriage when responsible parenthood or of accidental sterility makes it impossible to have children. In this case, however, the love that they express to each other is an integral love, containing as its source all the other values of the marriage, even if these values cannot be effectively realized. In the sexual practices where these essential values are separated by human design, however, either this love is lacking (as in autoeroticism) or from the outset it lacks the full meaning of sexual love. Thus premarital love is not a total giving in a permanent commitment, whereas homosexual love may be a permanent commitment in friendship but lacks that male-female complementarity essential to the specific character of sexual love with its intrinsic relation to the family.

The pastoral care of persons struggling with all these problems is beyond the scope of this book. To be consistent with the Scriptures and the tradition of the Christian community, however, they must be guided by this integrated complex of values, which can be formulated in the following *Principle of Personalized Sexuality*:

> *The gift of sexuality must be used in keeping with its intrinsic specifically human teleology, which is (1) the loving, pleasurable, bodily expression of the complementary union of a male and female and (2) the perpetuation and expansion of this personal communion through the family they beget and educate.*

This principle is rooted in the basic need to live socially and to preserve this society. Its specifically Christian interpretation can be summed up simply by repeating that its religious symbolism is to witness in this passing world of birth and death to the fidelity of love between Christ and his people, a love whose transcendent and everlasting character is also especially realized and witnessed by Christian celibacy.

10.2 CONTROVERSY ON CONTRACEPTION

Our approach to the topic of contraception accepts the painful fact that today the Christian community is profoundly divided over the teaching of the Church in regard to methods of limiting the generation of children. In many countries there is a deep gap between Church teaching and actual practice— between how this teaching is presented and interpreted by some priests and by others, among whom are theologians and married couples. Some are convinced that the outcome of this debate concerning family limitation can only be the ultimate defeat of the present official teaching; others, of its ultimate vindication and consistent enforcement. Evidently a process of discernment is still going on within the Christian community. Our aim is to present the different aspects of the question as fairly as we can and correctly convey the official teaching, since this is essential information for the well-informed Christian conscience (3.4, 8.1).

The rise of a new value system, in the form of the humanism of the Enlightenment in the eighteenth century and of the immense social changes brought on by the Industrial Revolution in the nineteenth century, led to a renewed Christian concern for the family institution. In the twentieth century this concern has been intensified by the rapid rise in the divorce rate and the decline of the birthrate toward zero growth. Humanists generally accept these changes as an inevitable part of technological progress, to which social mores must be adjusted by what is often called "the sexual revolution" (Greer, 1984).

Christians have reacted in different ways. Some reassert traditional norms (Quay, 1988). Some attempt to rethink these norms with the purpose of strengthening them (Cahill, 1985; Rigali, 1986). The chief point of controversy among Christians, however, has been whether the practice of contraception will further weaken marriage or can be used to strengthen marriage (J. Kelly, 1986).

Until 1930 the Christian churches generally regarded contraception as a threat to marriage, but in that year the Anglican Church at its Lambeth Conference declared in favor of some uses of contraception (Gallagher, 1981). Catholic theologians had generally opposed this view, and Pope Pius XI reacted sharply to this declaration in the encyclical *Casti Connubii* (1930):

> ...any use of marriage, whatever, in the exercise of which the act is deprived through human industry of its natural power of procreating life, violates the law of God and of nature, and those who do anything of this nature are marked with the stain of grave sin (p. 28).

Pius XI's teaching was frequently repeated with greater precision by Pius XII. For example, in 1951 in an "Allocution to Italian Midwives," Pius XII said:

> Matrimony obliges to a state of life which, while carrying with it certain rights, also imposes the fulfillment of a positive work concerning the state of life itself....On married partners who engage in the specific act of their state, nature and the Creator impose the responsibility of providing for the conservation of the human race. This is the characteristic service from which their state of life derives its peculiar value, the bonum prolis *(value of children)* (p. 28).

By this Pius XII did not imply that every couple has a duty to propagate the race, nor that the use of sex always entails such an obligation, but simply that marriage finds it proper completion in begetting and raising a family (John Paul II, 1981b; Caffara, 1985).

On the whole this official teaching was received without much public protest by Catholic married couples, but soon medical discoveries raised new questions. In the same year as *Casti Connubii* was published, 1930, Ogino and Knaus announced their discovery of a scientific way to predict the sterile period of a woman's menstrual cycle, thus making possible the regulation of conception by the exclusive use of this period for sexual intercourse—the *rhythm method*, or more accurately *calendar rhythm*, since its use depends on the calendar regularity of the cycle.

At first theologians disagreed as to whether this method was simply another form of contraception, although as early as 1853 there was official recognition of this possibility (Sacred Penitentiary, 1853, 1880). However, this controversy was ended by Pius XII in the 1951 address just quoted, in which he said that methods of controlling conception by restricting intercourse to the sterile period, even for the whole duration of a marriage, were licit when justified by serious medical, eugenic, economic, or social reasons. Thus, for the first time, clear papal authority was given to the principle of responsible parenthood and to the use of scientific methods to control conception.

Pius XII was convinced that this position was consistent with *Casti Connubii* because the use of the sterile period seems not to involve any positive alteration of the essential meaning of the marital act. This act still retains its natural teleology ordered to procreation, although it takes place at a time when the woman is not fertile. It must be admitted, however, that this ordination to procreation is only *remote* and *indirect*, since the act takes place when conception is impossible.

Many priests hailed and promoted calendar rhythm as a fortunate pastoral solution to the practical dilemmas faced by married couples. Enthusiasm began to wane, however, when it became evident that even normal irregularities in the menstrual cycle can invalidate the prediction of the sterile period, and when many couples reported that the necessary abstention and uncertainty were a source of marital tension.

Soon after this papal approval of calendar rhythm, the first progesterone drug (the "pill"), which prevents conception by preventing ovulation, became available in 1952. This new method led to a theological debate that, as William Shannon (1970; see also Valsecchi, 1968) has observed, went through two different phases. In the first of these phases a number of theologians, of whom Louis Janssens of the University of Louvain was the most prominent (Swift, 1966), argued that the use of progesterones is not contraceptive in the sense condemned by *Casti Connubii*, since it could be regarded simply as an aid to the use of the sterile period by extending this period under effective control.

The lack of consensus on the validity of this interpretation, however, and especially the discovery that progesterones not only suppress ovulation but also sometimes might be abortifacient by preventing implantation of the fertilized ovum after conception (Hume, 1983), led to a second phase of discussion. Some theologians now began to question the whole interpretation of natural law on which the teaching of *Casti Connubii* seemed grounded. They argued that most contraceptive methods (provided they were not abortifacient), were, from a moral point of view, not essentially different from the use of the sterile period (Birmingham, 1964).

In view of the number and prominence of the theologians taking this position, many Catholics began to use progesterones and many confessors tolerated this practice. Many Catholic healthcare professionals and educated, conscientious Catholic couples who had followed this theological debate with great attention believed this new view supported their own experience and reflections. Thus it began to appear that this discernment process going on in the Church might lead to a modification of the previous teaching (Cavanaugh, 1964).

Attempt to Find a Solution

At the same time, the broader social problems of world poverty greatly concerned Pope John XXIII as the Second Vatican Council approached and led him to organize a Pontifical Study Commission on Family Population and Birth Problems to examine the population policies of the United Nations and to recommend a course of action for the pope. This commission met once in 1963 and twice in 1964.

As the Second Vatican Council continued, Pope Paul VI enlarged this commission to 58 members, including three married couples, five laywomen, moral theologians, physicians, psychologists, demographers, sociologists, and pastoral marriage counselors. Its fourth session was held March 25-28, 1965, in Rome (Hoyt, 1969). The Council itself concluded with the issuance of the document *Pastoral Constitution on The Church in the Modern World,* which contained the very important section "Fostering the Nobility of Marriage" (nn. 47-52), in which for the first time (but not without some anticipation in the writings of Pius XII) a new, fully personalistic view of marriage was proposed, along with a renewed condemnation of abortion. The "duty of responsible parenthood" was affirmed and the possible dangers of prolonged sexual abstinence in marriage referred to, but the question of licit and illicit methods of birth regulation was reserved by Paul VI until the completion of the commission's work.

After the close of the Council, a fifth and final session of the commission, now again enlarged to include 16 bishops as an executive committee, was held in Rome for two months in the spring of 1966. The discussion centered on two questions: (1) Is contraception intrinsically evil? (2) Can the Church change its teaching?

The result was a sharp division: a majority favored a change in the traditional teaching to permit at least some forms of contraception, and a minority opposed this position. The final report, "An Outline for a Document on Responsible Parenthood," was sent to the pope on June 23, 1966. It was written by six members of the theological subsection of the commission and approved by nine of the bishops in attendance, opposed by three, with three abstentions. It was accompanied by a separate document called "Pastoral Approaches," along with what is often referred to as the minority report and a rebuttal by those favoring the final report (Hoyt, 1969; R. Kaiser, 1985; Murphy, 1981; Valsecchi, 1968).

Paul VI then took almost two years of further study, apparently through private consultation of bishops and theologians, before publishing the encyclical *Humanae Vitae* on July 29, 1968. Because four years of waiting had produced widespread expectation of change, and because many had already adopted practices contrary to the traditional teaching, the encyclical provoked still further controversy. The national bishops' conferences of many countries issued pastoral letters attempting to explain the encyclical in terms acceptable to their people and to indicate how it might be pastorally applied (A. Flannery, 1969; McGrath, 1976).

In the United States, numerous moral theologians openly dissented from the encyclical and claimed a right to dissent from official teaching on this and other moral issues (C. Curran, 1975, 1979; C. Curran and Hunt, 1969). Greeley (1973, 1976) published evidence to show that, although most U.S. Catholics accepted the changes effected by the Second Vatican Council without great difficulty, *Humanae Vitae* was a major factor in the alienation of some Catholics in the United States from their Church.

The reason this controversy so upset U.S. Catholics is that it seems that the strong language of *Casti Connubii* and the milder yet unequivocal language of *Humanae Vitae* involve the infallibility of the pope and the Church. The common view, however, is that these documents do not claim to make a definitive decision about a revealed truth of faith or morals, which is all that the First Vatican Council (1870) declared to be an object of infallible definitions—a declaration confirmed by the Second Vatican Council (1964a). That *Humanae Vitae* (and thus *Casti Connubii* itself) does not have of itself infallible authority is evident in several ways. Most clearly, however, several national conferences of bishops, without ever being corrected by Paul VI, declared in their pastoral letters to their people that *Humanae Vitae* was not an infallible pronouncement (A. Flannery, 1969). Considering, however, that it reaffirmed in a very solemn way a consistent position of previous popes, *Humanae Vitae* possibly contains revealed truths about human sexuality that may later be solemnly defined (Ford and Grisez, 1978). Nevertheless, that it does contain such revealed truths can only be a matter of theological opinion or personal conviction at present. Thus its authority is that of a major document of the Church's ordinary teaching. Pope Paul VI gave great care to this document after attempting to inform himself of all the relevant data through the commission's work and other consultation, and this teaching has been repeatedly reaffirmed by John Paul II and the World Synod of Bishops. Section 3.4 has already explained (1) the respect due to such ordinary teaching, (2) the doctrine it may contain that could be infallibly defined in the future by an extraordinary declaration of a pope or council, (3) the scope of theological debate that it still permits, and (4) the role it should play in forming the personal conscience of Catholics. Further details on this are developed in 10.7.

This controversy has not only continued but has also broadened its scope to extend to all the issues of traditional sexual morality, as evidenced by the issuance by the Sacred Congregation for the Doctrine of the Faith (SCDF) of a document "Declaration of Certain Problems of Sexual Ethics" (1975a) an instruction on "Pastoral Care of Homosexual Persons" (1986) and the instruction *Donum Vitae* (SCDF, 1987) in regard to artificial methods of generation and experimental research. Moreover, the Sacred Congregation informed Fr. Charles Curran that he could no longer be considered "a Catholic theologian teaching in the name of the Church," because of his dissent from Church teaching in regard to sexuality,

(Ratzinger, 1986). In the United States a study commissioned by The Catholic Theological Society of America, *Human Sexuality* (Kosnik, et al., 1977), was very critical of the thought of the Church as expressed in the document issued by the SCDF in 1975. By implication the authors would also be opposed to the latter documents issued by the SCDF. On the other hand, some American Catholic physicians, philosophers, and theologians (R. Connell, 1970; Ford and Kelly, 1964; Grisez, 1964; Kippley, 1974; W.E. May, 1977b, 1983; Ratner, 1981) vigorously supported the traditional position of the Church.

How can greater consensus be achieved in this matter? We believe that certain points are becoming clearer, and we present them as our response to the invitation of the World Synod of Bishops of 1980, which invited "theologians to work, joining their forces with the Church teaching authority, so that the biblical foundations and personalist grounds" of the teaching of *Humanae Vitae* "might be brought to light more fully."

Search for Consensus

The expectation of those who disagreed with the teaching of the encyclical was that its widespread disregard by married couples, the opposition of so many notable theologians, and the hesitations of the national hierarchies would inevitably result in its modification. This has not taken place, however, and to date the signs do not indicate that it will. The World Synod of Bishops meetings in 1980, under the presidency of John Paul II, to discuss the problems of the Christian family in the world today, after very frank and realistic discussion of these difficulties (Murphy, 1981), unanimously reaffirmed the teaching of *Humanae Vitae* in agreement with the pope, who had already repeatedly confirmed it. The apostolic instruction issued after the synod of 1980, *Familiaris Consortio* (John Paul, II, 1981b), affirmed and developed the traditional teaching. On the twentieth anniversary of the document, national and international meetings of theologians supported its conclusions as the result of the study and experience of those years. In addition, Pope John Paul II (1984b) commented extensively on *Humanae Vitae* in a series of biblical-theological allocutions explaining the traditional teaching as an expression of the teaching "on redemption of the body and sacramentality of marriage." These reflections of Pope John Paul II present the teaching of *Humanae Vitae* in the context of personalism. In our opinion this confluence of papal teaching, plus the unanimity of the representatives of the national bishops' conferences of the whole world, after years of controversy, has largely countered the impression of confusion left by the pastoral letters of these conferences following the publication of *Humanae Vitae*. This also constitutes another serious sign that strengthens the case of those (Ford and Grisez, 1978) who consider the doctrine of *Humanae Vitae* to be irreformable, that is, an infallible element of the ordinary teaching of the Church (see 3.4).

Nevertheless, this still leaves the task of asking *why* the critics of the Church's teaching have not prevailed. Some will explain the situation in terms of the politics of the Roman curia (R. Kaiser, 1985). Such explanations, however, as with the attempts to give a merely political explanation of the First and Second Vatican Councils, or the conflict between Peter and Paul in the early Church, are of little relevance in a sincere search for the guidance of the Holy Spirit who works in the Church even through human weakness. What are the *theological* factors to keep in mind?

Theological Factors

First and most important, the Second Vatican Council and the statements of the Church since the Council clearly situate the problem of sexual ethics in the context of the Christian Church's historical concern for the *family* as an institution. These statements, however, describe this institution in a more biblical and personalistic way than formerly (John Paul II, 1984b). What we have called the Principle of Human Dignity in Community (1.5, 8.2) and the Principle of Personalized Sexuality (8.3) are to be realized in the family. The family alone can form a new generation in the Christian vision of the meaning of sexuality, that is, a love between husband and wife that is "human, total, exclusively faithful, and fruitful" and the source of all other sexual values. According to the Scriptures, a sexual love that is not "human, total, exclusively faithful, and fruitful" is not what the Creator designed sexual love to be.

This is what *Humanae Vitae* (1968) and *Familiaris Consortio* (1981), in echoing the Second Vatican Council, mean by saying that the *unitive* and *procreative* meanings of marriage may not be separated, although they can be enriched by human co-creativity (John Paul II, 1984b). This conception of marriage is freed from obsolete influences present in some versions of natural law reasoning and, moreover, does not rest merely on philosophical theories. As 8.3 indicates, this view had its origin in biblical teaching as interpreted by Christian experience and reflection. In its present personalized form, however, this view is a new development deepened by modern appreciation for human historicity and subjectivity. Generally, even those theologians (including those who wrote the "majority report" of the papal commission) who defend contraception seek to do so by showing that contraception, when practiced to strengthen marital love and fulfill the obligations of responsible parenthood, is consistent with this Christian vision of the meaning of sexuality (Häring, 1969). Those who attempt to defend contraception by attacking this basic principle of the inseparability of the unitive and procreative meaning of sexuality have no hope of prevailing against the clear message of the Scripture and tradition.

Second, it does not further a consensus to connect this specific question of contraception too closely with those revisions of moral theology, such as proportionalism, that want to abandon exceptionless moral norms and deny the existence of intrinsically immoral acts (John Paul II, 1984a). The failure of the papal commission's majority report to deal squarely with the problem of whether a contraceptive act is intrinsically immoral, apart from its circumstances and the circumstantial intentions of the couple, possibly left Paul VI no alternative except to reject their counsel. Section 8.1 argues that the sweeping revision of classical Catholic moral theology as proposed by proportionalism does not stand up under critical examination as a progressive development. If the case for contraception rests on this proportionalist methodology, it is weak.

Why, then, have leading theologians dissented from *Humanae Vitae*? In a review of the history of the question, Francis Murphy (1981), a historian of the Second Vatican Council and outspoken critic of *Humanae Vitae*, summarized the reasons: (1) a failure to take into account the crisis of overpopulation; (2) a failure to listen to the witness of the Christian married laity who not only do not see contraception as wrong but have experienced it as positive benefit to their lives as Christian families; (3) a failure to follow up on the new personalistic approach of the council to sexuality; and (4) a failure to answer serious theological objections. We cannot present or answer these objections in detail here, but we will point out very briefly why the events of years seem to have greatly weakened the force of the reasons mentioned by Murphy.

Reasons for Dissent

As to the first of these reasons, it is true that *Humanae Vitae* does not itself deal adequately with the problem of overpopulation, but this question pertains rather to the social teaching of the Church, including that of Paul VI and John Paul II, which does deal with it seriously (see 10.3).

The second reason is the supposed failure of *Humanae Vitae* to hear and respond to the witness of Christian couples concerning their actual experience with contraception (Birmingham, 1964; Bromley, 1965). Thus Archbishop John Quinn at the 1980 synod stated that 76.5 percent of Catholic women of childbearing age in the United States use contraception and that only 29 percent of American priests regard this as sinful (Murphy, 1981). However, here as well there is a "minority report" of those couples especially those practicing Natural Family Planning who strongly reject contraception that must be heard (Kippley, 1974; Zimmerman, 1981).

What theological interpretation is to be given these majority and minority testimonies? Is the testimony for a change in traditional teaching an evidence of the Holy Spirit? Or is it the work of the Deceiver, who reigns in a world where war, racism, sexism, and the exploitation of the poor are also widely accepted and even promoted by believing Christians? Does this "new insight into the nature of human sexuality" have its source in the Gospel and reverence for the work of the Creator? Or is its source in the influence of the humanism that dominates the contemporary "free world" and teaches that technology, freed of all reverence for nature, is the answer to every human problem? Certainly the fact that the public opinion polls also show an increasing acceptance of abortion by believing Christians must caution against too readily accepting the popular and theological approval of contraception among American Catholics as clear evidence of the guidance of the Holy Spirit. "Beloved, do not trust every spirit, but put the spirits to a test to see if they belong to God, because many false prophets have appeared in the world" (1 Jn 4:1; see also John Paul II, 1981b).

If this rise in the practice of contraception had resulted in an increased stability of Catholic marriages, we might feel more confident that it is in conformity with the Gospel, but the divorce rate among Catholics corresponds to the national average. Of course, the witness of married Catholics can by no means be denied. It is very important to progress in understanding the full God-given meaning of sexuality. It is doubtful, however, that this witness has yet been clearly heard, not so much because the bishops are deaf but as yet no adequate process exists by which this witness can be expressed. Public opinion polls taken among nominal Catholics do not provide such a process.

The third reason—that Paul VI failed to adhere to the new vision of the Second Vatican Council—is stated by Murphy (1981) as follows:

> Insisting that the moral aspects of any procedure to be used in regulating the transmission of life depended on objective standards, the council refrained from entering the debate over contraceptive methods, deferring to the decision of the pope whose commission was studying this matter. But the council declared that moral evaluation of sexual conduct should be based on consideration of "man's person and his acts." In *Humanae Vitae* Pope Paul chose to ignore this innovation and returned to the traditional basis of "marriage and its acts" (p. 23).

However, Paul VI begins the doctrinal part of the encyclical by saying:

> The question of human procreation, like every other question which touches human life, involves more than the limited aspects specific to such disciplines as biology, psychology, demography, or sociology. It is the whole person and the whole mission to which the person is called that must be considered: both its natural earthly aspects and its supernatural, eternal aspects. And since in the attempt to justify artificial methods of birth control many appeal to the demands of married love or responsible parenthood, these two important realities of married life must be accurately defined and analyzed. This is what we mean to do, with special reference to what the Second Vatican Council taught with the highest authority in its *Pastoral Constitution on the Church in the Modern World* (n. 7).

Paul VI then very explicitly attempts in his subsequent argument to treat the question in terms of "human person and his or her acts." The Council said:

> Therefore when there is question of harmonizing conjugal love with the responsible transmission of life, the moral aspect of any procedure does not depend solely on sincere intentions or an evaluation of motives. It must be determined by objective standards. These, based on the nature of the human person and his or her acts, preserve the full sense of mutual self-giving and human procreation in the context of true love. Such a goal cannot be achieved unless the virtue of conjugal chastity is sincerely practiced (n. 51).

Thus the Council left for the pope to decide what these "objective standards" for the marital act might be, based on the nature of the human person, and it is just this that Pope Paul VI tried to do. To find any contradiction between *Humanae Vitae* and the *Church in the Modern World*, one would have to show that they present different views of the "nature of the human person," which is far from evident. What is evident is that Paul VI attempted to write his encyclical with the same dynamic and personalistic approach to Christian anthropology that the

Council itself had taken. One has only to read n. 50 of the Council's document to see that it also very strongly stressed that "marriage and conjugal love are by their nature ordained toward the begetting and educating of children"; although it then added, "Marriage to be sure is not instituted solely for procreation."

Finally, as to the fourth reason, the chief theological objections to *Humanae Vitae* are summed up by Murphy (1981) in his historical account as follows:

> Pope Paul's argument was based on an obsolete concept of biology that attributes to every act of coitus a possibility that happens only relatively rarely, namely, the transmission of life. The encyclical admitted that coital acts during infertile periods are legitimate. But, by their very nature, such coital acts are not directed toward procreation, and thus they do actually separate the unitive meaning of conjugal intimacy from the possible transmission of life. This means that at one point the encyclical itself unwittingly accepts a factual separation of the unitive and generative aspects of coital acts—those that occur during the woman's infertile periods. The second great difficulty pointed out by theological opponents of the encyclical is that it measures the meaning of the human act by examining its physiological structure. In a number of places in the document, biological organisms and the processes of nature are accepted as the determinants of moral meaning. They are said to represent God's plan and therefore to be morally normative (p. 24).

To consider the second of these objections first, we have already shown (2.2, 8.3) that the complaints against "biologism" or "physicalism" so often brought today against classical moral methodology arise from the dualism of philosophical idealism going back to Descartes and Kant, in which the human person as subject is placed in opposition to the body considered as object. Consequently, it is thought to be depersonalizing to consider that the human body in its biological structures and functions could in any significant way determine the moral character of the free, spiritual activities of the person. If one accepts the account of the human person given in Chapter 1, however, in which the human person is *embodied* intelligent freedom, human acts, even the most spiritual such as love, are determined not exclusively but nevertheless fundamentally by their bodily character.

Gustave Martelet (1969, 1981), reputed to be one of the drafters of the encyclical (W. Shannon, 1970), has shown that Paul VI clearly intended to avoid any possible accusation that he was teaching that the morality of a human act is determined exclusively by its biological structure. For this reason, in *Humanae Vitae* he stressed that the human *meaning* of the sexual act is primary. Pope John Paul II seeks to stress the same aspect in his writings on the subject. Although it is not the material but the formal aspect of a human act (i.e., its immediate intention as a means to the end) that gives an act its formally moral character, this immediate intention cannot rectify physical (ontic) structures if these, by their own intrinsic teleology, imply something contradictory to basic human needs.

The teaching of the Church is not that a contraceptive act is morally evil simply because of its biological structure, but because the human person who performs the act cannot reasonably perform this type of biological act as truly fulfilling human needs. For example, a mature person cannot reasonably perform acts of masturbation as if these really satisfied the true meaning of human sexuality; nor can married persons perform acts of coitus interruptus, sodomy, or mutual masturbation as if these really expressed the true meaning of sexual love. There can be, and has been historically, some disagreement as to what type of sexual acts are appropriate in married life, but there has never been question that some must be excluded by reason of their inability to express humanly (including biologically) the integral meaning of Christian sexual love.

The real difficulty of the critics is indicated by Murphy's (1981) sentence, "They [biological processes] are said to represent God's plan and therefore to be morally normative." It is just this, however, that so clearly distinguishes the Christian view, which finds the whole universe, including the human body-person, to be a purposeful expression of the Creator's wise love from the humanist view of the world which finds no teleology but only blind evolutionary forces in nature. This does not deny, as we have emphasized in discussing the Principle of Stewardship and Creativity (8.3), that human reason is co-creative with God. Persons have the right and duty to perfect their bodies. Artificial contraception is not wrong because it is artificial, but because it is art used not to perfect nature but to frustrate it.

"Open to the Transmission of Life"

The first of the theological reasons mentioned by Murphy is the really substantial one, and the only one for which a modification of the teaching of the Church might be possible—namely, the question of whether a morally significant difference exists between the regulation of conception by the use of the sterile period and by contraception. It is this distinction that most Christians who accept contraception find difficult. The point is not as Murphy wrongly claims, that "Pope Paul's argument was based on an obsolete concept of biology," but whether it makes sense to say that acts deliberately chosen during the sterile period are "open to the transmission of life" in some morally significant sense that contraceptive acts are not. On this precise question that discussion must stay focused if consensus is to be achieved.

The majority-approved final report of the Pontifical Commission (Hoyt, 1969) asked and tried to answer this question as follows:

> What are the limits of the dominion of man with regard to the rational determination of his fecundity? The *general principle* can be formulated in this matter: It is the duty of man to perfect nature (or to order it to the human good expressed in matrimony) but not to destroy it. Even if the absolute untouchability of the fertile period cannot be maintained, neither can complete domination be affirmed. Besides, when man intervenes in the procreative process, he does this with the intention of regulating and not excluding fertility. Thus he unites the material finality toward fecundity which exists in intercourse with the formal finality of the person and renders the entire process "human."

This is the essential point on which *Humanae Vitae* refused the arguments of the commission's majority. The commission had argued that contraceptive acts are justified because they can be regarded as "partial acts" whose morality is determined by the couple's sexual life in its *totality*. If this totality is ordered to both love and procreation, these values are not separated by the contraceptive character of the partial acts. The encyclical, however, insists that these values cannot be separated even in the single marital act, but that every act must remain "open to the transmission of life." If these intrinsically related meanings are not objectively present even in the single act, the act cannot express true marital love, and thus it is intrinsically contrary to the human meaning of sexuality.

An Obvious Question

This raises the obvious question: How then are marital acts deliberately confined to the sterile period really an expression of true marital love? *Humanae Vitae* explained the issue briefly in this way:

> In reality, these two cases differ greatly from each other. For in the former case, the married couple use an opportunity given them by nature; but in the other, the couple prevent the order of generation from having its natural processes. (*In priore, coniuges legitime facultate utuntur sibi a natura data; in altera vero, iidem impediunt, quominus generationis ordo suos habeat naturae processus.*) If it is undeniable that in both cases the married couple by mutual and certain agreement for plausible reasons desire to avoid offspring and seek the certainty that offspring will not be born, nevertheless it must also be admitted that in the former case only does it occur that the couple are able to abstain from marital intercourse in the fertile periods, when for just motives the procreation of children is not desired [author's translation] (n. 16).

In *Familiaris Consortio*, Pope John Paul II set forth a more personalistic explanation:

> When couples, by means of recourse to contraception, separate these two meanings that God the creator has inscribed in the being of man and woman and in the dynamism of their sexual communion, they act as "arbiters" of the divine plan and they "manipulate" and degrade human sexuality and with it themselves and their married partner by altering its value of "total" self-giving. Thus the innate language that expresses the total reciprocal self-giving of husband and wife is overlaid, through contraception, by an objectively contradictory language, namely, that of not giving oneself totally to the other. This leads not only to a positive refusal to be open to life, but also to a falsification of the inner truth of conjugal love, which is called upon to give itself in personal totality.
>
> When, instead, by means of recourse to periods of infertility, the couple respect the inseparable connection between the unitive and procreative meanings of human sexuality, they are acting as "ministers" of God's plan and they "benefit from" their sexuality according to the original dynamism of "total" self-giving, without manipulation or alteration.
>
> In the light of the experience of many couples and of the data provided by the different human sciences, theological reflection is able to perceive and is called to study further the difference, both anthropological and moral, between contraception and recourse to the rhythm of the cycle: It is a

difference which is much wider and deeper than is usually thought, one which involves in the final analysis two irreconcilable concepts of the human person and of human sexuality. The choice of the natural rhythms involves accepting the cycle of the person, that is, the woman, and thereby accepting dialogue, reciprocal respect, shared responsibility, and self-control. To accept the cycle and to enter into dialogue means to recognize both the spiritual and corporal character of conjugal communion and to live personal love with its requirement of fidelity. In this context the couple comes to experience how conjugal communion is enriched with those values of tenderness and affection which constitute the inner soul of human sexuality in its physical dimension also. In this way sexuality is respected and promoted in its truly and fully human dimension and is never "used" as an "object" that, by breaking the personal unity of soul and body, strikes at God's creation itself at the level of the deepest interaction of nature and person (n. 32).

Thus it is possible for a couple to perform the marital act in a sterile phase of the natural cycle with the aim of achieving three values: (1) the expression of mutual love through total self-giving (the unitive meaning), (2) rational family planning (the procreative meaning), and (3) freedom from sexual compulsion by the discipline of periodic abstention. On the other hand, when they perform a contraceptive act, they positively exclude the procreative meaning and distort the unitive meaning, which no longer has the character of total self-giving because it is separate from its essential relation to procreation. They also lose the ascetical growth in freedom.

In what sense is a marital act deliberately placed in the infertile period still "open to the transmission of life"? Certainly this act is not directly and *proximately* ordered to procreation (since it is sterile). Thus the order is only indirect and *remote*. This remote ordination, however, does not seem merely to be the circumstantial intention of the agents, but objective and intrinsic to the moral object. It consists in the fact that God through nature has provided that human reproduction should normally result not from single acts of intercourse, but from a permanent partnership bound together by frequent sexual acts, only some of which are directly and approximately fertile. The infertile acts, therefore, are naturally ordered to fertility, although only indirectly and remotely. In this sense, although only in this sense, can they be said to be open to the transmission of life.

How, then, is it true to say that the deliberately infertile *contraceptive* act is "closed" to the transmission of life? Certainly it is closed if employed for merely hedonistic reasons in marriage or if used outside marriage by reason of a morally wrong intention that changes the moral object. When it is employed as an act of marital love that expresses itself in responsible parenthood, however, is not such an infertile act still *remotely* ordered to procreation, just as is the act in the sterile period? Thus one can argue that the two acts differ only in the mode in which the sterility is effected, and the question again is how this difference in mode differentiates the human meaning of the acts. The difference in mode in one case is said to be "natural" and in the other "artificial." *Natural* here cannot mean "without human intervention," since both modes result from the intervention of human intelligence—in the one case to choose the time of the acts; in the other to alter in some degree the process of the acts. How can one determine whether this difference of mode is ethically significant? The answer must be given in terms of the principle, *art perfects nature,* and this improvement of nature must be judged in terms of the achievement of a God-given natural finality. Regarding finality in both modes, however, the marital act apparently is open to the transmission of life only in the sense of an indirect and remote ordination.

Paul VI, however, did not judge this remote ordination to procreation of contraceptive acts to be sufficiently evident or objective to provide for the inseparability of the unitive and procreative meanings of sexuality. This is because in such acts the relation of these two values seems to depend not on the act itself, but rather on a subjective attitude or circumstantial intention, thus opening the way to other uses of sex that the Christian conscience has always rejected. The encyclical enumerates these as (1) extramarital sex, (2) exploitation of women as sex objects, (3) governmental intervention in parental rights, and (4) attrition of the Principle of Totality and Integrity (8.2), which limits other medical interventions contrary to human integrity. Thus Paul VI, despite general pressures to take a more permissive stand, believed his pastoral duty was to draw the line as to which methods of responsible parenthood would clearly protect the essential character of marriage. The teaching of the Church in recent years has affirmed the thought presented by Pope Paul VI and elaborated on it.

That the pope's fears were not wholly imaginary is evidenced by the fact that, since the encyclical, debate on questions of sexual ethics among Catholic theologians has become increasingly radical. Some now defend as morally justified in certain circumstances the practice of masturbation, homosexuality, and extramarital intercourse, which the commission majority in 1966 vehemently rejected (C. Curran, 1982; Curran and McCormick, 1988; Kosnik et al., 1977).

Thus the question originally posed remains: "Is there a morally significant sense in which the act of intercourse deliberately engaged in only in sterile periods is essentially different from that act contraceptively modified?" Pope Paul's and Pope John Paul's answer is yes because although the act performed in the sterile period is only remotely and indirectly ordered to the transmission of life, it is so ordered by its natural and God-given teleology which the partners respect. This natural teleology is deliberately destroyed, however, in the practice of contraception, whether by a barrier method or by the temporary or permanent sterilization of one of the partners. This difference is morally significant because sexual love was designed by a wise and loving God as a mystery in which the partners participate freely and intelligently as lovers and co-creators in an activity basic to their fulfillment as human beings and as members of the human community. To alter the design of this divine gift of a means by which sexual love is fittingly expressed in such a way as to confuse its essential meaning is contrary to the integrity of the couple and inevitably leads to the corruption of human society.

In our opinion, this insight into the way contraception contradicts the God-given meaning of sexuality, as revealed in Scripture and tradition, expressed in *Humanae Vitae,* and reaffirmed in the face of much criticism by John Paul II in collegial action with the 1980 synod and in *Familiaris Consortio* (1981), is logically consistent and consistent also with the known data of human science and historical experience. The arguments brought against the teaching of the Church concerning the marital act have not demonstrated it to be fallacious nor provided an alternative consistent with the theological and scientific data. Undoubtedly, it is a stumbling block not only to humanists who deny its basic assumptions, but also to many Christians of goodwill to whom it seems far fetched and hopelessly unrealistic. But may this not be because the contemporary mind has accepted as "realistic" a social system based on an unlimited and anti-ecological manipulation of the natural order that is surrealistic and ultimately self-destructive? We should not be scandalized as Christians because such controversies about moral issues exist in the Church at the level of its ordinary teaching, nor that they continue to awaken theological debate. Such struggles are necessary for the growth of the Church and its efforts to meet the needs of the times. The remainder of this chapter discusses first the social applications of this teaching and then its pastoral applications.

10.3 RESPONSIBLE PARENTHOOD THROUGH NATURAL FAMILY PLANNING

To reiterate, the Second Vatican Council, *Humanae Vitae,* and *Familiaris Consortio* emphasize that to be truly human and moral, sexuality must express the freedom and responsibility of mutual love, including the intelligent planning of parenthood, so as to provide for the proper care and education of the children. The primary responsibility for such care belongs to the parents. They have the right to community assistance in this task, however, according to the Principle of the Common Good, Subsidiarity, and Functionalism (6.1, 8.2), both because the right to marry and have children is a basic human right and because a family makes a fundamental contribution to the common good of the community (John Paul II, 1981b).

Catholics, especially healthcare professionals, therefore cannot be indifferent to the population explosion and the ethical problems it raises. Also, they cannot solve such problems by blind trust in providence. All recent papal documents dealing with social problems address these issues (Paul VI, 1967; John Paul II, 1987a), and papal representatives have become involved in the work of the United Nations and other international organizations in an effort to plan for the global future. The popes generally have favored a position that, although it is not popular in the United States, is probably the majority opinion in the world at present (Dych, 1982; World Population Conference, 1974). Briefly, this view can be summarized as follows.

1. The growth rate in developed countries, including those with a high percentage of Catholics, has steadily declined for many years and will soon reach zero.
2. This crisis results from the ecological imbalance produced when developed countries introduced modern medicine into their colonies or dependencies without at the same time raising the standard of living proportionately.

3. The Malthusian view that population growth must exceed growth in food production has been proved false, and modern technology should be able to supply food for all, provided that the present abnormal population growth can be slowed.
4. The most effective program of responsible parenthood will have two features:
   a. It will be supported by strong economic development.
   b. It will promote those methods of birth regulation most acceptable to the value systems of a people, including methods acceptable for Catholics (John Paul II, 1981b).

Thus the popes, in disproving some methods of birth regulation, have not neglected to promote a definite social program that includes a reasonable answer to the population problem. Even those who would not agree with that answer should admit that it is more realistic than the two solutions most popular in the United States: (1) the "lifeboat" ethics discussed in Chapter 9, according to which the United States should maintain its own standard of living and let the rest of the world starve; and (2) the planned parenthood solution, which relies on promoting the use of contraceptives and abortion by the poor, while ignoring the need for a radical global economic readjustment. Both these solutions rest on the unrealistic assumption that the United States and the other developed countries can indefinitely continue their present style of life, based in large measure on the exploitation of underdeveloped countries.

If one accepts the view that population control has to be achieved by profound social changes rather than by the use of particular methods of birth regulation, then what methods are ethically acceptable in view of the Catholic and other value systems which emphasize the intimate relation between sexuality and procreation? How can couples limit the size of their families and still enjoy the sexual expression of their love in a way that will strengthen their permanent commitment to each other, give joy to their life together, and provide a healthy model of sexual love for their maturing children?

The Second Vatican Council (1965c) in the *Pastoral Constitution on the Church in the Modern World* (n. 51), *Humanae Vitae* (1968), and *Familiaris Consortio* (1981b) affirm the Christian value of periodic abstinence and the acceptability of natural family planning methods, that is, those making use of naturally sterile periods. The Council, however, also recalled the pastoral advice of St. Paul (1 Co 7:5) that while it is legitimate for a married couple by mutual consent to abstain from sexual relations for a time, especially for spiritual and ascetic reasons, prolonged abstinence can be dangerous to the marriage.

As already mentioned, such periodic abstinence first began to be practiced scientifically by the calendar rhythm method, which depends on the regularity of a woman's menstrual cycle. Because this cycle varies considerably in different women and for some is quite irregular, this method could not be practiced effectively by many couples. It sometimes led to insecurity and tension in married life and gave the whole theory of birth regulation through natural methods a poor reputation, with the result that many physicians are still not well-informed on the whole issue. Today, however, new techniques for detecting ovulation have been discovered, so that the irregularity of a woman's cycle has become irrelevant (E. Billings and Westmore, 1985; Gross, 1987). Moreover, knowledge of the cycle of fertility cannot only help couples limit pregnancy, it can also help them achieve it when desired (World Health Organization [WHO], 1984).

Modern Methods

Two modern and well-tested methods of determining the time of ovulation and the periods of fertility and infertility are the sympto-thermal method and the ovulation method, the latter often called the Billings method after the physicians who developed it. The *sympto-thermal method* uses complex criteria for determining the time of ovulation: changes in cervical mucus, changes in the position and softness of the cervix and the dilation of its opening, and a shift in temperature, all of which are caused by a rise in blood estrogen as a result of the ovulation process. Some sympto-thermal methods add a calendar calculation as in the older calendar rhythm method (Klaus and Brennan, 1981). This method's advocates believe the concurrence of these signs ensures greater effectiveness.

The *ovulation,* or *Billings, method,* on the other hand, uses only the appearance of mucus at the vulva, determined by the woman herself on the basis of a sensation of wetness and the color and elasticity of the secretion. This alkaline mucus of an appropriate viscosity provides a kind of natural valve (J. Billings, 1983) that facilitates the movement of the sperm into the uterus and fallopian tubes at precisely the time when ovulation has produced a mature ovum ready for fertilization, while at other times its absence leaves the sperm to be destroyed by the normal acidity of the vagina. In the presence of this facilitating mucus, the sperm can survive for several days, but probably not for more than six (Hilgers, 1980; Klaus and Brennan, 1981). The most recent studies seem to show that the Billings method is as effective for many as the more complex sympto-thermal method (WHO, 1987).

Recent natural family planning studies (WHO, 1984) report 97 percent *use* effectiveness and 98 percent *method* effectiveness, the latter figure taking into account those pregnancies that could be explained by a failure of the couple to abstain at a time when they knew by the method they might be fertile. Thus the method effectiveness rate is as good or better than any known contraceptive method except sterilization. User failures occur in all forms of contraception except sterilization (which also sometimes although very rarely fails) and in fact are not always failures, since interviews often reveal both conscious and unconscious motivation by couples to achieve pregnancy (WHO, 1987).

Recently, another method to identify fertility in women has been dis-covered. Ovarian and pituitary hormone production shows characteristic patterns during the fertility cycle. Urinary estrogen and pregnanediol measurements detect the beginning, peak, and end of the fertile period. Economical enzyme immunoassays and other tests that measure the urinary estrogen and preg-nanediol glucuronides have been developed. Seemingly, this will enhance the effectiveness of the ovulation method (Brown et al., 1987).

Proponents of these methods insist that while these are not difficult to teach any couple, their effectiveness depends on accurate instruction and the competence of well-instructed teachers (WHO, 1981). Learning the method from books is discouraged unless competent teachers are unavailable (Hilgers, 1980). These methods have not yet won general acceptance among physicians in the United States. Several reasons are put forward for this lack of acceptance, the most prominent being that U.S. physicians tend to trust the effect of pharmaceuticals rather than the natural processes of the person.

Advantages of Natural Family Planning

No methods of birth regulation are without some serious disadvantages, and natural methods have been criticized on several grounds. First, although they are highly effective under ideal conditions, natural methods have not been as widely tested in ordinary conditions as have progesterones and intrauterine devices. It has been shown, however, that the Billings method can be used with excellent success even by uneducated women (WHO, 1981). Second, some (Guerrero, 1973) have theorized that natural family planning may produce genetic defects, since if a pregnancy does occur, it is more likely to be at a time when the ovum or sperm are somewhat aged. Hilgers (1977) has shown that not only is there little evidence for such a theory, but strong reason to regard it as false, and a recent study (Brown et al., 1987; Gray, 1984) again disproves this theory. Third, and much more important, natural methods require a period of abstinence, which if they are to equal progesterones and intrauterine devices in effectiveness, may be as long as half the cycle (WHO, 1984). Moreover, there is evidence that such abstinence makes following the system more difficult (WHO, 1987).

In answer to this last and most serious difficulty, proponents of natural family planning first point out that because of improved methods, abstinence can often be reduced with safety to five or six days in a cycle. Second, they emphasize that contraceptive methods also have strong psychological drawbacks. Thirdly, the same studies from WHO that set forth the difficulties of NFP also reported overall satisfaction with the method, even though it required greater self-discipline to follow.

Positively, proponents of natural methods (Kippley, 1974; Zimmerman, 1981) argue that:

1. Such methods place responsibility on *both* partners, not merely on the woman, as do most methods, or on the man, as does vasectomy.
2. Many women who use such methods have reported an enhanced sense of personal dignity resulting from an awareness of their own body and its rhythms (Klaus, 1979).
3. Abstinence from intercourse can help a couple learn to have confidence in the strength of their love for each other and to express it in a variety of ways, without that preoccupation with "total orgasm," which is proving to be a source of tension for many men and women today.

270

4. Periodic abstinence removes something of the sexual routine and enhances the experience when it is actually decided on.

Although spontaneity is an element of lovemaking, a truly mature notion of spontaneity is not just being able to have intercourse at any time. Rather, it is knowing how to give oneself to another at the *appropriate* time, a time necessarily determined by the rhythm of some lifestyle.

Besides these possible subjective psychological advantages, natural family planning has several definite objective merits.

1. When properly practiced, it can be as effective as any method except sterilization and does not have the obvious disadvantages of a sterilizing procedure.
2. Unlike other comparably effective methods, that is, progesterones and intrauterine devices, it has no medical risks.
3. It is never abortifacient, as progesterones and intrauterine devices almost certainly are.
4. It is inexpensive, does not require regular medical checkups to avoid side effects, and can be effectively taught by simple practical instruction.

Finally, the mechanistic tendencies of our society are evidenced in reaction to natural family planning. The tendency is to evaluate methods of family limitation only from statistical efficiency, instead of questioning which methods result in greater marital love between man and wife.

Healthcare professionals need to be well-informed on natural family planning and have a serious professional obligation to promote it as a method indubitably in keeping with Christian values, as well as having important medical advantages for couples who use it consistently and satisfactorily. Catholic healthcare facilities and physicians should provide instruction in this method honestly and objectively. Also, they should give correct information about other methods so that couples will not think they are being treated as guinea pigs but have free and informed consent in trying to use natural methods for responsible parenthood. It is especially essential that Catholic scientists advance research on natural methods so as to overcome the crisis of conscience among Catholics. They also must provide others with a method of responsible parenthood and population control that does not tend to separate sexuality from family life, as has the spread of contraceptive practices.

10.4 STERILIZATION AND OTHER METHODS OF CONTRACEPTION

Sterilization

Humanae Vitae accepts the ethical concept of responsible parenthood through use of the sterile period but rejects as unethical other methods of family limitation that are widely accepted today:

Therefore in conformity to these principles of a human and Christian teaching on marriage, we must again declare that the direct interruption of generation already begun as a legitimate way of regulating the number of children, and especially abortion, even for therapeutic motives, are to be altogether rejected. Equally to be excluded, as the teaching authority of the Church has frequently declared, is direct sterilization of a man or a woman, whether this be temporary or permanent. Likewise is every act to be rejected which, either in anticipation of the conjugal act, or in its accomplishment or in the development of its natural consequences, proposes, whether as an end or a means, to render procreation impossible (n. 14).

In *Familiaris Consortio* (1981b), John Paul II states that it is "a grave offense against human dignity and justice for governments or public authorities to attempt to limit the freedom of couples in deciding about children. Consequently, any coercion applied by such authorities in favor of contraception, or still worse, of sterilization and procured abortion, must be altogether condemned and forcefully rejected."

For some, however, the birth control issue is a purely technical matter of calculating the evident advantages and disadvantages of particular methods, since they disregard the considerations that have occupied Catholic thinking. For example, a theologian such as Joseph Fletcher (1954) concludes that if persons have the right to control parenthood, they have the right to use any means that assists to this end unless it has serious medical disadvantages.

From this point of view, the most effective and apparently the least dangerous method of preventing pregnancy (although it is not 100 percent effective) is permanent sterilization of the man through vasectomy or of the woman by ligation of the fallopian tubes (Population Crisis Committee, 1985). This is termed *direct* sterilization because its direct purpose is contraceptive. Rather than a treatment for pathology, it is intended to render the subject sterile but not impotent. The latest figures state that 16.6 million adults have been sterilized in the United States (Hatcher et al., 1987).

When sterility results merely as a side effect of a medical treatment directly aimed at a specific pathology, it is said to be *indirect* and can be justified by the Principle of Totality and Integrity (2.4) because the direct purpose of the procedure is to restore health. Thus diseased sex organs can be removed surgically or can be treated by drugs or radiation therapy even if treatment results in sterility (Lawler et al., 1985).

Because direct sterilization is a form of contraception, it is intrinsically unethical and contrary to the Principle of Totality and Integrity because it sacrifices a basic human function without the necessity of preserving life. It is usually said that sterilization is much safer than oral contraception and intrauterine devices. Nevertheless, tubal ligation can occasionally result in tubal pregnancies fatal to the fetus and dangerous to the mother (H. Peterson et al., 1983). Although surgeons are having increasing success in repairing sterilization for people who change their minds (both vasectomies and tubal ligations), the risk that such attempts will fail remains high (Flickinger, 1985; Miskell, 1986). An increasing number of both men and women, especially those who have been sterilized at an early age or those planning to remarry, now wish to have children.

As a form of birth regulation, the chief disadvantage of sterilization is that it deprives the human person of a basic human capacity (W.E. May, 1987).

Individuals so deprived do not at the time want any more children and often report subjective satisfaction with the results. Nevertheless, the ability to reproduce, even when not actually used, relates the individual to the community and its future. The sense of power, of life, and of belonging that this engenders is reflected in the religions and philosophies of all cultures, as the Old Testament testifies by treating sterility in man or woman as a curse (1 S 1:5-6; Ho 9:14). The efforts of Indira Ghandi, politically disastrous to her regime, to enforce a sterilization program on a people of ancient culture illustrate both how tempting this method is to governments seeking a simple and permanent solution to the problem of population control and how deeply it is resented and feared where this sense of the human meaning of complete sexual power is still alive among the otherwise powerless.

Involuntary sterilization is an obvious violation of the Principle of Free and Informed Consent (John Paul II, 1981b). In 1979 the U.S. Department of Health, Education, and Welfare issued guidelines for federally funded institutions that ensured such consent for any sterilizations of persons confined to these facilities. These rules include a moratorium on the sterilization of all mentally incompetent persons under the age of 21 and a 30-day waiting period for all others. Nevertheless, there clearly can be considerable pressure for sterilization of even mildly retarded persons and of the poor, especially blacks and Hispanics, allegedly for eugenic reasons, but really to reduce the costs and trouble to parents and the public of "unwanted children" (Varga, 1984).

The highly technological culture in the United States is singularly insensitive to deep human needs, which are unconscious or suppressed by cultural influences. Simply because most sterilized persons respond on a questionnaire that they experienced only a feeling of relief and freedom as a result of their surgery is not necessarily a reliable indication of its deeper consequences. Social and psychological research on such effects is still very superficial, and the present ecological crisis warns of the gradual long-term risks of what at first appeared to be harmless and effective technologies.

Directive 20

The U.S. Catholic Conference (USCC) included the following statement in its *Ethical and Religious Directives for Catholic Health Facilities* (1971):

> Directive 20: Procedures that induce sterility, whether permanent or temporary are permitted when: (a) They are immediately directed to the cure, diminution, or prevention of a serious pathological condition and are not directly contraceptive (that is, contraception is not the purpose); and (b) a simpler treatment is not reasonably available. Hence, for example, oophorectomy or irradiation of the ovaries may be allowed in treating carcinoma of the breast and metastasis therefrom; and orchiectomy is permitted in the treatment of carcinoma of the prostate.

As a result of the controversy concerning the interpretation of this directive, the Holy See was questioned by the National Conference of Catholic Bishops

(NCCB) whether "medical sterilizations," that is, sterilizations desired because the woman would experience some physiological difficulty if she became pregnant, were to be considered direct or indirect sterilizations. For example, a woman with nephritis might suffer from uremic poisoning if she became pregnant. Would a tubal ligation be allowed to prevent a future pathology? The result of this dialogue between the Holy See and the U.S. bishops was a clarification of Directive 20. The response of the Holy See (SCDF, 1975b) was followed by two statements of the NCCB (1977, 1980). In regard to the nature of the act in question, the documents distinguished between direct sterilization and indirect sterilization:

> Any sterilization which of itself, that is, of its own nature and condition, has the sole immediate effect of rendering the generative faculty incapable of procreation, is to be considered direct sterilization, as the term is understood in the declarations of the pontifical Magisterium, especially of Pius XII. Therefore notwithstanding any subjectively right intention of those whose actions are prompted by the care or prevention of physiological or mental illness which is foreseen or feared as a result of pregnancy, such sterilization remains absolutely forbidden according to the doctrine of the Church (SCDF, 1975b) (p. 9).

> Thus sterilization may not be used as a means of contraception nor may it be used as a means for the care or prevention of a physical or mental illness which is foreseen as a result of pregnancy (NCCB, 1977) (p. 5).

On the other hand, procedures that induce sterility are not always forbidden (NCCB, 1977):

> Procedures that induce sterility are permitted when (a) they are immediately directed to the cure, elimination, or prevention of a serious pathological condition and are not directly contraceptive; and (b) a simpler treatment is not reasonably available (p. 5).

Underlying the statement of the Holy See concerning sterilization is the traditional interpretation of the Principle of Totality and Integrity. According to the traditional application of this principle, surgery may not be used to excise or damage a part of the body unless (1) the continued presence or functioning of a particular organ causes serious damage to the whole body; (2) the harm to the whole body cannot be avoided except by the surgery, which gives promise of being effective; and (3) one can reasonably expect that the negative effect will be offset by the positive effect (Pius XII, 1952).

Thus, according to its proper meaning, the Principle of Totality and Integrity applies to the physiological functions of the person and cannot licitly be extended to other levels of human function such as the social or the spiritual. In the past few years several theologians have sought to apply this principle to every aspect of a person's existence, including the relationship to family, community, and society at large (Häring, 1973; Nolan, 1968). When considering the effort to interpret the Principle of Totality and Integrity in such a way as to justify sterilizations for medical reasons, Charles Curran (1973) affirmed, "In evaluating such an approach, one must honestly recognize that such a proposal runs contrary to the explicit teaching of Pius XII."

The difficulty with extending the Principle of Totality and Integrity to social or psychic aspects of human life is that it erodes the distinction between the order of nature, in which a natural determinism exists, and the order of human culture (or social and psychological determinisms), which in the long run is under human control. As this book demonstrates throughout, this distinction between the order of nature and the order of human culture is debated today because (1) society is achieving more and more technical control over the determinisms of nature and (2) society is becoming increasingly aware of how imperfect our control is over cultural determinisms. Nevertheless, this difficulty in distinguishing precisely between nature and culture does not destroy the significance of the distinction.

Alleged Reasons

The document emanating from the Holy See also commented specifically on the reasons that had been put forward to allow direct sterilizations in Catholic hospitals. These reasons invoked (1) the common good, (2) the Principle of Totality and Integrity, and (3) dissent (SCDF, 1975b). Hence, the documents explained:

> 1. Neither can any mandate of public authority, which would seek to impose direct sterilization as necessary for the common good, be invoked for such sterilization damages the dignity and inviolability of the human person.

> 2. Likewise, neither can one invoke the Principle of Totality in this case, in virtue of which principal interference with organs is justified for the greater good of the person; sterility intended in itself is not oriented to the integral good of the person...inasmuch as it damages the ethical good of the person, which is the highest good, since it deliberately deprives foreseen and freely chosen sexual activity of an essential element.

> 3. The Congregation, while it confirms this traditional doctrine of the Church, is not unaware of the dissent against this teaching from many theologians. The Congregation, however, denies that doctrinal significance can be attributed to this fact as such, so as to constitute a "theological source" which the faithful might invoke and thereby abandon the authentic Magisterium, and follow the opinions of private theologians which dissent from it (p. 9).

Hospital Policy

Concerning the activities of Catholic healthcare facilities in the United States, the NCCB (1977) declared:

> Freely approving direct sterilization constitutes formal cooperation in evil and would be "totally unbecoming the mission" of the hospital as well as "contrary to the necessary proclamation and defense of the moral order." The Catholic health facility has the moral responsibility (and this is legally recognized) to

decide what medical procedures it will provide services for. Ordinarily, then, there will be no need or reason to provide services for objectively immoral procedures (p. 6).

Although the documents declared that formal cooperation was not allowed, they did state that material cooperation might be allowed under certain conditions (SCDF, 1975b):

> The traditional doctrine regarding material cooperation, with the proper distinctions between necessary and free, proximate and remote, remains valid, to be applied with the utmost prudence, if the case warrants. In the application of the principle of material cooperation, if the case warrants, great care must be taken against scandal and the danger of any misunderstanding by an appropriate explanation of what is really being done (p. 10).

Specific criteria for the use of material cooperation were set forth in the statements of the NCCB in 1977 and 1980:

> 1. If the cooperation is to remain material, the reason for the cooperation must be something over and above the reason for the sterilization itself. Since as mentioned above, the hospital has authority over its own decisions, this should not happen with any frequency (1977) (p. 7).

> 2. In making judgments about the morality of cooperation, each case must be decided on its own merits. Since hospital situations, and even individual cases, differ so much, it would not be prudent to apply automatically a decision made in one hospital, or even in once case, to another (1977) (p. 7).

> 3. The local Ordinary has responsibility for assuring that the moral teachings of the Church be taught and followed in healthcare facilities which are to be recognized as Catholic. In this important matter there should be increased and continuing collaboration between the Bishop, healthcare facilities, and their sponsoring religious communities. Local conditions will suggest the practical structures necessary to insure this collaboration (1980) (p. 175).

Material cooperation can be justified only in situations where the facility, because of some duress or pressure, cannot reasonably exercise its autonomy. The Catholic health facility must take every precaution to avoid creating misunderstanding or causing scandal for its staff, patients, or the general public and must offer a proper explanation when necessary. It should be made clear that the facility disapproves of direct sterilization and that material cooperation in no way implies approval.

Material Cooperation

What type of situation in the United States might warrant material cooperation of Catholic healthcare facilities with persons wishing to perform or who have performed direct sterilizations? Some believe that the failure of the *Ethical and Religious Directives* to allow for liberal use of material cooperation in regard to sterilizations is a serious mistake, if not an injustice (Bayley and McCormick, 1980). What are Catholic hospitals to do when staff physicians believe a sterilization is medically justified? Or when it might be possible to reduce the risk of two separate surgeries (e.g., cesarean birth and tubal ligation) by performing both at the same time?

The traditional norms of moral theology in regard to cooperation are explained in section 8.1. Although formal cooperation with ethically wrong actions is never permissible, remote material cooperation in actions that are objectively evil is not only permitted but sometimes might be required in a world where, without such cooperation, many good actions would be frustrated or eliminated altogether. If Catholic hospitals are to carry out their ministry, they cannot avoid engaging in some activities with evil but unintended effects. Some of these will involve working with persons who choose to perform acts that the hospital would not feel ethically justified in doing on its own behalf but that must be tolerated for the sake of the primarily good results of the cooperation. Thus, by paying dues to state hospital associations, Catholic hospitals give support and recognition to some hospitals in which abortions are performed. Their failure to belong to the association, however, would endanger their own ability to pursue their mission and would also weaken the work of the association to uphold medical and ethical standards. In belonging to the association, Catholic hospitals perform a good moral action, and their support of hospitals performing abortions is material and remote.

A Catholic hospital cannot approve a direct sterilization, since this would be formal cooperation. Consequently, it is not proper for a hospital to propose in its ethical code a list of "medical indications for which sterilization is permitted," since this amounts to an approval of elective sterilization. Cooperation also would not be permissible if the hospital's cooperation is material but immediate (8.1); that is, if the hospital would not formally approve of the procedure but would offer substantive help, such as supplying nurses or surgical facilities that makes performance of the prohibited procedure possible. Because of the many difficulties involved, William Smith (1977) has argued that cooperation by a Catholic hospital in direct sterilizations would never be sufficiently remote to be justified, even if the patient's and physician's actions were in good faith unless it were ordered through an injunction of a court.

In light of the allowance for material cooperation mentioned in the documents quoted earlier, we believe that exceptional cases may occur in which material cooperation of the Catholic hospital would be justified. For example, rather than lose an obstetrical/gynecological service, could tubal ligations be allowed in conjunction with emergency cesarean deliveries? Whatever decisions are made, only a case-by-case process should be followed. Also, the local bishop should be consulted because such decisions could cause scandal.

A more clear-cut case of remote material cooperation might occur if the direct sterilizations were not performed under the auspices of the Catholic hospital. Consider the following example.

The declining birthrate in the United States has led to a strong movement for hospitals to consolidate obstetrical departments so that a single center located in one of the hospitals can afford the highest quality care. Catholic hospitals cooperating in such an effort would not be allowed to cooperate in a center that performed abortions Wisely, any form of material cooperation in regard to abortions was explicitly prohibited by the *Ethical and Religious Directives* (n. 12). However, would a Catholic hospital be allowed to cooperate in forming a common obstetrical unit where direct sterilizations were performed under the auspices of a non-Catholic hospital? Would this be remote material cooperation? It seems this type of cooperation would be legitimate if the medical personnel and operating rooms were not related directly to the Catholic hospital, if it were clear that the Catholic hospital did not approve of the direct sterilizations, and if efforts were employed to overcome any scandal that might develop in forming joint ventures. If Catholic hospitals do not cooperate in joint ventures, they will be accused of wasting health resources and frustrating an effort to provide quality healthcare. Moreover, lack of cooperation of this nature might lead to a loss of obstetric service at the Catholic hospital. If a Catholic hospital or healthcare corporation is involved in setting up a prepaid health maintenance organization (HMO), the same reasoning would apply. The contract for memberships in such a plan should clearly state that the services of the Catholic hospital would not include direct abortions or sterilizations, regardless of services performed by other members of the HMO. Such restrictions are legal and have not rendered Catholic HMOs less marketable (Health Plus, 1987).

Other Contraceptive Methods

Sterilization is the most drastic form of contraception because it is permanent, but other methods also raise questions. *Oral contraception* in its various forms also is used extensively in the United States (Hatcher et al., 1987). As already noted, some theologians believe that oral contraception approximates natural methods because (1) it is not permanent, (2) it operates by artificially extending the natural period of sterility by suppressing ovulation, (3) it does not alter the sexual act psychologically or esthetically, and (4) it seems simple to use in a pill-consuming culture. The teaching of the Church, however, clearly states that hormonal pills separate the conjugal and reproductive goods of the marital act if used as a means of contraception. If used to treat a true pathology in the generative organs, they would not be considered illicit. The following ethical questions must be asked in evaluating oral contraceptives: Is there true pathology? Are the drugs really being used to correct this pathology, or is the resultant sterility the direct aim of the medication?

Oral contraceptives have two very serious drawbacks. More and more evidence shows many undesirable side effects; at least 60 varieties have been reported (see *Index Medicus,* "Contraception: Adverse Effects,"). Some are dangerous or even fatal to those suffering from circulatory disease, especially for women past 35 years of age. Despite apparent ease of use, therefore, contraceptive drugs have to be taken under medical supervision. The potential harm is offset in some physicians' opinion by the statistical evidence that these risks are considerably less than the risks of the pregnancies that the method prevents. A statistical comparison of the risks of pregnancy for all women (including, for example, minority women, who in the United States do not receive adequate maternity care) does not tell us much about the comparative risks for a woman given high-quality care. In any case, to risk death to bring a child into the world and to risk death to avoid one are not easily compared. Although many scientists seek to allay fears by comparing risk and benefit (Ory et al., 1983), the risks remain very real.

The second and much more serious drawback of oral contraceptives is that they may not act as a contraceptive suppressing ovulation but rather as an abortifacient by altering the uterine lining so that it will not receive a fertilized ovum (Hume, 1983; Speroff et al., 1983). The abortifacient action is more likely to occur with the present-day "minipill" contraceptives than with the original pills, which used estrogen as well as synthetic progesterone compounds (Hilgers, 1980). Some might argue that the woman who takes oral contraceptives intends the contraceptive effect and that therefore any abortive effects would be indirect. Even if the intention were contraception, however, a proportionate reason for use of the drug must exist equal to or greater than the serious risk of destroying an unborn child, a condition not easy to verify.

Several other devices are used for contraception purposes: intrauterine device, intrauterine diaphragm with cream or contraceptive jelly, condom, and reduced-dosage hormonal drugs (Hatcher et al., 1987). *Intrauterine devices (IUDs)* share the same disadvantages mentioned in regard to oral contraceptives: medical risk and possible abortifacient action (Hume, 1983). The incidence of uterine perforation and pelvic inflammatory disease (PID) make the use of an IUD a serious health risk (Hatcher et al., 1987). For this reason, malpractice risks associated with their manufacture and insertion have resulted in virtual abandonment of IUDs in the United States (D. Edelman, 1987). Moreover, as high as 20 to 25 percent of women using IUDs were involuntarily sterile after removal (Cramer et al., 1985; Daling et al., 1985). The Food and Drug Administration requires that the following information be issued with the IUDs: "IUDs seem to interfere in some manner with the implantation of the fertilized egg in the lining of the uterine cavity. The IUD does not prevent ovulation" (*Physicians' Desk Reference*, 1986). That is, its action is abortifacient.

The *diaphragm* with spermicidal jelly and the *condom* are probably medically safe and are contraceptives in the strict sense; that is, they prevent conception rather than destroy the conceptus. Similar to the diaphragm are the contraceptive *vaginal sponge* and the *cervical cap*. Their use is not without physical difficulties (Kelagham et al., 1982), and their effectiveness varies depending on the consistency of use (D. Edelman et al., 1984). They can, however, be objected to as esthetically displeasing; also, just as the sterilizing methods suppress the generative significance of the sexual act, these methods diminish its *unitive* significance. They resemble, to a degree, *coitus interruptus* (withdrawal before ejaculation), which all would admit cannot express total self-giving.

Still other contraceptive methods include *vaginal foams* and *jellies*, coitus interruptus, and *postcoital douche*. These are not recommended as contraceptives because they are not effective (Shirm, 1982). *Breast-feeding* can be a useful element in natural family planning for the general population, but there is no indication it will be an effective means to limit pregnancies for specific women (Hatcher, 1987). However, breast feeding should be strongly encouraged for both the health of the child and the full development of the mother-child bonding, which is important for the child's psychological growth and the mother's sexual fulfillment (Weichert and Gerard, 1977).

The pastoral principles for dealing with persons experiencing conflict over the various methods of birth regulation are discussed in 10.7.

10.5 ARTIFICIAL INSEMINATION AND IN VITRO FERTILIZATION

As already argued, besides for the continuation of the human race, persons need to have children also because human sexuality finds its complete expression of love not simply in orgasm but ultimately in family life. Many people are unable to have children because of impotence or infertility. This latter condition has been overcome to some extent through artificial insemination and in vitro fertilization with embryo transfer. We describe each process and offer a moral evaluation.

Artificial insemination is any process by which fertilization of an ovum takes place not as a result of the act of sexual intercourse, but as the result of sperm being introduced into the woman's vagina by means of an artificial process. The sperm used in artificial insemination may be from the husband of the woman who wishes to conceive; if so, the process is referred to as *homologous insemination,* or *artificial insemination by the husband (AIH)*. If the semen is from a man other than the husband, it is known as *heterologous insemination,* or *artificial insemination by a donor (AID)*.

Although the feasibility of artificial insemination of human beings was known in the last century, it was not practiced to any significant extent until the 1930s. Today it is not an unusual occurrence. People who have children in this way, however, usually do not care to reveal the fact, and thus it is difficult to collect accurate statistics. Judging from the number of scientific and popular articles written on the subject in the last few years in the United States and elsewhere, many thousands of children are conceived and born as a result of artificial insemination (Olshansky and Sammons, 1985).

The process of artificial insemination is comparatively simple (Strickler, 1975). Semen is collected, usually by masturbation, into a sterilized container. Sometimes the semen might be frozen and used at a later date, but more frequently it is used within a few hours. If the semen of a donor is used, some attempt should be made to screen him in order to avoid transmitting a debilitating disease, but recent surveys indicate that only one third of the donors are screened (Olshansky, 1985). The semen is introduced into the vagina as close as possible to the day of ovulation by means of syringe or plastic cap placed at the cervix. Recent studies show that conception results in approximately 60 percent of the cases; a higher percentage results if insemination is repeated over a number of cycles (Council of Europe, 1982).

In Vitro Fertilization with Embryo Transfer

In natural reproduction, one ovum is released into the fallopian tube each month at mid-menstrual cycle. During intercourse, millions of spermatozoa are deposited in the vagina. Many of them swim through the uterus, but only a few dozen reach the ampullary end of the fallopian tube. When a sperm penetrates the ovum, fertilization occurs. The resulting embryo remains in the fallopian tube for two or three days and then enters the uterus, where it implants and grows over the next nine months.

The process of *in vitro fertilization (IVF)* with *embryo transfer (ET)* bypasses the fallopian tubes. The ovum is removed from the ovary immediately before ovulation and is placed in a petri dish with sperm from the husband or another man. The fertilized ovum is transferred to the uterus; after a number of days it implants and then grows over the next nine months. Thus the process of IVF with ET has four distinct stages: the induction of ovulation, the retrieval of the ova, fertilization, and transfer of the embryo (Biggers, 1981; Seibel, 1988).

More often than not, agents that induce ovulation are used to promote maturation of several ova. Thus a number of ova are fertilized because the success rate of IVF is greater if more than one embryo is transferred to the uterus. If there are "extra" embryos, they are either frozen with the intention of using them later for the same woman, or they are destroyed. Some countries allow research on "extra embryos" (Warnock Report, 1985).

When IVF was first attempted, it was used only for women whose fallopian tubes were absent or damaged. Now it is used for other reasons, such as severe endometriosis. The procedure is also used for some sources of male infertility, such as low sperm count, or when the sperm of the man is incapable of living in the woman's cervix. Will IVF be used in the future to control genetic and sexual characteristics of the future human being?

To date, IVF and ET have not been very successful. Only 5% of the procedures result in live births, although the results seem more encouraging if more than one procedure is attempted. Birth defects are no more frequent than those occurring in natural generation, and it seems that the process itself is not the cause of the birth defects (Seibel, 1988). Each attempt costs anywhere from $6,000 to $10,000 and is usually not covered by private health insurance or HMOs (*New York Times*, July 27, 1988).

From a legal point of view, the children resulting from artificial insemination and in vitro fertilization with embryo transfer have been in an ambiguous position. In some countries, laws considered heterologous insemination (AID) as a form of adultery, and thus the children would be considered illegitimate. At present in the United States, it seems that children born of gametes of the parents would be considered legitimate without question (Strasberg-Cohen, 1982). Some state laws consider a child generated from a donor's sperm as illegitimate. Moreover, if the child were generated from a donor's sperm without consent of the husband, his obligation to support the child might be successfully challenged in court.

Theological Evaluation

In evaluating both artificial insemination and in vitro fertilization, the Church returns to the basic notions of human sexuality: that the family is the goal of human sexuality and that the unitive and procreative aspects of the act of generation must not be separated by a deliberate human act. To act otherwise is to act contrary to the natural and moral order revealed by God (John Paul II, 1984b). Moreover, the Church follows a moral method that stipulates that every human act has its own morality and that the intention does not justify an immoral act. "The desire for a child is a good intention, but the good intention is not sufficient reason for making a positive moral evaluation of *in vitro* fertilization between spouses" (SCDF, 1987). Thus the moral goodness or badness of a human act or a series of human acts may not be subsumed or overlooked by evaluating only the intention of the person or the consequences of a series of human actions.

In regard to artificial insemination using the sperm of a man other than the husband (AID), Pope Pius XII clearly stated (1949b):

> Artificial insemination in marriage, with the use of an active element from a third person, is equally immoral and as such is to be rejected summarily. Only marriage partners have mutual rights over their bodies for the procreation of new life and these rights are exclusive, nontransferrable, and inalienable-....Between marriage partners, however, and a child that is the fruit of the active element furnished by a third person—even though the husband consents—there is no bond of origin, no moral or juridical bond of conjugal procreation (p. 118).

Pius XII (1951) seemed to include in his condemnation artificial insemination using the sperm of the husband (AIH) because he stated:

> The marital act, in its natural setting, is a personal action. It is simultaneous and direct cooperation of husband and wife which by the very nature of the agents and the property of the act is the expression of mutual giving which in the words of Scripture, results in the union of "one flesh" (p. 171).

Several Catholic theologians, however, thought the statement of Pius XII was ambiguous, and maintained that artificial insemination with the husband's sperm would be acceptable if it did not involve masturbation (Griese, 1987; Haring, 1973).

However, in a more recent statement concerning "Interventions upon Human Procreation" (SCDF, 1987), which considers both forms of artificial insemination (AIH and AID) and in vitro fertilization with embryo transfer, the Church made the moral evaluation of AIH more explicit. In this document, four principles summarize the teaching of the Church in regard to both artificial insemination and in vitro fertilization with embryo transfer:

1. Human procreation must take place in marriage.

> The procreation of a new person, whereby the man and the woman collaborate with the power of the creator, must be the fruit and the sign of the mutual self-giving of the spouses, of their love, and of their fidelity. The fidelity of the spouses in the unity of marriage involves reciprocal respect of their right to become a father and mother only through each other (p. 23).

2. Using the sperm or ovum of a third party is not acceptable.

Recourse to the gametes of a third person, in order to have sperm or ovum available, constitutes a violation of the reciprocal commitment of the spouses and a grave lack in regard to that essential property of marriage which is its unity....Moreover, this form of generation violates the right of the child; it deprives him of this filial relationship with his parental origins and can hinder the maturing of his personal identity (p. 24).

3. Generation of new person should occur only through an act of intercourse performed between husband and wife.

Fertilization is licitly sought when it is the result of a conjugal act which is per se suitable for the generation of children to which marriage is ordered by its nature and by which the spouses become one flesh....Spouses mutually express their personal love in the language of the body which clearly involves both spouses' meaning and parental ones....It is an act that is inseparably corporal and spiritual. It is in their bodies and through their bodies that the spouses consummate their marriage and are able to become father and mother (p. 27).

4. The fertilization of the new human person must not occur as the direct result of a technical process which substitutes for the marital act.

Homologous artificial fertilization in seeking a procreation, which is not the fruit of a specific act of conjugal union, objectively effects an analogous separation between the goods and the meaning of marriage (p. 27).

Conception *in vitro* is the result of the technical action which presides over fertilization. Such fertilization is neither in fact achieved nor positively willed as the expression and fruit of a specific act or the conjugal union (p. 30).

Surrogate Motherhood

As a corollary of the second principle just mentioned, the Church rejects surrogate motherhood, the practice of a woman agreeing to carry a child for a married couple or for a person other than her spouse, because it involves the gamete of a third party. The document states (SCDF, 1987):

Surrogate motherhood represents an objective failure to meet the obligations of maternal love, of conjugal fidelity, and of responsible motherhood; it offends the dignity and the right of the child to be conceived, to be carried in the womb, to be brought into the world and to be brought up by his own parents; it sets up to the detriment of families a division between the physical, psychological, and moral elements which constitute those families (p. 25).

The Supreme Court of New Jersey determined in the famous "Baby M" case that surrogate contracts are not valid and that the mother should retain visitation rights, no matter what agreements were made before the birth of the baby (*New*

York Times, Feb. 3, 1988). Although the decision applies only to the state of New Jersey, it serves as a guide for decisions in other states. One commentator on the Baby M case remarked that surrogate motherhood calls on a woman to be everything a mother should not be (Callahan, 1987a).

Reaction to Church Teaching

The statement of the Church in regard to methods of generation (SCDF, 1987) also considered the matter of research on human embryos (see Chapter 9). Although some reactions to the document accused the Church of being behind the times, others welcomed the document as a needed warning directed to the reproductive changes that science has introduced into human society without benefit of public discussion (National Catholic Reporter, 1987). An example of the reproductive changes that have been introduced involves a woman in South Africa who became pregnant with the embryos formed in vitro from gametes of her daughter and the daughter's husband; thus she would be the mother of her own grandchildren. Also, a feminist sperm bank in California regularly inseminates lesbian women, and another sperm bank in the same state seeks to specialize in the sperm collected from Nobel Prize winners.

Some Catholic theologians objected to the teaching of the document in regard to artificial insemination and in vitro fertilization when married couples were concerned (McCormick, 1987; Vacek, 1988). The arguments contrary to the Church's statement were based either on dissent, on consequentialist reasoning, or on the desire to evaluate only the consequences of the process and not the actions by which the results were produced.

Assisted Procreation

The recent document of the Church in regard to human procreation did not prohibit all forms of artificial assistance to the marital act. Although in vitro fertilization and embryo transfer (IVF and ET) in all forms were prohibited, the way was left open for assistance to the act of intercourse properly performed.

Repeating the teaching of Pope Pius XII (1956b) the document maintained (SCDF, 1987):

> Moral conscience does not necessarily proscribe the use of certain artificial means destined solely either to the facilitating of the natural act or to ensuring that the natural act normally performed achieves its proper end. [Thus,] if the technical means facilitates the conjugal act or helps it reach its natural objectives, it can be morally acceptable (p. 32).

> A medical intervention respects the dignity of persons when it seeks to assist the conjugal act either in order to facilitate its performance or in order to enable it to achieve its objective once it has been normally performed (p. 33).

Two methods of fertilization, *low tubal ovum transplant (LTOT)* and *gamete intrafallopian transfer (GIFT)* have been advanced by some scientists and theologians as merely assisting the natural process and thus being in compliance with the teaching of the Church. Originally, LTOT involved the retrieval of one or more ova and their transfer to the uterus, with fertilization taking place through normal intercourse (McCarthy, 1983). Although LTOT was deemed acceptable by the Archbishop of Cincinnati (Griese, 1987), it was not very successful. Thus LTOT was modified in 1985 so that both ova and sperm are inserted into the Fallopian tube, the sperm is collected in a perforated silastic sheath used in a complete conjugal act performed immediately before the sperm and ova are inserted. The revised process is called T.O.T (Tubal Ovum Transfer) or T.O.T.S. (Tubal Ovum Transfer with Sperm). In this form it has not as yet received ecclesiastical approval, but some maintain it is acceptable because it is performed as a sequence to an authentic conjugal act (McCarthy, 1988). In the GIFT method of fertilization, the ovulation-inducing medications and the retrieval of ova are similar to those of IVF. The sperm, which is retrieved from a perforated condom used during normal intercourse, is then "capacitated"; that is, specific changes in metabolism and in the plasma membrane are induced to allow fertilization to occur. The spermatozoa are washed in a special insemination medium to separate them from the seminal plasma, which is believed to contain several factors that make fertilization less likely, and are capacitated by one of several methods. The methods of capacitation involve centrifuging of the spermatozoa and collecting the sperm that seem to have more potential for fertilization (Seibel, 1988). Rather than have the fertilization occur in a Petri dish as in IVF, however, in the GIFT Process the ova and spermatozoa are kept separate until inserted into the fimbriated end of the fallopian tube where fertilization may occur. If the sperm utilized in the GIFT Process is obtained by means of a perforated condom, then GIFT and TOT are similar, the GIFT process involving more elaborate preparation of the sperm. But if the sperm is obtained outside the act of intercourse then GIFT must be rejected because it does not specify the primacy of the conjugal act (McCarthy, 1988).

Clearly, if fertilization occurs in the TOT or GIFT process it occurs in its natural site, not in vitro, which obviates one objection to IVF and ET. But does this process obviate other objections? Presupposing the sperm is collected immediately after an act of intercourse is the generation of a new human being the specific effect of that act of human intercourse? Does not the technology directly cause the fertilization and thus substitute for the marital act rather than simply assist the natural fertilization process? Can the act of intercourse using a perforated condom be considered "morally one" with the act by which the ovum and sperm are placed in the fallopian tube? Is the act of intercourse involved in TOT and GIFT "per se suitable for the generation of children?" (SCDF, 1987). Is the capacitation of the sperm and its placement after the act of intercourse in the fallopian tube together with an ovum retrieved beforehand from the woman "facilitating the conjugal act to reach its natural objectives?" Or does this process rather "substitute for the conjugal act?" (SCDF, 1987).

To date the Church has evaluated neither the TOT nor the GIFT processes (Ratzinger, 1987). We ourselves question that TOT and GIFT are acceptable processes because the technology involved seems to replace the conjugal act as the sufficient cause of the uniting of the sperm and ovum rather than simply to assist it. No matter which attitude one has toward TOT and GIFT, the problem of human infertility must be acknowledged as serious. Methods used to overcome this difficulty will be evaluated differently by those with a merely humanist view of reality than by those with a Christian viewpoint. Thus it will make a difference whether one views the human body as subject to any manipulation as long as the result is desirable, or whether one considers the human body as a gift from God that has a definite purpose to fulfill in our overall pursuit of human destiny.

10.6   TREATMENT OF RAPE VICTIMS

Rape is one of the more common social crimes. Because many rape victims hesitate to expose themselves to shame and notoriety, and because false charges of rape are often filed, it is difficult to ascertain with any degree of accuracy the number of rapes committed in the United States each year. When crimes of violence are tabulated, however, the percentage of rapes increases each year. There is evidence that rape is motivated by hostile impulses—a desire to assert the aggressive power of the rapist and to humiliate the victim—more than a desire for sexual pleasure (Lifshitz, 1986). Strange to say, some people would actually defend rape in some cases and justify it within marriage on the ground that it meets masculine needs. Without or within marriage, however, to perform the sexual act against the will of the partner is contrary to the meaning of sexuality as an expression of mutual love (E. Bayer, 1982). Pope John Paul II (1980c) pointed out the sinfulness of the husband who even in thought considers the wife a mere sexual object, without regard for her free personhood. Such behavior is a part of wife abuse, which is at last being exposed to public concern.

A victim of rape should be given the most sensitive and charitable care possible. Such victims often complain justifiably that they are treated by the police and medical personnel alike as though they were responsible for provoking the attack, thus compounding the grave injustice from which the woman has suffered. Many cities now have formed rape treatment task forces, not only to help educate police and medical personnel concerning humane treatment of rape victims, but also to prevent the crime by alerting the public to the signs of impending attack and to the measures that might ward it off (Sparks, 1988). Hospital procedures developed by such task forces are designed to accomplish four things:

1. To offer the psychological support and counseling that the woman needs to work through the trauma of the attack and its aftermath. Often this will require follow-up treatment with a counselor or psychologist.
2. To provide medical care for injuries or abrasions that might have occurred.
3. To gather evidence to be used if the rapist is apprehended and prosecuted. This usually consists of a rather extensive examination of the vagina, pelvic area, and clothing.
4. To provide treatment to prevent possible venereal disease and pregnancy.

This last point, preventing pregnancy, raises special ethical problems. Since the woman probably is in the sterile portion of her cycle and because the trauma of rape has an antiovulatory effect (Mahkorn and Dolan, 1981), the chances of conception after rape are very low statistically. Becoming pregnant is a very serious concern to the victim, however, and she deserves every help that medical professionals can give her, provided that help is ethical. Of course, in many cases, it will be possible to ascertain that conception is not at all likely, for example, if the woman is taking contraceptive drugs or if an examination of cervical mucus shows she is not in a fertile phase. If pregnancy is a possibility, since the victim is in no way responsible for the possible pregnancy, she has the right to avoid it. A woman who has consented to intercourse takes responsibility as a free person to use the sexual act in keeping with its intrinsic significance of love and procreation. On this responsibility the arguments of *Humanae Vitae* against contraception are based. The rape victim, however, has no such responsibility because she has not consented to the sexual act. Thus she has assumed no responsibility to give proper meaning to the sexual act that has been unjustly forced on her.

Therefore some Catholic moralists today admit that a woman who is in real danger of rape may, before the attack and if the danger is real, take a drug to prevent conception or even insert a diaphragm (E. Bayer, 1985). After the rape, through her own action or that of a medical person, she may do what is possible to render the sperm inoperative, to prevent it from joining the ovum, or to delay the production of ova.

From the discussion of abortion in 9.2, however, it follows that once the woman has conceived, she cannot take any action that would abort or destroy a fertilized ovum directly or request others to do so, nor may they cooperate with her in doing so. Although she has the right to protect herself from the effects of the aggression, she does not have the right to do so at the expense of the life of an innocent fetus. There is no proportion between the fetus' right to life and her right to be free of the injury done to her, serious as this is. Finally, a woman does not restore her personal dignity and integrity by destroying the life of another person who is her own child, but rather by caring for that child and thus demonstrating to herself and others her great dignity as a person, a woman, and a caring mother.

Problems arise, however, when methods to prevent conception are proposed that not only prevent conception, but that also may be abortifacient. As already noted, such methods are illicit if the woman is protecting her rights at the expense of the rights of a child already in existence. This is true even in the period before the implantation of the fertilized ovum in the uterus because, as 9.2 argues, most probably the zygote is truly human even before implantation, and this probability favors the rights of the fetus. On the other hand, when *doubt* exists as to whether conception has in fact taken place, the probability should favor the rights of the woman. This means, therefore, that as long as it is truly doubtful that the woman has conceived, she can take means to prevent conception, even if these means might in some cases actually be abortifacient if conception has taken place without her knowing it. Once it becomes certain or highly probable that conception has occurred, however, she must then recognize the rights of the fetus to life and avoid any serious risk of abortion. Thus using a method that not only prevents ovulation but also inhibits implantation of the embryo after the sperm is no longer active (72 hours) would be an abortifacient procedure.

Formerly, when discussing licit methods of attacking the sperm before conception, Catholic moralists recommended (with some limitations as to time) dilation and curettage (D & C), vaginal douche, or intrauterine douche (O'Donnell, 1957). Today, from both the medical and moral points of view, none of these methods seems to be acceptable.

The vaginal douche may be used for cleansing and sanitizing purposes to prevent veneral disease but is unlikely to prevent conception. Conception takes place ordinarily in the fallopian tubes, not in the vagina or uterus, and recent studies show the sperm enters the tubes 5 to 30 minutes after intercourse (Fordney-Settlage et al., 1973). Thus, the vaginal spermicidal douche might attack some of the sperm remaining in the vagina but would be ineffective for most of them. The intrauterine douche is considered too dangerous because the fluid it introduces could flow through the fallopian tubes into the peritoneal cavity and perhaps cause serious infection. Competent gynecologists do not employ this procedure today.

The theologians who formerly allowed D & C realized that the scraping of the womb made it impossible for an already implanted zygote to survive or for a fertilized ovum to be implanted. They argued, however, that the principle purpose of this action was to eliminate the sperm, and if this were done soon enough after the attack, the Principle of Double Effect could be used (Healy, 1956). Given the new evidence of the motility of the sperm, it no longer seems reasonable to say that D & C is a specific remedy to remove the sperm when the significant sperm is probably already out of the uterus.

Antifertility Treatment

Most rape treatment protocols recommend that antifertility drugs be administered by injection or orally over a few days. At one time diethylstilbestrol (DES) was a favored drug for treating rape victims. Its use was debated by Catholic theologians (D. McCarthy, 1977; O'Donnell, 1976). Because of acute side effects for the woman and possible birth defects in the fetus if the treatment is not successful, however, DES is no longer used for this purpose (Stenchever, 1987). At present, the recommended treatment is ethinyl estradiol, marketed in the United States as Ovral; a dosage of 100 micrograms is given within 72 hours of rape, with the same dosage repeated 12 hours later. The rape protocols state that Ovral or other hormones should not be administered until a test is given to determine whether the woman is pregnant. If the test is positive, the pregnancy occurred before the rape, and nothing should be done to injure the embryo (Braen, 1988).

Ovral and other high-dose progestins recommended in rape protocols inhibit ovulation and thus prevent conception. However, these hormones also affect the uterus, so that a fertilized ovum cannot implant in the endometrium. Thus, if given when there is a chance of limiting ovulation or sperm mobility, there would be no objection to using such hormones when the intention of use is not abortifacient. If given at a time when their effect could only be abortifacient, however, these drugs would be illicit.

The Committee for Bioethical Issues of the Bishops of Great Britain and Ireland considered the treatment for rape victims and stated (1986a):

> 1. The effect of administering hormones—large doses of estrogen or estrogen-progestogen combinations—will differ according to the stage of the menstrual cycle when they are given. If administered early in the cycle, they should prevent ovulation and therefore conception. If given about the time of ovulation, they could immobilize the sperm in the genital tract and thereby inhibit fertilization. If given after ovulation, their effects upon the female reproductive tract are such that the survival of any embryo will be put at risk, whether directly or by prevention of implantation or by inducing early menstruation as a result of a sudden fall in the steroid level.

> 2. A woman who is the victim of rape is entitled to defend herself against the continuing effects of such an attack and to seek immediate medical assistance with a view to preventing conception.

> 3. Catholics may seek and administer hormonal postcoital contraception after insemination by sexual assault, provided (i) that there are no grounds for judging that ovulation preceded or will coincide with the administration of postcoital contraception, and (ii) that the postcoital contraceptive is administered urgently, within about a day, after the assault (p. 637).

When commenting on this document, the Committee on Bioethical Issues (1987b) stated:

> Concern for the unborn and loyalty to Catholic teaching should not lead anyone to conceal the truth that for women in the predicament of rape there are possibly some effective self-defensive choices which, in some circumstances, they and/or their medical advisers might take in full conformity with all the truths which the Catholic Church upholds about strict respect, not only in attitude but also in each and every choice, for human life and for the procreative significance of sexual communion (p. 238).

In conclusion, we would summarize the responsibilities of Catholic healthcare facilities when caring for rape victims in the following manner:

1. Catholic healthcare facilities should prepare and carefully observe a protocol for the treatment of rape victims in which the first concern is respect for the dignity of the woman, regardless of her character or socioeconomic condition (Gregorek, 1988). This should include both medical and counseling help to reduce the harm she has unjustly suffered and should shield her as much as possible from embarrassment.
2. The protocol should provide for the collecting of adequate and accurate information for the police so that the aggressor can be brought to trial and conviction.
3. The protocol should also include medical tests to determine if the woman is pregnant. If the tests are positive, nothing should be done that would cause harm to the embryo.

4. If it is determined that the woman is not pregnant and not using contraceptive medications or devices, the following norms are offered as guidance in administering antifertility medications.

   a. Antifertility medications should not be administered if the sperm are probably no longer active. Otherwise, the purpose of the action would be abortifacient. Thus, the antifertility medication must be used within two to three days of the attack.

   b. If ovulation has not occurred within a current menstrual cycle, antifertility medications may be administered to prevent ovulation.

   c. If it is certain ovulation has occurred within the menstrual cycle, antifertility drugs may not be used because their effect could only be to inhibit implantation.

   d. If there is doubt as to whether ovulation has occurred or not within the present menstrual cycle, antifertility drugs may be used with the purpose of preventing ovulation. The doubt in question concerns the fact of ovulation, not the fact of conception.

   Under these guidelines, the woman is not attacking another person but prudently seeking to avoid conception. Although there is remote risk that implantation might be affected, the risk is not substantial (Bishops of GB and I, 1987b). If physicians or rape victims wish to avoid all risk to a potential third party and thus would not wish to administer or receive antifertility hormones, their consciences should be respected by the Catholic healthcare facility.

5. Facilities should be aware that, depending on state laws, they may be liable to legal suit if they fail to provide a rape victim with the opportunity to avoid pregnancy. Consequently, if a Catholic facility believes in conscience that it is unable to provide treatment that can be established as adequate in the local courts, it should make sure that victims can be promptly referred to their own physicians for whatever antipregnancy treatment they themselves choose.

10.7   PASTORAL APPROACH TO MEDICAL SEXUAL PROBLEMS

Pastoral Implications of *Humanae Vitae*

Catholics experiencing difficulties of conscience in sexual ethics in relation to healthcare usually are referred to a priest, often the chaplain in a healthcare facility. Chapter 14 discusses the chaplain's role in ethical counseling. It is also important that all Catholic healthcare professionals understand the changes in pastoral practice prompted by the Second Vatican Council, some of the most controversial of which relate to sexual ethics. Consequently, this section deals at some length with the way in which the teaching of the Church on contraception and sexuality is being pastorally applied and the implications this has for the instruction of Catholics in sexual ethics, a task in which members of the healthcare profession often play an important role.

Many of the critics of *Humanae Vitae* (Paul VI, 1968), the subsequent *Declaration on Certain Problems of Sexual Ethics* (1975a), and the *Pastoral Care of Homosexual Persons* (1986) issued by the Sacred Congregation for the Doctrine of the Faith have complained that the pastors of the Church seem content to pronounce moral judgments but do not provide much pastoral help for dealing with problems Christians experience in everyday life. When we read *Humanae Vitae* and *Familiaris Consortio*, however, as well as the pastoral letters of the various national episcopal conferences explaining *Humanae Vitae* (Horgan and Flannery, 1972), we are struck by the firm way in which the Magisterium maintains Christian marital ethics as traditionally understood, but we are also struck by the fact that the popes and bishops constantly seek a compassionate approach to sexual problems.

Previous popes had denounced contraception in very strong language as a "shameful stain on marriage," "moral ruin," and "a grave sin." For a time confessors were instructed by some theologians to question every married couple they suspected of practicing contraception (Creusen, 1932). Although this pastoral extreme was later somewhat moderated, the ordinary practice up to the controversy over oral contraceptive drugs was to refuse absolution and communion to those who would not promise to abandon this practice. At that time the Church's discipline was aimed at halting the spread of contraception. In the United States this policy was surprisingly successful, as proved by the Catholic birthrate for a long time remaining significantly above the national average.

Eventually, however, this battle was lost (M. Moore, 1973). As already mentioned in 10.2, in the United States *Humanae Vitae* produced a catastrophic negative reaction among Catholics that partially offset their positive reaction to the reforms of the Second Vatican Council. Church attendance fell greatly, and it seems the great majority of younger married Catholics ignored its conclusions in practice (Greely, 1976). Such statistics cannot determine whether Paul VI was doctrinally mistaken because, as 3.4 explains, opinion polls and the conformity in practice to the standards of American culture are not very good signs of the *sensus fidelium*, or faith witness of the Christian people (John Paul II, 1981b). Experience with the effects of a contraceptive society have not weakened the Church's teaching.

Perhaps the original difficulty in accepting *Humanae Vitae* was caused, in part at least, by Pope Paul VI taking what appeared to many to be an *ambiguous* stand: too hesitant, then too intransigent; too firm on principles, too vague on how they could be pastorally applied. One must admit, however, that any change in moral discipline is likely to meet such difficulties. What is this change in pastoral practice? It consists in the fact that Paul VI no longer insisted explicitly that those continuing to practice it should be refused absolution or denied communion (Delhaye et al., 1969; Gallon, 1968; Godden, 1968; Martelet, 1969). Thus *Humanae Vitae* gives the following instruction to married couples:

> We do not at all intend to hide the sometimes serious difficulties inherent in the life of Christian married persons; for them, as for everyone else, "the gate is narrow and the way is hard, that leads to life." ...Let married couples, then, face up to the efforts needed, supported by the faith and hope which "do not

disappoint...because God's love has been poured into our hearts through the Holy Spirit, who has been given to us"; let them implore divine assistance by persevering prayer; above all, let them draw from the source of grace and charity in the Eucharist. And if sin should still keep its hold over them, let them not be discouraged, but rather have recourse with humble perseverance to the mercy of God, which is poured forth in the Sacrament of Penance. In this way they will be enabled to achieve the fullness of conjugal life...(n. 25).

And to priests:

To diminish in no way the saving teaching of Christ constitutes an eminent form of charity for souls. But this must ever be accompanied by patience and goodness, such as the Lord himself gave example of in dealing with men and women. Having come not to condemn but to save, he was indeed intransigent with evil, but merciful towards individuals. In their difficulties, many married couples always find, in the words and in the heart of a priest, the echo of the voice and the love of the Redeemer (nn. 28-29).

Some national episcopal conferences (Delhaye, 1970; A. Flannery, 1969; Horgan and Flannery, 1972) simply urged their people to obey the encyclical. This was the position of many Third World bishops (India, Ceylon, Philippines, Mexico) as well as those of Spain, Scotland, and Ireland. Others (Italy, Switzerland, Germany, England, Japan, United States) urged confessors to deal with those practicing contraception in a very compassionate way and to avoid anything that might make these couples give up the regular use of the sacraments. Finally, the French, Belgian, Dutch, Austrian, Scandinavian, and Canadian bishops openly raised the question as to what attitude the confessors should take toward those who believed that it would be morally wrong to give up the practice of contraception in their present circumstances, concluding that it was not always necessary for the confessor to refuse absolution. The Austrian bishops pointed out that the pope had refrained from speaking of contraception as a "grave sin" and advised: "If someone should err against the teaching of the encyclical, he must not feel cut off from God's love in every case, and may receive Holy Communion without first going to confession" (A. Flannery, 1969).

Since Paul VI seems to have tolerated these more liberal interpretations of the pastoral application of the principles he enunciated in *Humanae Vitae,* and since the subsequent popes have not denounced them, they are not evidently inconsistent with his own pastoral purposes in issuing the encyclical (McCormick, 1973b; Zalba, 1970). But how can they be understood theologically? The most radical interpretation would seem to be that of the Austrian bishops, namely, that although individual contraceptive acts are *objectively* "disordered," this moral evil may be only venial, unless aggravated by hedonism, irresponsibility, and so forth (W. Shannon, 1970).

Some Objections

There are three obvious objections to this view about the gravity of the moral evil of contraception.

1. Popes Pius XI and Pius XII, whose condemnation of contraception Paul VI reaffirmed, clearly considered it an objectively grave or mortal sin (10.2). As Valsecchi (1968) and others have emphasized, however, these popes were principally considering the hedonistic use of contraception. Paul VI, however, had before him the commission report of theologians who attempted to make a case for the use of contraception, not for egoistic motives but precisely to promote marriage and family. It would seem, therefore, that his omission of any attempt to characterize the gravity of contraception in such cases is significant.

2. If contraception is not a mortal sin, why didn't the pope say so and quiet the whole controversy? It seems to trivialize the encyclical to say that it is dealing only with venial evils. This objection, however, overlooks that the pope is not merely interested in the issue of gravity, but in proposing a Christian view of sex in the face of an increasing erosion of Christian values (John Paul II, 1984b; MacDonald, 1975; Schall, 1968). Even if in such cases contraception is only a venial sin, the principle of chastity that it violates is of very grave importance. Moreover, the pope undoubtedly believed that once the principle is violated, even in small matters, the way is open to hedonistic uses of contraception and then to still graver evils. Finally, the pope may have believed that contraception is per se a mortal sin, but he did not wish to bind the faithful to this opinion because he saw it as less clear and certain than his principal message and thus prudently refrained from committing himself on this point.

3. Much more serious is the objection that there is no reason to believe that the pope intended in the encyclical to abandon the traditional teaching of moral theology that any deliberate sin against the right moral order in sexual matters is per se a grave or mortal sin, since it violates the God-given order in a matter of great importance not only for the individual but for the race. This is the well-known maxim, *in regard to the Sixth Commandment there can be no light matter*. It would seem, therefore, that Paul VI supposed that this maxim would make it clear to priests that if contraception is per se wrong, it is a mortal sin against the Sixth Commandment.

Today, however, this axiom is disputed by some moral theologians (Patrick Boyle, 1987). A. Meier (1966) and Kleber (1971) have shown that historically this maxim has had a checkered career. As already argued (3.4, 8.1), a sin is mortal because it is an act by which one turns away from friendship with God, either *directly* or *indirectly*, by turning away from friendship with a neighbor, since to hate one's neighbor is contradictory to loving God, who loves both alike. Persons destroy friendships with neighbors, however, only by wishing them or doing them a *serious* harm. Thus contraception is not a mortal sin unless it is of the nature to cause serious harm to oneself or another.

Theologians have never considered sexual sins as direct acts against God. They are not (ordinarily) sins of malice, but of weakness, since they are done for pleasure, not to harm others (with the exception of rape, sadistic acts, or those performed to humiliate or out of revenge). They become mortal when aggravated by such malicious purposes, but this is exceptional.

How, then, can most sexual sins be mortal? What serious harm do they do? Humanists generally argue that they are harmless. Christian theologians, however, have generally believed that just as sexual acts can do great good, they can also do great harm. Classical moral theology argued that adultery is mortal because of the injustice it does one's spouse, to whom fidelity was promised. Fornication was said to be mortal because of the danger of harm to the illegitimate children who might be born. In general, it was argued that these acts violated the divine order in a very serious matter, namely, the good not of the individual (as sins of gluttony and drunkenness) but of the race. It is difficult to see, however, that every inordinate sexual act really threatens the survival of the race. Thus it was finally argued that if exceptions are allowed, the whole order of sexual morality will be endangered because sexual pleasure is so great that, if indulged, it will move beyond all limits (Connery, 1977).

Thus the ultimate reason given by classical moral theology for rating as mortal *every* sexual sin was a "slippery-slope" argument based on the tendency of human beings to regress to an egoistic level. However, this argument is firmly rooted in the sad experience of the ambiguity of human sexuality (USCC, 1988). Sexual need can become an addictive egoism that is destructive to self and others, or it can introduce the person to genuine love and creativity. The adolescent, once initiated to sexual pleasure by masturbation or fornication, lacking the social discipline and support of marriage, will probably have great difficulty in keeping under control the addictive drive to repeat such experiences. It is the acquisition of this addictive egoistic hedonism that is the harm caused by illicit sexual acts. Such sexual addiction, of course, does not do the physiological harm that drug addiction causes; however, in another sense it may be more harmful because it distorts what is most intimately personal in the human being, the capacity for self-giving in love.

It is not so clear, however, that sexual acts performed within marriage that are less than ideal cause this type of serious harm. Classical theologians held that when married couples perform the normal sexual act not as an expression of love but in a merely selfish way, they sin, but only venially because such acts still take place in the context of committed love (Noonan, 1965). Could not the same reasoning be applied to the contraceptive act when it is used to express love and in an effort to fulfill the duties of responsible parenthood? This act is disordered because of its departure from the natural process on which *Humanae Vitae* insists, and thus in some measure it opens the way to hedonism and the other possible consequences mentioned in the encyclical. But is this danger so great as to be qualified as mortal sin?

This argument deserves further study, but considering the weight of the counterarguments, *it does not provide a safe basis for pastoral practice.* Therefore, the issue can be more securely and practically treated in terms of *subjective* or *developmental* morality, to which we turn next.

A Developmental Approach

When it is healthy, human life is a process of growth and development. The Christian view of human life emphasizes this developmental thrust and understands it also as a process of liberation from the bondage of sin and retrogression. However, ethical life has often been considered in purely static, legalistic terms of laws observed or broken. Thus it was assumed formerly that if the pastors of the Church had condemned something as sinful, no one who had been informed of this condemnation could be subjectively justified in acting against it. Today it seems extreme to draw such a conclusion.

First, there is the possibility of an erroneous conscience resulting from the criticism of Church teaching emanating from humanistic sources and from some Catholic theologians (Dominian, 1984; Kosnik et al., 1977). Thus, the Belgian bishops in their pastoral statement (Delhaye, 1970) assert that Catholics may be in good faith when they say they cannot in conscience follow the practical conclusion of the encyclical when it forbids them to use contraception in fulfilling their obligations of responsible parenthood.

Second, some persons, as the French bishops noted in their pastoral letter, may yet find themselves practically perplexed in conscience (Horgan and Flannery, 1972; O'Callaghan, 1970). As Sahuc (1970) has explained, such couples find themselves faced with the duty of simultaneously (1) preserving their marriage by sexual expression of love, (2) being responsible parents, and (3) refraining from the practice of contraception, which seems the only practical way they know of to meet the first two obligations. In the hierarchy of values, the first two are clearly of greater weight than the third. Consequently, they rightly choose to seek the greater good at the expense of the lesser evil. The French bishops in their pastoral letter adopt this lesser-evil solution in cases of conflict of duties (to which several other of the pastoral letters also refer) and assert, "Contraception can never be good. It is always disorder, but this disorder is not always culpable."

Some commentators on the French pastoral letter have pointed out that it seems to contradict a passage in *Humanae Vitae:*

> To justify conjugal acts made intentionally infecund, one cannot invoke as valid reasons the lesser evil, or the fact that such acts would constitute a whole together with the fecund acts already performed or to follow later, and hence would share in one and the same moral goodness. In truth, if it is sometimes licit to tolerate a lesser evil in order to avoid a greater evil or to promote a greater good, it is not licit, even for the gravest reasons, to do evil so that good may follow therefrom; that is, to make into the object of a positive act of the will something which is intrinsically disordered, and hence unworthy of the human person, even when the intention is to safeguard or promote individual, family, or social well-being. Consequently, it is an error to think that a conjugal act which is deliberately made infecund and so is intrinsically dishonest could be made honest and right by the ensemble of a fecund conjugal life (n. 14).

The French bishops, however, were certainly aware of this passage. They are not denying that contraception is intrinsically wrong and always disordered; they agree to this. In the abstract or essential order, of which the pope is speaking, there cannot be an irresolvable conflict of duties. Nevertheless, in the concrete or existential order, persons may not be able to discover what that solution is, and it is in such perplexity that they are bound to choose the greater good at the expense of the lesser evil. A counselor dealing pastorally with persons in such perplexity can ordinarily help them to a correct solution. When persons in good faith remain perplexed, however, then the confessor, without approving the doing of evil for the sake of good, should not reject their decision to do what seems best to them. In addition, when a counselor deals with someone who is *not* wholly in good faith, but who is debating between two evil acts, the counselor (without approving either act) may assure the person it is better to choose the lesser evil. Thus the counselor might point out that contraception is certainly less evil than abortion if he or she sees that the person is likely to choose the latter.

Third, since the evil in question is at worst a sin of weakness, many people admittedly are caught in addictive life patterns and lack perfect freedom of decision. Much of this bondage is the result of moral education and social support in a society where Christian ideals are little understood and often contradicted by social institutions. One need only think of the prostitute who seems to have no other way of making a living, the man in a bad marriage, the lonely celibate who is caught in a habit of masturbation, or the homosexual who cannot marry. It is true that all such persons can live chaste lives if they are open to God's grace. However, here and now such persons, although sincerely desiring to live as Christians and striving not to harm others or to go deeper into depersonalization, lack the strength to pull themselves out of their situation all at once. Can every new act of impurity be judged a mortal sin? Previous theologians would have said that in such cases culpability is reduced, perhaps to the point of venial sin. The important question is whether such persons can be helped to begin to free themselves to the point that a way of life conformed to the Christian ideal of sexuality can be freely chosen. Thus, from a pastoral point of view, a counselor has to decide how to help such persons move closer to the norm, without further burdening or discouraging them (Delhaye, 1975; Lawler et al., 1985; NCCB, 1976; Shehan, 1973). The practice of confessors formerly was to insist (1) that such persons promise to give up the sin here and now, (2) that they not commit the sin again before going to communion, and (3) that they come again to confession and renew their promise before going to communion if they had backslid. The rationale was to keep the objective norm clearly before the sinners' minds and to get them to renew regularly their sincere promise of amendment, with no risk of receiving communion insincerely.

Today, with a more nuanced understanding of the psychology of sin, many confessors would consider this method to be *sometimes* counterproductive in helping the penitent move forward. It would seem that such persons can have true contrition if they are sincerely trying to eliminate from their lives the worst and most harmful elements of what they are doing, which lie at the limits of their actual freedom. Thus the prostitute will start looking for another way to support herself, the masturbator will begin to seek a less introverted lifestyle, and the homosexual will cease promiscuity. It can then be judged that the continued immoral acts are subjectively venial and need not keep these persons from communion—provided that they keep trying to keep the law of Christ in its totality and continue to come regularly to confession, striving to be freed from bondage step by step. Above all, the confessor needs to communicate to these persons that God has not rejected them, nor has the Christian community of the

Church, but that the confessor wants to help them in every way possible and does not demand a heroic moral transformation all at once. This attitude is not essentially contrary to that of good confessors in the past, but the pastoral strategy is somewhat different.

The pastoral directives in *Humanae Vitae* seem to open the way to some such pastoral procedure in dealing with those who practice contraception not for egoistic reasons but in an effort to fulfill their marriage obligations. Paul VI clearly wanted confessors to keep couples receiving the sacraments while educating them to seek a more natural method of regulating family life. The bishops seem to have understood this, as evidenced either by their explicit pastoral instructions or at least by their toleration of the widespread employment of such an approach by their priests. Unfortunately, in the United States too many Catholics, educated in a somewhat mechanical morality, have become alienated from the Church because they believe they cannot without hypocrisy continue to receive the sacraments unless they promise to cease contraceptive practices absolutely, whereas those who continue to receive are alienated from the pope because they believe they are defying him.

Good pastoral care will work to heal these wounds and divisions by creating an atmosphere in which the conscience of individuals, accepted at a particular stage of their lives and their spiritual and moral development, is truly respected. At the same time, such care must encourage individuals to open themselves to the guidance and support available in the community of the Church and of society (B. Ashley, 1981).

Synod of Bishops

The World Synod of Catholic Bishops meeting under the presidency of Pope John Paul II in 1980 in their "Message to Christian Families," after reaffirming the teaching of *Humanae Vitae*, said:

> We wish to say to you, brothers and sisters, that we are fully aware of the frailty of our common human condition. In no way do we ignore the very difficult and trying situations of many Christian couples who, although they sincerely want to observe the moral norms taught by the Church, find themselves unequal to the task because of weakness in the face of difficulties. All of us need to grow in appreciation of the importance of Christ's teaching and his grace and to live by them. Accompanied and assisted by the whole Church, these couples continue along the difficult way toward a more complete fidelity to the commands of the Lord (n. 20).

Among the propositions adopted by the synod as the basis of a future pastoral document to be issued by the Holy See, they suggested that priests should use the "law of gradualness," recognizing a need frequently for "patience, sympathy, and time" in educating couples to an understanding of the papal teaching, but at the same time insisting on the normative nature of this teaching. John Paul II (1981b) commented on this in his own terms by saying:

Directing their attention to those things which concern pastoral ministry for the good of couples and of families, the fathers of the synod rejected any type of "dichotomy" between a pedagogy, which takes into account a certain progression in accepting the plan of God, and the doctrine proposed by the Church with all its consequences in which the precept of living according to the same doctrine is contained; in which case there is not a question of a desire of keeping the law as merely an ideal to be achieved in the future, but rather of the mandate of Christ the Lord that difficulties constantly be overcome. Really, the "process of gradualness," as it is called, cannot be applied unless someone accepts the divine law with a sincere heart and seeks those goods which are protected and promoted by the same law. Thus, the so-called *lex gradualitatis* (law of gradualness) or gradual progress cannot be the same as *gradualitas legis* (the gradualness of the law), as if there were in the divine law various levels or forms of precept for various persons and conditions (n. 34).

This commentary of the pope must also serve as a commentary on what we earlier have called a "developmental approach." The moral norms taught in *Humanae Vitae* apply to all couples, whatever their situation, not merely as an ideal but as an obligation, since the objective effects of using sexuality in a manner contrary to the nature of the human sexual person are not overcome just because couples do so in good faith or under great pressure. The "law of gradualness" or of development is not a gradualness of the moral law, but of persons in their subjective development as Christians coming to a practical understanding and effective acceptance of these objective obligations in their own lives through their own experience, reflection, and prayer, assisted by compassionate yet principled pastoral guidance. John Paul II (1981b) has emphasized these same points in his *Apostolic Exhortation on the Family,* which fulfills the request of the synod.

Education for a Sexual Future

The "sexual revolution" projects a future in which the Christian vision of human sexuality will appear ridiculous and unrealizable. For Christians, however, human sexuality is governed by norms of *hope,* a hope on which a truly human future must be built.

To build a healthier future, it is essential to help Christians develop a fully human understanding of their sexuality (SCDF, 1975a). Catholic healthcare professionals and healthcare facilities can play an important role in this developmental task. We suggest three contributions for which there is urgent need.

1. The first responsibility of Christian healthcare professionals and facilities in the area of sexuality is to promote and cooperate with sound programs of education for chastity. Sound sex education is primarily spiritual and ethical, not medical, but healthcare professionals have an essential role to play in it because of its close connection with bodily life. Although many sex education programs today provide excellent biologi-

cal and psychological information, they also promote the value system of humanism that Christians find quite inadequate. Such programs, however, can hardly be criticized without providing superior ones. A Christian program should begin with helping parents succeed in their natural role as the principal sex educators. Today many parents suffer from (a) the predominant influence of humanist values and (b) incorrect, distorted views of Christian values that stress negative, repressive aspects of sexual morality based on fear, rather than a positive but realistic view based on a true understanding of God's gifts and their own stewardship. A sound program of Christian education for chastity should provide the following types of instruction:

a. Understanding of the unitive-procreative meaning of sexuality in sacramental marriage

b. Knowledge of mental hygiene and essential biological knowledge about sexual differences and equality, lovemaking, intercourse, pregnancy, and birth

c. Information on why people have a need for children and on the problems of sterility, adoption, and limits on the right to have children

d. Information on the problems of responsible parenthood in today's society, natural family planning methods and alternative methods, and ethical evaluation of all birth regulation methods

e. Explanation of the rights of the unborn child

f. Discussion of the problems of genetic defects and the Christian attitude toward defective persons

g. Consideration of the problem of homosexuality and similar difficulties in psychosocial development. Such programs can be considered preventive medicine, since they might go a long way to reduce the frequency or severity of many of the problems described in this chapter. However, they will not have a widespread effect unless they are also joined to social programs aimed at improving the climate of society.

2. Sound education for chastity must be based on continuing research and open discussion. When sexual issues are involved, such objectivity is difficult to achieve. Some physicians and nurses have really had to struggle to obtain a hearing for natural methods of delivery and breast-feeding, since such an approach appeared as a conservative attack on medical progress. Similarly, in ethical questions dealing with sexual matters, modern culture has a strong bias toward voices announcing the coming of new "freedoms" and a suspicion of those who are concerned to retain and strengthen traditional values of modesty and chastity and the disciplined restraint these require. To arrive at an atmosphere in which both sides can be fairly heard when discussing sexual issues is extremely difficult. A Catholic healthcare facility should develop a Christian identity committee where such discussions can take place in a truth-seeking atmosphere.

299

3. Catholic healthcare professionals who play a role in public and social agencies that deal with sexual problems should take care that these agencies do not content themselves merely with promoting birth control. Responsible parenthood must be an important objective of any such agency, but this objective should not be conceived in merely negative terms. Rather, the principal goal of all such work should be to strengthen and promote the family as the basic institution of society. Only in an atmosphere of good family life based on faithful love can the next generation develop toward a mature, fully human sexuality.

CHAPTER 11

Reconstructing Human Beings

OVERVIEW

In recent years, medical technology has moved from the mere capability of repairing the human body to new capabilities of remodeling the body through surgical reconstruction, and even by genetic intervention, which will alter not only an individual, but also all his or her descendants. Some of these new capabilities are already practical, others still futuristic. This chapter deals in some detail with certain present problems associated with modifying the human person but also touches on the futuristic ones for purposes of illustration.

A basic axiom of medicine has always been the Greek dictum, *art perfects nature*, which implies that a human person can be healed (or patched up) and developed to maturity, but he or she cannot be essentially remade. Today, however, the situation has changed. We must face the questions: Is it right for persons to become their own creators? Can and should human nature be remade? Can genetic engineering hasten the processes of evolution by eliminating troublesome wisdom teeth or appendices, or at least by some type of surgery at a very early age, before trouble arises? Might the technology of the future greatly reduce the complexities of the digestive system, which so often becomes diseased? Can human beings be fed in some simpler way, perhaps by a more effective intravenous method? Might all human beings be sterilized and reproduce artificially? Francoeur (1972) has answered that because "we can, we must" and calls this the "technological imperative." Jonas (1979, 1984), however, cautions against the tendency to accept scientific progress as an unalleged benefit.

After discussing briefly the ethical norms guiding the development of the human body (11.1), this chapter discusses organ transplants (11.2), a partially successful means of patching up the body, and transsexual surgery (11.3), remaking of the body. The chapter then discusses ethical issues prompted by that genetic engineering (11.4) and concludes with a discussion of genetic screening and counseling (11.5).

11.1   MODIFYING THE HUMAN BODY

The first steps toward remaking the human body have already been taken (L. Shapiro et al., 1986). Three levels of physical remaking seem possible:

1. Surgical procedures would replace existing organs with transplants, biological constructs, or artificial organs that are not mere substitutes for natural organs but that expand old or introduce new functions into the body. To reiterate, the digestive system might be replaced with a new way of nourishing the body, much of the reproductive system might be eliminated, and children might be produced in a test tube and incubated in an artificial womb.

2. Embryological development might be influenced by drugs or surgery (M. Harrison et al., 1981) so as to mold the development of the phenotype (the actual body) while not changing the genotype (inherited characteristics). Thus the phenotypic sex of a child could be determined at will despite the genotype by altering the course of development very clearly in embryonic life. There are possibilities of expanding the human senses to make seeing or hearing possible beyond the present or upper range of sight and vision.

3. Ultimately genetic engineering might be employed to produce any gene combination in the fertilized ovum, thus creating human beings by "recipe" (Robertson, 1985). Already the development of the technique of "recombinant DNA" (deoxyribonucleic acid) has made it possible to produce new species of bacteria with useful (and perhaps dangerous) combinations of genetic traits. Related to this is the production of clones from the somatic cells of a parent or artificial reproduction of multiple individuals all having the same genetic composition (LaBar, 1984).

The basic ethical issue here is seen by some theologians to be the question of the extent of human dominion over nature (Hendry, 1980). This is a classical way of posing the issue, but it is perhaps too much influenced by the Greek image of God as a jealous monarch who becomes angry when Prometheus infringes on his prerogatives. Others would see such attempts to improve on human beings as an insult to the work of the Creator, whose masterpiece is humankind, or at least as a fatal temptation to pride (Ellul, 1965, 1980).

Today, however, in considering radical human development, two theological points must be stressed.

1. God is a generous Creator, who in creating human beings also called them by the gift of intelligence to share in his creative power. Consequently, God does not want human beings to leave fallow the talents he has given them, but encourages them to improve on the universe he has made.

2. Such improvement is possible because theology can accept the idea that God has made an evolutionary universe in which the human race has been created through an evolutionary process that is not yet complete. Thus God has called humankind to join with him in bringing the

universe to its completion, and in doing this, he has not made them merely workers to execute his orders or to add trifling original touches on their own. Rather, God has made them genuine co-workers and encourages them to exercise real creativity.

Granted this view, however, it is not so clear that the remaking of the human body on new lines is really the appropriate place for humankind's creativity. Remolding the environment and creating human culture takes time enough. No doubt with greater knowledge some of the business of evolution may be tidied up by removing such vestiges as wisdom teeth or appendices if, indeed, this would be a real improvement. Someday genetic disease may also be eliminated and even human health advanced eugenically. Before technology attempts to produce Superman, however, it needs to heed the paradox proposed by MacIntyre (1979), who first imagines what types of human beings he would like to produce. They would have the ability to live with uncertainty; to keep rooted in the particularity of everyday life; to form nonmanipulative relations with others; to find their fulfillment in their work; to accept death; to keep hopeful; and be willing to die for their freedom. He then concludes, "The project of designing our descendants would, if successful, result in descendants that would reject that project."

It is important to remember, however, that human creativity depends on a human brain. Any alteration that would injure the brain and thus a person's very creativity would indeed be disastrous mutilation, especially if this were to be transmitted genetically, thus further polluting the gene pool with defects that might be hidden and incalculable.

It is generally admitted that knowledge of this wonderful brain is still in its beginnings (G. Edelman, 1987; Institute for Theological Encounter with Science and Technology [ITEST], 1975; Rosenfield, 1987). The complexity of the brain is beyond any other system imaginable, and this complexity is reduced to a relatively very small organ capable of self-development from the embryo and of self-maintenance, but not of self-restoration. The human brain may be near the limit of complexity and integration possible in organic, living systems. In this case any radical improvement may be illusory, whereas even slight alterations may be very damaging. Thus, to say the least, radical attempts to alter the structure of the human brain must be viewed with the utmost caution, since the risk of producing only persons of lowered intelligence is very high.

This is certainly not so true of other organ systems, and it is possible to imagine that someday in other environments it might become necessary, for example, to replace the human lungs with other ways of obtaining oxygen. In principle it would seem that such changes would be ethical (1) if they gave support to human intelligence by helping the life of the brain and (2) if they did not suppress any of the fundamental human functions that integrate the human personality. Thus alterations that would make it possible for a human being to directly sense the external world at least as effectively as he or she now does with "five senses" would be contrary to the Principle of Totality and Integrity (2.4), as would alterations that would make it impossible for human beings to experience the basic emotions, since emotional life is closely related to human intelligence and creativity. Again, alterations that would make human beings sexless and incapable of parenthood would also be antihuman. The following conclusions can be drawn:

1. Genetic engineering and less radical transformations of the present normal human body would be permissible if they improve rather than mutilate the basic human functions, especially as they relate to supporting human intelligence and creativity. Transformation would be forbidden, however, (a) if human intelligence and creativity are endangered and (b) if the fundamental functions that constitute human integrity are suppressed.

2. Experimental efforts of this radical type must be undertaken with great caution and only on the basis of existing knowledge, not with high risks to the subjects or to the gene pool. The use of surgery and genetic manipulation to improve human bodies is ethically good, provided that they take full account of such risks and are not carried away by a false ambition to work technical miracles without regard to their real meaning for human living. In particular, Christians should be concerned that such innovations do not weaken the fundamental relations within the family or the sense of the child as a unique gift of God.

3. The Principle of Stewardship and Creativity throws light on many of the problems of human reconstruction. Natural law should not be conceived of as a fixed pattern of human life to which human beings are forever confined. Rather, the Creator has made human beings free and intelligent, and it is precisely this intelligent freedom that is human nature and the foundation of natural moral law. Human intelligence, however, is not disembodied; it depends on a brain and a body that have a specific structure. In caring for their total health, persons not only have the right but the obligation to understand their psychological and biological structure and to improve themselves even in ways that may seem novel to past generations. Such improvement is good stewardship of the share in divine creativity with which God has endowed humankind.

11.2   ORGAN TRANSPLANTATION

Any surgical procedure involves some reconstruction of the human body, but there is a striking difference between procedures such as setting a broken bone or sewing up a wound or removing a tumor, which assist a natural healing process or remove a diseased part, and a procedure by which an organ originally belonging to another is transplanted into the human body in place of one of its own parts that has become dysfunctional. The latter procedure involves the rights not of one person but of two and thus raises a new moral question.

Two types of organ transplants are possible, one involving an organ or tissue taken from a dead person and given to a living person and the other involving an organ taken from one living person and given to another living person. Transplanting an organ or tissue from a dead person to a living person presents no ethical problem. With few exceptions, religious groups as well as humanistic ethicists have recognized the worth and ethical validity of such transplants (Jonsen, 1985; Pius XII, 1956a; Simmons and Fulton, 1973). If some serious question arises concerning this type of transplant, it stems from factors other than the transplant itself. For example, concern was expressed about the worth of heart transplants, most of it arising either from the great expense of money and personnel involved in a medical procedure that brings little substantive value to human society in general (Lawrence, 1980; Ramsey, 1970; Thorup et al., 1985) or from fear that in some cases the organ donor had not actually expired (P. Williams et al., 1973). These concerns are no longer prominent, however, because of better survival rates in recipients and greater ability to ascertain the criteria for total brain death (Black, 1984). Pope Pius XII (1956a) summed up Catholic teaching on transplants involving an organ from a dead person:

> A person may will to dispose of his body and to destine it to ends that are useful, morally irreproachable and even noble, among them the desire to aid the sick and suffering. One may make a decision of this nature with respect to his own body with full realization of the reverence which is due it....this decision should not be condemned but positively justified (n. 646).

Far more difficulties arise, however, with organ transplants between living persons. Before 1950, the morality of transplanting an organ from one living person to another was discussed by Catholic theologians from a theoretical point of view (Cunningham, 1944). Although an interesting question, it was somewhat impractical because transplants between living persons were contemplated but not yet possible. Many theologians who considered the subject did not approve of it. These theologians argued that the Principle of Totality and Integrity would justify mutilation or injury to one part of the body provided it was done to preserve the person's own health or human life. The principle would not justify a transplant to another person, however, because one person is not related to another person as means to end or as part to whole. Thus one person's bodily integrity could not be sacrificed for another. Although they could not use the Principle of Totality and Integrity, other theologians sought other ways to justify transplantation (G. Kelly, 1956).

Whatever the theoretical discussions, organ transplants from living donors were performed in the early 1950s. Because of genetic similarity, identical twins were the first subjects of kidney transplants. Although many early transplants were not always successful because the transplanted organ often was rejected by the reaction of the recipient's immune system, it was clear that organ transplants were a reality (J. Murray, 1986). Scientists began to argue that unless there was freedom to undertake such experiments, medical progress would be hampered (Fox and Swazy, 1978). Thus, ethicists and moralists gave the problem closer scrutiny.

Gerald Kelly (1956), a leader in this development, wrote:

> It may come as a surprise to physicians that theologians should have any difficulty about multilations and other procedures which are performed with

the consent of the subject but which have as their purpose the helping of others. By a sort of instinctive judgment we consider that the giving of a part of one's body to help a sick man is not only morally justifiable, but, in some instances, actually heroic (p. 323).

In developing the rationale for a more liberal opinion, Kelly maintained, "It is clear from reason and papal teaching that the Principle of Totality cannot be used to justify the donating of a part of one's body to another person. Moreover, since man is only the administrator of his life and bodily members and functions, his power to dispose of these things is limited." However, Kelly sought to delineate as clearly as possible the limits of this dominion, especially concerning organ transplants.

Thus, Kelly asked, is there any other way in which this seemingly worthwhile and Christian action could be justified? He suggested that the principle of fraternal love, or charity (see our Principle of Common Good, Subsidiarity, and Functionalism, 6.1 and 8.2), would justify the transplant provided that there was only limited harm to the donor. Although it was not unanimously accepted, some theologians agreed with this opinion and developed it more clearly. Distinguishing between anatomical integrity and functional integrity, they stated that the latter, not the former, was necessary to ensure human or bodily integrity (McFadden, 1976). *Anatomical integrity* refers to the material or physical integrity of the human body. *Functional integrity* refers to the systematic efficiency of the human body. For example, if one kidney were missing from a person's body, there would be a lack of anatomical integrity, but if one healthy kidney were present and working, there would be functional integrity because one healthy kidney is more than able to provide systemic efficiency. If a cornea were to be taken from the eye of one living person and given to another, however, the case would be different. Not only would anatomical integrity be destroyed, but functional integrity would be destroyed as well. The loss of sight in one eye severely damages vision, especially depth perception. Thus in this case, more than anatomical integrity is involved.

This distinction between anatomical and functional integrity that we have incorporated in our formulation of the Principle of Totality and Integrity (2.4) explains why blood transfusions and skin grafts are acceptable and why theologians have approved elective appendectomy if the abdominal cavity is open for another legitimate reason. In these situations loss of anatomical integrity may occur through loss of blood, skin tissue, or an internal organ, but no loss of functional integrity occurs.

Thus the concept of functional integrity is the key factor in addressing the morality of transplants between living persons. Certainly, a risk is involved if a donor surrenders an organ to another person, even if the donor has two of them. Aside from the risk involved in the surgical procedure, such donors take the risk of serious illness themselves if the one remaining organ becomes damaged or diseased. The risk, however, although serious, is deemed to be justified by the fact that donors share in the common good of the community to which they contribute by helping another, that is, by love (Ramsey, 1970).

306

Clearly, organ donation is not an obligation; rather, it is something chosen in the freedom of charity. Motivated by the same charity, one could decide not to offer an organ. Such a decision would not be unethical. For this reason, it is imperative that a donor's free and informed consent be obtained (3.4). Given the fact that the more successful transplants are between members of the same family, familial or social pressure to offer oneself as a donor may at times be severe (Bernstein and Simmons, 1975; Greenberg et al., 1973; Mack, 1980), but the courts (rightly, we believe) refuse to compel such donations. Because of the motivation that should underlie the donation of an organ by a living person, it is clear that selling organs is unethical. The federal government has prohibited the sale of all organs in the United States, but sale of organs by living donors in some countries is a common practice (Gorovitz, 1985).

We agree with Kelly and others that organ transplants between two living persons are licit if the donor's functional integrity is maintained, but we would caution that great care should be taken in weighing the merely potential benefit against the actual risks. Consent should not be given unless the prognosis for both the donor and the recipient is good. In some cases it is necessary to weigh the value of a brief prolongation of life for the recipient against the lifelong risk to the donor.

In addition to the rationale put forward by Kelly and others to justify transplants between living persons, some Catholic theologians go a step further and seek to justify these procedures either by expanding the Principle of Totality and Integrity or by treating the whole process as a curative action, even though two people are involved and one will be injured (Nolan, 1968). In so doing, they destroy the limits so carefully delineated by Kelly and others to protect human integrity. According to these theories, the human unity predicated on body and soul is destroyed, and the body becomes something used by the person, some of which is at the disposal or "over against" the person and thus may be sacrificed by the person for any higher good. Falling heir to Cartesian dualism that renders appreciation of the body-soul unity of human nature impossible, one author even concludes that both eyes may be donated "for the good of another person." Section 2.4 lists the reasons why we believe such views do not do justice to the Christian view of the integrity of the human person (Ramsey, 1970).

The development in the last 40 years of the moral teaching of theologians concerning organ transplants between the living is of more than antiquarian interest. First, it shows clearly that the opinion of theologians can evolve. Second, it shows that by refining accepted principles, and not denying them, a way can be found to prove new positions. Third, it demonstrates that many ethical problems are solved by starting with intuitive judgments and then examining the principles in light of the solution proposed in the intuitive judgment.

In summary, the transplanting of organs or tissues from a dead person to a living person does not offer any intrinsic ethical problem. Transplanting organs from one living person to another is also ethically acceptable provided that the following criteria are met:

1. There is a serious need on the part of the recipient that cannot be fulfilled in any other way.

2. The functional integrity of the donor as a human person will not be impaired, even though anatomical integrity may suffer.

3. The risk taken by the donor as an act of charity is proportionate to the good resulting for the recipient.

4. The donor's consent is free and informed.

Other Issues

In addition to the ethical issues that flow from the nature of an organ transplant, issues solved by an understanding of the Principles of Totality and Integrity and Common Good and Community, several additional ethical issues are associated with transplantation of organs. These additional issues concerning the allocation of scarce resources (1, 2, 3) are also solved by applyig the Principle of Common Good and Community. The last two issues are solved by the Principle of Human Dignity in Community (4) and the Principle of Legitimate Cooperation (5). Surprisingly, these other issues have arisen primarily because of the success of organ and tissue transplants. This success is mainly the result of the use of cyclosporin and other drugs that suppress the activity of the recipient's immune system (Boffey, 1984). The following new ethical issues require our consideration.

1. The first ethical issue is *how to allot available organs to recipients fairly* (Jonsen, 1985). Because so many different organs and tissues are now subject to transplant—not only heart and kidneys, but lungs, liver, pancreas, spleen, skin, and bone marrow as well—there is a continual shortage of suitable organs and tissue for transplant. At present, the system of obtaining organs and allotting them is not well defined. Regional transplant centers, funded in part by the federal government, publicize the need for organ donations; maintain waiting lists, including those who need transplants; and assist physicians in allotting the available organs. Recent legislation has set guidelines for national sharing of available organs based on genetic matching between donor and recipient (McDonald, 1988). In general, the organs are allotted to those in most grave need who at the same time have some chance of survival if the transplant is successful. Thus medical criteria are the basis for allotment. Because all potential recipients are registered, a "first come, first served" allotment is followed in theory.

As mentioned, buying and selling organs as commercial products is unethical because of the motivation that justifies the transplant in the first place. The federal government has supported this ethical principle by prohibiting the sale of organs for transplant. In many other countries, however, the sale of organs is neither prohibited nor unusual (Bermel, 1986).

Should available organs in the United States be allotted only to citizens of the United States, or should citizens of other countries be allowed to benefit from the transplantation program? Congressional hearings reveal that approximately 8,000 Americans await treatment for kidney transplants because wealthy citizens of other countries are able to pay to receive a transplant (U.S. Congress, 1984).

The Task Force on Organ Transplantation of the Department of Health and Human Services (DHHS, 1986) recommended that a quota system be established to place foreign nationals on a waiting list. To date, this has not been accomplished, and many transplant centers look on foreign nationals as a source of profit; thus, if foreign nationals can pay, they are usually accepted as candidates for transplant. This issue illustrates the problems that arise because the United States does not have any adequate national health policies to handle such problems. Although we do not maintain that foreign nationals should be totally excluded from transplant programs in the United States, there should be norms, or even federal regulations if necessary, that eliminate monetary factors as the major criterion for transplant candidacy and that strengthen medical need as the basic factor for candidacy.

2. A second ethical issue flowing from the success of the organ transplant program concerns the *financing of organ transplants*. Should organs be made available to all citizens of the United States, or only to those who can afford the procedure? And if the federal government would fund all organ transplants, must any limits be set on the program? The medical, hospital, and postoperative costs for transplants are well above the means of the average family (M. Benjamin, 1988). At present, the federal government funds most of the costs of kidney transplants and funds heart transplants if the potential recipient qualifies for the Medicare program (DHHS, 1986). Few potential heart recipients qualify for this program. Some private health insurance plans fund heart transplants, but the tendency is to limit this type of benefit. At present, for liver transplants and other procedures that are still considered experimental, the recipients or their families are required to raise funds themselves, often through public appeals, which sometimes are not successful though some private insurance companies are beginning to fund liver transplants at selected medical centers. Moreover, many states limit Medicaid expenditures to "basic" healthcare benefits and will not fund such procedures as liver transplants or bone marrow transplants (Welch and Larson, 1988). In response to the growing desire for organ transplants and the need to have some public policy in regard to funding of organ transplants, Callahan (1987b) suggests that consideration be given to limiting access for the elderly to transplants and other life-prolonging procedures.

Although there are no easy solutions to the funding issues that arise from the success of organ transplants, two thoughts should be prominent as we seek ethical criteria for a solution. First, are we as a nation devoting enough resources to healthcare? Although the present expenditures exceed 11 percent of the gross national product (GNP) (Grimes, 1988), is there any indication that this sum represents the limit that should be devoted to healthcare? Clearly, although the percentage of the GNP devoted to healthcare in the last 30 years has increased dramatically, so has the complexity and sophistication of medicine and healthcare. To compare healthcare of 1990 with healthcare of 1960 is to compare apples and oranges.

Second, an overall health policy must be formulated if we are to have a just and fair access to healthcare for all citizens. As Callahan (1987b) points out, at present no national policy deals with access to healthcare, but decisions are made as though our policy is to keep everyone alive as long as possible. In the immediate future, some policies must be determined for the United States that not only will afford basic care to all people who at present do not have adequate care, but that will also establish some equitable limits to public funding of sophisticated technology and innovative therapies. The difficult part of framing new policy in this regard is that some people will not live as long as they would if no new policy existed. For example, if Callahan's ideas were followed, some elderly people would not live as long because they would not be eligible for organ transplants financed through public funds. On the other hand, some people now are dying sooner than they would because our present policies are inequitable (Lurie et al., 1986).

   3. A third issue arising from the success of transplant surgery is the *desire to increase the supply of organs suitable for transplant*. Clearly, as organ transplantation has become more successful, the issue of organ supply has become more of a national priority (R.W. Evans et al., 1986). How can organs be procured without violating the rights of families and dying patients (Caplan, 1985)? In addition to increased public appeals made by voluntary groups, the Joint Commission for the Accreditation of Healthcare Organizations has requested each hospital to frame a policy that stipulates the procedure for requesting organ donations from the family of a dying or deceased person (American Hospital Association, 1986b). At present, the Anatomical Gift Act has been approved in each state (Sadler et al., 1968); this allows a person to sign his or her driver's license and indicate the desire to donate organs after death. However, the custom in most states requires the family to confirm such a donation; if the family were to disagree with the statement the patient made before death, it is unlikely that physicians or hospital administrators would approve surgery to remove organs for fear of ensuing malpractice litigation.

Basing arguments on the common good and that a transplant after death would not harm the donor in any way, Boyle and O'Rourke (1986) maintain that a presumption in favor of organ donation should be established. In the Boyle/O'Rourke plan, those who have religious or other reasons for denying the donation of organs could make their desires known before death, in much the same way people now reveal their desires to donate organs. If no objections are verified, however, the organs could be removed for transplant, even if no positive statement granting this permission was made beforehand by the deceased person. Although changing the presumption in regard to organ donation by the deceased may seem rather radical, it corresponds to the practice in some other countries (Prottas, 1985). Basically, we are in agreement with Boyle's proposition and think that it not only would increase the supply of organs for transplant, but would impress on the public the need to emphasize community needs in the provision of healthcare.

4. Another effort to increase the supply of organs has been made by some who challenge the present *criteria for brain death*. Must the person's total brain be dead before organs are removed? In the case of anencephalic infants, for example, the higher brain (cortex) will never develop, but the brainstem is still functioning. Although these infants will die shortly after birth, some maintain they are not "alive" and thus have their vital organs removed, causing the death of debilitated infants (Holzgreve et al., 1987). Determining that a person is incapable of recovery of higher cortical functions is quite different from saying that a person is dead (Arras and Shinnar, 1988). The physical evidence clearly shows that the development of the cerebral cortex does not constitute a "marker event" between prehuman and human development (Australian Research Commission, 1985). Moreover, absence of the higher brainstem would not constitute death. For example, the President's Commission for the Study of Ethical Problems in Medicine and Biomedical and Behavioral Research (1981) stated:

> First...it is not known which portions of the brain are responsible for cognition and consciousness; what little is known points to substantial interconnections among brainstem, subcortical structures, and the neocortex. Thus, the "higher brain" may well exist only as a metaphorical concept, not in reality. Second, even when the sites or certain aspects of consciousness can be found, their cessation often cannot be assessed with the certainty that would be required in applying a statutory definition (p. 40).

Although the anencephalic infant may not develop in a manner that fulfills the full potential usually associated with "person," there is no scientific justification to consider anencephalic infants as dead. Rather, they should be considered living human beings until total brain death occurs. True, an anencephalic infant is a severely debilitated human being and a human being who will not live for long. Because there is no effective means of overcoming the pathology from which the anencephalic infant suffers, therapeutic care may be withheld. A real and dramatic difference exists, however, between allowing a person to die because a serious pathology cannot be overcome and directly killing an innocent human being.

Brain death criteria for infants have not been established accurately (B. Robinson, 1981; Rowland et al., 1983). Even the recent attempts to offer guidelines for brain death in children are not extended for application in the premature infant (Annas et al., 1987). Thus, even transplant centers that seek to allow anencephalic infants to die before transplanting organs have experienced difficulty making this determination (Blakeslee, 1987). As death approaches, an anencephalic infant may be placed on a respirator to ensure that blood will continue perfusing the organs even after death so that the organs will be apt for transplant, as is done in the treatment of an adult who will be an organ donor. Thus anticipating the death of infants and keeping their body fluids flowing after brain death through use of a ventilator would not be unethical. However, no organs should be removed until brain death has been certified from clinical signs, as difficult as this might be if the infant is on life-support systems.

5. A final ethical issue concerns the *use of tissue taken from fetuses for transplant purposes* (Lehrman, 1988). Living cells taken from aborted fetuses are being transplanted into other human beings with serious diseases. People with Alzheimer's disease and Parkinson's disease, for example, have received transplants of brain tissue from recently aborted fetuses. Fetal tissue is more adaptable for research, and perhaps for therapy, because fetuses do not have a well-developed immune system. Thus the tissue garnered from fetuses is less likely to be rejected in another person's body and seems to grow faster than tissue taken from other sources (McCullagh, 1987). The best material for research seems to come from fetuses in the second trimester of life. Many scientists and other citizens have expressed concern about ethical issues involved in this form of research because the raw material for research comes from fetuses killed in elective abortions (Andrusko and Bond, 1988; Wolinsky, 1988).

Clearly, the research in fetal tissue has not caused the legalization of elective abortions. One and one-half million abortions per year were occurring in the United States long before research with fetal tissue was initiated. However, although no intrinsic connection exists between research on fetal tissue and elective abortions, those involved in this form of research have an ethical responsibility to make sure that the distance between the two realities is kept clear. There should be no indication that researchers are encouraging or promoting elective abortion. To accomplish this, two steps should be taken:

1. No monies should be paid for fetal tissue taken from aborted fetuses. There are federal laws against the sale of organs for transplantation (McDonald, 1988); it also seems federal laws should prohibit the sale of fetal tissue for research as well.

2. A second manner of disassociating with the destruction of living human beings is to foster the availability of fetal tissue derived from culture processes. The ethical issue resulting from the source of supply for fetal tissue might be solved if the source material for the culture is derived from spontaneous as opposed to elective abortions.

Some ethicists and scientists compare fetal research to organ transplants from cadavers (Mahowald et al., 1987). Thus they maintain that the use of aborted fetuses is acceptable if the mother gives consent. However, further consideration belies this assumption. When a family surrenders through proxy consent organs from a cadaver for heart or liver transplant, they have not been involved in causing the death of the person in question. Thus, although there is no direct connection between researchers and abortion, one must not assume that informed consent solves the ethical issues resulting from the use of tissue from aborted fetuses (Burtchell, 1988).

At present, the federal government will not subsidize research using fetal tissue, and some states have prohibited this type of research.

11.3   SEXUAL REASSIGNMENT

Sexual reassignment is a type of reconstructive surgery by which the sexual phenotype of a male is altered to resemble that of a female, or vice versa (H. Benjamin, 1980; Fisk, 1973; J. Meyer, 1974). Such surgery, along with hormonal treatment and psychotherapy, is often used to treat transsexualism when psychiatric treatment fails. Transsexualism is described in the *Diagnostic and Statistical Manual of Mental Disorders* (DSM III) as involving the following five criteria (American Psychiatric Association, 1980):

1. Sense of discomfort and inappropriateness about one's anatomical sex
2. Wish to be rid of one's own genitals and to live as a member of the other sex
3. The disturbance has been continuous (not limited to periods of stress) for at least two years
4. Absence of physical intersex or genetic abnormality
5. Not caused by another mental disorder, such as schizophrenia

Transsexual surgery involves radical mutilation: castration and construction of a pseudo-vagina for the male, mastectomy and hysterectomy (sometimes also the construction of a nonfunctional pseudo-penis and testes) for the female, along with hormonal treatments with possible serious side effects (Markland, 1975). This raises the ethical question of whether the attempt to change a person's biological sex is ever a legitimate aim of medical care (B. Brody et al., 1981).

Catholic moralists have always admitted that in cases where a child is born with ambiguous genitalia, the parents should raise the child as belonging to that sex in which he or she is most likely to be able to function best. Also, there seems to be no objection to the use of surgery or hormones to improve the normal appearance or function of such persons in accordance with the sex in which they are to be or have been raised. The reasoning behind this traditional position is that a person must "live according to nature" insofar as this is humanly knowable.

Recently, however, knowledge of sexual development has vastly increased, and sexual ambiguity is seen as far more complex and common than formerly thought (Monteleone, 1981). The biological determination of sex depends on the presence or absence of the Y chromosome in the one-cell zygote, which in the beginning constitutes the human person (see 9.1). When present, the Y chromosome produces TDY (testicular determinant Y) as early as the 8-cell stage of development, and the person begins to move toward maleness; otherwise all zygotes develop as females. All embryos originally have undifferentiated gonads and two sets of sexual ducts, the Wolffian and Müllerian, but at seven weeks the male gonads differentiate and begin to produce hormones that destroy the Müllerian ducts and cause the development of the male genitalia. Otherwise, the Wolffian ducts are absorbed and the gonads and the Müllerian ducts develop into the female sexual system. At the same time, the differing hormonal balance in the two sexes causes certain differences in the male and female brain, in particular preparing the female brain to regulate the menstrual cycle. It has been established for some animals, but not certainly for human beings, that these

313

neurological differences also result in behavioral differences in the two sexes (Gemuth, 1988).

All these biological determinations are at work before birth. After birth it is probable, but not yet proved, that there are *biophysical* events at the unconscious level, similar to the imprinting demonstrated in animals, that also promote sexual differentiation, such as the way the mother cares differently for a female than for a male child. Finally, at the conscious *environmental* level, the person learns his or her own *gender identity* and assumes a *gender role* in society. In this long and complicated process many things can go wrong at each stage, with the result that in the human population a whole spectrum of conditions exists between the normal masculine and feminine conditions. "Normal" here means a condition determined by that sexual teleology designed by God to culminate in successful heterosexual marriage (see 8.3).

Among these possible abnormalities, *homosexuality* is a highly varied condition, probably having many etiological factors. In this case a person who is phenotypically unambiguously male or female and in no doubt about his or her gender is conscious of greater sexual attraction to those of his or her own sex than to others and who, consequently, is unable to enter into a satisfactory marriage. *Transvestism* is a condition in which a person, usually heterosexual in orientation, is more comfortable sexually while wearing clothing symbolic of the opposite sex. This is probably a form of fetishism (S. Levine and Lothstein, 1981). *Transsexualism* differs from these because of *gender dysphoria syndrome,* that is, an anxiety, sometimes reaching suicidal depression, as the result of the obsessive feeling that one's "real" sex is the opposite of one's phenotypic sex.

The argument of psychotherapists and surgeons who undertake sexual reassignment as a remedy for this syndrome is that the victims find no relief in other therapies, are insistent on surgery even to the point of threatening suicide, and are generally satisfied with its results (Springer, 1987). Ethicists who follow a utilitarian or proportionalist methodology can approve such surgery if they are convinced that the good effects outweigh the bad. The methodology used in this book (see Chapter 8) can approve of it only if this can be shown to be simply an extension of the classical position that in cases of sexual ambiguity, it is permissible to choose the more probable sex, as already explained. Can this be demonstrated?

Reasons to the Contrary

At present, we do not believe this case can be demonstrated for several reasons. First, it has not yet been established that the cause of gender dysphoria syndrome is biological (Hoenig, 1985), although this theory has been suggested by some (Monteleone, 1981; M. Peterson, 1981). No such cause is evident at the genotypic or phenotypic level, and as yet the evidence is tenuous that the reason transsexuals believe from early in their lives that they have "a soul different from my body" is caused by some developmental accident in the central nervous or hormonal systems. At present, it remains more probable that the determining causes are at the psychological level of development, although there may be some biological predispositions (Holden, 1979). Consequently, the gender ambiguity in question is primarily psychological and should be treated psychotherapeutically. A recent study of the problem (Lothstein, 1982) shows that the condition is much more common in males than females and that of those males applying for sexual reassignment surgery, only about 10 to 25 percent can be diagnosed as having *primary* gender dysphoria, that is, of the type that "has an obvious, documentable, lifelong, profound disturbance of core gender identity." J.K. Meyer (1974) went so far as to state, "I have seen any number of men who would like to live as females and vice versa; I have not seen one with a reversal of core gender identity." Other candidates for surgery can only be diagnosed as suffering from *secondary* gender dysphoria, which is stress-related and results from "failures of other gender identity adaptations, such as transvestism, effeminate homosexuality, gender ambiguity." Thus the arguments for biological rather than a psychological etiology of this syndrome will hold (if at all) only for a very restricted group of patients.

Second, contrary to what is often stated, when candidates for surgery are required to undergo psychotherapy in preparation for surgery, many are found to be ambiguous about really wanting it and in the end decide against it. Moreover, most transsexuals who have been carefully diagnosed appear to be suffering from serious psychological problems, sometimes subtle and not immediately recognized, other than their gender dysphoria (S. Levine and Lothstein, 1981). Even after surgery they continue to need at least some psychotherapeutic support, although their frequent difficulty in forming stable personal relationships makes this follow-up difficult.

Third, although when this type of surgery was first introduced there were enthusiastic reports of its success, as experience accumulates there is less agreement that it does much good. The latest survey of studies evaluating the outcome of transsexual surgery concludes that that previous studies have indicated more people being satisfied with the overall results of the surgery by a 2 to 1 margin (Walinder, 1984). However, the surveys that offer the previous favorable reports are criticized for their lack of objectivity, and "the paucity of control groups make attribution of either improvement or deterioration to the surgical intervention scientifically untenable" (Abramowitz, 1986). Johns Hopkins University, noted for its leadership in research in this field, announced the suspension of its program for further reassessment as a result of a report by J.K. Meyer and Reter (1979), which concluded that this type of surgery offers no advantage over psychotherapy. Another study in regard to Medicaid funding of sex-reassignment surgery affirms this conclusion (Jacobs, 1980).

Fourth, from a theological point of view, it is clear that surgery does not really solve these persons' problem because it does not enable them to achieve sexual normality or to enter into a valid Christian marriage and have children. Since many of these individuals are somewhat asexual (S. Levine and Lothstein, 1981), their problem is not primarily sexual satisfaction but the relief of the burden of anxiety, which can usually be at least considerably lightened by psychotherapy. Some (Lavin, 1987) raise the question of whether in severe cases the possible relief of anxiety might outweigh the other disvalues involved.

However, we would invoke the Principle of Totality and Integrity (2.4, 8.2) to show that the good of the person cannot be achieved at the expense of the destruction of a basic human function, in this case the sterilization of the person, except to save the person's life. Furthermore, the studies reported by no means give assurance that sexual reassignment solves the more general psychological problems from which most of these victims suffer.

We conclude that, based on the present state of knowledge, Catholic hospitals or healthcare professionals are not justified in recommending or engaging in this type of surgery. Certainly compassion should be extended to this small but greatly suffering group of human beings, but it should take the practical form of psychotherapy and pastoral guidance. It is unfortunate that the widespread publicity given to sex-change surgery and the exaggerated reports of its success have created an increasing demand among troubled people, most of whom would not be accepted for such surgery by any reputable clinic.

How should such cases be dealt with pastorally? The fundamental aim of the therapist, as well as of the pastoral counselor, in these cases should be to restore the patient's sense of personal self-worth. He or she must be helped to see, as should homosexuals and those suffering from other sexual problems, that today's culture is grievously mistaken in its exaggerated stress on sexual identity and activity as a primary determinant of human worth. They must be assisted to find interests—spiritual, intellectual, and social—that will enable them to escape their preoccupation with their sexual identity and discover their more fundamental value as human persons. As for persons who have already undergone surgery, we believe they should be counseled not to attempt marriage and should be supported in their efforts to live chastely with the assistance of the sacraments and the respect and fellowship of the Christian community.

11.4   GENETIC INTERVENTION

Gift or Order

The issue of the parents' need and right to have children or even to *order* the sort of child they want is also at the base of many new problems that loom on the horizon concerning genetic engineering, or to use an expression with less pejorative connotations, *genetic intervention*. This is the effort to repair genetic defects at their genotypic source in the genes and chromosomes rather than in their phenotypic effects and, further, to control and produce at will new combinations of genetic traits in offspring (W. Anderson, 1985; Glover, 1985).

One of the simplest forms of such engineering would be to determine at will the sex of the fetus by selecting sperm that do or do not have the Y chromosome that determines maleness and then using selected sperm for artificial insemination or in vitro fertilization and implantation (Robertson, 1985). Section 10.5 discusses the ethical issues involved in such methods. Even if a technique could be invented that would promote or suppress the production of one or the other type of sperm in the male parent without interfering with the normal process of sexual intercourse, the social and ecological consequences of such intervention could be counterproductive.

Biologists are convinced that evolutionary selection has developed the process of sexual differentiation by a genetic mechanism of the sort we find in the human species because this ensures an approximate 50/50 distribution of the sexes. Some additional mechanism not fully understood even produces a slightly higher number of male zygotes to offset the higher mortality of males. Studies made in the United States (Holmes, 1985) show that most young couples now want two children, preferring a boy first, but once the boy is assured, then a girl. Although this preference is probably cultural and subject to cultural modification, it possibly also has a sociobiological foundation in the greater mortality of males. These studies predict that if sex selection was widely adopted, there would first be a marked rise in male births, but then a leveling to a 50/50 distribution. It seems, therefore, that the promotion of sexual selection might not be seriously deleterious to society, although it certainly would have risks and would have few, if any, social advantages over leaving it to nature. Its only advantage would be that parents would have freedom of choice, provided that overall they use this choice to have equal numbers of boys and girls.

Ethically speaking, is this free choice of a boy or a girl an advantage to the *child?* After all, parents should not let their subjective preferences operate at the expense of their children in this matter, just as it is unethical for them to insist that the child be a doctor or a lawyer if this is not truly for the best interests of the child. It might be argued that it is somewhat advantageous for a boy to have a sister, and vice versa, rather than a sibling of his or her own sex, but if would be difficult to prove that such an advantage, if it exists, is of major significance. On the other hand, as argued in 10.3, Christian teaching shows that it is highly significant to children that they be accepted by their parents as a divine gift to be loved for what they uniquely are and not merely because they conform to the parents' hopes or expectations. At present, society is becoming more aware of the immense injustice and harm done to women by cultural patterns and structures that constantly say to a girl, "You should have been a boy." Sex selection by the parents either will reinforce this male preference pattern or, if parents can be reeducated to equal preference, will still say to the individual child, "You are loved because you conform to your parents' preferences." This seems an injustice to the child and further reinforces the cultural message that children exist primarily to fulfill the needs of the parents rather than for their own sake. This implication is already built into many cultural structures, and people have an ethical responsibility to fight against it. The healthcare profession should discourage such attitudes, not promote techniques to further them.

Complex Forms of Intervention

The same consideration applies to more complex forms of genetic reconstruction. Although some progress has already been made in genetic recombination at the level of simple organisms, the possibility of using such methods to correct genetic defects or to create new genetic structures in human zygotes or embryos is still remote (W. Anderson, 1985; Laura, 1985).

If the purpose of such techniques is therapy for an individual fetus, the only ethical issue is the proportion of probable benefit to risk. The issues already discussed, however, concerning in vitro fertilization and artificial insemination and implantation arise if these techniques can be used to produce a healthy embryo only at the expense of creating several embryos from which one will be selected and the others allowed to perish (see 10.5) (Lejeune et al., 1984).

What if the purpose is not therapy of an existing fetus, but the production of superior human beings? Two methods have been proposed. One is to replicate many genetically identical individuals by cloning. In such a process, nuclei from the somatic cells of a "superior" individual would be transplanted into a denucleated ovum, which would then develop into an identical twin of the donor. This would require in vitro fertilization and implantation into a foster mother's womb (Bashim, 1984; Watson, 1971). Another method is to recombine genes in the nucleus of a zygote, for example, by using viruses that have the capability of incorporating a section of a chromosome derived from one nucleus and fixing it in a chromosome of another (transduction) (W. Anderson, 1985; B. Davis, 1970). Theoretically, it may become possible to synthesize chemically new genes that have never existed in the gene pool or to produce them by artificial, controlled mutation. Thus it might also be possible to produce a human being according to "recipe," with the height, complexion, physiological traits, and mental abilities desired. Although this is still very remote (Kass, 1985), we would not rule it out ethically merely on the grounds that it would be usurpation of God's creative power, since we believe that God wishes to share this creative power with human persons insofar as they are capable of using it well (Principle of Stewardship and Creativity, 8.3).

Grave ethical difficulties, however, do arise over whether society has either the knowledge or the virtue to take the responsibility for creating these superior members of the race (Callahan, 1981; John Fletcher, 1985; Gustafson, 1973; Kass, 1987). Attempts to define *superior* eugenically are so ambiguous as to be arbitrary (Rifkin, 1984). Because human beings are evolutionary and historical beings, *superior* does not mean a being superior in one age and culture, but rather a being with capabilities of meeting the challenges of new and unpredicted situations. Genetic variation assists this flexibility, whereas the production of many identical human beings or favoring certain supposedly superior types amounts to a restriction on this genetic variability. At most, a eugenic policy would have to be content with introducing into the gene pool some new, apparently valuable traits or increasing somewhat the percentage of their presence. Furthermore, all the difficulties already raised about the way in which such techniques tend to separate the child from its relations to parents and family arise once more.

The following conclusions can be drawn:

1. It is more feasible, technically and ethically, to improve the human condition by improving the environment and development of the individual, that is, the *phenotype*, than by modifying genetic endowment,

that is, the *genotype*. Priority in research and investment of medical resources should be given to the former effort. Genetic research is extremely important, however, to understand the interactions of genotype and phenotype (Rose, 1984).

2. Presently proposed methods of genetic reconstruction of human beings involve in vitro fertilization and other procedures that are ethically objectionable because they separate reproduction from its parental context and involve the production of human beings, some of whom will be defective because of experimental failure and who probably will be destroyed. This contravenes the basic principles of ethical experimentation with human subjects (see 9.5; Callahan, 1981; Ramsey, 1970; Sacred Congregation for the Doctrine of the Faith, 1987).

3. Proposals to improve the human race by sex selection, cloning, or genetic reconstruction are ethically unacceptable in the present state of knowledge. Unless limited to very modest interventions, they would restrict the genetic variability important to human survival, and they would separate reproduction from its parental context.

4. If the foregoing problems can be overcome, it will be ethically desirable to develop and use genetic methods for therapy of genetic defects in existing embryos, keeping in view the risk-benefit proportion (Office of Technology Assessment, 1984).

In addition to discussion about efforts to reconstruct human genes, much discussion has focused recently on the possible effects on the ecological balance and the possible medical and commercial uses of experiments with and large-scale production of new life forms by the technique of *recombinant DNA* (deoxyribonucleic acid). This involves the modification of the genetic code of existing life forms by introducing into their chromosomes fragments derived from the chromosomes of other life forms, thus producing organisms with combinations of genetic and inheritable traits never before found in nature. For example, it is possible to produce food plants that can directly utilize atmosphere nitrogen and thus eliminate the use of fertilizers, or to produce rather inexpensively the heretofore extremely scarce interferon, a natural substance believed to have many important medical uses, including cancer therapy. The U.S. Supreme Court, in *Diamond v. Chakrabarty*, held that a live, man-made microorganism is patentable, thus opening the way to its commercial development (Ehrman et al., 1980). Those who favored patenting such biological inventions argue that this will promote research, as it has for drugs. The analogy, however, also suggests the possibility of serious abuses for profit. The same basic ethical principles that govern any form of research apply here (9.5), with the additional precautions that what is involved are not merely individual human subjects, but the total environment, and that possible widespread epidemics could result if something goes wrong (National Institutes of Health [NIH], 1987). The greatest worry, but one which should not be exaggerated, is whether some new life form, against which there is no existent immunity in the human, animal, or plant ecosystem, may multiply beyond bounds, as has so often occurred when alien species are introduced into an ecosystem already in balance.

11.5   GENETIC SCREENING AND COUNSELING

The medical specialty of diagnosing inherited or genetic defects and their treatment, as well as the task of screening populations for these defects and counseling couples who are or may become parents of defective children, is developing rapidly. Special clinics dedicated to this are being founded throughout the United States (Capron, 1984; John Fletcher et al., 1985; Lappe, 1984).

Three basic discoveries have made it possible to predict at times inherited traits of a child before birth (Carmi, 1983; S. Reed, 1980; Watson, 1987): (1) Gregor Mendel's theory of the laws of the combinations of units of inheritance, (2) these units or *genes* being located in the chromosomes of the nucleus of every cell, and (3) genetic code consisting in variations in a fundamental substance, DNA, out of which the genes are composed. Techniques of diagnosing these defects at early stages of child development are being perfected. These include *amniocentesis*, by which the genetic condition of the unborn child can be determined in some respects by examining the amniotic fluid in which the fetus floats in the womb. Another technique is *chorionic villi sampling*, in which a plastic catheter is inserted through the cervix to biopsy villi, the hairlike projections in the placenta. This is rapidly growing tissue, and results of chromosome tests are available in a few days (Holder, 1985; Kahn, 1987). The chorion villi test may be performed about eight weeks earlier than amniocentesis. Also, techniques to counteract some of the deleterious consequences of genetic defects are being worked out, and there is even the prospect of methods for correcting the defective genes themselves by DNA recombination (W. Anderson, 1985).

Why such advances are medically important is evident from the following statistics. There are approximately 3,000 different diseases in the single-gene disorder group, all of which are caused by different abnormal genes (Ngyan and Sahat, 1987). Today, 33 percent of infant deaths are related to genetic causes. More than 100 genetic conditions can be diagnosed prenatally. Parent carriers of defective genes may have as much as a 50 percent risk of generating offspring with a genetic defect. The polygenic conditions, such as diabetes mellitus, gout, and some allergies, occur in 1.7 to 2.6 percent of all live births. There seems to be approximately a 5 percent incidence of genetic disease in all live births (Kahn, 1987; Osmundsen, 1973; Taysi, 1983).

In view of these facts, some scientists, in the name of preventive medicine, advocate prenatal or postnatal *genetic screening* of the whole population for four purposes: (1) to advance scientific research, since such research is necessary to achieve full understanding and control over human inheritance; (2) to assist responsible parenthood so that carriers of genetic defects may not pass them on; (3) to make possible early therapy before the malfunctioning of defective genes has caused extensive damage; and (4) to give the parents the option of aborting the child when the defect is serious and no therapy is yet known (Macklin, 1985; Murray et al., 1984).

We have already given reasons why this last purpose is ethically unacceptable, but the first three are certainly legitimate. They do, however, raise serious questions (Capron, 1984). First, the research purposes of genetic screening must be regulated in the same way as any other type of research on human subjects (see 9.5). Thus, since amniocentesis involves risk of spontaneous abortion (although the risk has been reduced with the help of sonography to less than 1 percent), it cannot be used unless there are also proportionate benefits for the fetus. At present, therapeutic help for a genetically deficient fetus is limited, but more progress in this field is noted each year (Hendren and Lillehi, 1988; NIH, 1987). Some ethicists maintain that amniocentesis benefits the fetus because it helps the parents prepare more adequately for the birth (Dube, 1983). In sum, amniocentesis is indicated only when a pregnancy is thought to be at increased risk for a particular disorder (Kahn, 1987). Recently, Roy (1984) has pointed out a more profound ethical issue that may result from prenatal screening:

> Prenatal diagnosis delivers the knowledge required to exercise the kind of quality control over the unborn that amounts to a control over birth....The earlier long-standing belief of a theocratic reproductive culture in the equality of all human beings based on the identity of their origin and destiny has given way to an emphasis on the empirical inequalities of human beings (p. 16).

Most screening techniques used postnatally only involve the withdrawal of an insignificant amount of body fluid or tissue and are harmless. Nevertheless, informed consent is required in all such cases, and it is highly questionable that it is legitimate to enact laws that require compulsory screening for research purposes alone. Even when consent is given, care must be taken about how the information is used (Crauford and Harris, 1986). If the results are made known to subjects, there is danger that they may misunderstand or exaggerate the seriousness and possible consequences of their condition or the condition of their children. If the results are known to others, there is danger of stigmatization, that is, that victims will be regarded by others as humanly inferior or dangerous. For example, it is unfair to label those blacks who are carriers of the sickle cell trait, or those Jews who are carriers of the Tay-Sachs syndrome, as diseased or defective. Second, the use of screening to promote responsible parenthood is in general a laudable purpose, since couples undoubtedly should not bring into the world children for whom (with the reasonable assistance of society) they cannot adequately care, and since the care of defective children presents special burdens. Consequently, prospective parents have the duty to seek the scientific information useful to such decisions, and society has the duty to assist them in obtaining such information (John Fletcher, 1982). As already noted (10.3), the right of married couples to beget children is conditioned by their capability to provide for them.

Caution is necessary, however, in the face of programs of *negative* eugenics advocated by certain enthusiasts (Glass, 1975; Modell, 1982; Osmundsen, 1973) who argue that modern medicine has upset the ecological balance by saving the lives of more and more defective persons who formerly would have died before they could reproduce. Thus the load of defective genes in the gene pool is increasing, and a much higher level of genetic disease may soon occur in the population. As Lappe (1972) has written:

> The consensus of the best medical and genetic opinion is that whatever genetic deterioration is occurring as a result of decreased natural selection is so slow as to be insignificant when contrasted to "environmental" changes, including those produced by medical innovation (p. 421).

If only those persons who themselves suffer from a particular genetic disease are prevented from reproducing, this still does not eliminate heterozygous carriers who will continue to transmit defects dependent on recessive genes (Thompson and Thompson, 1988). At present, technology is far from being able to detect all these carriers. Even if science had this ability, such elimination would extend to many people. This would probably also mean the elimination from the gene pool of many desirable traits because the same persons carry both good and bad traits, which sometimes are genetically linked in ways still very obscure. Thus programs of negative eugenics based on present knowledge would achieve their goals only very slowly, over many generations, and might have side effects worse than the evils they remedy. Moreover, as defective genes are eliminated from the gene pool, they are constantly being replaced by mutations caused by environmental factors.

It seems, therefore, that such information cannot be used to compel persons to refrain from reproduction, but it may be supplied to them to enable them to make responsible personal decisions (John Fletcher, 1982). Even here, however, some public caution is needed. Some states have adopted compulsory screening of newborn infants to detect those afflicted with phenylketonuria (PKU), a genetically based metabolic disease that results in mental retardation and can be treated by diet (Andrews, 1985). After these programs were instituted, it was discovered that some persons who test positively do not develop mental retardation, and that the dietary treatment to which they were subjected may even have been harmful (Barden et al., 1984). Thus genetic testing programs have to be carefully designed. The Research Group on Ethical, Social, and Legal Issues in Genetic Counseling and Genetic Engineering (Hastings Center Institute, 1972) has suggested guidelines, which can be summarized as follows:

1. The attainability of the program's aims should be pretested by pilot projects and other studies, and the program should be constantly evaluated and updated.
2. Community participation in planning and executing the program should be secured to educate the public as to the true significance and legitimate use of the information obtained.
3. The information obtained should be made available according to clearly stated policies known to those participating before they consent, and their privacy should be carefully protected.
4. Screening programs should be voluntary. The rights of parents to make their own decisions about the use of the information in family planning should be protected and care taken to avoid stigmatizing them or their offspring.
5. Information about screening should be open and available to all, with priorities given to well-defined populations suffering from frequent defects.

6. Programs should not be instituted unless the tests used are able to give relatively unambiguous information, and this should be precisely recorded.

7. The general principles with regard to experimentation with human subjects, such as informed consent and protection from risks, should be observed.

8. Persons to be screened or who have their children screened should be informed before they consent about the nature and cost of therapy and its risks or if no therapy is available.

9. Counseling to help the subjects understand and deal with the information should be provided.

We would also add that it is important to consider whether the cost in money and personnel in administering such programs give them high priority in view of the rarity of most of these conditions. It must be recognized, however, that in some cases (e.g., PKU) the testing per subject is quite inexpensive, whereas the cost of caring for even a few mentally retarded children in institutions may be very high.

Genetic Counseling

If such screening programs are to be voluntary, the main concern is to counsel parents as they attempt to decide how to use this information in planning their families (Baumiller, 1983; Capron, 1984; John Fletcher et al., 1985; Garver and Marchese, 1986; P. Harper, 1981).

Genetic counseling may be characterized as a process of communication that attempts to deal with the human problems associated with the occurrence, or the risk of occurrence, of a genetic disorder in an individual or family (Atkinson and Moraczewski, 1980). This process involves an attempt by one or more appropriately trained person to help an individual, couple, or family do the following:

1. Comprehend the medical facts, such as the risk of occurrence or recurrence of a disorder, the possibilities for diagnosis, the probable course of the disorder, and the available therapies.

2. Appreciate the ways in which hereditary and environmental factors contribute to the disorder, and the extent to which specified relatives are at risk for being affected or for producing an affected child.

3. Understand the options for dealing with a positive diagnosis, such as methods of contraception or sterilization, abortion, institutionalization, adoption agencies, and other social services.

4. Choose the course of action that seems appropriate to the clients in view of their own values and goals, and act in accordance with that decision.

5. Make the best possible adjustment to the disorder in an affected member of the family or to the risk of a recurrence of the disorder.

A family comes to a genetic counselor because of fears about possible defects in children already in existence or about their responsibilities for future pregnancies. These fears may have arisen because of positive test results in mass screening, or because of a record of genetic disease in parents, previous children, or close relatives (John Fletcher, 1982).

Some argue that if serious reasons exist to believe a fetus is gravely defective, the parents should be persuaded to agree to abort the child if this suspicion is confirmed by amniocentesis (Silber, 1981). Otherwise, they argue, it is difficult to justify the risks of the amniocentesis procedure. If abortion is ethically unacceptable, the counselor should not recommend prenatal screening that is potentially dangerous to the infant unless this is justified by the possibility of intrauterine therapy proportionate to the risks or of some benefit to the infant because the parents will be better prepared to care for the child. A recent survey of fetal surgery expresses that the main value of antenatal diagnosis lies in prompt postnatal treatment of major malformations before complications develop (Hendren and Lillehi, 1988). The desire to satisfy the parents' curiosity concerning the sex of the child does not seem to be a sufficient reason for subjecting the infant to even minimal risk of harm.

Again, some counselors would suggest that even when amniocentesis cannot determine genetic defect with certainty, the parents are free to decide whether they wish to take the risks or to abort; the law seems to suggest this option (Dickens, 1986). This means that if parents decide to abort, they are also risking the destruction of a normal child because such tests are not infallible, nor do they perfectly predict the degree of phenotypic impairment. We believe that counselors should not recommend abortion as a solution. If the parents declare a firm intention to abort, the counselor should not cooperate in any way with them. The reason is that the rights of the fetus to life should be protected by counselors—exactly as they would protect the rights of a child already born— against the infringement of these rights by the parents, no matter how well-intentioned they may be. A counselor, however, in doing whatever possible to avoid abortion, should exercise great prudence, avoiding threats, pressures, and recriminations, since these will only aggravate the situation. Indeed, undue persuasion may lead to a malpractice claim (American College of Obstetricians and Gynecologists, 1985; Annas, 1985a; Holder, 1985). In sum, if abortion is in question, the counselor should respect the conscience of the parents while doing everything possible to protect the child.

Is it permissible for a counselor to give information to parents whom the counselor only suspects may resort to abortion? In the present ethical climate this suspicion always exists, and it has deterred Catholic healthcare facilities from instituting genetic counseling centers. Parents, however, have a right to such information, which has good as well as bad uses, and the counselor who supplies it cooperates only materially and remotely if the parents use it for a purpose the counselor considers unethical. Moreover, counselors may be legally liable if they do not inform parents that an unborn child may be suffering from a genetic defect and that it is possible in some cases to make sure of this by amniocentesis or other prenatal tests (Annas, 1979), even though parents might use this information to obtain an abortion. In our opinion, Catholic healthcare facilities have a duty to provide such counseling in accordance with Christian moral standards, since otherwise parents will be forced to obtain information from centers where abortion will be an accepted and even encouraged solution (McCormick, 1984a).

For reasons already given in 9.2, we reject such arguments as that of Glass (1972), who writes:

> It is not equally a right of every person to be born physically and mentally sound, capable of developing fully into a mature individual? Has society, which must support at great cost, the burden of genetic misfortune resulting from mutation, chromosomal accident, and prenatal harm inflicted by trauma or virus no right at all to protect itself from the increasing misfortune? Should not the abortion of a seriously defective fetus be obligatory? Should not the loss of a defective child be recompensed by the opportunity to have another, a sound child by prenatal or postnatal adoption (p. 252)?

It certainly is a right for a child to be free of every defect that medicine has the power to prevent or correct. It is paradoxical, however, to believe that this right is protected by destroying the child who has not been saved from defect. Glass is really talking about the concern of the parents and society to save themselves the burden of defective children. Parents may have the responsibility not to generate such children, but having generated them, they also have the duty to care for them. They cannot lighten their burden by destroying an unborn child any more than an infant or adolescent. Underlying such arguments is the basic conviction that it is better never to be a defective person. This is an assumption of some humanists, but it is not consistent with a Christian view of the value of a person or the true meaning of human life.

It remains true, however, that couples have the duty of responsible parenthood, and society has a legitimate concern to support and encourage this responsibility. The genetic counselor, therefore, has the function of helping prospective parents prepare themselves for the possibility that a fetus will be defective and to plan ways to provide for this eventuality. The counselor also has the task of helping them decide whether they will or will not have children.

Parental Responsibility

In the past, some would have argued that a person or a couple at risk of begetting a defective child or children, or of transmitting defective genes to future generations, should fatalistically marry and beget children and "leave it to God." This fatalism, as already pointed out, has not been as damaging to society as some eugenic enthusiasts have thought, since it does not upset the ecological balance established by evolutionary selection. Even today, when medical advances have upset this balance by counteracting this selective process, such fatalism can only very slowly increase the social burden about which Glass is so concerned. Nevertheless, Christian teaching does not favor fatalistic attitudes, but rather advocates parental responsibility.

Prospective parents, therefore, have to consider these factors: (1) their own need to have children as the completion of their mutual love, (2) their own capacity to care for these children, and (3) the risk that each particular child may suffer from grave handicaps requiring special care, including the possibility that this child will be faced in turn with the question as to whether he or she should pass on defective genes to the next generation. Some significant risks of defect exist for *every* child and could not be eliminated even by the most radical use of abortion. Thus in all cases parents must decide whether they have the capacity to care for a potentially defective child. Furthermore, the counselor and society have the duty to assist the parents in accepting and meeting reasonable risks. For counselors or society at large to encourage in parents the attitude that they should not have children unless the children are perfect and require the least care possible is as reprehensible as to encourage parents to reproduce fatalistically.

Certainly, the correct professional attitude for genetic counselors is to give the parents reliable, objective information as to the probabilities of defect and its consequences and the type of therapy and care that will be required. Counselors should also help them (directly or by referral to others professionally competent) to deal with personal, economic, and social factors that determine the parents' capacity to meet the demands of care if a child has a particular defect. They should also inform the parents about the social resources that may be available to help. On the basis of this objective information and counseling support, the individual or couple must make their own decision about whether their need for children justifies taking the risks involved. Such decisions must be made not merely by some persons, but by everyone, since begetting new life is essentially a risky business. The reason that genetic counselors are needed today is that now more information is available about the risks involved in reproduction and more help is needed in dealing with the complexities this information discloses.

As already argued in 10.5, the need and right of a couple to have children is not absolute. Thus, if the risks are high, such as 25 percent, of begetting a child so defective as to require care that the parents cannot supply, even with reasonable and available social assistance, then they have the responsibility to consider not begetting children. Genetic counselors, therefore, while respecting the consciences and psychological freedom of their clients, will help persons at high risk make this difficult decision. Moreover, these parents should be informed properly about the various methods of birth regulation, especially natural family planning, and the ethical evaluation of these methods (10.3).

Problems also arise with regard to adults who have a genetic defect that will eventually become a serious handicap or lead to early death, for example, Huntington's chorea, which in middle life results in progressive neurological degeneration (Crauford and Harris, 1986). On the one hand is the responsibility of the person not to pass this defect on to children, and on the other, the personal difficulty of living under a sense of doom. Undoubtedly, as people become more aware of the existence of genetic defects, it will become impossible to keep such knowledge from them. It would seem that all individuals should have the freedom to decide whether they wish a diagnosis. Nevertheless, we would argue that individuals who seriously suspect they have such serious defects would be wise to have the matter settled by a reliable test and to adjust their life plans accordingly (N. Rice and Doherty, 1982).

At the same time, the right of persons to make decisions about reproducing genetic defects should be respected both by the Church and by society, and they should not be stigmatized because of their decision. The reasons are these:

1. The balance of factors cannot be reduced to objective certitude, especially because weighing of personal needs and capacities is involved.

2. The value of personal responsibility in the use of sex and living of family life greatly outweigh the damage done society by the increased genetic load, which cannot be significantly lightened in the short run and about which insufficient information exists to lighten significantly in the long run.

3. If the parents prove mistaken in their decision, society can and should assume the responsibility for adequate care of the children, a burden that is not great compared to many other health problems.

Clearly, if society promotes adequate education about genetic hazards, in a population where the birthrate is low and falling, it is probable that negative voluntary eugenics will become a part of the general social pattern. Genetic counseling will promote this. Catholic genetic counseling will also promote it without encouraging abortion or neglecting the parents' freedom of decision, while actively promoting a more optimistic and life-affirming attitude toward the inevitable risks of parenthood.

CHAPTER 12

Psychotherapy and Behavior Modification

OVERVIEW

Many ethical issues surround the topic of mental health and the methods used to promote and restore it. In this chapter we discuss the concept of mental health, studying its physiological and psychic etiology (12.1). Then we consider the two main methods of restoring mental health, insight and action therapy (12.2), and the many ethical issues arising from these therapies (12.3). Behavior control is another form of human behavior modification that involves many ethical issues (12.4). Chemical dependency (12.5) and sexual dysfunction (12.6), combinations of mental and physiological impairment, are fittingly considered at the conclusion of this section, since the methods used to overcome these impairments are applications of insight and behavioral therapies.

12.1 THE CONCEPT OF MENTAL ILLNESS

In dealing with ethical problems in psychiatric medicine, a very special problem arises: What is the difference between mental illness and ordinary physical illness? Chapter 2 clarifies this point by presenting a four-dimensional model of human personality. In this model the *psychological* dimension is closely interrelated with the *physical* dimension but also clearly distinct from it, as well as from the ethical and spiritual dimensions. The failure in the history of medicine to make these distinctions has been a source of vast confusion, and this remains a source of current controversy (Brody and Engelhardt, 1980; Glymour and Stalker, 1983; Perl and Shelp, 1982).

Thus a group of antipsychiatry psychiatrists has made a strong, if exaggerated, case against the whole concept of mental illness and the medical model of psychiatry. The most eloquent is Szasz (see also Laing, 1976; Torrey, 1972). In books such as *The Myth of Mental Illness* (1961; 1974, 1987), Szasz has argued that the concept of mental illness is completely invalid and that the greater number of psychiatric illnesses are really social maladjustments between the behavior of a nonconformist individual and the demands of a social system. The cause of these maladjustments is found in the modern social system, which is unable to deal with individual differences. Szasz has even compared modern psychiatry and mental hospitals to the medieval religious Inquisition, that is, to an institution whose purpose supposedly was to enforce conformity of more highly individualized personalities to a rigid and oppressive social system through a cruel process of interrogation and torture. One group of psychiatrists call themselves "radicals" and see the whole mental health establishment as an instrument of oppression (Erwin, 1978; Haafhems et al., 1986).

Further evidence that these accusations are not without serious foundation is shown in the actions of some governments (Medvedev and Medvedev, 1971; Stover and Nightengale, 1985) that have confined dissidents to mental institutions under the pretext that anyone who criticized the regime must be insane. More recently, the American Psychiatric Association (APA) indicated that ethical problems can arise in treatment of patients by appointing a task force to study the use of seclusion and restraint in psychiatric therapy (APA, 1985).

The novel of Ken Kesey (and even more the movie based on it) *One Flew Over the Cuckoo's Nest* (1962) dramatized the way in which patients, even those self-committed to a mental institution, can be reduced to robotlike conformity by the "system." The tragedy of this story was that the "monster" Nurse Ratchett was in fact a dedicated, well-meaning, and highly professional person who quite unconsciously had become a manipulator of people. Clearly in such cases it is not the individuals who are sick, but a system that fits both patients and healthcare professionals into a mutually destructive gestalt.

This accusation is further strengthened by realization of the effect of the "total institution" on human beings (Goffman, 1962; Rothman, 1980), which indicates the dangers of a closed social system where people so live within a rigid set of man-made ideas and behaviors that they are cut off from contact with a reality beyond and different from their limited perception. This often leads to a distorted, *paranoid* way of perceiving and interpreting the world. The only omission in the analysis of Goffman is that not only an asylum, a prison, or a hospital can become a "total institution." Modern society itself, with its technological organization, its mass media of brainwashing, and its all-seeing surveillance, can act as a total institution, so that there is no escape except (as in Kesey's novel) to sail out to sea in a boat.

This problem climaxes in the current problem of penology (H. Schwartz et al., 1984; L. Schwartz, 1982). In former times, punishment was thought to be distinguishable from therapy. The legal system assumed that a crime, unless committed by persons so mentally disturbed that they did not know they were committing a wrong (i.e., a breach of law), was the responsibility of the agent. The proper way to deal with crime was by death, corporal punishment, or imprisonment. These were considered both as punishments and as *deterrents* to future crime by the criminal or others because fear of punishment would be an element in the rational calculation of anyone tempted to commit a crime.

In recent years, however, another theory that has gained increasing acceptance maintains that many or even most crimes should not be considered punishable facts for one of two reasons (Hull, 1983; Menninger, 1968):

1. The person is suffering from some psychological maladjustment whose roots are unconscious and uncontrollable.
2. The person has been led by social injustices and by acceleration in a subculture to follow a set of standards in judging what is right and wrong different from the laws of the dominant culture.

In such cases the person has not in fact committed any *ethical* wrong, and the proper means of social control is not punishment, but in the first case, treatment, and in the second, reeducation.

Consequently, in today's society the line between punishment and treatment has become questionable. Criminals are incarcerated not to make them fear future incarceration if they commit crimes again, but to cure them of mental illnesses and to educate them to conformity with accepted social standards of behavior, sometimes with little protection of their basic human rights (Many, 1980). On the other hand, the patients in mental institutions, even those who at first voluntarily accept confinement, come to believe that their condition is no different from that of prisoners, since they are subjected to treatment they do not understand and over which they can make no real choice.

Thus Richard M. Restak has argued in *Pre-Meditated Man* (1975) that most of the problems of bioethics are not really ethical in the ordinary sense, but *political,* that is, questions of power as to whose will concerning human behavior is to prevail. The line between normal behavior and abnormal behavior thus turns out to be only a question of who is deciding what *they* want *us* to do (Szasz, 1982).

This obliteration of distinctions is a social reality today and a very dangerous one. The warning should be heeded, but the outcries against the system should not be allowed to confuse the problem of medical care still more (Ingleby, 1980; Robitscher, 1980). First, it is necessary to hold firmly to the fact that a form of human behavior that is dysfunctional and caused by organic and physiological defects does exist (Kaufman, 1985; Snyder, 1973). Lesions of the central nervous system, as well as a wide variety of physiological disorders, can make it difficult or impossible for human beings to sense and perceive the world correctly, to live in a state of emotional balance and sensitivity, to think clearly, and to make decisions free from uncontrollable impulses. Moreover, increasing evidence suggests that there may be a genetic basis for some mental illnesses, particularly for schizophrenia and manic-depressive psychosis (Kegley, 1985). However, the tendency to consider genetic causes as the source of all mental illness must be resisted (Lewontia et al., 1984).

The problem here, of course, is not that these physical disabilities (except in the most severe cases) automatically lead to highly abnormal behavior. Rather, it is a matter of tension between the innate capacities of the individual and the demands of the environment. For example, a patient with a respiratory disorder may be relatively comfortable under some atmospheric conditions and intensely uncomfortable under others that would not greatly distress a normal person. This disparity may also prevail among people with an inadequate or impaired capacity to adjust to certain environmental and social stresses. Clearly this suggests that the mental health of a society is to be achieved not only by treatment of the individual, but also by political and social readjustment of the environment to more adaptive lifestyles. It would seem that modern society should have the social control to tolerate varied human capacities.

Recognition of this fact has led recently to the policy (made possible by the use of psychotherapeutic drugs and under the pressure of economic considerations) of sending as many patients as possible back into the community, supported by outpatient treatment. Although this policy is basically sound, it has sometimes been abused, thus leading to serious neglect and further social disorders (Marcos and Cohen, 1986).

The general conclusion, therefore, is that a large number of people in society require psychiatric care that is impossible without hospitalization. Extreme caution must be taken within practical limits to protect the human rights of the patient, especially regarding both voluntary and involuntary commitments and retention, the right of treatment during the patient's stay (Rubenstein, 1983) and even the right to refuse some forms of treatment (Casswell, 1986).

Thus psychiatric care must include an effort to help patients develop skills to cope with the social situation in which they must live after leaving the hospital, a situation they ordinarily cannot alter much. The patient's family must share in this process to assist in the patient's reentry into normal living, or a halfway house should be available to facilitate this difficult transition. It is essential, moreover, that Christians recognize and respond to the need for a profound social transformation of culture so that it will be able to meet the needs of so-called deviants who are precisely the "little ones" to whom Jesus went out.

A mental disorder with apparently no organic defect or only a secondary one might be more accurately called a *mental illness* or *emotional disturbance*. Here it does seem misleading to continue to use a medical model if this means the same model as is used for organic diseases (Sider, 1983). Psychotherapy as such is a different form of therapy than that used for physical disease. To treat patients by talking with them or guiding them in recalling and reenacting past experiences is very different from treating them with drugs.

Mental illness, therefore, in the strict and proper sense, results from faulty development and use of human cognitive and affective capacities (Culver and Gert, 1982). Physical and physiological impairments may contribute to this faulty development and function because they inhibit the adaptive capacity of the person (Sider, 1983).

Thus psychotherapy is sometimes more similar to education or reeducation than to the medical model of treatment (Ursano and Silberman, 1988), if "education" means not the mere acquisition of information but rather the learner's own growth toward self-understanding and control, which the therapist facilitates but does not originate. Psychotherapy is based on the assumption that the mentally disturbed person has at least some capacities for normal mental life, but that these capacities have not been properly developed, are malfunctioning, or are being poorly used. In other words, the mentally sick person has the capacity to cope with life situations satisfactorily, but he or she has not learned how to use this capacity effectively or is inhibited from such use by abnormal fears and faulty perceptions of reality.

12.2   PSYCHOTHERAPEUTIC METHODS AND GOALS

Methods

There is, however, an important difference between psychotherapeutic or mental health education and other types of education. *Education,* in the usual sense as a function of an academic institution, is the development of human capacities at the rational or conscious level. Psychotherapy deals with psychic processes less conscious and less free than rational thought, just as education at the spiritual level deals with psychic processes that transcend the level of discursive rational thought. Physical education as such deals with the training of processes that are physiological rather than psychic.

At present, there is a plethora of psychotherapeutic methods (Petrila, 1986; Ursano and Silberman, 1988), but two very different conceptions of human psychological development are reflected in the two main current schools of psychotherapy. Perry London, in *Behavior Control* (1969), calls these "insight therapy" and "action therapy." In practice these therapies overlap, but they have different theoretical and clinical sources. The *insight therapies* derive largely from Freud and the psychoanalytical school, although they have now moved on to include a great variety of therapeutic methods other than psychoanalysis, especially to include the social group aspect of behavioral disorders (Engel, 1981). What characterizes these therapies is that they aim at helping individuals *understand* ("have insight into," "get in touch with") their own behavior and its affective sources and thus learn how to deal with life situations in an effective way. It is assumed that mental disorder means simply that (1) patients lack this insight or the skill to deal with their emotions and interpersonal relations; or (2) as with the obsessive person, they have much insight and little skill; or (3) as with the psychopathic person, they have much skill and little insight because during the course of their psychosocial development they have been traumatized or wrongly guided. Thus psychotherapy of this type deals with lack of coordination between the rational level (and in the case of the therapy of Jung et al. [1964], perhaps also with the spiritual level; Arraj and Arraj, 1984) and the psychological level of the personality. Normal persons have this coordination between rational and subrational processes, whereas neurotic or psychotic persons do not.

On the other hand, *action therapy* is the outcome of the behaviorist school of psychology, which rejects or bypasses the whole notion of the subconscious because it does not consider the notion of consciousness to be of any great help in psychological theory (Agras and Berkowitz, 1988). Even those who do not go to these theoretical extremes understand human behavior in terms of *operant conditioning.* Human beings behave as they do because they live in a physical and social environment that has educated them to behave in a certain way. This education consists in an ordered series of rewards and punishments (positive and negative reinforcements) that favor some forms of behavior and eliminate others.

In such a view, mental illness is behavior that is unacceptable to society and that also may be internally so self-inconsistent as to cause painful conflict in the organism. Action therapy, therefore, is a process of reconditioning the person to a more self-consistent and socially acceptable type of behavior. Its methods do not depend on growth in insight from subjects, who need not know how their malconditioning has arisen or even how the therapy works; these methods are aimed simply at removing undesirable behavior patterns and developing new ones.

It should be noted, however, that action therapies include not only reeducation by means of external rewards and punishments (e.g., by administering painful electric shocks), but also extend to reeducation of the person's fantasy life by desensitization, as when a patient overcomes a phobia by imagining painful situations and gradually comes to feel less anxious about them. Thus methods that rely on suggestion are considered action therapy, although they may appear similar to methods in insight therapy.

The controversy between these two points of view still continues and is often obscured by bitter polemics, but it probably reflects two aspects of human psychology that are not necessarily contradictory. Action therapy reflects the fact that human behavior, which at first may be conscious and deliberate, quickly takes on a pattern and becomes automatic and subconscious. Thus, when a person is learning to drive a car or play the piano, each motion is conscious and deliberate, but once the habit is acquired, these actions can be performed without conscious attention. This applies also to motivation, because in general it is easier and more pleasant to perform in a habitual manner and more difficult and even painful to go against a habit or routine response. The advantage of such automatization of behavior is obvious; it frees one's attention from the details of routine behavior and permits concentration on decisions about new or unusual situations, problems to be solved, and new skills to be acquired. Without this capacity to form habits, a person's energies would be wasted on the routine acts rather than concentrated on the adaptive and creative ones.

Furthermore, in psychosocial development the formation of such habits in the child precedes the time when the human person is mature enough to have full self-consciousness and control. No wonder, then, that children who have been badly trained by their social environment arrive at the stage of self-control with many faulty, and perhaps disastrously restricted or inconsistent and conflictual, patterns of behavior whose origin and even existence they do not understand. These may even lie in the unconscious part of the psyche. Thus children may have developed irrational fears by associating fear reactions with harmless stimuli, but they no longer understand why they are afraid.

The action therapies, based on a highly developed theory of learning through conditioning, seek to reeducate the patient by extinguishing undesirable patterns of behavior and establishing or strengthening desirable ones. Included are not only external behaviors, but also undesirable emotional reactions, especially the hampering and disorganizing type of fear called *neurotic anxiety*.

The insight therapies agree that the human being has many automatisms and that aberrant adult behavior is basically caused by faulty conditioning in early childhood, when the organism is highly impressionable and the power of the ego to resist environmental influences is low. The emphasis of insight therapies, however, is on the emergence of the ego or self as controlling behavior in an adaptive manner in the face of the natural and social environments. Consequently, if the therapist simply corrects faulty habits in the client, this only treats the symptoms. The real problem is to help patients develop a strong ego and to understand how they came to have faulty habits so they will be able under their own choice to form better ones. Thus it requires at least some measure of exploration of the past and a growing insight into one's own personality structure (Kolb and Bradie, 1982).

Apparently, therefore, the two therapies can complement each other (Karasu, 1982). In fact, the latest behavioral theories go beyond Skinner and postulate an interaction between environment, behavior, and cognition processes to explain human behavior (Bandura, 1986). Moreover, clients who have acquired insight into their own behavior and unconscious motivation may still need to be taught how to recondition themselves and to be aided by others in so doing. Freud and the psychoanalytical school too quickly assumed that a person who understands why he or she acts irrationally will then spontaneously be free to act rationally. This failed to take into account that psychological restructuring in the form of breaking old habits and forming new ones is a complex task. In this case learning theory is extremely important. On the other hand, the goals of action therapy seem too limited because they are based on a narrow, behavioristic conception of human life. Such learning theories have been developed from animal experimentation and have proved themselves most practical in dealing with subnormal intelligences, just as insight therapies are most successful with highly intelligent, verbal, and creative personalities. Learning good habits is not all there is to having an integrated personality. It is also necessary to develop an autonomous ego.

Thus, insofar as it is distinct from medical therapy, psychotherapy is not so much a process of healing a defective organic structure, as of reeducation, not at the level of fully rational behavior, but at the level of automatic, conditioned, or subconscious behavior. Its purpose is to free the individual from undesirable patterns of behavior, especially those that are inconsistent, so that rational free life becomes more possible.

Goals

This definition, however, raises a serious question: What is "normal" behavior when mental health is concerned (Clements, 1983; Sider, 1983)? The action therapist Joseph Wolpe (1966) quotes R.P. Knight (1966) with approval, saying that the criteria of successful psychotherapy of any type can be summarized as follows:

1. Relief of undesirable symptoms (e.g., excessive anxiety)
2. Increased productivity in the person's work
3. Adjustment and satisfaction in sexual relations
4. Better interpersonal relations

5. Increased ability to endure the stresses of life

Robert Harper (1959), after surveying the bewildering array of therapies then current (the situation has not much altered since that time; see Petrila, 1986), concludes that most therapies have to settle for the following results to consider themselves successful:

1. The weak ego of the patient is supported by the stronger ego of the therapist.
2. The lack of realism of the patient is corrected by the more realistic attitude of the therapist.
3. The patient learns to see that many things he fears are not so terrible.
4. The patient learns to be more patient in solving problems, less impulsive and panicky.
5. The patient acquires a greater or new faith or "life-myth" from the example of the therapist, who represents a hope for health.
6. The patient gets a more objective perspective on his or her problems from discussing them with the therapist or therapy group.
7. The patient focuses his or her floating anxieties on the outcome of the therapy process, so that he or she feels less isolated and helpless.

At present, psychotherapeutic methods do not have a clear record of effectiveness (Wilkinson et al., 1986). Psychoanalytical methods are extremely time-consuming and expensive. The action therapists have argued that the insight therapists have very little objective proof that their methods succeed better than natural processes; furthermore, the success they have seems largely independent of the mode of therapy and mainly dependent on the personal relation with a therapist who is a sensitive, realistic, and caring person.

The action therapists claim to have a better and more demonstrable record of success, but on examination this success mainly appears in rather restricted areas of neuroses, and its permanence is often questioned. Furthermore, action therapy fails to achieve the ultimate aim of developing a strong autonomy in the patient. At present, it must be concluded that this type of problem is very complex and knowledge about it and ability to cure it still very limited. Nevertheless, therapy undoubtedly is sometimes successful. Perhaps this is not so different from any other area of medical care, or of ethical and spiritual guidance. It can never be stressed too much that all modes of therapy are only of service to facilitate the inherent power of human beings as organisms and persons to heal themselves.

Clearly, the goals listed by Wolpe and Harper are rather modest. Other therapists speak in terms of "the mature personality." These terms, however, as well as the popular "autonomous person," are ambiguous (Edwards, 1981). If *mature personality* means that therapy extends to total development of the human person—that is, to the development of what once was called "the virtuous man," who is morally excellent and also spiritually profound and creative—this clearly goes beyond the psychological level and encroaches on the ethical and spiritual level. It is true that some therapists, particularly those of the Jungian and existentialist schools (Rollo May, 1983), have come to be not only therapists in the usual sense, but also something similar to gurus or spiritual guides. Their work more closely resembles that of a philosopher, educator, or spiritual director than that of a healthcare professional. Although not denying the great value of the work of some of these persons, it seems that some limit must be put on the task of psychotherapy. Its work is complete when the person becomes psychologically normal (i.e., in a state of normal adult health). After this form of normality is attained, the individual should achieve even more growth throughout the whole of human life; however, guidance of this growth seems to exceed the work of psychotherapy and to demand ethical and spiritual counselors.

How, then, can this line be drawn? A look at the insight therapies provides the answer. Psychoanalysis, for example, is terminated when patients are sufficiently *free* to manage their own lives realistically, independent of the therapist, and are no longer hampered by unconscious motivations or self-deluding excuses that would prevent them from perceiving the world as it is; they can make free choices and carry them out effectively (Menninger, 1958). In short, the patient now has a self-determining ego, which realistically recognizes its own emotional complexity, its innate needs, and its limitations. It also realistically recognizes the practical and human situations of life to which it must accommodate itself to satisfy its needs. This does not mean that all clients who terminate therapy will live their lives well in an ethical sense. A psychologically healthy person can, theoretically at least, also be an ethically bad person and a spiritually undeveloped person, but this is caused by his or her own free choices, not from compulsions imposed by personal background or social situation. At the point when the client can live by free choice, he or she no longer needs the therapist or therapy. Of course, a client may later regress under new stresses and have to return to treatment.

This notion of autonomy or freedom as defining the term *therapy* is not so acceptable to action therapists. Influenced by behaviorism, they often reject the notion of freedom altogether. Thus B.F. Skinner and his followers carry on systematic war against the whole notion of human free will (Skinner, 1971, 1976, 1985). As many critics (Gaylin, 1973; Machan, 1974) have pointed out, however, Skinner and other behaviorists unconsciously contradict themselves. They assert that the therapist can assist the client to behave more realistically, that is, as the therapist behaves. This makes sense if the therapist is *free* to choose between alternative modes of behavior for himself or herself and for the client, whereas the client, although still *not* yet free, wants to become free. This makes no sense, however, if both are equally unfree and merely conditioned by their environment (as Skinner's theory asserts).

Therefore even extreme behavioristic therapy really aims at freeing the patient (Dworkin, 1976). It does not merely substitute one determinism for another. Rather, it substitutes a type of determinism that is instrumentally consistent with self-determination at a higher level for a type of determinism (neurosis) that is incompatible with such self-determination. Thus skill in typing is a conditioning consistent with the freedom of the writer to create an original composition and is preferable to a neurotic compulsion to repeat a fixed pattern of words, which would be incompatible with creative writing.

Therefore mental health is psychological freedom based on a realistic perception and understanding of the world, and it involves self-understanding, self-consistency, and self-control. By *self-control*, however, we mean a *realistic* self-control, that is, one based on a realistic recognition and practical provision for one's intrinsic needs as a human being. *Mental health must be considered before the ethical questions of moral right and wrong, since only when a person is free can there be a question of moral choice and moral responsibility.*

In view of the multidimensional and integral character of human personality, however, it is important to emphasize that no human being is totally free. Human freedom is limited (1) by innate biological structure, determined genetically, and by various accidents of development, with its innate needs or drives; (2) by unconscious conditioning of the sort already described and that therapy deals with; and (3) by one's knowledge of the world and self, set largely by the culture in which one lives, and the scope of one's experiences and education. Psychotherapy deals principally, but not exclusively, with limitations of human freedom that arise from the level of unconscious conditioning (Holt, 1980).

It is best to conceive this limited freedom in terms of the *area* in which a given individual is free. Thus studies on members of extremist groups such as the Ku Klux Klan began with the assumption that racists are people of authoritarian personality type. To the surprise of the researchers, it turned out that these people, who appear to be imprisoned by political views that approach a paranoid view of reality, were on the average perfectly normal from a psychological perspective. Perhaps determinism here was more at the level of socialization rather than of unconscious conditioning and can be corrected only by ethical education, not by psychotherapy.

At the psychological level, the area of freedom is very limited in the psychotic person who is out of touch with reality. Most psychotic persons, however, probably have some areas of freedom, at least sometimes; this is why they can be reached by psychotherapy or chemotherapy (as the case may be), which aims to gradually extend these free areas. Neurotic persons are decidedly more free but have some areas of unfreedom that do not occur in normal persons. The normal person also has a limited area of freedom, but its limits lie near the level of the necessary determinisms of automatic and routine behavior that are compatible with normal freedom.

Also, the areas of freedom among normal individuals undoubtedly differ widely. Highly creative and adaptive persons have much greater freedom in their lifestyle than normal, but limited, unimaginative, rigid people who operate best only in routine situations. Even here there is a question of whether therapy (e.g., of the Jungian type) may lead such people to greater freedom. Modern therapy has tended to move from the treatment of sexual neuroses, common as a result of the Victorian refusal to recognize basic biological needs, to the treatment of anxiety, common in this century as a result of excessive demands on a work-oriented society, which fails to recognize human needs for leisure and human intimacy (Masters and Johnson, 1976; Masters et al., 1986). Thus therapy deals more and more with neuroses of emptiness or lack of meaning as a result of society's failure to recognize the creative and spiritual sides of personhood. In all these cases, psychological therapy can only go so far to awaken the person's full capacity for freedom.

Freedom demands not only trust between persons but also within social groups. Recently, more and more methods of *group* therapy are becoming common, not only because of the shortage of therapists but because mental illness is partly a disturbance of social relations and can be adequately treated only through learning social communication skills. In particular, family therapy, in which a family is treated as a dynamic system whose malfunction is reflected in the psychological problems of individual members, gives promise of a radically effective approach to many mental problems that originated in the family.

Such methods raise some special ethical issues, chiefly those of confidentiality and of adequate professional control. The frank communication required within the group can easily lead to an abuse of the privacy of individual members; if the therapist does not remain fully in charge and sufficiently sensitive to the needs of every member, some especially fragile participants may be more hurt than healed by the experience (Schmid et al., 1983). The therapist has the responsibility not to permit the psychological condition of any member of the group to be destabilized to a degree that the therapist is not willing or not able to see that it is worked out before the process is terminated, even if this means additional one-to-one sessions with the disturbed patient or at least proper referral for further therapy.

12.3 ETHICAL PROBLEMS OF PSYCHOTHERAPY

Punishment

On the basis of the distinctions just made, the first point about the ethics of psychotherapy is to reject any use of psychotherapy as *punishment* (although it must be admitted that the neurotic patient may at first perceive it as punishment no matter what the therapist intends). Punishment and reward (in the proper sense of the terms) belong only to *ethical* acts, that is, free, responsible acts. This, of course, requires penological reforms by which the courts decide first on the facts of a criminal action and then separately on the *moral* responsibility of the person who has committed the act. In this second decision, expert testimony from psychiatrists should be admitted, but it should be directed toward determining whether the defendant's freedom was so limited by psychological factors as to remove his or her freedom with regard to this particular class of acts. This expert testimony should be fully subject to the adversary process so that the lay jury can determine whether there are solid grounds to doubt the freedom of the defendant (Berlin, 1983; Fingarette and Hasse, 1979).

Therefore psychiatrists called on in court for expert testimony, insofar as the present confusion of the law permits them (Bedau, 1980), should be primarily concerned to make clear to the jury why in their expert opinion the chronic or temporary psychological condition of the accused person did or did not render him or her so unfree that the accused cannot be held responsible for the act he or she is accused of; or if the accused is partially or remotely responsible for the act, then in what degree or in what respect (Halleck, 1984). Also, when a defendant is acquitted on the basis of lack of responsibility, then the court, in an entirely different process, should decide the question of involuntary commitment for treatment or of confinement to prevent the person from harming himself or herself or others. Such confinement, however, should not be dealt with as if it were punishment, since it would be unjust to punish someone for acts for which he or she was not responsible.

The question then arises whether psychiatrists should play any role in the process of punishment itself (Fersch, 1979; Monahan, 1980). It seems that their role should be limited to two functions.

1. Psychiatrists could diagnose prison inmates who develop mental illnesses and require occasional treatment exactly on the same basis as for medical ills. Ideally, if inmates require hospitalization for either medical or mental health reasons, they should receive it outside the prison; such time should not count for the fulfillment of their term of punishment.

2. Psychiatrists could act as consultants to penologists in setting up prison routines that make for good mental health and discipline, but they should not be engaged in staffing these services (Tancredi, 1983).

At present, much controversy surrounds proposals to rehabilitate prisoners by behavior control programs, which in effect are action therapies designed to recondition the criminal to social behavior by a planned series of rewards and punishment (S. Axelrod and Apsche, 1983; Pincus, 1984). This can be conceived in three ways: (1) as voluntary education, in which case it is certainly ethical to give prisoners an opportunity to engage in it as they would in any type of socially acceptable education program; (2) as therapy; and (3) as part of prison discipline. In the last case, it is part of the prisoner's punishment and should have some supervision from the courts, which should not permit cruel and unusual punishment, that is, something other than prescribed by law as appropriate to the crime. As therapy that the prisoner must undergo involuntarily, it should not be permitted without a court order committing the prisoner to such therapy.

In actual practice today, these matters are greatly confused. The psychiatric profession, however, has a responsibility to clear them up and to refuse cooperation with gross violations of the distinction between therapy and punishment, just as physicians have refused to act as executioners by administering capital punishment by lethal injections (W. Curran and Cassells, 1980; Malone, 1979). This is even more true if therapy is used as a means of suppression of political or social dissent, which amounts to a punishment for political crimes (Aviram and Schnit, 1984).

Granted that therapy has been carefully distinguished from punishment (which is no part of the therapeutic profession), what of the problem of the patient's informed consent? In this case, as in other medical questions, the patient's free and informed consent clearly is required if he or she is capable of such consent, for reasons already made clear in 3.4. The special problem is that mentally disturbed patients (1) may be unable to understand the purposes or risks of the treatment and (2) may not be truly free to make a decision when they refuse treatment. Some ethicists, basing their opinion on the principle of autonomy, would require that the therapy be withheld if there is no informed consent (Engelhardt, 1982). We would agree with Clements (1983), however, who maintains: "Since the life sciences have norms of functioning, there is in fact an alternative ethical system to the patient autonomy system. This alternative gives a philosophically respectable basis for ethically choosing patient good or best interest over patient choice."

Therapists should not assume, however, that patients who initially refuse treatment have no freedom. Every effort should be made to assist patients to arrive at a truly free decision if there is some hope that this can be achieved by giving them time to think it over, become calm, work through their fears, or discuss the matter with others. Any kind of therapy is much more likely to be successful and is at much less risk of traumatizing side effects if patients enter it voluntarily. Consequently, healthcare professionals have the responsibility to take the time and make the effort to permit patients to make their own free decisions if possible. If patients freely decide *against* therapy, it should not be given, and if at any time during treatment they freely withdraw consent, therapy should not be continued (Perl and Shelp, 1982).

Risks

Patients self-committed to a hospital may find themselves in a situation where in fact freedom to withdraw from highly traumatizing treatment is no longer practically possible. Every psychiatric institution, however, must be dedicated to the proposition that it is therapeutic only to the degree that it really respects and seeks to enlarge the patient's capacity for freedom. If it lessens this capacity, it is countertherapeutic; it is making the patient ill rather than well.

On the other hand, when it is rightly judged that free consent, at least in the area of treatment, is impossible, then commitment must be made by the patient's guardian, with scrupulous observance of due legal process. The guardian (usually a member of the family) may be biased, either because of selfishness, ignorance, and more often through unconscious factors, which may very well be part of the client's own breakdown (Pleak and Applebaum, 1984).

If the treatment is carried out without the patient's consent, a primary objective of this treatment must be to bring the patient as soon as possible to the level of mental integration, where at least some self-determination becomes feasible. This means that the use of drugs or psychosurgery simply as a method of controlling patients or tranquilizing them cannot of itself be a legitimate therapeutic objective. Undoubtedly, those who have to care for patients who are out of control are strongly tempted to pacify them so they "don't make trouble." This is permissible to defend the patient against harming himself or herself, the therapist, or others, but such self-defense is not *therapy;* it is only preliminary to therapy. Unfortunately, some mental hospitals have become hardly more than custodial facilities (Rothman, 1980). It is for this reason that recently a number of patients or guardians have successfully brought lawsuits based on the right to treatment (Applebaum, 1982). It is essential, however, that in such matters the courts require genuine therapy and not merely more tranquilization.

Is merely custodial care ever permissible? It must be granted that in some cases no therapy proves beneficial and no responsibility in justice exists to give more than ordinary care to the patient. This state of affairs, however, should be more reluctantly admitted in the case of mental illness than of organic illness, since mentally ill patients remain conscious and probably retain some minimal freedom. Consequently, they still need human communication and interaction, as well as spiritual care.

Even extremely psychotic patients who have only minimal freedom seemingly are still capable of treatment through active therapies. Although they are not free, they still can learn. Thus it is possible to replace more destructive patterns of behavior with those that are more constructive and more compatible with freedom. Again, the aim here must not be primarily to control patients so as to make them less troublesome, since in the process such patients might become more bottled up or their rigid behavior might increase. The aim must be to prepare the way for freedom.

For patients whose psychosis is less all-embracing and for neurotic patients, not only action therapies but also the insight therapies are feasible. The use of insight therapies, however, raises a whole series of ethical problems (APA, 1981; R. Moore, 1978).

The first of these is the process of *transference* (Marmer, 1988; Menninger, 1958). Psychodynamic therapy depends in some measure or other on a patient's becoming dependent on the therapist for the duration of treatment. This dependency mirrors the child-parent relationship and involves not only trust but, at least sometimes, also an element of erotic love. Without this profound dependency, patients are not freed from their anxieties and inhibitions sufficiently to let themselves become conscious of their true motivations. The termination of therapy is marked by a patient's having become sufficiently autonomous and under self-control that he or she no longer needs the therapist. As with matured human beings, such patients may still love their parents but do not need them.

This vulnerability of patients obviously invests the therapist with special ethical responsibilities. The first of these is that therapists must not violate the trust placed in them (Schmid et al., 1983). This requires that a therapist carefully maintain professional secrecy, be truly concerned for the patient, prompt in appointments, and reasonably available for consultation. It means also that therapists are honest with patients and do not lie to them or break promises. Furthermore, the therapist must avoid all manipulation of the patient in the sense of seeking personal gratification from the treatment rather than seeking the patient's benefit. This does not demand that the therapist have a superhuman objectivity; rather, it simply means that the therapist is worthy of trust.

Clearly, this excludes the therapist from having sexual relations with the client (although some have defended this as possibly therapeutic; see Gartrell, 1986). The idea that the therapist could engage in such relations merely for the patient's sake seems unrealistic, and the risk that the patient will then or later view it as exploitation is all too real. The Principles of Ethics adapted by the APA are clear in specifying that sexual relations between psychiatrists and their patients are unethical (section 2.1) (APA, 1981, 1986a, b).

Some have raised the question as to whether it is permissible for patients to enter into therapy if they risk falling in love with the therapist. It should be emphasized that the danger here seems no greater (and perhaps more consciously avoided) than the danger of the patient's falling in love with his or her medical doctor. The relationship is rather that of parent to child than of lover to lover, and its excessive erotic investment is the mark of the illness from which the patient is already suffering rather than its consequences. This risk seems no greater than the patient's coming to hate the therapist and seek to harm him or her, as has sometimes happened.

A second issue sometimes raised by Catholics is whether the process of *abreaction* is not dangerous, since the patient in free fantasy revives the memory of former temptations or sins, of illicit sexual activity, or of hostility and destruction. Is it legitimate to again put oneself in the "occasion of sin" where sinful consent is possible? Similarly, some object to the process of abreaction, especially in the case of nondirective therapy, because the therapist may permit the patient to engage in objectively wrong actions. Such dangers may occur in therapy, but they are usually the result of poor therapy. The purpose of psychoanalytical abreaction is precisely to return to some sin or mistake of the past where the patient failed to resolve a problem correctly and to help the patient now face it in a clearer light. It is not likely that patients engaged in the therapeutic process will actually consent to what they consciously reject just because their rejection now becomes fully conscious. Also, good therapists do not encourage their patients to act out their neuroses (Ornstein and Kay, 1983). Even in psychodrama or venting of feelings, the reenactment is precisely a dramatic one, that is, a "make-believe" in which it is essential to the therapeutic process that it *not* be a real, freely willed activity. If the patient acts out a neurosis, it is generally recognized that this reinforces the neurosis rather than liberates the patient from it.

Value Systems

Perhaps the most controversial issue of psychotherapy is whether the therapist is permitted to change the patient's value system (Block and Chodoff, 1981; Rokeach, 1973). The common answer is that a therapist should not change this system but should try to adjust the patient to the system. This answer, however, is somewhat disingenuous. As the existentialist psychoanalysts have pointed out, distortions in the patient's value system often underlie the disorder. Furthermore, the source of many problems is the patient's superego, which is partly the value system of the parents or society that has been incorporated in the child's unconsciousness. Here is the source of all the issues raised by the antipsychiatrists. Is therapy simply the adjustment of patients to the disordered value system of the society in which they live?

On the other hand, if the psychological and ethical dimensions of human personality are distinct, as we have argued, it clearly cannot be the role of the therapist to indoctrinate the patient in a value system.

In answer to this difficulty, we must say that there are certain values on which the very relation of client to therapist depend, and these must be reinforced by therapy (Clements, 1983). Thus, the therapist must help the client to become more trustful, more honest, more hopeful, more courageous, more patient, and more realistic. Such values are common to most recognized ethical systems, whether religious or philosophical. The therapist must adhere to these values and should not be reluctant to strengthen them in the client. If clients submit voluntarily to therapy, they *freely* accept these values no matter how unfree they may be in other respects. This is the small area of mental health and moral virtue that must become the basis of recovery. Therapists teach these values primarily by their *example* in their relations to clients as they attempt to establish satisfactory therapeutic transferences. Consequently, the importance of a genuinely personalist education for psychiatrists is even more important than for other physicians (Light, 1980; see also 4.3).

The effort of the therapist is thus to extend the area of freedom for patients. As patients become freer, they must make some free ethical decisions and will do so according to their own *conscious*, rational system of values. At this point, the therapist is nondirective in the sense that it is not the therapist's task to give the patient ethical advice, but only to help the patient be free of illusion and neurosis in making decisions. This requires great delicacy and objectivity on the part of the therapist. It may mean the therapist sometimes thinks that the client's decisions are not ethically good, objectively speaking. In such a case, the therapist may point out that the client's decisions are questionable or refer the client to an ethical counselor (clergyman, lawyer, friend), but the therapist should be careful not to take any responsibility for the client's decision. Thus the therapist ought to refer the client to ethical or spiritual advisers if it becomes apparent that the client's value system is inconsistent or inadequate.

A deeper problem, however, is raised by Philip Rieff (1968) in his book *The Triumph of the Therapeutic* and by others. Is it possible that the whole system of insight therapy as it originated with Freud has a built-in system of values or ideology that it inculcates? Thus many have accused psychoanalysis of being essentially a product of the middle class in opulent capitalist countries. They argue that it has taken on the political function of adjusting this middle class to a social system riddled with inherent contradictions. Freud (1930) himself saw all of civilization as the imposition of social controls on human beings' infinite and even contradictory drives. Consequently, every social system is a delicate balance between the repressive controls necessary for social life and work and the explosive drives of the id. In capitalist countries, as Rieff shows, the abundance of goods and the impersonal shape of social organization contribute to a much greater permissiveness, a society in which all types of behavior (between "consenting adults") is tolerable. Others, such as the proponents of radical sexual therapies, argue that as this permissiveness spreads, it will lead to social revolution.

Rieff predicts that we are embarking on a "therapeutic society" in which the "therapeutic man" will become typical. Such a person, whom Rieff pictures as the type successful psychoanalysis actually produces, is one who lives for a constant succession of intensely satisfying experiences, without any drive to realize some plan of life or some ultimate goal. This person is highly autonomous in the sense that he or she feels no guilt about seeking personal satisfaction in every situation, leaving the others involved to take care of themselves. This person is capable of satisfying intimate relationships but does not depend on any particular person for achieving these; thus he or she can move from one relationship to another without any sense of loss or guilt for infidelity.

If Rieff is correct, and certainly very different interpretations of the goals of psychoanalysis are given by Erik Erickson (1968), Erich Fromm (1975), Rollo May (1983), and others, the inherent ethic of psychoanalytical theory is to produce autonomous, hedonistic, goalless, conscienceless persons—the very sort ethicists have always condemned as selfish, loveless, and empty. Such persons are individualistic in the extreme, uncommitted to any social goals except the achievement of freedom to do what they please. Rieff's interpretation of psychoanalysis emphasizes Freud's belief that civilization, that is, social life, is always repression, not fulfillment, of fundamental human needs—a necessary evil. If this is the whole picture, it is difficult to see how a Freudian ethics could ever be compatible with either a Christian value system or a Marxist one. It is essentially an ideological defense of the style of life of those who profit from capitalism and who use their analysts to quiet their guilt.

Recently, Alan Bloom, in *The Closing of the American Mind* (1987), described the present generation of college students in terms similar to those employed by Rieff. Dominated by relativism, Bloom finds his subjects highly self-centered and devoid of commitment to family, religion, or country. Although Bloom attributes the causes of this malaise to many different factors, he does maintain: "Once Americans had become convinced that there was a basement to which psychiatrists have the key, their orientation became that of the *self*, the mysterious, true, unlimited center of our being. All our beliefs issue from it and have no other validation."

These accusations offered by Rieff and Bloom are very serious ones. They demand that:

1. The community of therapists must make a serious examination of social conscience and a purification of the theory, training, and practice of therapists, who must become conscious that the goals of therapy must be related to higher social and spiritual goals.

2. Clients should trust their therapists not as omnipotent fathers, but only for their limited skill. Clients also should receive guidance at the ethical (political and social) and spiritual levels from others as soon as they become sufficiently free emotionally to do so (Van Kaam, 1986).

Thus persons undergoing therapy should not change their system of values, divorce their partners, give up their religious vocation, or change their religion or their professional vocation merely under the influence of psychotherapy. The tendency to erect one of the many forms of therapy (including the various mystical cults now so popular) into a religion is a violation of the lines between the psychological level of personality and the ethical and spiritual levels doomed to end in disillusionment.

In recent years, some of the Protestant and Catholic clergy and members of religious orders have discovered the value of psychotherapy and have come to place an excessive faith in it to meet all the needs of people for counseling, to the detriment of their confidence in the value of their own special roles as ethical and spiritual guides (Murnion, 1984). They have become preoccupied with getting in touch with their feelings, getting freed up, or developing a capacity for intimacy, and some have deserted the celibate life, the priesthood, or the ministry to become psychotherapists themselves so that they might "really" help people. A similar phenomenon has been experienced by the U.S. Jewish community, where psychotherapy has become a widespread substitute for the religious discipline of the Torah, the therapist has taken the place of the rabbi, and Freud the place of Moses.

Undoubtedly, religious people and the clergy in particular have sometimes been in real need of therapeutic experiences to correct an excessively repressive religiosity that disregarded their human emotional needs. Too often such persons have been discouraged from obtaining needed psychotherapy by the false notion that although morally good people may be physically ill, they cannot be mentally ill. Nevertheless, profound self-understanding and choice of one's life vocation require an exploration of the self that goes even deeper than psychology can penetrate and where ethical and spiritual guidance is of great value. What is needed are ethical and spiritual guides who genuinely appreciate the contributions of psychotherapy to human wholeness, but who pursue their own roles with a sense of their own mission. There is an important analogy between psychotherapy and spiritual purification, but it is an analogy, not an identity (Van Kaam, 1985).

It would be very unfair to blame either Freud or his disciples for these unfortunate consequences of an excessive faith in the power of psychotherapy in its present state of development. Freud's great contribution to understanding human behavior is established; a fruitful historical development has already taken place, building on his work and giving it greater balance. Current psychoanalytical theory is concerned with the social as well as the individualistic aspects of human personality and is contributing to other models of human maturity than that depicted by Rieff. Consequently, there is no reason to doubt that in the future psychoanalysis could help Christians to be more truly Christians, or Marxists to be more truly Marxists, by becoming freer to choose their own system of values and to interpret them in a way consistent with the facts of human experience.

12.4 BEHAVIOR CONTROL

In addition to the use of insight and action therapies, it is possible to alter human thought, feeling, and behavior by means of drugs, surgery, and psychological conditioning. All are considered forms of behavior control. Behavior control might be described as "getting people to do someone else's bidding." In this sense, behavior control has existed since the beginning of time. In the more restricted sense, however, the sense in which we use the term in this section, behavior control is any *medically indicated* treatment, procedure, or process that is intended, with or without a person's consent, to cause a person to discontinue a personally or socially undesirable activity (Agras and Berkowitz, 1988; Kerlanger,

1986). As this description indicates, behavior control is not necessarily contrary to a person's intention or desires, but it signifies that some force over and above internal human motivation has been used in the interest of changing an activity pattern. The purpose of this control may be therapeutic (e.g., the use of drugs can sometimes actually correct a physiological malfunction producing abnormal behavior), or it may simply be aimed at controlling antisocial actions (H. Clark, 1987).

For example, a person trying to overcome the habit of alcoholism may use Antabuse (disulfiram) to help conquer the habit. Although the use of this drug is in accord with this person's desire, it is still a form of behavior control. From an ethical point of view, behavior control has become a serious problem because of the increased efficacy of surgical procedures in controlling behavior, the vastly increased panoply of psychoactive drugs that modify emotional responses, and the increased tendency to impose conforming societal norms. These procedures are not only comparatively new; they are swift and efficient and their effect on a human person can be deep and lasting. Thus they have greater potential for good or evil than many of the techniques of scientists and physicians in the past centuries. Also, a temptation exists to attempt the solution of problems by altering the person rather than attempting to transform the social environment.

Three major forms of behavior control are prevalent today that are associated, either closely or remotely, with medical care. They are shock therapy and psychosurgery, psychoactive drugs, and psychological conditioning. After describing the three forms of behavior control associated with medical care, we present some ethical principles that may be applied to evaluate their use.

1. *Shock Therapy and Psychosurgery.* Since the 1930s, there have been experiments with many types of treatment of psychological dysfunctions by means of profound stress on the central nervous system through chemicals or electricity. Generally, this form of treatment is known as *electroconvulsive therapy,* and because of the undesirable side effects of some of these treatments, the only one generally retained is *electroshock.* Many therapists and therapeutic institutions reject electroshock, but it is still considered by others as worthwhile therapy (National Institutes of Health [NIH], 1985), especially for involutional depression, where it often has dramatic results in patients who otherwise require protracted hospitalization. Electroshock and other treatments have been justified on various theoretical grounds, but what is most certain is that these procedures produce temporarily a severe loss of memory and general state of psychic disorganization (Valenstein, 1980). Apparently this makes it possible for some patients to break out of fixed patterns of fantasy and feeling and to begin to respond in a more normal way (Abrams and Essman, 1982).

Psychosurgery is surgical destruction of certain parts of the brain for the purpose of treating psychiatric conditions. Arguments on the ethics and merits of psychosurgery vary from severe condemnation to considerable enthusiasm (Black and Szasz, 1977; Kleinig, 1985; Valenstein, 1986). The psychosurgery procedure that attracted the most attention was the *prefrontal lobotomy* performed in the

1930s and 1940s on people with severe psychotic disorders. This procedure, which in some cases could be performed under local anesthesia, consists essentially in severing the white nerve fibers that connect the frontal lobes of the brain with the thalamus. The result of this surgical procedure is a blunting of human emotional responses.

Because lobotomy is an irreversible and drastic procedure, it was performed only on persons with severe behavior problems such as acute aggression or severe despondency. Often the result of this procedure was an almost complete lack of emotional response by the patient. According to some experts, the emotional response could be restored to some degree, especially if proper treatment were given after the procedure. However, emotional responses would never be as strong nor as disturbing as before the surgery. Because of the dramatic effect of this form of behavior control, the procedure fell into disuse when psychoactive drugs became more effective for the treatment of severe psychosis. In recent years, psychosurgery has become once again more common throughout the world. Modern procedures using, for example, ultrasound, electrical coagulation, or implanted radium seeds, are more localized and less destructive. A more sophisticated form of controlling human activity, but one that can be classified as psychosurgery, is *electrical stimulation of the brain (ESB)*. This involves implanting electrodes in the human brain and controlling actions and responses by means of electrical stimuli. This form of behavior control was developed by Jose Delgado (1969; Schwitzgebel and Schwitzgebel, 1973).

Despite some indications that present-day psychosurgery is helpful for severely depressed patients and despite the potential use of ESB in helping people with organic brain disease, many scientists and physicians denounce all forms of psychosurgery (Carroll and O'Callaghan, 1984; Gostin, 1980). Chief among these critics is Peter Breggin (1972, 1979), a practicing psychiatrist whose scathing denunciation, based mainly on ethical considerations, was reprinted in the *Congressional Register* (March 30, 1972). Legislators became so involved in this medical-moral issue that two bills to prohibit psychosurgery, or limit it severely, were introduced in Congress. On the other hand, those who argue for the use of this form of therapy do so for the following reasons: (1) it has sometimes proved very successful in the treatment of patients with epilepsy or Parkinson's disease for whom drugs do not satisfactorily control the disorders; (2) it sometimes is the only remedy for intractable pain; and (3) it may be necessary in treatment of certain violent, uncontrollable seizures (some of which are epileptic), since otherwise the patients injure themselves or have to be confined in isolation.

2. *Psychoactive Drugs.* A drug is psychoactive when it has some psychological effect: alters thoughts, imagination, perception, or emotions; causes alertness, drowsiness, or feelings of anger; and so forth. Such drugs are also called *psychotropic,* and the study of these drugs is called psychopharmacology. Some psychotropic drugs have proved highly effective in psychotherapy in (1) tranquilizing patients in manic states or in uncontrollable anxiety; (2) reducing the condition of mental confusion and dissociation, especially in schizophrenia; and (3) lifting certain types of depression (J. Silver and Yadofsky, 1988). These effects may be

347

symptomatic, rather than truly curative, but at least they may hasten the natural recovery from an episode. Moreover, they may help return a person more quickly to a more normal way of life and thus prevent the regression that often results from prolonged institutionalization. Also, they make it possible to use other types of therapy. The fact that such remarkable results have been obtained by drugs strongly suggests that the physiological causes of mental illness are very important.

This raises the hope that as these underlying organic causes are understood, more successful therapies and preventives for mental illness can be developed. It is also clear, however, that drugs can never be the total answer to the problems of mental health, which also involve the factors of social environment and psychological development (Lewontia et al., 1984).

Some forms of psychoactive agents have been used since the beginning of civilization. Alcoholic beverages were invented at the same time as cereal agriculture. Opium in one form or another has been used as a pain reliever for centuries. Aspirin, the first of the wonder drugs, has been used for more than 100 years to treat pain and anxiety.

Extreme ethical concerns over the use of psychoactive drugs, however, did not develop until recently after several pharmacological compounds were developed or synthesized that alter mental and emotional functioning (Snyder, 1986). Some of these drugs which are readily available to the public at large, have demonstrated value to treat specific mental illness, but others such as lysergic acid diethylamide (LSD) are not associated with therapeutic use (W. Clark, 1985; Stevens, 1987). Given the wide range of known drugs, there seems to be one available to suppress or evoke any emotional state or symptom.

The extent to which psychoactive drugs are used in this society is itself an ethical concern (Klerman, 1981). Antipsychotic, antidepressant, and antianxiety drugs are used not only by people who are severely ill and unable to manage their emotions without medication, but also by relatively normal people attempting to control anxiety, tension, depression, insomnia, and other states arising from the stress of life in modern society (Martorano, 1982). Prescriptions for psychoactive drugs account for 20 percent of all prescriptions written in the United States. Studies made in the 1980s indicate that about 10 to 15 percent of adults use one form of psychoactive drug or another, and women are twice as likely as men to use these forms of behavior control (Baldessarini, 1985). In addition, many use nonprescription or over-the-counter drugs for relief of headache, backache, tension, insomnia, anxiety, and other "lesser" maladies of life. Much anxiety among parents has been caused by the controversy over the use of drugs in public schools to control hyperactive children. Although the psychotropic drugs available for behavior control at present comprise an impressive array, the potential for the future is even more awesome (Baldessarini, 1985). Klerman (1981) says, "As knowledge of the relationship between brain and behavior increases, it is likely we will develop knowledge of the neurochemical and neuropharmacological bases of memory, learning, mood, aggression, appetite, and sexual lust." Thus, not only must psychoactive drugs be evaluated as therapeutic agents, but also future ethical evaluation must consider their potential to improve capabilities and enhance personal pleasure and enjoyment of life (Schroeder, 1985).

    3. *Psychological Conditioning.* We have already discussed operant conditioning (12.2) as a mode of psychotherapy. It can also be used as a form of behavior control by medical personnel. In fact, Skinner (1971, 1976, 1985) argues that in the future it will replace all other forms of ethical education and social control. Here we need only point out two aspects of his proposal that have important ethical implications.

First, Skinner denies that human beings possess the power of choice of alternate modes of activity, since he is convinced his experiments have demonstrated that all human behavior is deterministically shaped from birth by environmental forces. According to Skinner, "Freedom and dignity are myths that are preventing us from seeing how continually and subtly we are being shaped by our environment."

Second, in the process of operant conditioning, Skinner asserts that no need exists to inform people their behavior is being changed. Moreover, changes in behavior can be determined for the masses by an elite group of managers. As Gaylin (1973) has pointed out, it is evident that Skinner assumes without question that his own humanist values will be inculcated. In other hands, of course, antihumanistic values might just as effectively be enforced (Lifton, 1982). For Skinner, all education is operant conditioning. As Häring (1975) observed, "Skinner seems absolutely unable to distinguish between manipulating persons and their minds and, on the other hand, engaging in genuine liberating dialogue. The categories of freely acquired convictions and respectful dialogue are totally absent in his technical manipulative world view."

Nevertheless, it may be reasonably argued that conditioning techniques may be preferable to the use of overt force when social control must be exercised over persons of defective intelligence who lack the capability of free choice or over those who incorrigibly resist necessary control (e.g., prisoners, violent mobs). Much more research is necessary, however, to determine the real effects of such methods (S. Axelrod and Apsche, 1983; Halleck, 1984).

Ethical Guidelines

Given these examples of behavior control and modification methods that are prevalent and becoming more common every day, we suggest several ethical principles that should govern their use, all of which are applications of the more general Principle of Human Dignity in Community (1.5, 8.2), which requires that social control enhance the dignity of the members of the community, not reduce them to mere means of political manipulation (Ingleby, 1980).

    1. No form of treatment may be used that will destroy human freedom. Pius XII (1952) stated this well when he wrote:

> In exercising his right to dispose of himself or his faculties and organs, the individual must observe the hierarchy of the scale of values and within an identical order of values the hierarchy of

349

individual goods to the extent demanded by the laws of morality, so, for example, man cannot perform upon himself or allow medical operations, either physical or somatic, which beyond doubt do remove serious defects or physical or psychic weaknesses, but which entail at the same time permanent destruction of or a considerable lasting lessening of freedom, that is to say, of the human personality in its particular and characteristic functions (n. 361).

Thus any form of psychosurgery, personality manipulation, and use of psychoactive drugs that would remove or severely limit human freedom or destroy human personality could not be permitted and may need legal control (Guydish and Kramer, 1982; NIH, 1985).

2. If the purpose of the behavior control is therapeutic, the benefit to the patient must be the purpose of the action and the damage or risk must be accidental to the therapeutic action. A frontal lobotomy, for example, should be performed only as a last resort and with some indication that there will be an overall benefit for the patient. Above all, lobotomy and ESB should not be considered as ordinary treatments for prisoners and others who have displayed antisocial behavior. As a general rule, signs of organic brain pathology should be present before psychosurgery is approved.

3. If the purpose of the treatment is therapeutic, the long-range effect of the treatment must be considered as well as the short-range alleviation of some particular difficulty. Simply because a particular therapy alleviates or eliminates a symptom does not mean that it is ethically acceptable. Most of the drugs currently available for the relief of anxiety and tension carry some danger of dependency, habituation, and addiction (Freedman, 1981; Lehmann, 1979). Such dependency diminishes human freedom and dignity and thus is to be avoided. Therefore the very theory prevalent in the United States of using psychoactive drugs to treat psychological difficulties when the disorder lacks a physiological or organic basis must be questioned. Would it not be better to treat the causes of anxiety or depression through counseling or increased self-awareness rather than to depend on pills, which merely treat the symptoms? Questions such as this are fundamental in developing a philosophy of healthcare, and they are too often neglected in search of easier, but less beneficial, solutions.

4. If behavior controls are used, the rules of free and informed consent apply, including the right to refuse treatment (Gallant, 1983; Gilbert, 1981; R. Levine, 1983). Thus operant conditioning, psychoactive drugs, and psychotherapy should not be inflicted on competent people or imposed on them (Annas, 1980; Turnquist, 1983). If they are incompetent, the norms for proxy consent for therapeutic treatment should be followed (Eth et al., 1984). Moreover, children, prisoners, and people with a limited sense of awareness should not be subjected to experimental behavioral control, nor should proxy consent be given unless the treatment is truly therapeutic for them (Sprague, 1978).

5. The Principle of Professional Communication (5.2) regarding confidentiality must be applied with special care in psychotherapy, since the trust of the patient in the therapist is of fundamental importance, even in group therapy or where peer review of the psychiatrist's performance is necessary (Arnstein, 1986; DeKraai and Sales, 1984; Schmid et al., 1983).

6. Experimental research on behavioral control should conform to the norms explained previously in the section on human experimentation (9.5).

7. Use of behavioral control procedures to improve human capabilities such as memory, intelligence, and sexual abilities would seem to be licit if free consent is given, if there is no other way to achieve the same goal, and if the action is in accord with the integrity of the human person. In itself, human betterment, or human improvement, is ethically acceptable and beneficial. Care must be exercised, however, to make sure that the basic integrity of the human person is not violated and that addiction does not result in the course of seeking self-improvement.

8. Using alcoholic beverages or even psychoactive drugs for relaxation or pleasure is not in itself ethically wrong provided that freedom is not notably restricted. Such substances used moderately might provide needed and legitimate relief from the everyday strain and tension of life. Because there is a great tendency to abuse the use of drugs, however, even to become dependent on or addicted to them, and because of the potential bodily harm resulting from some drugs, great care is required in the use of any behavior-modifying substance for recreational purposes.

12.5   ADDICTION OR CHEMICAL DEPENDENCY

Generally speaking, addiction is habituation to some practice harmful to the subject. Although the term *addiction* usually refers to habituation to drugs, one can also be addicted to other detrimental substances or activities, such as alcohol, tobacco, coffee, and excessive food, as well as too much sleep, too much work, and pursuit of sexual pleasure (Francis and Franklin, 1988). Many people use all these things in ways that do not destroy human equilibrium, but some persons, for a variety of reasons not fully understood, become addicted to them. Their whole life is more and more absorbed by a single activity that distorts the personality, consumes physical and psychic energy, and often results in an intense self-centeredness, personality deterioration, and inability to communicate with others. Addiction or dependency on drugs and alcohol are more likely to result in such extreme symptoms. Thus this section addresses those addictions that are often referred to as *chemical dependency*.

One component of chemical dependency, and the most obvious, is its *hedonistic* character, although persons who are in other respects very ascetic may fall victim to it, precisely because they lack healthy pleasures in their lives. In the face of every difficulty of life, every tension or frustration, the chemically dependent person runs away from the loss of normal satisfaction and achievement by indulgence in the physical pleasure, relaxation, and euphoria of the addicting experience (Vaillant, 1984). However, this search for pleasure alone does not constitute addiction; rather, addiction also involves the increasing sense of guilt and helplessness that begin to accompany each overindulgence. The result is that the incipient addict begins to indulge not for the sake of pleasure itself, but to blot out the guilt and remorse for the consequences of previous indulgences. Furthermore, this vicious circle is reinforced by the use of psychological coping mechanisms of rationalization and denial that victims need to suppress guilt and pain, so that they become increasingly unable to perceive the real consequences of behavior. Alcoholic persons, for example, frequently suffer from blackouts, repression, and delusional euphoric recall that so distort their memory that they actually have a very incomplete picture of what is happening to them.

Persons of very different personality types can become addicted, but a common feature is excessive *dependency* needs, sometimes masked by outward aggressiveness and competitiveness. Moreover, as addiction progresses, it tends to produce a pattern of behavior that overrides all temperamental differences.

At one time addicts were thought to come mainly from the poorer classes (Barber, 1967), and undoubtedly addiction is common among some socially depressed groups. Recent research demonstrates, however, that chemical dependency can affect people of all backgrounds. Often gifted, talented, wealthy, and successful persons succumb to this severe personality problem (R. Smart and Murray, 1985).

Chemical dependency or addiction may be broadly classified as physiological or psychological. *Physiological addiction*, which causes a modification or need in the addict's physiological system, usually requires increasing doses of the addicting substance to obtain the same physiological effect. Moreover, in physiological dependence, withdrawal from the object of dependency, for example, heroin, results in severe physiological disturbance, even death, because the body has become so adapted to the presence of the substance in the system (Kosten et al., 1985a). In physiological addiction, however, the psychological component remains essential; thus persons who lack this component can sometimes use even so highly addictive a drug as heroin without exhibiting the typical features of addiction. *Psychological dependency* itself results from a learned conditioned behavior pattern that leads the victim to anticipate the pleasure and release of tension, even when the substance does not notably modify the physiological system (Khantzian, 1985).

Chemical dependency, especially drug addiction, is one of the most highly publicized and most morally condemned social problems in the United States. However, some important facts and questions are sometimes overlooked because of the widespread moral condemnation of such abuses. First, is chemical dependency more a personal or a cultural problem? Studies have shown that chemical addiction is especially serious in the United States (Yamaguchi and Kandel, 1984). Is this because chemical addiction is merely a symptom of some larger American problem such as poverty, anomie, or spiritual deprivation (Kosten et al., 1985b)?

Second, does the strict government control of addictive substances, especially drugs; the special moral disapproval; and the severe penalties for sale and use foment rather than solve the problem? Would chemical addiction be less of a problem in the United States if it were considered a medical or social problem rather than a moral and legal one (Rounsaville and Kleber, 1985; Szasz, 1977)? Removing the moral stigma from addiction to alcohol has been helpful in assisting many people to overcome this addiction (Mendelson and Mello, 1985). Would a similar response to the use of drugs, plus legalization of narcotics for sustaining treatment of addicts, be beneficial over a long period (Ansabel, 1983)? While avoiding a naive optimism about easy solutions for chemical dependency, we must seek to learn from the experience of other nations in this regard, and above all these problems must be considered in the total context of American culture and its socialization process (Bissell and Royce, 1987).

Is this to say that the sense of moral guilt felt by the addict is merely neurotic? On the one hand, therapists speak of addiction as a "disease" in order to reduce its moral opprobrium and to achieve a more sympathetic attitude on the part of nonaddicts. On the other hand, an important part of therapy is to get addicts to accept moral responsibility for the harm they have done themselves and others through addiction. This ambiguity can be cleared up if two points are kept in mind. First, chemical dependency is always a psychological disease because it involves an abnormal behavior pattern accompanied by the neurotic coping mechanisms already described. It can also be a physiological disease because it sometimes produces physiological dependency and usually produces widespread organic changes that greatly aggravate the condition. Second, *voluntary* acts must be distinguished from *free* acts. Addictive behavior is voluntary in the sense that it proceeds from an inner compulsion, but it always involves a restriction of freedom, since the addict becomes less and less able to perceive alternatives of action or to choose among them. In times of addictive need, the practical conscience of the addict is concerned totally with the need for a drink or a fix. He or she acts voluntarily, compulsively, but without free choice.

Thus actual consumption of addictive substances by addicts is seldom in itself a morally cupable act, and the guilt felt afterward is unrealistic and neurotic. Even the acquisition of the addiction often proceeds so gradually and subtly that it is difficult to judge that the addict knowingly and deliberately chose addiction. Nevertheless, it would be a mistake to think that the *whole* guilt felt by addicts is illusory. If it were, it would be difficult to explain why admission of responsibility has proved so important a part of therapy. The truth seems to be that the real moral responsibility of the addicted person lies in the obligation to ask and receive help from others when this is offered, since therapy cannot be effective until the addict accepts help. Acceptance does not take place all at once but passes through stages of (1) *admission* into treatment, (2) *compliance* with treatment (with hidden defiance and resistance), (3) *acceptance* or recognition of real need for health (with unrealistic anticipations of cure), and (4) *surrender,* that is, realistic acknowledgment and acceptance of the responsibility for lifelong change. Thus it is a mistake to reduce this complex situation either to a purely moral question or to a purely sociological or medical one. To deny all moral responsibility or capacity to change is to degrade addicts as persons, yet to pass judgment on their degree of responsibility is to misjudge the many ways in which they are victims of forces beyond individual control.

However, treatment outcome studies in alcoholism indicate that a variety of treatment programs yield benefit and may be cost effective; however, few studies exist that differentiate which programs are best for which types of patients. "So far the outcome literature reflects that patient factors such as having a stable family, stable job, less sociopathy, less psychopathology, and a negative family history for alcoholism are more powerful predictors of positive prognosis than is type of treatment" (Francis and Franklin, 1988).

It is not necessary here to describe therapeutic methods in detail. They involve detoxification and at least a month of intense group psychotherapy, accompanied by a thorough indoctrination in the nature and effects of addiction. This intensive treatment must be accompanied by at least two years of outpatient follow-up. It is important that the family of the addict share to some degree in the therapy, and that both the addict and family members participate in support societies such as Alcoholics Anonymous and Al-Anon (for spouses). The element of mutual help involved both in group therapy and in these support groups seems to be one of the most important features of any treatment, since the addict is able to face painful reality and yet recover a good self-image only through support of others who have experienced the same problems.

Students of addiction emphasize that the earlier in the addiction that therapy takes place the better, but they also point out that family and employers often contribute to the problem by covering up, excusing, or attempting to endure addictive behavior, hoping that the addict will finally come to his or her senses. This spontaneous self-insight by addicts is very rare, and family, friends, and employers have a serious ethical responsibility to face the facts realistically and intervene decisively and persistently until the addict accepts treatment. Intervention is best done by those who can be supportive rather than judgmental, but who can also face the addict with detailed evidence of the seriousness of his or her condition.

Healthcare professionals sometimes are impatient with and contemptuous of alcoholics and other addicts, whom they regard as delinquents rather than as victims of illness. Such attitudes are intensified by unwarranted pessimism about the effectiveness of therapy. This is especially unfortunate because healthcare professionals themselves have an especially high rate of chemical dependency, caused not only by their relatively easy access to drugs but perhaps also by the *ethos* of the profession. This maximizes guilt feelings over breach of professional standards while doing little to support persons who may have high dependency needs, which they mask under professional self-assurance and pride.

Therefore, it is important for professionals to acquaint themselves thoroughly with the nature and therapy of addiction, the ways of intervening to get addicts to accept treatment, treatment centers to which they can be referred, and ways to support them in their new life (Bissell and Royce, 1987).

Perhaps an even more effective way for healthcare professionals to combat chemical addiction is through preventive measures. They can play an important role in combating the mentality in the United States that seems to predispose people for substance abuse and addiction (J. Miller, 1983; National Institute of Drug Abuse, 1986). According to this mentality, every pain, every sorrow or frustration, can be overcome with a pill, potion, or injection of some type. Pharmaceutical firms constantly push drugs through advertising, and healthcare professionals often are used by such agencies to promote unnecessary drug use. Christian professionals will not share in this promotion because they realize that human pain, frustration, and sorrow simply cannot be suppressed. Human beings grow as persons by facing the difficulties and struggles of life realistically, "bearing one another's burdens" (Ga 6:2) as free people, not as slaves to a pleasure ethic. In saying this, we are not proposing an exaggerated stoicism as the Christian ideal, but a realistic effort to overcome the real causes of suffering rather than an escape into unconsciousness. Alcoholics Anonymous, which has led the way to the most successful methods of therapy for chemical dependency, has always emphasized that the addict cannot recover without a reaching out for a Higher Power and a willingness to repair damage done to the neighbor and to be of service to the neighbor.

12.6   SEX THERAPY AND RESEARCH

Therapy

The inability to engage in satisfactory sexual expression is widespread (F. Anderson and Rubenstein, 1978) and often is a contributing factor to marital discord, although perhaps it is as often an effect as a cause. What should be not only an expression but also a source of deepening love and commitment, rich in tenderness and joy, can be a source of profound depression and alienation. Couples frustrated and puzzled by sexual dysfunction are sometimes exploited by marriage counselors or sex therapists who are unqualified or irresponsible, since these disciplines are relatively new, rapidly expanding, and lacking in well-established professional or legal controls (APA, 1986b). Healthcare professionals can be of great help in preserving and improving family life if they are well-informed about the goals and effectiveness of sex therapy and the availability of reliable practitioners to whom couples may be referred.

According to Masters and Johnson (1970, 1976), the most prominent therapists and researchers in this field, the most common forms of sexual dysfunction for men are premature ejaculation, impotency, and secondary potency difficulties; for women, the most common forms are vaginismus and orgastic dysfunction. Contrary to the beliefs of some psychoanalysts, sexual dysfunction need not be a sign of a deep or severe psychic pathology; it can be the result of various relatively superficial maladjustments that impede spontaneity. As Kaplan (1974) states, sex therapy "differs from other forms of treatment for sexual dysfunction in two respects: first, its goals are essentially limited to the relief of the patient's sexual dysfunction and, second, it departs from traditional technique by employing a combination of prescribed sexual experiences and psychotherapy." Thus sex therapy has a more limited objective than psychoanalysis or marital therapy. These latter two forms of assistance seek to help people with sexual dysfunction, but they concentrate more on the underlying conflicts and destructive interpersonal behavior that may give rise to such dysfunction. In sex therapy, however, the dysfunction is treated directly, and the therapy is complete when the couple is able to achieve a satisfactory sexual response.

During the past 30 years, centers for sex therapy have been widely established in the United States, but the original and most renowned center was founded in 1959 at Washington University in St. Louis by William Masters and Virginia Johnson. In 1974, this center, which offers therapy and trains professional therapists, was named the Reproductive Biology Research Foundation; later the name was changed to the Masters and Johnson Foundation. Other centers for research treatment of sexual dysfunction exist at Cornell University and other university hospitals, but few centers combine research and therapy. In addition, many healthcare professionals, psychiatrists, psychologists, and special therapists offer sex therapy in private practice, as do the practitioners of dubious competency already mentioned.

At the larger centers, the common sexual dysfunctions of married people are treated through an integrated combination of instruction and actual sexual experiences in which the couple explore a more relaxed, personalized approach to sexual relations freed from anxieties about "performance." The instructions are usually given by a man-woman team, and the actual experiences are engaged in privately by the couple in their home or a hotel near the therapy center. At the beginning of therapy, a thorough history is taken and a complete physical examination given. After therapy, which typically consists of about 10 days of instruction, a follow-up is made to see if the couple has successfully integrated the new approach to sexual relations into their ordinary living. More than 80 percent success is usually reported by such centers, which is remarkable considering the relatively short period of therapy compared to that required to meet other types of marital problems in marriage counseling.

As a general rule, most centers and private therapists accept only married couples for treatment. At one time Masters and Johnson made use of paid surrogate partners for single persons and in special cases for married persons, but they have discontinued this much-criticized practice.

Christian Principles

The Principle of Personalized Sexuality (8.3, 10.1) indicates the importance for married couples to be able to express and deepen their love by satisfying sexual relations. The clinical experience of sex therapists today seems to show that when couples have good interpersonal relations, effective communication of attitudes and feelings, and a positive and anxiety-free attitude toward bodily intimacy and sensual enjoyment, sexual dysfunction is rare and special training unnecessary. In today's culture, however, many men and women find interpersonal communication, even at nonsexual levels, difficult and are inhibited in the spontaneous expression of their feelings both by inhibiting fears and by exaggerated competitive attitudes. Thus much of the need for sex therapy could be obviated by adequate preparation for marriage.

From a Christian point of view, this education ought to express the intimate relation between the various meanings of sexuality as sensual satisfaction, as love and completion between man and woman, and as the source of the continuing life of the family and society, and it should show how permanent self-giving is the heart of the matter.

When couples learn to communicate with each other honestly and lovingly, sexual adjustment is usually easy because intercourse is itself essentially a form of intimate communication. Effective sex education cannot be merely abstract but must include an experiential growth that enables persons to understand their own sexuality and to learn to relate to others as sexual persons through encounters appropriate to their age and personal maturity. Persons also need help, however, so that these growth experiences do not lead them down the dead-end paths of autoeroticism or a depersonalized search for satisfactions unrelated to the deeper meaning of sexuality as marital commitment.

Therefore, sex therapy undoubtedly may be necessary and ethically acceptable for married couples who need to overcome difficulties of miseducation or personal sexual development, provided that the prescribed sexual actions are performed with the married partner, and in view of the expression of marital love through complete sexual union and not as a substitute for it. It is desirable that a sufficient number of Christian healthcare professionals prepare themselves to provide such therapy in the context of a truly personalized attitude toward sexuality, lest such technical knowledge should be abused so as to further weaken family life rather than to promote and strengthen it.

At present, no definite set of ethical standards exists for professionals involved in sexual therapy, although a group of prominent practitioners sought to develop such guidelines (Masters et al., 1977, 1980). However, *The Principles of Medical Ethics* of the APA (1981; 1986) would seem to apply to sexual dysfunction counselors. Given the importance of the human activity involved, the need for definite moral standards is obvious. First, the same confidentiality required of anyone offering therapeutic treatment must be observed. Second, the persons involved should not be asked to perform actions that are immoral or contrary to their conscience. Thus use of surrogate partners as well as activities that are intentionally and directly masturbatory or otherwise deviant must be rejected. Third, therapists must not engage in sexual activity with patients. Unfortunately, studies show that these moral standards are sometimes violated (Gartrell, 1986). Violations of these principles will not only harm the patients, but will also destroy respect for sexual therapy and those who pursue it as a profession.

Unfortunately, sex therapists also often seem to approach their task from a purely scientific-technological point of view. One noted psychiatrist (Kaplan, 1974) completes her study of some of the literature with the lament, "There is a conspicuous absence of the word *love*." We cannot help but wonder, therefore, whether this approach may still further the depersonalization of human sexuality from which our culture suffers. Christians working in this field should exert leadership in the opposite direction.

Research

What has just been said of sex therapy also applies to sexual research and experimentation, including diagnostic procedures that may be used to determine the normality of sexual response, for example, to diagnose homosexual tendencies. Such research is legitimate and necessary to understand better the nature of human sexuality and the physiological or psychological pathologies to which it is subject. Such research, however, must be in accord with the principles already laid down in 9.5 for psychological experimentation with human subjects, which means that the experimental experiences must be designed to be therapeutic or truly educational for the subject and not depersonalizing or reinforcing of patterns inconsistent with the total health—moral and spiritual, as well as biological and psychological—of the human person (Bower and de Gaspanis, 1978).

Such conditions exclude sexual acts between unmarried partners, and especially the use of prostitutes, and certainly between the therapist and patient, although Riskin (1979) attempted to defend this. These conditions would seem also to exclude the use of subjects who are immature or otherwise lacking in mature control of their sexual impulses and behavior, unless the experiment itself tends to strengthen this control. The type of experiment, often reported, that exposes subjects to viewing photographs to measure sexual arousal is highly questionable because it involves risk of consent to illicit acts. Since, however, there could be a proportionate reason for such a risk, this type of experiment is not absolutely excluded. For example, the use of pictures for diagnostic purposes or for some benefit to the patient in conditioning experiments and therapy (e.g., in some operant conditioning therapies for homosexual orientation or compulsive anxiety) may be justified if the temptation involved is moderate and the subjects are warned that the purpose is not pornographic but simply to test initial reactions.

Thus sexual therapy and sexual research can be carried on in an ethical manner. Basically, both sexual research and sexual therapy aim at helping people to express their love for one another more fully. However, great care and sensitivity must be observed in the practice of sexual therapy and in the experiments prompted by sexual research. In either case, the fundamental integrity of the persons involved must be respected. Thus actions that are in themselves immoral are not justified. Moreover, the activities involved in either research or therapy should be carried on in view of the fact that human love is not accomplished or developed through technique or knowledge alone. A deeper awareness and mutual communion must be present to enhance human love. Not only are these admonitions derived from an integral view of human nature and human love, but they also take into account a long-range view of human dignity. What have we gained if we learn everything there is to know about sexual activity but in the pursuit of pleasure learn less and less about fulfilling human love?

CHAPTER 13

Suffering and Death

OVERVIEW

This chapter considers suffering and death, two concomitant realities of healthcare and medicine, from a Christian perspective. We begin by considering the response of healthcare professionals to suffering and death, analyzing the phenomenon of fear of death from the viewpoint of Christian spirituality (13.1; 13.2). In our present era we use two different sets of clinical signs to determine that human death has occurred (13.3). Thus the ethical evaluation of brain death is considered. Christian care for the dying and dead person requires truth telling (13.4) and respecting the remains of the person after death has taken place (13.5); these responsibilities are discussed next. Finally, we consider the ethical distinctions between suicide, euthanasia (13.6), and allowing to die (13.7).

13.1 MYSTERY OF DEATH

From time immemorial, human beings have viewed suffering and death and asked, Why? Why would a loving God allow people to suffer? Why would God allow a child to be born with Down's syndrome, or allow the father of a large family to undergo a mental breakdown, or allow a mother to be taken from her growing family when others, aging or without children, are left untouched? People both wise and callow have questioned the meaning of suffering and death since the beginning of time. In the Jewish and Christian traditions, some insight has been gained over the centuries concerning these concomitants of human existence (C. Lewis, 1943; Nouwen, 1972). Some of the knowledge and understanding is found in the Scriptures; much of it is in the oral tradition of churches and families. However, suffering and death remain mysteries—mysteries that will never be unraveled clearly and completely in this life—because they are bound up in the intimate life and love of God. Admitting that suffering and death are mysteries that cannot be solved fully in this life may seem to be a denial or delimitation of the human desire and power to know the truth. Actually, it is not a denial of human potential and aspiration. Rather, it is an admission that human beings are incapable of knowing everything, and that God plays a very important part in the life of any individual person or any group of persons.

To say that suffering and death are mysteries does not take them out of the realm of human investigation, nor does it mean that we should stand in helpless awe of sickness and death. After all, some of the great moments in human history are the result of human beings' efforts and success in conquering illness and disease. There is, however, a point beyond which human beings cannot go. Suffering shall never be eliminated, and each person must die. These ultimate truths are testimony to the power of the Creator, with whom humankind cooperates in the genesis and continuation of the human race, but who in the last analysis is the ruler of the world, the Lord of the universe.

"Death was not God's doing; he takes no pleasure in the extinction of the living. To be—for this he created all" (Ws 1:13-14). "God had not wished to include suffering and death in man's destiny" (Pius XII, 1944). From where, then, came suffering and death? St. Paul says, "Through one man sin entered the world, and with sin death, death thus coming to all men inasmuch as all sinned" (Rm 5:12). This original sin was essentially a sin of pride, the will to be like God not by using God's gifts to come closer to God in community, but to use these gifts to set up the human individual in self-centered domination of the world apart from God. It is this misuse of God's gifts from the beginning of the human race to this day that has prevented humankind from overcoming the natural causes of suffering and death. This misuse also introduced into the world countless unnatural causes and transformed natural death, which might have been a joyful completion of this life and a serene passage into a greater life, into a blind, terrifying mystery.

Although people have turned their backs on God, he has not turned from them but has offered them forgiveness and restoration. In his mercy, however, God cannot deny their human freedom but has called them to return to him, not simply by restoring them to their innocent beginnings, but by a long history of struggle and learning from experience, an experience in which suffering is inevitable. For the Christian and for all who travel the same road in less clear ways, God has revealed in Christ the direction of their journey and the power of grace by which it can be traveled (O'Meara, 1973). In baptism, according to St. Paul (Rm 6:1-11), through the cross of Christ humanity has died and been reborn in a new creation that will be completed in the resurrection of the body in eternal life. Human beings live now in such unity with Christ that all the events of their lives take on meaning from his life and death. Consequently, both the joy and the suffering of this life have a Christian meaning: its joys are signs of the hope for everlasting life in his kingdom, which is already present here on earth in promise; and its sorrows are a sharing in his cross through which a victorious resurrection is to be achieved.

Jesus came to conquer suffering and death. In what sense has he succeeded? People still get sick and continue to suffer, and death is inevitable. He conquered sickness, suffering, and death in the sense that he gave them a new meaning, a new power. By believing in Jesus as Savior, by joining suffering and death to his, humankind overcomes the evil aspect of suffering and death. Through his sacrifice, human beings are able to conquer the evil associated with suffering and death (Schillebeeckx, 1981b). Although the results of original and actual sin are still present in life, they no longer dominate it. Rather, suffering and death are transformed into the very actions that help humankind fulfill its destiny.

At one time death was defined as separation of body and soul. Although this definition is true, it is no longer adequate. In their attempts to specify more clearly what it means to die, modern theologians have concentrated on death as a personal act of a human being, an act that terminates earthly existence but also fulfills it (Sacred Congregation for the Doctrine of the Faith, 1979). Thus the person is not merely passive in the face of death, and death is different for the just than for the sinner. In the view of Rahner (1965), a view accepted and developed by many theologians, death is an active consummation, a maturing self-realization that embodies what each person has made of himself or herself during life. Death becomes a ratification of life, not merely an inevitable process (Boros, 1965). It is an event, an action in which the freedom of the person is intimately involved. Dying with Christ is an adventure; it is a consequence of, but not a condemnation for, sin. This is a new approach to death, yet it is thoroughly in keeping with the Christian tradition. Indeed, this view of death seems to describe more clearly the experience of Christ, who offered his life rather than have it taken from him, who completed his love and generosity in the final act of obedience to the Father: "It is consummated" (Jn 19:30). Not only pastoral care personnel, but also those in other fields of the healing profession, will enrich their own lives and the lives of their patients if they are able to communicate this notion of death.

13.2   FEAR OF DEATH

Because healthcare professionals are human, they tend to retreat from any phenomenon that causes fear or wonder. Death is such a phenomenon; it involves awe, fear, and mystery. For this reason, healthcare professionals, just as other people, are tempted to avoid facing the evil of death (Cranford, 1985). The result of this fear has been catalogued by perceptive physicians and philosophers (E. Becker, 1973; Cassell, 1976; Aries, 1981; Hilfaker, 1985). When healthcare professionals are controlled by fear, they often deceive patients as to their true condition and neglect their need for understanding or comfort. Moreover, the occasion for personal spiritual growth is lost for both the patient and the healthcare professional, and the opportunity to help another human being prepare for death and eternal life is lost as well. Studies show that too many healthcare professionals retreat and cut themselves off from the dying patient completely (Landau and Gustafson, 1984). To put it another way, dying is not only a biological process, but also a psychological process that involves the healthcare professional as well as the patient.

To overcome fear and to help people die well, the healthcare professional must learn to handle the emotional strain that accompanies suffering and death and to deal with the ethical dilemmas sometimes encountered (R. Mack, 1984). Although many helpful books on these topics are available, some clinical training in this area is also necessary. Every hospital staff should include people who specialize in the care of the dying. Their purpose is not only to help the dying patient work through fear, anger, and depression, but also to help the members of the healing team participate in the event of death in a way that is healthful for themselves, (Gadow, 1980; Ingelfinger, 1973; P. Maguire, 1985). Otherwise, healthcare professionals, no matter how well-educated or technically expert, will suffer psychological harm from their constant involvement in death. Is the high rate of alcoholism, suicide, and divorce among healthcare professionals in some way connected with stress over their inability to express their grief and sadness at the constant sight of death (Bosk, 1979)?

Given the power and prestige of the healthcare profession, acknowledging the importance of God in human life, the mystery of his presence as evidenced through suffering and death, is an important step in humanizing that profession. To accept limitation is to accept one's humanity. Healthcare professionals who assume a position of unlimited power in the process of healing have an outlook that is unrealistic. They think of themselves as the persons who cure, rather than realizing that it is God who cures and healthcare professionals who cooperate in this work by using the forces of nature.

Those who must deal with the dying have three options: (1) they can ignore the dying patient and thus become hardened and jaded; (2) they can relate to the dying patient in a sincerely personal manner without knowing how to deal with their own feelings; or (3) they may relate to the dying patient in a healthy way, recognizing the psychological strain that patient and professional undergo together (Fleyner, 1977). Taking this last option can teach a professional to value the experience of helping another fellow human being suffer and die in Christ, either with explicit Christian faith or perhaps simply with an openness to the mysterious future, which is the effect of Christ's grace in those who do not know him except under some other name or symbol. Few healthcare professionals, however, will be able to achieve this healthy, healing attitude without special training in the art of working with the dying.

In learning this art of the care for the dying, three points should be kept in mind. First, because suffering and death are obstacles to the fullness of life that Christians affirm, we have not only the right but the duty to try to overcome or mitigate them. Thus Christians should strongly favor medical research to conquer disease and to preserve and prolong life, for example, the crusade to eliminate heart disease and cancer or to make the environment more healthful. Medicine as a profession, as a science, and as an art has a Christian birthright.

Second, efforts to overcome the evils of sickness and suffering by medical science have not eliminated the healing role of prayer, which is also a part of the Christian heritage. Jesus healed physical as well as spiritual ills and commanded his followers not only to preach but also to heal and drive out demons (Mk 3:14-15). The reference to demons indicates the forces of evil that must be overcome for complete human healing in all the dimensions of the human person, spiritual and ethical, as well as psychological and physical; these forces are greater than merely human intelligence, even with the aid of science, can ever hope to achieve. Thus, to complete human healing necessitates turning to Jesus Christ, who has conquered sin and death and who is the source of all healing powers, even those provided by modern medicine. Therefore healthcare professionals striving to help the suffering and the dying need to pray for and with them.

Third, although sickness and suffering have entered the human world through sin, they are not themselves sinful, nor is the one who is suffering always the same one who has sinned. Jesus suffered because of the sins of others, and this is also true of innocent persons today. Because people are all part of one human community, they bear not only the consequences of their own personal sins but also the consequences of others' sins. Thus people often injure their own health and have to suffer the consequences, but they also suffer from a bad environment produced by others, and through the neglect of others they may lack the means to maintain and recover health. Thus healthcare professionals should see the sick as victims rather than as responsible for their own condition, unless in fact this responsibility is obvious. Even if they are in fact responsible, sick persons must then be helped to understand the forgiving mercy of God by which the road of hope is always open. The real problem of caring for the suffering and dying, therefore, is to help them realize that they can bring good out of evil by making their painful and frightening experiences a means of personal growth and a witness of courage to others who someday will have to meet the same test. The current situation of patients with acquired immunodeficiency syndrome (AIDS) emphasizes the importance of helping patients to approach death with a sound theological outlook. Although the situation of AIDS patients may be hopeless in regard to their physiological condition, the mercy of God is always open for them (U.S. Catholic Conference [USCC], 1987). Caregivers should help AIDS patients realize that they have not lost their human dignity (Kübler-Ross, 1987).

Christian healthcare professionals will best succeed in this difficult task if they themselves understand suffering and death in terms of the suffering, death, and resurrection of Jesus Christ, which provides the only help in living hopefully with this mystery. Many healthcare professionals feel utterly defeated by the death of patients whom they have cared for and by the helplessness of even their best efforts in many cases to restore normal health. Only Christian hope has an answer for that despair.

Clearly, it takes more than words to accomplish this transformation of suffering and death. One must be willing to surrender to God through the person of Jesus Christ every day if one wishes to give new meaning and power to suffering and death. The small deaths one dies every day prepare a person for the larger and more important deaths and finally for the ultimate moment of meaning and power.

The perfection of Christian suffering and death is to accept it with hope and joy. This is not possible unless one works at it faithfully, relying on the unfailing grace of God. To communicate to patients effectively the meaning and power of death, healthcare professionals must have some experience of its reality

363

themselves. Thus healthcare is more than a job, more than knowledge and technique. Basically, in its fullness it is a way of life that sees beyond the hurt, the sickness, the anguish; a way of life that enables one to look beyond the drudgery of daily reality, beyond the suffering in the hospital ward and the emergency room; a way of life that centers in God's love for his children, his ability to bring good out of evil, the suffering of Christ for all human beings, and his victorious resurrection.

13.3   DEFINING DEATH

When biologists speak of the death of any living organism, they refer to that inevitable and critical moment when an organism ceases to function as a specific, unified, homeostatic system and becomes disorganized into a mere collection of heterogeneous chemical substances (President's Commission for the Study of Ethical Problems in Medicine and Biomedical and Behavioral Research, 1981). Sometimes, however, even after this moment, some tissues or cells of the former organism may continue temporarily to carry on some independent minimal life functions. From a biological point of view, the death of a human organism is similar to any death and is determined in much the same way, by various signs that the unifying life functions have ceased. However, few people believe that human death is nothing more than a biological event. Human death has a mystery about it because at death we loose touch irrevocably with a person who previously was able to communicate and to share our human community of thought, of love, of freedom, and of creativity (Kung, 1984). Human death is not merely a decay of an organism, it is the departure of a member of the human community. People all over the world have interpreted this departure of someone known and loved as the separation of a spiritual soul from its body. Science is unable to close the door on such an explanation. Christians believe that the departed will return in their bodily personhood in a transformed existence, as Jesus did (Lk 24:36-43).

In any case, people often have the painful responsibility of determining when the death of another has occurred, because the time of death influences many other human decisions, such as inheritance, legal and moral rights possessed by the dying person, spiritual care for the dying person, and possibility of organ transplantation.

Dying is a process, but death is an event (Black, 1983; Capron, 1986). We can be certain this event has not yet occurred as long as a person can communicate through speech or gesture. When such communication ceases, we can only judge by signs that are no longer distinctly and specifically human. We do not dare conclude, however, that death has occurred merely because such specifically human signs are no longer evident, as becomes very clear when we observe someone wake from sleep or coma.

Consequently, we are morally obliged to treat anybody who is apparently human (even in the fetal state) as a human person with human rights until we are sure that this body has become so disorganized that it no longer retains its human unity. To know this, we must be reasonably sure of three facts: (1) that the body does not now exhibit specific human behavior, (2) that it will not be able to function humanly in the future, and (3) that it no longer has even a minimal capacity for human functions because it has lost the basic structures required for human unity. This third condition is required because medical experience has shown that persons who have been in apparent coma nevertheless have sometimes recovered human consciousness. Such resuscitation is possible as long as the essential structures of the human organism remain and the causes that inhibit their normal function can be removed. This is why some speculate that in the future the human body may be frozen and revived centuries later.

At the same time, there is no reason to deny that after true human death some cells or even organs of the human body may for a time (perhaps indefinitely if artificially supported) continue to exhibit some life functions. These functions are not those of the human organism as a unified entity, but merely a residual life at a level of organization comparable to that of plants and lower animals. Thus the essential point about determining human death is not to decide whether any life is present, but whether human life in the sense of a unified human person is still present (Grundstrand, 1986).

Some signs of human death were always easy to identify in the past. If rigor mortis or putrefaction occurred, even nonprofessionals were able to recognize that the human organism was irreversibly destroyed. Other less conclusive signs of human death were the absence of breathing and heartbeat, although it was known that these might sometimes be revived by such methods of resuscitation as were then available. When such efforts failed, death was judged certain. Physicians were required to pronounce the patient dead on the basis of such evidence and certify the time of death for legal purposes such as inheritance. Thus cessation of spontaneous heart and lung function became known as the *clinical* signs of death.

In recent times, two developments have led to the proposal of a new set of clinical signs for determining human death (Canada Law Reform Commission, 1981; Cassell et al., 1972; President's Commission for Study of Ethical Problems in Medicine and Biomedical and Behavioral Research, 1981). First, machines have been perfected that artificially aid the function of the heart and lungs or that enable a person to be resuscitated after the heart and lungs have ceased to function for a short time. Often people recover full and spontaneous heart and lung function as a result of being temporarily assisted by such machines, proving that the essential structures of the unified human organism had not been destroyed. On the other hand, it seems possible that such machines may be able to maintain heart and lung function at least temporarily, even after this unity of the organism has ceased to exist, since the heart completely separated from the body can continue to beat, just as tissues in a test tube can continue to exhibit some residual life if nourished by an appropriate solution.

Thus such artificially sustained heart and lung action is not proof that human life still remains, yet as long as they are sustained, it is impossible to verify the traditional signs of human death. Therefore the question arises: Are there other clinical signs that can be used, not to constitute a new definition of death, but rather as alternative criteria to establish the same essential fact, namely, that human life is no longer present because unified human function is not present and cannot be restored (Agich and Jones, 1985; New York Task Force on Medical Ethics, 1986)?

The second, and perhaps more important, reason for seeking new clinical signs of death has been the recent advancement of techniques of organ transplantation, especially of the kidney and heart. Such transplant are more likely to be successful if the organs are retrieved from a body through which blood continues to circulate. Thus transplant surgeons prefer to keep the cadaver of a dead donor on a respirator. How, then, is it possible to be sure that the donor is in fact dead (Areen et al., 1984)?

Brain Death Criteria

First, the traditional cardiovascular clinical signs are basic and sufficient and should be retained when determining death. The new brain-death criteria, assessing function of the whole brain, should be employed only when traditional signs cannot be used because the dying person is dependent on a respirator or other form of artificial maintenance. If brain death is permitted to become the exclusive criterion for human death, no one would be judged dead without elaborate tests in a hospital. Present moral dilemmas about how to determine death are caused largely by excessive reliance on technology, and that excess should be moderated rather than encouraged.

Second, the new brain-death criteria must be ascertained by well-trained professionals. Human error and even carelessness must be anticipated and avoided. How can such errors be prevented when human life is at stake? Most criteria for brain death require more than one clinical observation of the patient. In the first set of criteria used to certify brain death, the Harvard criteria, the observations were separated by 24 hours. At present, 6 to 12 hours between observations is considered sufficient. Moreover, persons applying the clinical criteria for brain death must be trained to recognize such conditions as hypothermia and drug-induced coma, which may produce a condition from which the patient can recover (Canada Law Reform Commission, 1981). Other safeguards require that the physician who certifies death should not be a member of a transplantation team, that might be overanxious to pronounce the donor dead. In some cases, the opinion of more than one physician is required before brain death is determined. One way or another, fail-safe procedures must be built into the process of using brain functions as the clinical signs to ascertain human death.

Third, and most serious, is the question about the nature of brain death itself (Pontifical Academy of Sciences, 1985; President's Commission for the Study of Ethical Problems, 1981). It is critical that the criteria used to certify brain death establish that the person is dead, not merely dying or in a deep coma. Although the medical profession has accepted the general idea of using the brain as the main criteria in some cases to establish human death, exactly which specific signs should be used to determine that human death has occurred have not been agreed on by all (Byrne et al., 1979; Molinari, 1978; President's Commission for the Study of Ethical Problems, 1981). For the most part, the criteria center on clinical observation, such as response to pain, cerebral function, brainstem reflexes, and testing for apnea. These clinical observations are confirmed by use of an electroencephalogram (EEG) or blood-flow studies. The variance in opinion as to the validity of brain-death criteria primarily results from theoretical issues. Thus one group of physicians maintains that cessation of neuronal activity in the brain is not sufficient to signify human death unless the cessation is proved to be irreversible and indicates destruction of all cerebral function (Byrne et al., 1979). This argument seemingly has been obviated by studying the circulation of blood in the brain by means of an angiogram or isotopes rather than by using an EEG to study neuronal activity. If the angiogram establishes that blood no longer circulates into the brain, the brain is dead because no way exists to restore activity to the brain when circulation ceases. The lack of blood circulation in the brain may also be proven through newer methods of imaging (Levy, 1987). Hence, when the whole brain is dead, the person is dead, since the organ that is the source of unified activity no longer functions, even though there may still be signs of residual cellular activity in the brain and other parts of the body.

Although it is not our purpose to settle any differences of opinion in regard to medical matters, we conclude that when total and irreversible function of brain activity is clinically proved, the person in question is dead because the form (soul) is no longer able to inform the matter (body). To date, many states have approved this method of discerning human death in so-called Definition of Death Legislation, and the need for national legislation in this regard has been recommended (President's Commission for the Study of Ethical Problems, 1981). The legislation of the various states requires that the signs indicate that total, not merely partial, death of the brain has occurred.

Partial Brain Death

Would it be possible to declare a person dead if only some part of the brain, that is, the higher or neocortical centers on which specifically human thought processes apparently depend, did not develop fully or ceased to function (Braunstein et al., 1978; Younger and Bartlett, 1983)? This view is defended by some who wish to use anencephalic infants as organ donors before total brain death occurs or who maintain that such infants may be aborted in the third trimester (Chervenak et al., 1984; Holzgreve et al., 1987). The philosophers Robert Rizzo and Paul Yonder studied this question and declared (1973):

> We must ask whether the death of the cerebral cortex or neocortex signals human death, even though other parts may be still functioning for a time....We offer the hypothesis that human death should be related to the cessation of functions distinctly human since breathing, heartbeat, and circulation are vegetative processes shared by other animals....

> From all clinical evidence the death of the neocortex marks the end of the physiological basis for human consciousness, that is, a consciousness unique in its powers of reflection. It signals the end of the brain as a dynamic integrated

whole and presages in most cases the imminent death of other cerebral systems (p. 226).

Despite some support for the position that cortical death constitutes human death (Zaner, 1988), this position presents several difficulties. First, if people who have spontaneously functioning hearts and lungs but no other vital signs are declared dead, what about people who have weak signs of "human life" (R. Veatch, 1975)? If those in a deep and irreversible coma are declared dead insofar as human life is concerned, what about people who are mentally retarded or senile? Do they show sufficient signs of human life to be kept alive? Or should only minimal care be given to those who no longer have the functioning signs of human life that are associated with activity in the cortex of the brain? Persons who argue for the elimination of retarded, senile, infirm, and debilitated persons in certain circumstances believe partial brain death should be accepted as a proper clinical sign for human death (Harris, 1985). However, society must go very slowly in accepting such a definition unless it is willing to bury people when they are still breathing and their hearts are pulsating spontaneously.

If the criteria of *partial* brain death were to be used as sufficient evidence of death, ethical responsibility would require certitude about two facts. *First,* the essential structures necessary and sufficient to constitute the unified organism of the human person would have to be found in the cortical function of the human brain, separated from the rest of the body. This certainly is plausible from what is now known. *Second,* most of the brain would have to be considered unnecessary for the specifically human functions of thinking and willing, but existing only to maintain and move the body and supply the higher brain centers with nourishing materials. This also is plausible, but the present state of knowledge on this is far from certain (President's Commission for Study of Ethical Problems in Medicine and Biomedical and Behavioral Research, 1981). It is generally recognized today that the brain is a system of subsystems that are intimately interdependent. Although it is possible to localize such functions as speech and sight in particular parts of the brain, this is not proof that only one such part is involved in the function or even that it is its primary center, since inhibition of a merely secondary or auxiliary part of a system may impede its function (Benton, 1976; Gaddes, 1985). Thus, at present, such localization of human functions is merely tentative.

In sum, we accept total brain death as a sufficient criterion for human death, but we do not believe that partial brain death is sufficient. We do not believe that death should be certified as long as patients are able to maintain spontaneous breathing and heartbeat, since this constitutes strong evidence that the brain, as the seat of the essential unity of the human body, is still living, even if it is not evidencing its higher functions. Although there may be reasonable doubts, the benefit of the doubt should be given to the rights of the person.

13.4   TRUTH TELLING TO THE DYING

"What to tell the patient" has been considered one of the more difficult and delicate ethical questions for healthcare professionals. The Principle of Professional Communication, formulated in 8.1, is relevant here. Not long ago, some physicians and other healthcare professionals thought that the less patients knew about their condition, the better would be the chances of recovery (Oken, 1961). Moreover, some healthcare professionals would even withhold information of impending death, fearing that such knowledge might lead a person to despair (Cope, 1968). In some parts of the world, this is still the practice of many physicians (Palouzie, 1985). Because of an awakened moral sense by healthcare professionals and a sharper realization that patients have legal and moral rights that must be respected (American Medical Association [AMA], 1973; P. Gillon, 1985b), however, today there is a much greater tendency to be open and honest with patients concerning their condition. In general, patients have the right to the truth concerning their condition, the purpose of the treatment to be given, and the prognosis of the treatment (Horan and Halligan, 1982). The "Patient's Bill of Rights" of the American Hospital Association (AHA, 1972) states:

> The patient has the right to obtain from the physicians complete current information concerning diagnosis, treatment, and prognosis in terms the patient can be reasonably expected to understand (n. 3).

The *Ethical and Religious Directives for Catholic Health Facilities* (USCC, 1971) declare:

> Everyone has the right and duty to prepare for the solemn moment of death. Unless it is clear, therefore, that a dying patient is already well prepared for death as regards both temporal and spiritual affairs, it is the physician's duty to inform him of his critical condition or to have some other responsible person impart this information (n. 8).

Clearly, information concerning serious sickness or impending death is to be furnished even if the individual does not ask for it. Legal precedent as well as moral concern prompts this realization. Thus physicians and other healthcare professionals may not defend their lack of communication on the grounds that the patient did not wish to know and did not ask questions. In some hospitals, a patients' representative helps patients understand their situation, especially when surgery is anticipated. Whenever possible, the leader of the healthcare team, the physician, should be involved in explaining the situation to the patient.

Although healthcare professionals usually respect the rights of patients insofar as providing the proper information is concerned, difficult situations often arise and healthcare professionals hesitate to tell patients their true condition. For example, if patients with serious cases of cancer know their true condition, they might become despondent and lack the desire to live, thus contributing to their illness (R. Goldberg and Tull, 1983; M. Knight and Field, 1981). People who are dying might become despondent, morose, and even suicidal if they know their true situation. With this in mind, the "Patient's Bill of Rights" states:

> When it is not medically advisable to give such information to the patient, the information should be made available to an appropriate person in his behalf (n. 8).

369

This statement is well-intentioned but also unsatisfactory and incomplete. It indicates that when healthcare professionals think that knowing the truth might harm the patient, they can fulfill their obligation by telling some friend or member of the family about the patient's condition and the prognosis. The statement does not indicate, however, what the member of the family or the friend is supposed to do with the information. To ensure Christian treatment for the patient, therefore, another dimension of the situation must be explored.

Even though medical personnel might fear untoward results if patients are informed of their true condition, this does not mean that patients should not be told the true facts. Healthcare professionals should remember in these cases the words of Dr. Eric Cassell (1976): "The depression in patients that commonly occurs after the diagnosis of a fatal disease seems to stem in part from the conspiracy of silence. The physician can be a great help by simply making it clear to the patient that he is available for open and direct communication." Thus the medical team, along with a friend of the patient or a member of the family, should work together and dispose the patient so that he or she will be able to accept the truth. Interviews with seriously ill or dying patients reveal that they do not wish to be kept continually in doubt about their condition (Llewelyn and Fielding, 1983); on the other hand, they do not want it revealed to them in an abrupt or brutal manner, according to Dr. Elisabeth Kübler-Ross (1969):

> When we asked our patients how they had been told, we learned that all the patients know about their terminal illness anyway, whether they were explicitly told or not, but depended greatly on the physician to present the news in an acceptable manner (p. 183).

Howard Brody (1981) assesses the practical situation aptly when he states:

> ...telling a patient something takes place over a span of time and is not a one-shot affair. Thus, the shading of phrases used, whether the truth is delivered all at once or in small doses, and the kind of follow-up are all important parts of the ethical decision, as well as "tell" or "don't tell." A decision to reveal a grave prognosis, which may be "ethical" in itself, may become "unethical" if the physician tells the patient bluntly and then withdraws, without offering any emotional support to help the patient resolve his feelings. In fact, the assurance that the physician plans to see it through along with the patient, and that he will always make himself available to offer any comfort possible, may be more important than the bad news itself. In many of the "sour cases" that are offered as justification for withholding the truth, it may well be the absence of this transmission of compassion, rather than the telling of the truth, that produced the unfortunate result (p. 40).

Because physicians are not always able to convey information concerning serious illness or impending death in a fitting manner, every healthcare facility has the moral obligation to include on its staff a person who is trained in the dynamics of helping patients accept sickness, suffering, and death in a Christian manner. The value of these pastoral care persons' working closely with healthcare professionals is evident. Crisis counseling is not an arcane art, but on the other hand, one must be adequately prepared to perform it well. Well-meaning but untrained people can do other than good when trying to help in crisis situations.

Kübler-Ross (1978) maintains that to help others face death, one must be at peace with death oneself. The normal training for religious ministry does not prepare a person in this specialty. Several hospitals in the United States, however, have training programs to meet this need. The need for this service in hospitals is clear and has been recognized, but help in facing sickness and death is also necessary for people in a noninstitutional setting, such as for the poor and elderly (Still and Todd, 1986).

In summary, increased knowledge of psychology and greater regard for the subjective process that accompanies sickness and dying has changed the ethical question in regard to truth telling. As Kübler-Ross declares: "The question should not be 'Should we tell?' but rather, 'How do we share this with the patient?'"

13.5   CARE FOR THE CORPSE OR CADAVER

When a human being dies, the body is no longer vivified by the life-giving principle or soul by which it was constituted a substantial element of the human person. The cadaver of a person, then, is not a *human* body in the proper sense of the word. Insofar as is possible, the remains of a person should not be referred to as though the human person existed *in* the human body or was, so to speak, limited by the human body. Language of this nature is misleading because it implies a duality in human existence; in a certain sense, the living human person *is* the living human body. When persons die, they exist in a new form, in a sense incomplete, because they no longer have a body (Rahner, 1965). While existing in this life, the human person is a substantial unity of spirit (form) and body (matter), not an accidental juxtaposition of two distinct entities. The remains of a human body may resemble the body of a living person, and this resemblance may be prolonged through embalming; however, the remains are not a *human* body, but a mass of organic matter, decomposing into constitutive, organic elements.

If the corpse of a human person is not a human body, why are people so concerned about proper care for the remains of the deceased person? Why treat it with the respect and reverence that it usually receives? Respect and reverence are due the remains of a human being because of the sacredness of the human soul, which once informed the now inert mass still bearing the person's image. To mourn that the person will no longer be presenting the same human manner as before, certain reverential spiritual actions are performed that express the love of the people who remain. Respect for the dead body, then, signifies respect for human life, respect for the Author of life, respect for the person who once existed in human form and who now exists in a different modality. Thus the actions and ritual that people follow when caring for the body of a deceased person have a meaning beyond their mere utility.

Although the ritual of wake, funeral, and burial has been criticized for its gross and inhuman excesses (Mitford, 1975), fundamentally this process has a meaning and worth in accord with the Judeo-Christian tradition. Having friends share the burden through liturgical services is also a source of strength and support for bereaved people. Thus the legitimate customs of people at the time

371

of death are not signs of superstition or blind fear; rather, they bespeak a noble belief about life, its purpose, and the enduring strength of human love.

In accord with the respect due to the remains of a human person, no organs should be removed from a corpse, nor should the body be dismembered in any way, unless a sufficient reason justifies such an action. Usually the next of kin or the person to whom the corpse is committed for care has the legal right to determine if organs may be removed from the body and if an autopsy may be performed (*Pierce v. Swan Point*, 1872). The right of the next of kin in regard to caring for the human body is not absolute. It may be superseded by statements made by the person while still alive, for example, through the Uniform Anatomical Gift Act, or by the needs of society, for example, when an autopsy might help stave off a contagious disease. In the future, the need of organs for donation in society may change our assumptions in regard to family rights to donate organs of the deceased (Boyle and O'Rourke, 1986). In Europe, donation of organs meets less juridical opposition (Prottas, 1985).

The Uniform Anatomical Gift Act is "designed to facilitate the donation and use of human tissues and organs for transplantation and other medical purposes and provide a favorable legal environment for such activities" (Lehrman, 1988; Sadler et al., 1968). At present, all 50 states have enacted the Gift Act, thus enabling persons who are of sound mind and 18 years of age or older to give all or part of their bodies to persons or institutions authorized to practice or perform research medicine or to engage in tissue banking, with the gift to take effect at death. This law also recognizes the right of the next of kin to donate the body or any part for the same purpose, but in most states the law declares that if there is a conflict between the donor and the next of kin, the wishes of the donor have precedence. The person or institution to whom the donation is made need not accept the gift. If the gift is accepted, following removal of the part named, the body is transferred to the next of kin or other persons under obligation to dispose of the body. If the whole body is retained for research at a medical school, it will often be cremated on completion of the research. In such cases, there may not be a wake but a funeral service; a memorial mass, for example, is usually celebrated without the corpse being present if the person was Catholic.

Protection from civil and criminal proceedings that might result from the removal of organs or experimentation on the corpse is granted by the Gift Act to all persons concerned, including physicians, next of kin, funeral directors, and medical examiners. However, in practice, if the next of kin refuses the request for organ retrieval, even if the deceased person had signed an anatomical gift donation card, hospitals and physicians will usually follow the decision of the next of kin because they fear malpractice charges. Persons interested in donating a part of all of their body at death should inform their families of their desire so that if possible conflicts will be avoided.

From a Christian point of view, the practice of donating organs and one's body for scientific research is ethical and even to be encouraged if a true need exists. Thus, as Pius XII (1956a) advised:

> The public must be educated. It must be explained with intelligence and respect that to consent explicitly or tacitly to serious damage to the integrity of

372

the corpse, in the interest of those who are suffering, is no violation of the reverence due to the dead.

Another ethical question, however, does not admit such an easy solution: Is it immoral to accept or solicit payment for the gift of certain organs? Although some have defended such practices, other authors (Ramsey, 1975; Transplantation Society, 1985) maintain that abuses could arise very quickly if cadaver organs were sold or contracted for money. Ramsey points out that blood replaces itself, whereas human organs do not. With this latter opinion we agree. If society is to live in a humane manner, generosity and charity, rather than monetary gain and greed, must serve as the basis for donation of functioning organs. The National Organ Transplant Act (McDonald, 1988) prohibits the sale of human organs, although reasonable payments for expenses incurred by the health facility or donor are allowed.

Autopsy

Autopsy is the examination of a cadaver performed to provide greater medical knowledge concerning the cause of death. Occasionally, the benefit of an autopsy will be to provide knowledge about a rare or contagious disease. In such cases, the good of the community would overrule the rights of the next of kin, and if the next of kin were not willing, the court could order that an autopsy be performed. In cases of violent death or unattended death, an autopsy is required by law, no matter what wishes are expressed by the next of kin.

Usually, however, the purpose of an autopsy is not to trace the etiology of a rare disease nor to discover unknown or violent causes of death. More frequently, autopsies are performed to help health professionals achieve a higher level of efficiency in the care of the living (Bowman, 1983). The autopsy rate of a hospital is usually a good sign of concern for excellence and offers a gauge of professional integrity and interest in scientific advancement (Altman, 1988). Through autopsies, the diagnosis and treatment a person received can be evaluated and staff members encouraged to observe a high level of proficiency. For this reason, autopsies should be encouraged and people should be encouraged to look on them as an ordinary part of the medical care process. Needless to say, the human remains of a person should always be treated with utmost respect during an autopsy.

In the Judeo-Christian tradition, respect for the dead was usually displayed through burial of the corpse in the ground or in a mausoleum. Cremation of the remains, although not a common part of this tradition, has never been considered as disrespectful treatment. For a long time, however, cremation was forbidden in the Catholic Church because anti-Christian groups in the eighteenth century advocated cremation as a means of denying symbolically the immortality of the human person and the Resurrection. Thus, not because it was immoral in itself, but rather because of what it might signify, cremation was not an acceptable form of caring for the remains of a person in the Catholic Church.

Because cremation is no longer associated with a denial of religious truth, today, although burying the dead is encouraged as the usual procedure, the total remains or an amputated member may be cremated if there is a serious reason (SCDF, 1963): for example, if the custom of the country favors cremation, if there is danger of disease, or if suitable grave sites cannot be obtained at a reasonable cost. If the request involves no certain sign of disrespect for Christian faith, cremation may be requested by a dying person or the next of kin. Those who direct that their bodies are to be cremated, then, may be given the sacraments of the Church, as well as liturgical rites of burial, provided that the latter are not performed in the actual place of cremation.

Because of what it represents, the remains of a human person should be treated with respect and reverence. Healthcare professionals should never allow their frequent experience of human death to inure them to the great mystery and sacredness of human life. The danger in the practice of medicine at any level of its experience is that people become blasé or insensitive about suffering, death, and human remains to cover their own feelings of fear, inadequacy, or lack of faith. Although such feelings are often unconsciously motivated, they are nonetheless destructive of humane Christian healthcare. Moreover, it bespeaks a personality defect on the part of the healthcare professional that requires a new orientation toward the act and experience of death.

13.6 EUTHANASIA AND SUICIDE

The word *euthanasia* is derived from two Greek words that mean "good death" or "happy death." For centuries, the term referred to an action by which a person was put to death painlessly, usually to avoid further suffering from an incurable disease or to end an irreversible comatose condition. *Webster's New International Dictionary* (5th ed.), for example, defines *euthanasia* as "a mode or act of inducing death painlessly as a relief from pain." Euthanasia in this sense is often called "mercy killing" or even "death with dignity." In the more traditional meaning of the term, it could be performed with or without the consent of the person to be put to death. In the Judeo-Christian tradition, euthanasia without the consent of the patient would be murder and with consent of the patient would be both suicide and murder. Today, the proponents of euthanasia generally defend it in this latter form, where the patient's consent is given or at least presumed. Thus our ethical analysis needs to begin with the question of whether suicide is ever permissible, or whether it exceeds the limits of rightful control over one's own life. The high rate of suicide in the medical profession gives this question a special significance for bioethical reflection (Pitts et al., 1979).

It is important to be clear, as Novak (1971) has pointed out, that the issue here is not whether persons who commit suicide are to be morally condemned. No doubt most persons who take their own lives do so because they are so emotionally disturbed that they act compulsively, or at least their perception of objective reality is so distorted by their anguish and depression that their freedom of choice is greatly restricted. Consequently, either their act is not to be evaluated ethically at all, or at least it may be assumed that they act in good faith and are subjectively guiltless. Many experts in suicidology today seem to take it for granted that all suicides are compulsive and irrational (Durkheim, 1951; Menninger, 1938). Can this assumption really be made, or is there the possibility that the decision about whether to live or to take one's life may be a genuine ethical issue for some people who have the capacity to make a free and sane choice (Mayo, 1986)? Only in such cases does it make any sense to talk about the *morality* of suicide.

The Greeks and Romans both condemned and defended suicide (Choron, 1972; Noyes, 1973), as did Eastern cultures (Holck, 1974). The Epicureans, who considered pleasure and peace of mind the highest human goods, argued that it was better to kill oneself than to endure life if it had become more painful than pleasurable or peaceful. The Stoics, who believed that virtue or self-control was the highest good, argued that it was permissible to kill oneself if suffering or torture might force one to lose self-control or act ignobly, or where a choice had to be made to perish in a shameful way or "die with dignity." Dualists, such as some Platonists (but not Plato himself), agnostics, and Manicheans taught that the soul, which is the real person, is burdened by the body in this life or in many reincarnations; thus suicide might be justified as a laying down of this burden. Even in Christian Europe men and women have been regarded as heroic if they committed suicide for the sake of honor. Recently, some Catholic Irishmen and Buddhist Vietnamese have used suicide by self-starvation or self-immolation as a protest against injustice.

The monotheistic religions of Judaism, Christianity, and Islam have always opposed suicide, however, because they regard life as God's gift, which his children are to use as faithful stewards. Moreover, these monotheistic religions, unlike others, hold that eternal life is not the survival of a disembodied soul, nor endless reincarnation, but resurrected life with God. Consequently, Christians cannot escape accounting to God for stewardship of the bodies given them on earth, nor can they reject the body that will always be part of them. This view was already anticipated by the great Greek philosopher Plato, who argued that suicide is a rejection of duty to one's body, to the community of which the person is a part, and to God who gave the person life. In a very different way, another great philosopher, Kant, argued that suicide is the greatest of crimes because it is a person's rejection of morality itself, since a person must be his or her own moral lawgiver (see section 7.3). To kill oneself is to treat oneself as a thing (a means) rather than as a person.

Other Opinions

Today, however, this classical stand is being questioned (Engelhardt, 1986c; J. Rosenberg, 1983; Sluis, 1979). The Protestant moralist Joseph Fletcher (1960) has said, "The real issue is whether we can morally justify taking it into our own hands to hasten death for ourselves (suicide) or for others (mercy killing) out of reasons of compassion." Fletcher answers this in terms of his own situationism, according to which the only command of God is to "act lovingly." This leads Fletcher to an ethics of intention that justifies any means if it is effective for achieving loving ends because, "If we will the end, we will the means."

Consequently, it appears to him that there are many situations in which persons can will their own death for the good of others (as a war prisoner fearing torture that may cause him to reveal the hiding place of others) or in which others may be put to death out of compassion for their sufferings, assuming that they would want this to be done for them (McEllhenney, 1973).

Catholic theologians generally reject situationism, but those who hold for the principle of proportion, as developed by Knauer and others, are arguing that the moral law against suicide and euthanasia admits exceptions. Thus the Catholic moralist Daniel Maguire, in *Death by Choice* (1974, 1984), maintains:

> What he [Knauer] means is that the taking of innocent life is wrong if there is no commensurate reason for taking it....At the theoretical level, then, Knauer's ethical theory allows for euthanasia, suicide, or abortion under his dominant rubric of "commensurate reason." He slips out from under the old rule against intentionally taking human innocent life and comes up under the position that commensurate reason is what counts (p. 69).

Maguire maintains that Knauer and McCormick "are not willing to go as far as their theories"; that is, they consider mercy killing and suicide to be wrong because no proportionate good could come from allowing exceptions. However, Maguire is willing to follow the theory to its ultimate conclusions, and he states, "The morality of terminating life, innocent or not, is an open question, although it is widely treated as a closed one (p. 112)." Maguire believes termination of life can be moral or immoral according to the circumstances that give it moral meaning. He also claims that the traditional argument that suicide violates God's dominion over human life is not persuasive, since if God gives us a share in his dominion over our life in most matters, as he clearly does, why not over our death as well?

In general, these Christian thinkers believe that to make an absolute rule against suicide is, under some circumstances, to fail to respond compassionately to useless human suffering or to draw subtle distinctions that indicate the Pharisaic legalistic mentality repudiated by Christ. Humanists, emphasizing the autonomy of the individual, tend to favor the right of all persons to determine when their own life shall cease (Engelhardt, 1986c; Narveson, 1983). What values and countervalues, then, need to be balanced to decide in particular circumstances whether suicide is permissible (Battlin and Mayo, 1980)? The usual advantages often mentioned can be summarized as follows:

1. Suicide gives the human person full autonomy since he or she can choose to live or die, to be part of society or reject it.
2. Suicide enables a person to leave life with dignity, instead of enduring useless suffering, being a burden to others, and so forth, or suffering mental disease or unjustified disgrace and dishonor.
3. Suicide may enable one to avoid temptation to treacherous or ignoble acts that destroy one's personal integrity or that may be harmful to others, such as the revelation of secrets under torture.
4. Suicide relieves one's family, and also society, of burdens, so that their resources can be used for something better.

5. Suicide can be an act of heroic sacrifice for others, such as the kamikaze pilots in World War II.
6. Suicide can be a protest against social injustice, such as the Buddhist monks who burned themselves in protest against tyranny in Vietnam or the Irish Catholic hunger strikers.

The following disadvantages are also frequently mentioned:

1. Suicide is an intrinsic evil for a person to reject living out life to its full, since there is opportunity for personal growth as long as conscious suffering or conscious endurance is possible.
2. Suicide is contradictory to the very basis of morality, since by this act the person gives up all other moral responsibilities.
3. Suicide is not a road to immortal life, since that life is mysterious, and whether this is the proper way to enter it is not known.
4. By suicide the individual withdraws himself or herself from the community that has given him or her life and deprives it of a unique member.
5. Suicide is a rejection of God because it is a rejection of God's gift of life.
6. Suicide deeply hurts a person's loved ones and discourages them in their own task of living.

When these various values are weighed one against another in concrete cases, the reasons given to justify suicide are either social or personal. As regards the social reasons that persons might believe they have a duty in justice or charity to kill themselves for the good of others, Chapters 8 and 10 argue that society has no right to require some of its members to directly sacrifice their life for others, although it can require that they perform some positive action for the common good, which may involve the risk or even the certainty that they may incur death. Thus those who kill themselves because they believe this will benefit others are following an exaggerated sense of moral obligation, while at the same time they are failing to fulfill their social obligations to continue to participate in the life of the community.

It is probable that the personal reasons for suicide often underlie the social arguments. Basically, persons kill themselves because "there is no other way out" (Siegl and Tuchel, 1985). The question, therefore, is whether this can ever be reasonably said to be true. There is no doubt that one can *feel* this way easily enough, but can one conscientiously judge that it is really the case? Essentially, human persons are historical beings oriented to the future. As long as there is hope for a future, suicide is clearly unreasonable. When hope in the future is closed off, suicide may appear a rational thing to do. In a Christian scheme of values, however, hope in God grounds the future. By God's providence even the most painful situations not only can be endured, but also may be extremely important events in the completion of earthly life. In a humanist or Marxist system this may not be true, but Christians ought to wait on the God who gave them life, since he knows best how to prepare them for the mystery of eternal life with him.

Thus attempts to balance the various values of suicide lead back to the conclusion that suicide is intrinsically and always wrong, since in all circumstances it constitutes an abdication of one's responsibility to live out life in community with other persons and with God (Grisez, 1977). With this in mind, the statement of the Catholic Church, *Declaration on Euthanasia* (SCDF, 1980a) condemned suicide in the following words:

> Intentionally causing one's own death, or suicide, is equally as wrong as murder; such an action on the part of a person is to be considered as a rejection of God's sovereignty and loving plan. Furthermore, suicide is also often a refusal of love for self, the denial of the natural instinct to live, a flight from the duties of justice and charity owed to one's neighbor, to various communities or to the whole of society (p. 512).

As for the argument that if God shares with us a stewardship over life, why not over death, it should be noted that our stewardship over life presupposes that we *preserve* our life, not destroy it. Suicide is a rejection of God's gift of life and therefore of God the giver, not a use of that life in the service of the purposes for which God gave it.

Rejecting a Distinction

"By euthanasia is understood an action or omission of an action which of itself or by intention causes death in order that all suffering may be eliminated" (SCDF, 1980a). This statement of the Church emphasizing that euthanasia may result from an act or an omission of an act calls into question the distinction between *active* and *passive* euthanasia, which we used in previous editions of this book (2nd ed., p. 379). With others (Reichenbach, 1987), we equated passive euthanasia with allowing to die when there was no moral obligation to prolong life. Thus we considered active and passive euthanasia to be morally different. However, we now perceive that the term *passive euthanasia* was used by many to signify withholding treatment *regardless* of the moral obligation to prolong life. Therefore it seems more accurate to consider euthanasia, whether active or passive, as intending the death of a person in order to end suffering and bringing about that death by positive action (inducing death) or by omission (withholding treatment), when there is a moral obligation to prolong the person's life. Thus, as we use the term in this edition, the distinction between active and passive euthanasia does not constitute a moral difference. Active and passive euthanasia are both violations of another person's humanity. Using the term euthanasia with this connotation corresponds more exactly to the terminology of the recent Church teaching, and it also obviates the objections raised by some ethicists that if passive euthanasia is acceptable, active euthanasia should be acceptable as well (Brewin, 1986; Rachels, 1983). However, we continue to maintain that a clear moral distinction exists between euthanasia and allowing to die when there is no longer any moral obligation to prolong life (O'Donnell, 1987). The reasons that justify the decision that there is no longer a moral obligation to prolong life are discussed in the next section.

When persons freely choose to die and ask to be killed, they are not only committing the crime of suicide but also compounding it by making another a partner in the crime. To yield to such a request is false compassion (J. Sullivan, 1952). To have true compassion for the person who has made such a decision is to realize that the person feels hopeless, alienated from community, and doubtful of God's love. Mercy entails staying by such a person's side and through friendship helping him or her to recover hope. The mercy killer in such a case is really adding a final rejection to the many rejections that have already driven the person to that point of despair (Iglesias, 1984b).

On the other hand, if the sufferer is no longer really free to make a truly human decision but is pleading to be put out of the pain or depression that has taken away his or her capacity to think straight, the mercy killer is simply a murderer putting to death someone no longer able to protect himself or herself (Gula, 1987).

If the motives of mercy killers are examined, their claim that they did it for the sake of the victim cannot be easily accepted. The real motive may well be that the relative did not want to accept the responsibility of helping the dying person to the end. Often the killer says, "I loved my mother, I couldn't bear to see her suffer!" It is true in such a case that the killer could not bear to see her suffer, but the quality of that love is not so certain. No doubt, however, sometimes mercy killers are themselves not free enough from tortured feelings to make a sane decision. Medical personnel hardly have such excuses. By consenting to help their patients die, they may simply be evading the painful and threatening task of adequate spiritual care for the dying, which is discussed in Chapter 14.

As for the type of euthanasia used by the Nazis, in which patients were put to death without their consent because they were senile, insane, or defective, or as genocide, few in the United States today would defend such a practice, but some are beginning to discuss the morality of euthanasia for people in a comatose condition (Humphrey, 1982; Scott, 1983).

Generally, the medical profession has rejected euthanasia absolutely (AMA, 1988b), as is evidenced by the Hippocratic Oath as well as by more recent codes of medical ethics, such as The Geneva Declaration (1957) and the Helsinki Statement of the World Health Organization (1964). However, the tendency of the medical profession in the United States to prolong the act of dying even after the patient does not benefit from life-prolonging therapy has caused many people to opt for euthanasia as a certain manner of ending life when medical therapy is no longer beneficial (Crisp, 1987; Feinstein, 1986). The fear of prolonged dying has also led to creation of the living will (Marzen, 1986), and when the living will proved to be unsatisfactory, to creation of the durable power of attorney for incompetent people (Peters, 1987). Although the living will and durable power of attorney are not unethical and may even be helpful in some cases, they do not of themselves eliminate the decision-making problems that arise at the time of death (S. Johnson, 1987). As we discuss next, ethical treatment of patients at the time of death depends on a clear understanding of the ethical norms for withholding and withdrawing life support from persons with fatal pathology. Generally, the Christian churches have rejected euthanasia (Meilander, 1982). Repeating the consistent teaching of the Catholic Church (B. Ashley, 1987), the *Declaration On Euthanasia* (SCDF, 1980a) states:

379

It is necessary to state firmly once more that nothing and no one can in any way permit the killing of an innocent human being, whether a fetus or an embryo, an infant or an old person, or one suffering from an incurable disease, or a person who is dying. Furthermore, no one is permitted to ask for this act of killing for himself or herself or for another person entrusted to his or her care, nor can he or she consent to it either explicitly or implicitly. Nor can any authority legitimately recommend or permit such an action. For it is a question of the violation of the divine law, an offense against the dignity of the human person, a crime against life, and an attack on humanity (p. 511).

13.7   ALLOWING TO DIE

God gave us the gift of human life to show forth his goodness and love (Gn 1). We in turn show our love for God by respecting and fostering the gift of human life. As Jesus taught, love for God leads us not only to love ourselves, but to love others as well (Mt 22:37). One way to show our love for God, for ourselves, and for others is to prolong human life. Prolonging life is also one of our fundamental human needs. Although human life is a great good on which many other basic goods depend, Sacred Scripture indicates that it is not the ultimate good (Senay, 1981). At times the choice of another good may justify the indirect surrender of human life. In these circumstances, one does not choose death. Rather, one chooses another good, foreseeing that death will result as an unwanted effect of that choice. Jesus on the cross, for example, chose to do the Father's will and freely gave his human life for the salvation of the world. Martyrs surrender their lives rather than deny God in their hour of crisis. Thus Christians have always maintained that life could be surrendered indirectly, if continuing to live would impede the response of love for God. Making choices in this manner is an example of the Principle of Double Effect (8.1; Mangan, 1949).

Philosophical reasoning and Church teaching indicate that life need not be prolonged at all costs (Linacre Center for the Study of the Ethics of Health Care, 1979). The traditional manner of expressing the reasons that justify removing or withholding life support and thus allowing a person to die is to state that life need not be prolonged if the means to prolong life are (1) ineffective or (2) constitute a grave burden (G. Kelly, 1951; National Conference of Catholic Bishops [NCCB], 1986). Although these two reasons for withholding and withdrawing care are traditional in the literature of medicine and ethics (President's Commission for Study of Ethical Problems in Medicine and Biomedical and Behavioral Research, 1981), they must be clearly understood before they may be used accurately. For example, "ineffective means" for what goal? Or "grave burden" in regard to what goal? It seems Pope Pius XII (1957) answered these questions by stressing that the spiritual purpose of life should be the goal to which medical care is ultimately directed and by which its effectiveness is evaluated. In an often-quoted statement, he declared:

> Normally [when prolonging life is in question] one is held to use only ordinary means—according to the circumstances of persons, places, times, and cultures—that is to say, means that do not involve any grave burdens for oneself or for another. A more strict obligation would be too burdensome for

most people and would render the attainment of higher, more important good too difficult. *Life, health, all temporal activities are in fact subordinated to spiritual ends* (p. 2).

A more complete statement of the reasons that justify withholding or withdrawing medical care thus would be the following: the means to prolong life may be withheld or withdrawn if these means are ineffective to help a person strive for the spiritual purpose of life, or if they impose a grave burden on the person in regard to striving for the purpose of life (Schindler, 1988).

To understand clearly the ethical difference between euthanasia and allowing to die, several other distinctions must be understood clearly:

1. One confusing factor in determining medical care when death is in question is the use of the terms *imminent death and terminal condition.* These phrases often are introduced as though they determine a patient's medical care. According to some (May, 1987), only if death is imminent, may care be withdrawn. For example, in the Karen Quinlan and Paul Brophy cases, the lower courts refused permission to remove life-support mechanisms because they said "death was not imminent." The lower courts, and some other interested parties (Diamond, 1986), used the terms "imminent death" or "terminal condition" to indicate that a person would not die in the foreseeable future because life support had already been applied. Using the terms in this manner begs the question. The important question is not how long the patient might live with or without life-support systems, but whether there is a moral responsibility to initiate or continue life support. The Supreme Courts of New Jersey and Massachusetts when reversing the lower courts in the Quinlan and Brophy cases realized that "imminent death" was not the ethical issue. Rather, they considered whether or not the therapy was effective and whether or not it imposed a grave burden on the patients. As already indicated, the determination of whether or not life support is a moral responsibility is not solved by asking, "how long will the patient live if life support is utilized, but rather by asking the question: Is the life support effective, or does it impose a grave burden." The answers to these questions require an evaluation of the life support as it contributes to the spiritual goal of the individual patient, "from consideration of circumstances of persons, places, times and cultures" as Pius XII said.

2. The terms *ordinary* and *extraordinary* are often used when discussing whether or not life support should be utilized or not (O'Rourke, 1988). These terms must be used carefully or confusion will result because the terms are used differently by physicians and ethicists. Physicians use "ordinary" to describe an accepted or standard medical procedure. A procedure or medicine that is new or untested or still in the experimental stage is called "extraordinary." Thus, from the physician's point of view, something that was once extraordinary, such as cardiac angioplasty, may become ordinary because its therapeutic worth is proven. From an ethical perspective, on the other hand, a means to prolong life is "ordinary" and is morally obligatory, whereas a means that is "extraor-

dinary" is morally optional. Ordinary means to prolong life from the ethical perspective are "all medicines, treatments, and operations which offer a reasonable hope of benefit for the patient and which can be obtained or used without excessive expense, pain, or burden; extraordinary means are all medicines, treatments, and operations which cannot be used or obtained without expense, pain, or other burden" (Pius XII, 1957; Connery, 1980). When determining whether a particular medicine, procedure, or mechanical device is an ordinary or extraordinary means of medical care, one must consider the condition of the patient as well as all the social and familial circumstances. Hence, an a *priori* list of ordinary and extraordinary means of life support from the ethical perspective cannot be constructed. Before evaluating the means to prolong life as ordinary or extraordinary in the ethical sense one must consider the condition of the patient.

The recent Church statement *Declaration on Euthanasia* (SCDF, 1980a), as well as several ethicists (McCormick, 1984; Showalter, 1984) maintain that the terms *ordinary* and *extraordinary* are misleading and that they should be replaced by the terms *proportionate* and *disproportionate*. Although we recognize the potential confusion that may arise from inexact use of ordinary or extraordinary means, we believe that they are as accurate as any other terms when used with a view to particular patients and with the realization that from an ethical perspective, they have a different meaning than when used from a medical perspective. As Paul Ramsey (1970) declared when discussing the terms ordinary and extraordinary "These are meaningful specifications but there is uncertainty in applying them."

3. The meaning of the term *effective means to prolong* life is subject to debate. As we have indicated, we believe that this term refers to prolonging life in such a manner that the person in question is able to strive for the spiritual purpose of the life (O'Rourke, 1988). In order to strive for the spiritual purpose of life, one needs some degree of cognitive-affective function. Others, however, would maintain that a means is effective as long as it prolongs human life only at the minimal level of vegetative function, with no hope of restoring the capacity necessary for spiritual function (Barry, 1986). Thus some ethicists maintain that there is a moral obligation to prolong the life of people even if the medical diagnosis states that the person is in an irreversible coma or persistent vegetative state and will not regain cognitive-affective function, as long as there is no physical pain for the patients (May, 1987). This difference of opinion surfaces vividly in regard to the use of artificial nutrition and hydration for patients in a persistent vegetative state (Lynn, 1986). Many maintain that artificial nutrition and hydration should be evaluated as one would evaluate any other medical treatment, such as a respirator (AMA, 1986). Thus, if cognitive-affective function cannot be restored, the artificial nutrition and hydration may be withheld or withdrawn because there is no moral obligation to continue using ineffective

medical means (Annas, 1985; Cranford, 1984; O'Rourke, 1986; Rosoff, 1988). Others would maintain that artificial nutrition and hydration may be withheld or removed only if the therapy constitutes a grave physical burden (May, 1987; New Jersey Catholic Conference, 1986). Some proponents of this latter opinion maintain that artificial hydration and nutrition are not medical treatment, but rather constitute comfort care that should be given to everyone (Pontifical Academy, 1985). Even if artificial hydration and nutrition are considered comfort care, however, they may be withdrawn if they are ineffective or impose a serious burden upon the patient. The distinction between medical care and comfort care does not obviate the declaration that something is not morally obligatory if it is ineffective or imposes a grave burden to pursuing one's spiritual goal. Persons who are in a state of permanent cognitive-affective deprivation apparently do not experience pain (American Academy of Neurology, 1986); thus artificial nutrition would not be effective as comfort measures. Moreover, the serious burden arising from care whether medical or nursing may be spiritual or social as well as physical (Brophy, 1986). Therefore the indignity of existing in a state of persistent cognitive-affective deprivation would be a serious burden, as would the burden that a family would endure in caring for a person in such a condition. In this regard, it is significant to note that Pope Pius XII indicated that a grave burden "for oneself or another" might render a means to prolong life extraordinary. In hospices and nursing homes for religious, artificial nutrition and hydration are seldom used when there is little hope of restoring cognitive-affective function, yet such institutions are considered the epitome of comfort care for the dying. To date, the authority of the Church has not given a definitive statement regarding the use of artificial hydration and nutrition for patients who are permanently unconscious. We believe our opinion is based upon the traditional teaching of the Church regarding the use of life prolonging therapy, but we remain open to further development of Church teaching.

4. When considering the term *grave burden*, we may consider the burdens that arise from social, psychological, and spiritual circumstance, as well as those that arise from physical circumstances. A father who contracts cancer may determine that, rather than spend his life savings on surgery and hospitalization, he will devote his savings to the education of this children, allowing the cancer to take its natural course. A person undergoing dialysis may determine that the therapy is too burdensome from a social point of view. A person who might survive if on a ventilator 24 hours a day may decide that living in that condition would put too much strain on his or her family and ask to have the respirator removed. The person who makes a decision of this nature does not intend death, nor does he or she cause death. Rather, the person chooses a moral good incompatible with life, and death results from the underlying pathologies, the effects of which the person may have

previously circumvented (O'Donnell, 1987). One has the moral right to avoid a serious burden even if one foresees that death might ensue indirectly as a result of choosing to avoid the burden.

The nature of the decision was expressed in the *Declaration on Euthanasia* (SCDF, 1980a) in the following manner:

> It is also permissible to make do with the normal means that medicine can offer. Therefore one cannot impose on anyone the obligation to have recourse to a technique which is already in use but which carries a risk or is burdensome. Such a refusal is not the equivalent of suicide; on the contrary, it should be considered as an acceptance of the human condition or a wish to avoid the application of a medical procedure disproportionate to the results that can be expected or a desire not to impose excessive expense on the family or the community.

The practical difficulties concerning when to withhold or withdraw life-support equipment will always be present. Although there is no moral difference between withholding and withdrawing life support (President's Commission for the Study of Ethical Problems, 1983d), the emotional difference is a reality and should never be overlooked. The difficulty of decision making is especially acute when treatment for newborn infants with birth defects is in question. Without falling into a quality of life ethic, parents and healthcare professionals must realize that in some cases continuing life support of the newborn "would render the attainment of the higher more important good too difficult" (McCormick, 1974; Bryce, 1985). On the other hand, aggressive care of handicapped and genetically deprived infants should be instituted, with the ethical questions, is the care effective? will it impose a grave burden? being asked as treatment continues (Rostain, 1986). The attitude expressed in the original Baby Doe regulations of the Federal Government (Federal Register, 1983) that the life of every infant must be prolonged as long as possible no matter what impairment, is ethically unacceptable.

Who Decides

Who makes the difficult and delicate ethical decision that life should or should not be prolonged and that a certain means is ordinary or extraordinary? Some place the burden primarily on the physician (Tomilson and Brody, 1988); some believe it should be the duty of the courts to protect the rights of incompetent patients (Horan and Grant, 1984); others propose that ethics committees become involved in the discussion (Ruark and Raffin, 1988). Clearly the physician is involved in the decision in an integral manner and has the responsibility of considering the condition of the patient and determining the medical prognosis, that is, whether the means in question will cure, help appreciably, or have no effect on the dying patient (R. Gillon, 1985a). However, there are other circumstances to be considered in addition to the medical effectiveness of the means. What about expense, pain, spiritual and social burden? Only the patient or the family can decide concerning these circumstances. Thus the essential right to make a decision as to what would be an ordinary means and what would be an extraordinary means from an ethical point of view belongs to the patient (Pellegrino, 1981; J. Rosenberg and Towers, 1986). With the guidance of the physician, often in consultation with family members, the patient decides what actions should be performed and which should be omitted. The physician-patient relationship is expressed aptly in this manner (Pius XII, 1957):

> The rights and duties of the doctor are correlative to those of the patient. The doctor, in fact, has no separate or independent right where the patient is concerned. In general, he can take action only if the patient explicitly or implicitly, directly or indirectly, gives him permission (p. 3).

The statement of the AMA House of Delegates (1973) corresponds with this thinking:

> The cessation of the employment of extraordinary means to prolong life of the body when there is irrefutable evidence that biological death is imminent is the decision of the patient and/or his immediate family. The advice and judgment of the physician should be freely available to the patient and/or his immediate family (p. 4).

The most difficult problems arise when the patient is incompetent to decide concerning proper medical treatment (Annas, 1983; Cassel, 1984; Gutheil and Applebaum, 1985; Paris, 1986). Special care must be taken to defend the right to life of such persons. Some physicians are tempted, for example, to judge too easily that newborn children who suffer from a serious handicap are not to be treated (Bopp, 1985; J. Freeman, 1986). On the other hand, parents who have just been informed that a newborn is handicapped may too quickly decide to allow such children to die (Annas, 1979; Dubler, 1985; McLane, 1986). Patients who are severely depressed may also refuse treatment that they would have accepted in a better frame of mind (Steinbrook and Lo, 1986). There is evidence also of serious neglect of patients in long term care facilities who are allowed to go untreated (J. Warren et al., 1986). Consequently, great caution is always necessary in "letting die" decisions for incompetent persons.

This has led some (C. Baron, 1984; Robertson, 1983) to argue that the rights of incompetent patients are best protected by an appeal to the courts, where the adversary process ensures greater protection. It is also debated whether the courts should accept "substituted judgment" or "best interest of the patient" as the criteria for its own decisions (DeLancy, 1986). To date, in a whole series of cases, *Quinlan, Saikewicz, Perlmutter, Spring, Eichner (Brother Fox), Conroy, Jobes,* and *Brophy,* the courts have approved the withholding of treatment even if death might result (Kamisar, 1985; R. McIntyre, 1986). In our opinion, only in cases of conflict where one of the parties believes that the rights of the patient are imperiled, there should be recourse to the courts. Ordinarily, however, the physician should counsel the guardians by giving a medical opinion as to risks and benefits, and the guardians should make the decision on the basis of the patient's best interest, that is, to decide what is beneficial for the patient, given the circumstances that prevail. Best interest of the patient should respect the patient's reasonable wishes, if these wishes are known. However, the prior wishes of the incompetent patient should not be considered as the sole criterion for determining treatment because in the face of prevailing circumstances, the patient's prior wishes may be unreasonable. "Where the proper and independent duty of the family is concerned, they are usually bound only to the use of ordinary means (Pope Pius XII, 1957)."

Pain

Dying patients are often in pain, and questions arise about the proper medical treatment. The following considerations are offered to help make ethical decisions concerning pain control.

1. Pain is not an absolute human evil. Although suffering is to be alleviated whenever possible, it is not of itself a moral evil nor without supernatural and human benefits when rightly used (see also chapter 13.1). Some will scoff at this view of life, but the Christian tradition holds that great spiritual good can come out of suffering when this is joined to the suffering of Jesus. Christian teaching in this regard is often misrepresented, but it does not imply a masochistic desire for pain, nor does it stand in the way of medical progress. As one group of Christians who have investigated the situation (Amulree et al., 1975) maintain, "A terminal illness can be transformed into a time for which everyone concerned is grateful."

2. Alleviating pain by means of medicine or even by surgery does not constitute euthanasia, even if the suffering person's life might be shortened as a result of the medical or surgical procedure (Pius XII, 1957; SCDF, 1980a). In this case, the direct object of the act is to relieve pain; if life is shortened, it is an accidental, even though foreseen, result. This view is expressed succinctly in the U.S. Catholic Conference's *Ethical and Religious Directives for Catholic Health Facilities* (1971): "It is not euthanasia to give a dying person sedatives and analgesics for the alleviation of pain when such measure is judged necessary, even though they may deprive the patient of the use of reason, or shorten his life" (n. 29).

The opportunity to use suffering as a means of spiritual growth is not destroyed if pain-killing drugs are used. Rather, the individual and those who care for him or her have the right to use such drugs in a way that will permit the best use of the patient's remaining energies and time of consciousness, so that the patient can complete life with maximal composure.

3. In recent years, medical and psychological breakthroughs have occurred in regard to severe pain. Medically speaking, pharmaceutical and surgical procedures make it possible to control and alleviate severe pain in the hospital and at home. Severe and excruciating pain, then, is

hardly a realistic excuse for direct euthanasia or suicide. Moreover, an even more startling discovery in the control of pain has been made by people in the hospice movement (Krakoff, 1985; Perkins and Jonsen, 1985). Case studies demonstrate that pain is alleviated and controlled when human concern and care are given to the elderly. The ultimate human pain seems to be loneliness and the feeling of dying alone. If these feelings are overcome, it seems that pain is not such a prominent factor, even for those who are dying of debilitating disease (Kübler-Ross, 1969, 1978; Torrens, 1985).

Pastoral Norms

In summary, the following pastoral norms for decision making in regard to allowing to die can be formulated:
1. A physician may admit that a patient is incurable and cease trying to effect a cure; however, physicians should not cease trying to find a remedy for disease itself.
2. As long as there is a slight hope for curing patients or checking the progress of their illness, the physician should use the available remedies at hand, if this is the desire of the patient or proxy. However, the patient or proxy may refuse treatment if it is ineffective or constitutes a serious burden to the patient. The burden may be psychic, social, or spiritual, as well as physiological.
3. The patient, considering his or her medical prognosis as well as other spiritual and temporal circumstances of life, should determine in consultation with the physician whether a particular means is ordinary or extraordinary from an ethical point of view.
4. If the means are ordinary, they must be used; if the means are extraordinary, they may be used but need not be. Minimal means of maintaining the patient's comfort and well-being are always considered ordinary means (SCDF, 1980a).
5. If the patient is unable to make the pertinent decisions, family members, in consultation with the physician, should have the right and obligation to determine whether the means in question are ordinary or extraor-dinary and whether extraordinary means will be used. In making this decision, the family should decide as the patient would and for the benefit of the patient, not solely for the benefit of the family.
6. Such documents as the *Christian Affirmation of Life* and the *Living Will* may be used by patients as a means of informing family and physician and as a help in preparing for death (O'Rourke, 1974). We do not, however, favor that such documents be given legal status. Although such documents are not in themselves wrong, they do not solve the problems of decision making, and potentially they may led to disrespect for human life and inhumane care for the dying (Lebacqz, 1977; Stephens, 1986).

Part 5

PASTORAL MINISTRY IN HEALTHCARE

This book deals with persons seeking health, with the healthcare professionals who serve them in this search, and finally with some of the many difficult ethical decisions professionals and health seekers have to make together. This concluding Part 5, which consists of a single chapter, deals with one member of the healthcare team whose professional status is often not recognized, yet who has a very special, integrative role to perform on that team and in its ethical decision making, namely, the pastoral care minister.

CHAPTER 14

Pastoral Care and Ethical Decisions

OVERVIEW

Much of the material in this section may seem to be liturgical rather than ethical. It sums up the ethical purpose of this book, however, because medical ethics is concerned not with rules about forbidden procedures, but with a healing process that respects the sanctity of the individual person and seeks to restore the person to full participation in community. We first show that pastoral care is needed on the health team not as an adjunct to psychotherapy or social work, but precisely in its service to human persons in their search for spiritual health (14.1), which we argued in Chapter 2 is essential for total health, and also in service to the hospital staff itself (14.2). We then discuss the ways in which pastoral ministry can make this contribution to healthcare through spiritual counseling (14.3) and the celebration of Word and Sacrament (14.4). In this way, a truly caring and therapeutic community can be formed in which the crises of ethical decisions can best be met. Finally, in 14.5 we conclude by discussing the ways in which the religious minister can assist professionals, patients, and their families in the actual process of ethical decision.

14.1 RELIGIOUS MINISTRY AND THE HEALTHCARE TEAM

Need for Pastoral Healthcare

If Christian ministry is to be Christlike, care for the sick undoubtedly is an essential part of it. At least a third of the Gospel according to St. Mark, aside from the passion narrative devoted to Jesus' own suffering and death, is devoted to accounts of how Jesus healed the physically and mentally sick. His care for the sick seems to have been the clearest evidence to others of his mission from the Father and of the life-giving truth of his preaching.

Studies devoted to the history of pastoral care (Clebsch and Jaekle, 1964; Holifield, 1983) conclude that, traditionally, religious ministry has four functions: (1) to heal, (2) to sustain, (3) to guide, and (4) to reconcile. Whereas by healing and sustaining they have in mind something broader than physical and psychological healing and encouragement in times of sickness, it is obvious that ministers cannot heal and sustain if they are not intimately concerned with problems of physical and psychological health. Furthermore, we show in later sections that guidance and reconciliation are in some respects especially effective when they occur in times of health crisis.

The hospital in Western culture (6.3) originated in the pastoral care of the sick and only with the rise of humanism in the eighteenth century began to subordinate that concern to purely medical care. Even in the nineteenth century, however, the nursing profession in its modern form was the creation of Florence Nightingale, herself inspired by the Christian ideals of the Anglican Church and her work inspired by the tradition of the Catholic nursing sisters. Today, however, in many hospitals, pastoral care is left to occasional visiting ministers who are treated much as any other visitor. In others, a chaplain is provided, but he is regarded by the medical staff simply as a convenience to the patients such as the hospital barber or proprietor of the gift shop. It is becoming much more common, however, even for public hospitals to include a department of pastoral care as a recognized part of their therapeutic work. The members of such a department are still often regarded as somewhat less than professional colleagues of the medical staff, who think of them according to outmoded stereotypes (Richards and Johnson, 1980).

The first reason for this situation is the secularization of the medical profession, which believes itself neutral to religious concerns. This is the case even in many, perhaps most, Catholic and other church-related hospitals, where a large part of the medical staff may not be members of the sponsoring church. Even when a Catholic hospital has a largely Catholic medical staff, these healthcare professionals may still conceive their own tasks as rigidly separated from the concerns of pastoral care. Our interpretation of this secularization, on which we insist throughout this book, is that it is neither neutral, nor genuinely pluralistic, but sincere fidelity to humanism as an equivalent religion.

Thus the question arises as to whether a purely secular hospital serving principally humanist patients (who make up probably at least 40 percent of the American public) should have a pastoral care department and, if so, what its character should be. We believe that such a healthcare facility would still need a pastoral care department, although it probably should have a different name more in keeping with they symbolic system of humanism. The purpose of such a department would be to help patients deal with these existential (spiritual) problems that arise so acutely in times of illness or dying. The recent spate of books and articles on death and dying, many written from a purely humanist point of view, are evidence of this concern (D. Maguire, 1974; Rachels, 1983; Regan, 1986). Also, this need cannot be met adequately by psychotherapists or social workers. Some psychotherapists have developed an existential psychology to deal with human problems at this deeper level; for reasons already given in Chapter 12, however, this exceeds the professional competence of therapists, who are not ordinarily prepared to deal with philosophical issues concerning the meaning of life and with questions of ethical evaluation.

391

Since today most hospitals are pluralistic, a counselor working from the viewpoint of humanism must also be prepared to assist patients of other faiths. To do so, the humanist counselor must be able to take an honestly ecumenical approach, not scorning the value systems of Catholics, Protestants, and Jews. To do this adequately, a humanist spiritual care department would probably have to include some professionals committed to the major faiths.

The same standards, on the other hand, should hold also for church-sponsored healthcare facilities. In a Catholic hospital, pastoral care should be thoroughly Catholic, but as the Second Vatican Council has taught, being truly Catholic requires accepting pluralism and ecumenism. Thus Catholic hospitals should provide counseling for the large number of humanist patients who say they "have no religion," are "not interested in religion," and so forth. Such counseling should respect the system of values by which humanist patients live and should avoid proselytical or denominational pressures. At the same time, it should not neglect the need of such patients to deal with the problems of suffering, death, alienation, and loneliness on their own terms. The pastoral care departments in large church-sponsored hospitals need to provide professional counselors who are themselves humanists and thus able to help humanist patients.

A second reason for the ambiguous situation of pastoral care in many hospitals is that in fact the chaplain or others occupied in pastoral care lack specialized professional training to work with the sick. Although all ministerial education includes general skill in pastoral healthcare, assignments to a chaplaincy or pastoral care department in a modern hospital require specialization. Catholic hospitals only recently have begun to move away from the period when the local bishop supplied the hospitals of his diocese with a chaplain priest, often one unable to accept a regular pastoral assignment because of age or illness, but who could reside at the hospital and administer the sacraments. Catholic hospitals are now hiring only those chaplains certified for special training and competency in healthcare.

The development of *clinical pastoral education* (CPE) as the result of the pioneering work of Anton Boisen (1936, 1945) and its accreditation through a national association involved a shift to a more psychotherapeutic approach to the sick (Cobb, 1977; Derrickson and Ebersolo, 1986; Hiltner, 1969). This shift agreed in some respects with the traditional Protestant emphasis on pastoral counseling, but it produced a certain tension in ministerial identity for those who found it hard to reconcile the moralistic and evangelistic emphasis of their tradition with modern psychotherapy's stress on guiltless self-expression.

Because of their emphasis on sacramental ministry, in which counseling was often largely restricted to hearing confessions, Catholics were slower to accept the new psychotherapeutic approach. However, after the Second Vatican Council, CPE began to be a regular part of priestly formation in many seminaries, and the National Association of Catholic Chaplains (NACC) began to develop its own programs and certification in specialized pastoral ministry. Here again the tension between traditional types of ministry and psychotherapeutic emphasis has not yet been completely resolved (Duffy, 1983).

Although CPE or its equivalent has served to make ministers of pastoral healthcare more professional and has thus somewhat improved their status with medical staffs, it has also raised the question as to whether pastoral care is simply another form of psychotherapy and social work. Until pastoral care people themselves have a clearer theology of pastoral care and a surer sense of their specific identity, they will have difficulty being accepted as professionals by hospital administrators and medical staffs (Arnold, 1982; O'Connor, 1986).

In seeking this identity, clergy often claim that in some sense they deal with the whole person or the patient as a person, whereas other healthcare professionals are more concerned with special parts of the person. On the contrary, some physicians believe that it is the medical doctor who is the only complete healthcare professional, who must therefore head the healthcare team and make the final decision in all matters. Thus the physician deals with healthcare as a whole, while other members of the team, including the minister, deal only with special or incidental aspects of the patient's health problem (6.4). Thus such a physician considers the ministry of the clergy to the patient merely partial, auxiliary, or incidental and resents as presumptuous and intrusive any claim on the clergy's part to deal with the whole person.

This controversy about whole and part can be clarified by realizing that different wholes are in question. In viewing the patient under the aspect of *physical* health, the physician is the chief of any healthcare team and *de jure* has the ultimate decision in presenting to the patient an evaluation of a possible course of treatment, although *de facto* a nurse, dietician, physical therapist, or pharmacist may actually know more about the patient. The ultimate decision, however, remains with the patient or those responsible for the incompetent patient (John Fletcher, 1983a).

Patients as whole persons in making their decisions about how to use the services of the healthcare team must take into consideration other aspects of personality than physical health. Consequently, patients need the help and counsel of the psychotherapist, the ethical counselor, and the spiritual guide. In taking such counsel, it is clear that to the patients, physical health is only a *part* of the problem; in this problem the ethical and spiritual aspects are more inclusive than the psychotherapeutic or physical aspects of the person's health (see Chapters 1 and 2). From this point of view, patients, after receiving the physician's advice, may need to take ultimate counsel with their minister, priest, or some other equivalent spiritual guide. Sensitive physicians are quick to realize this and are happy not to stretch their responsibility beyond their professional competence for physical or, perhaps, mental health.

Nevertheless, ministers, insofar as they stand for the personhood of the patient in its totality and its ultimately spiritual character, have the obligation to defend the patient as a person in conflict situations, both against unjust actions of the staff and imprudence or negligence of the family or other guardians.

Thus, on behalf of the whole person, the first task of the healthcare ministry is to help patients understand the several dimensions of any health decision. Thus in a hospital it is reasonable that the pastoral care department play a significant role in receiving and dismissing patients. Entering patients need to look forward to their experience in the hospital as one over which they have genuine control, and they should leave it feeling they are prepared to go on with normal life. Ministers can help patients achieve this sense of self-control at a time when patients often feel they are helpless.

The foregoing tasks of the healthcare ministry, however, important as they are, remain secondary to its specific and central task of helping patients grow through their experience of sickness and convalescence or of death. But before discussing this principle work of healthcare ministry, we must discuss the responsibility of the pastoral care people for the other members of the healthcare team.

14.2   MINISTRY TO THE HOSPITAL STAFF

Not only the patients are persons, but so also are the members of the administrative and medical staffs and all the auxiliary personnel. Today it is well recognized in hospitals that the mental health of the staff is an important factor in the therapy of the patients (Fath, 1985). In fact, in any healthcare facility the effectiveness of healthcare depends in large part on the type of interpersonal relations that exist among its staff. Ultimately, this is a spiritual problem, since physicians, nurses, and others engaged in the very difficult vocation of caring for the suffering and confronting the crises of life and death are engaged in their own spiritual struggle (see Chapter 13).

Staff members need help to maintain their sense of dedication, their courage, and their human compassion against all temptations of routine, cynicism, callousness, and ambition. If the Christian Church from a long and often bitter historical experience has accepted the motto *ecclesia semper reformanda* ("the Church needs constant renewal"), this must be equally true of hospitals and the healthcare profession. Only on the basis of this constant effort to renew Christian humanism within the staff is there any real hope of sound ethical judgment in the care of patients.

A distinction needs to be made here between the *chaplain,* who is most properly an ordained minister (in Catholic institutions, a priest or perhaps a permanent deacon) and to whom the role of pastor of a community belongs by office, and other pastoral care professionals who are not ordained but who nevertheless have a genuine ministry, often entrusted to them by the local bishop. Where the pastoral care department is fully developed, its *director* may be the chaplain. This is not always the best arrangement, however, since the task of director of a department is administrative rather than immediately pastoral and can often be best fulfilled by a member of a religious order or a properly trained layperson. The director has the responsibility of assigning the tasks of the department to different members, which include the ordained chaplain's specifically priestly or diaconal functions, whereas counseling and other functions are shared with nonordained members under the director's coordination and supervision. All members of the department should be guaranteed the relative autonomy proper to their respective professional roles, including that required by the canonical duties of ordained ministers. This does not mean that in a pluralistic hospital the chaplain can be the pastor of the hospital community or of the hospital staff in any strict sense of the word, but he does seek to minister to all isofar as they are open to his help and to provide for the others to the degree possible.

The pastoral care department as a whole will be concerned with bringing to the hospital's attention administration issues of interpersonal relationships within the staff that affect the workings of the institution and the good of the patients. Most pastoral care ministers soon learn of many of these interpersonal issues informally through members of the administrative and medical staffs who come to them for counsel and encouragement.

Although pastoral care people usually attempt to help those who come to them with such interstaff difficulties with as much tact as they can muster, accusations of interference in medical or administrative matters can easily result. For pastoral care people to react to such criticism by confining their concern to private counseling often seems like neglect of responsibility to the institution and the patients it serves.

We would suggest this might be handled as follows:

1. The chaplain or director of the pastoral care department or some representative of that department who is especially competent should be included on the ethics committee of the hospital. This will provide a channel for raising ethical issues.

2. The staff should be thoroughly informed of the religious and counseling services that the pastoral care department is ready to provide to them. It is important here, for example, that a Catholic hospital let the personnel know they are welcome at the Eucharist and for personal confession or counseling. However, it is also important (and often neglected) to let non-Catholics know that the department has considered their needs, studied them, and made some provision for them in a way that is convenient and free of embarrassment.

3. The director should have a recognized procedure by which discussion can be facilitated with the administration, with the medical staff, with whatever group represents the nurses, and with the union or other representative body of the hospital employees, concerning issues of interpersonal relationships that the members of the pastoral care department may have observed are affecting patient or institutional welfare. Naturally, administrators may be reluctant to give the director this formal access to groups in the hospital with which the administration may be at odds. Unless such recognized access exists, however, the director or chaplain will not be able to play that role of arbitrator and peacemaker, which must be a primary and spiritual ethical concern of any truly human institution. Ethics is always concerned about the tension between justice and social harmony. It is absurd to speak of an institution's concern for medical ethics if it does not recognize the need for this type of peacemaking as a truly ministerial function.

If the pastoral care department is to fulfill this role, its members must have a profound respect for those who dedicate their lives to the healing profession and should acknowledge that Christian ministry to the sick is not a monopoly of the pastoral care department. For Catholics, the Second Vatican Council (1965c) reemphasized the ancient concept of "the universal priesthood of the believers," according to which Christ's ministry is not confined to ordained clergy. In its threefold function of teaching, shepherding, and worshiping this ministry is shared in a variety of ways by every member of the Christian community so that all Christians are ministers along with Christ, who himself is the Servant of the Father (O'Meara, 1983). Consequently, all Christians also share in pastoral ministry to the sick. Jesus made this one of the responsibilities for love of neighbor on which all persons are to be judged (Mt 25:31-46).

In a very special way, therefore, the physicians, nurses, administrators, and all the members of a hospital staff are not merely carrying out a secular service but a genuine Christian ministry of healing, deriving its authority from Christ's own healing work and witnessing to his continuing presence in the world. Thus the priest chaplain and the whole pastoral care department not only should refrain from monopolizing the religious aspect of healthcare, but should also carry on an educational effort to help the hospital staff appreciate the spiritual and ethical values of their own professional work.

With this respect for their co-ministers should also come an increased sensitivity by pastoral care people to how some medical professionals are warped or destroyed as persons by the tensions under which they work. From such insight should come a creative effort to suggest and develop ways in which justice, charity, and peace can heal the "wounded healers" (Emerson, 1986; Nouwen 1972).

Finally, it is important that the pastoral care department itself provide a model of true humanity and good interpersonal relations (Fath, 1980). Not infrequently, the chaplain is the most difficult person on the staff, not because he plays the role of prophet, but because he is a warped personality constantly defending his own clerical status. Needless to say, in such cases the administration should not let respect for the clergy stand in the way of seeking a reeducation or a replacement of the chaplain.

14.3   SPIRITUAL COUNSELING IN HEALTHCARE

Trust

We have discussed some of the functions which the religious minister can perform as an integrator of healthcare in the interests of the total health of the human person, but we have not yet discussed the specifically spiritual role of the minister. The reason that some have confused pastoral care with psychotherapy is because they are uncertain about what "spiritual ministry" really means or how it can contribute significantly to the patient's healing. To discuss this problem, we first begin with the question as to how spiritual counseling differs from psychological counseling as these occur during a person's stay in a hospital or long term care facility.

Persons who are ill are faced with potentially serious problems:

1. They may fear suffering and death.
2. They may face the uncertainties of diagnosis and prognosis and fear about the pain of embarrassment of various testing or treatment procedures unfamiliar to them or all too painfully familiar.
3. They may face the tedium of a long stay in the healthcare facility under circumstances they find either boring or excruciating.
4. They suffer separation from their regular work, friends, and family and are not comfortable in the new situation.
5. They may be worried and perhaps feel guilty about the various responsibilities at home that they cannot handle.
6. They suffer from a sense of deprivation of privacy and of freedom, almost as if they were imprisoned.
7. They may feel puzzled about *Why has this happened to me?* and may interpret their sickness as punishment for moral guilt. They may also anticipate further guilt through failure in courage and hope.
8. They may feel alone and deserted in meeting all the foregoing, and their sense of dignity, worth, and membership in the human community may be diminished by real moral guilt for which God's forgiveness is truly needed.

Spiritual ministers in their own proper role are called on to help patients in these struggles and may also be called on to help members of the health team who are faced with similar problems both in their personal lives and in their professional involvement with patients. The first task of the spiritual guide (as of any counselor and any real professional in the sense we define profession in Chapter 4), is to establish *trust,* but this trust differs from that on which most professional relations are based because it has a type of ultimacy. People often seek out a minister to confide in when they can no longer trust their lawyer, physician, or even their psychiatrist.

Yet many patients do not even trust a minister, and when the chaplain visits them they are thinking, What is his game? Is he trying "to save my soul," to make a convert out of me? Is he looking for an offering? Or for a confession? Thus ministers must build up trust on the foundation not of words but of behavior. A minister must keep promises, maintain contact, and be available to help in whatever difficulty is bothering the patient or to look for someone who can help. A minister must also be nonjudgmental, empathetic, and very careful about confidentiality. Finally, a chaplain's care is expected to extend beyond the patient to the patient's family.

Nevertheless, as in other counseling, this trust has its limits, and ministers must make clear to those they serve that a spiritual counselor has limited powers (Clinebell, 1984). Otherwise, the trust between chaplain and patient will soon appear to be violated. Thus chaplains should explain that (1) they cannot work miracles at will, or change structures, or get the patient out; (2) they cannot be continuously present and can give only limited time to any one patient; and (3) that their role is primarily that of a listener, counselor, and celebrant of the sacraments. All this should become clear in the implicit or explicit counseling contract. It is up to counselors to set these limits tactfully and to remember that they are dealing with patients who may very well have undergone considerable psychological regression, which makes them as dependent and demanding as a child in relation to its parents. The minister should give the patient permission for this dependency, but a limited permission. If such limits are not set, the minister will soon find that the patient interprets much that the minister does as a betrayal of trust.

This trust between a spiritual guide and the spiritual pilgrim, between a shepherd and the straying sheep, takes its special character first from the charism of the minister as an *ordained* person. The spiritual guide is an "apostle," that is, one sent by the Church in the name of God on whom the Spirit of God has been invoked by the prayers of the Christian community. Even when guides are not ordained, their ministry must somehow be authorized by the Christian community if it is to be given that special trust that should characterize it. Physicians and psychotherapists in their white coats are often invested with an analogous charisma, as explained in Chapter 4, in speaking of the priestly character of the whole healing profession, but this is only an analogy to the charism of the spiritual guide.

A minister, particularly if young and humble, may find the reverence shown him by a client because of this charism very embarrassing and even unreal. The young minister would prefer simply to be on friendly terms with a patient, not to be invested with a halo of mysterious power.

Timothy seems to have had the same problem judging from the advice Paul gave him, "Do not let people disregard you because you are young, but be an example to all the believers in the way you speak and behave, and in your love, your faith, and your purity" (1 Tm 4:12). If ministers have set appropriate limits to their role, however, this charismatic function will not expand absurdly. Within these limits, however, they should accept honestly the task of speaking for God and in his name, however awesome that claim may be (Kelsey, 1982).

This requires spiritual counselors to reflect constantly on two realities: first, that God is acting through them to accomplish what is quite beyond their own abilities and, second, that unless they acknowledge their own human limits, they will be placing obstacles in the way of God's work. Ministers who have this correct perception of their own role will not attempt too much, put themselves under impossible strains, or feel guilty at an inability to solve all problems of all patients. On the other hand, they will feel and communicate to patients unlimited hope in the loving power of God and a sense of each patient's dignity in God's eyes and their own (McBrien, 1987).

Some ministers are so secularized that they feel more comfortable in a psychotherapeutic role than in a spiritual one and thus fail their patients by refusal to speak in God's name. They avoid talking with patients about spiritual issues, praying with them, or inquiring about their need for the sacraments as if these were forbidden or offensive topics. Patients may very well read this as a lack of faith on a minister's part and thus as a threat to the patient's own faith, which is already sorely tried by doubts and anxieties raised by the patient's condition. Ministers who find themselves in a quandary about their own pastoral identity should attempt to resolve this ambiguity through spiritual guidance and perhaps psychotherapy if they are going to fulfill their responsibility of helping patients in *their* quandaries (Thayer, 1985).

Discernment

The minister, as with a psychotherapist, is a listener and a reflector through whom the realities of the patient's situation become clearer to the patient and more manageable. Furthermore, as with the psychotherapist, the minister listens not just to what the patient seems to be saying superficially, but to what the patient, perhaps unconsciously, is trying to say nonverbally and symbolically (Wicks et al., 1985). The psychotherapist, however, is listening for the message that rises from the patient's subconscious emotional drives, whereas the minister as a spiritual therapist is listening for a message that comes from a still deeper level, from that place the Scripture calls the "heart," that is, from the spiritual interior of the person's being where the person is committed to some sort of ultimate values and to some fundamental insight into reality (H. Egan, 1984). In most patients, as in most everyone, this commitment and vision is dim and confused indeed; yet it is the source of all personal life, where people really live and where they really die (Culligon, 1983). "Out of the depths I call to you O Lord, O Lord hear my voice" (Psalm 130). It is this voice *de profundis* to which the minister must listen. Moreover, a spiritual guide is not looking, as is the psychotherapist, for the psychic energies and motivations that flow from human instinctual needs, but for the work of the Holy Spirit in the patient, the signs of faith, hope, and charity, and the spiritual forces of sin and alienation that oppose these. This is the spiritual level of human functioning discussed in Chapter 2 (Fichter, 1981; Thayer, 1985).

The patient may raise these questions directly by saying, "Why has this happened to me, Father? Have I sinned? Am I going to be punished? What will happen to me if I die?" or "I don't seem to be able to pray now that I am sick," and so forth. Today in a secularized society, however, such questions are seldom asked *directly*. Even if they are, the chaplain may very well suspect that they do not really come from the spiritual level of personality but are merely the pious language that some people (especially those who are from a fundamentalist religious background) use in speaking of purely physical or psychological problems (Browning, 1987). Also the patient may think that this is the way you are supposed to converse with a minister, who is supposed only to talk that type of religious language. Therefore the counselor has to listen to religious questions inherent in pseudoreligious language (Hoff, 1984). In both cases counselors must go deeper to find the really spiritual level in the patient.

This requires patience, and it is usually a mistake to begin asking spiritual questions of a patient with whom the needed level of trust has not yet been established. On the other hand, experienced spiritual counselors learn how to cut through other levels of small talk and psychological talk to the issues with which they have to deal (Estadt, 1983). Simple directness is ordinarily not resented by patients. Catholics are usually not alarmed and even expect for "Father" to ask them if they want to go to confession or receive communion and to make some further tactful inquiry if they refuse. *Directness* is not bluntness or insensitivity. It is rather a form of respect for a patient, a refusal simply to play games.

This respect for the person demands that the minister not take advantage of the patient's weak condition (D. McNeill et al., 1982). It is unethical to try to force conversion of patients, accuse them of sin, make demands for prayer or faith, and so forth. It may seem incredible that some ministers carry on such a preaching attack on patients, but many patients will report unpleasant experiences of being confronted by zealous ministers in a hospital and being embarrassed or pressured. Reports of such experiences have done much to prejudice physicians and nurses against the ministerial profession.

The minister who exerts this pressure fails to trust in God's providence, by which God is using the patient's experience of illness as an occasion of possible spiritual growth. The Spirit of God is already at work in the sufferer in ways that are not labeled religious. The minister must recognize this growth process and cultivate it, helping patients to understand this in their own terms (G. Egan, 1986).

A specific responsibility for ministers is not only to deal with the patient's spiritual problems, but also to help him or her become vividly aware of the real presence of God and of the Church as the People of God in the patient's life in this very event of sickness where the patient may feel abandoned and isolated. Ministers are themselves a visible sign or sacrament of this presence, incarnating God, as it were, in a tangible, human, imperfect, but real form.

Also, it is not enough that ministers provide this witness of God's presence only to members of their own church. Too many ministers assume that they have responsibility only to their own parishioners or to those of their own denomination and that others will resent their presence. Usually, however, this is not the case. Most laity are less ecclesiastically defined than we think. For them any minister, even a rabbi, is still a "man of God" and as such ought to have some interest in them as "children of God." Even the humanist is seldom content with the silence of humanism in the face of the ultimate questions and is resentful if the religious minister writes him off as a nonbeliever.

Thus, as a spiritual adviser, the minister's primary task is really a very simple one. It is to say, as much or more by presence, attitude, and nonverbal symbols as by the exhortatory Word, that God is present to sick persons in their fear or suffering, that God as loving, caring Father, as co-suffering Lord Jesus, as Healing Spirit is present and acting, but this presence is in *mystery*. That is, it exceeds human rational empirical comprehension because it leads to an open future. This implies a spiritual awe before the *mysterium tremendum*. The sick person, as did Job, feels guilty and yet is not clear how he or she is guilty. There is a sense of *judgment*. The minister should not deny this. Indeed, a minister symbolizes this judgment. The minister also overcomes judgment, however, by being a sign of mercy and reconciliation (W. Barry and Connolly, 1982).

Sickness may be the time of genuine conversion in which persons truly find God for the first time in their lives or after a long time of forgetfulness and separation. The minister must affirm the reality of this invitation of divine mercy, but that is not the whole of the minister's responsibility. Conversion is the beginning of a new life, but that life has to be lived authentically or it will be lost again. Consequently, one of the chief aims of spiritual counseling is to assist converts to begin to grow daily in the Christian life and to plan practically to continue that growth once they have returned to the routine situations of everyday life (Gusmer, 1984).

It is important also that the minister, in helping sick persons realize God's presence, also make vivid to them that the minister is a sign of the concern of God's people, of the Christian community or church, for a suffering brother or sister. Sickness is in Old Testament terms a type of "uncleanness," and the patient may experience a "leprosy" of loneliness, alienation, and "excommunication" as an outcast from life and the human community. This is especially true of patients with acquired immunodeficiency syndrome (AIDS). The minister removes this excommunication and reunites the lonely one with the community that is praying for him or her. Recall how Jesus, healing a leper, sent him to a priest to be readmitted to the Jewish community (Mk 1:44). Recall as well, how Jesus might indicate that the cured person should "sin no more," but he never asked people how they became sick or how they contracted their pathologies.

14.4   CELEBRATING THE HEALING PROCESS

Word and Sacrament

The specific spiritual task of pastoral care, however, is not exhausted simply by the counseling situation. It must not be confined to talking about the presence of God, but it must deepen into *experiencing* that presence in prayer, worship, celebration, and communion (Leech, 1985).

Today, when most chaplains and other ministers as well are training in CPE, they sometimes feel a tension between the model of the chaplain as a pastoral counselor, whose main task is to engage in a therapeutic psychological process with the patient, and the former model of the pastor as the one who reads the Scriptures, prays with and exhorts the patient, and administers the sacraments (Holst, 1985). These two models seem opposed to each other. In particular, one seems aimed at removing feelings of guilt and giving feelings of interpersonal warmth and confidence and getting clients "in touch with their feelings," whereas the other tends to generate guilt and to impose a formalized religious response that covers up a patient's real experience.

Actually the two models, when they are well understood, are complementary and can reinforce each other. We have already shown how pastoral counselors by their own presence are already a *sacrament*, that is, a sign of the presence of God. The Word of God first came to human beings not in the text of the Bible that records his coming, but in the incarnation of Jesus Christ, the man who came to the sick and suffering, shared their suffering, and healed them by his contact (Schillebeeckx, 1981b). Ministers, because they are sent by Jesus, are the living witnesses, "other Christs," and a sign of Christ's care for the patient. Therefore, everything that the minister does to witness this tender concern, this ability to empathize, to listen, and not to judge, is a sacrament of Jesus' presence.

Even humor and light banter, if their purpose is precisely to establish real communication, resemble the wit that Jesus constantly displayed in his preaching and parables. Above all, the down-to-earthness—the freedom from stuffiness, self-righteousness, and elitism that can be the curse of the clerical state—is in imitation of Jesus, who did not hesitate to eat with sinners in simple fellowship.

Thus, when ministers read the Scripture with patients, they should already have placed the Scripture in a human relational context in which the Word of God can be truly understood. Prayer also must grow out of this living context; that is, it should be natural for two people who have come to share a common concern to give it prayerful expression. A minister should not be praying in front of an embarrassed patient who feels as if something is "being laid on him" in which he has no part. An opening for prayer will come, however, only if the patient senses that the minister's concern for him or her goes *deep*, deeper than the mere professional interest. The Scriptures used should be chosen just because they help to make real the presence of Jesus, especially in his power to forgive, heal, and lead one into the fullness of life (Kirwan, 1984).

The Catholic priest is more likely than the Protestant minister or the rabbi to be concerned about the administration of the sacraments in the hospital setting. These, too, must be understood not as some ritual intruding into a real situation, but as a ritualization of a process of healing that is already occurring. The primordial sacrament is the touching Jesus used when he healed the leper. It indicates the intimate presence, the care, the community, the power of life between Jesus and the sick and outcast. When a chaplain does what is so natural, namely, to hold the hand of sick persons to give them reassurance that the minister is there, that they are not alone, that is the primordial sacramental rite on which all the other sacraments are based—*human bodily contact* as a sign of *spiritual presence*.

Anointing the Sick and Reconciliation

In administering the sacraments, using the new rites that the Catholic Church and other liturgical churches have recently improved precisely for this purpose, ministers must try to enhance this character of human contact already present in the counseling situation. What ministers have done as good pastoral counselors, they now deepen and intensify by a sign that combines the verbal word of Scripture with the nonverbal sacramental act.

The new rite of Anointing of the Sick brings this out clearly (see Paul VI, Apostolic Constitution on the Sacrament of Anointing the Sick, 1972; Empereur, 1982). It is not merely for the dying, as formerly, but for any person seriously ill. *Serious* should be judged here not merely in physical terms, but also in psychological terms. Thus, when anyone is sick enough that the minister suspects that the thought of possible death with its deep anxiety has entered his or her mind and produced fear and the threat of despair, then the spiritual and perhaps physical healing of the sacrament is needed and should be given. Whenever there is question of major surgery or of any disease that patients know sometimes leads to death and thus raises this fear in their own minds, ministers can anoint. They should not anoint when the illness is one in which recovery is assured and that consequently does not appear to contain any serious threat.

What is the meaning of this rite? First, it is not merely something done by a priest to a patient. Even when ministers are alone, they are there to represent not only God, but also the Christian community (Rahner, 1963). In fact, God is the center of the Christian community, so the minister is there to represent the Trinitarian community into which all Christians are incorporated in the Second Person Incarnate by their baptism. The anxiety of sick persons is that by their illness they are outcasts, aliens to this community. Patients experience this by their isolation from usual daily life and by the threat of death that might take them away forever. What such patients need is the reassurance that their people and their God are still with them. The priest supplies the sign of this by *touching* a patient. This touch means "presence," "acceptance," and as such is common to all the sacraments. It is a special type of touch in this case, however, a *healing* touch because it is the "anointing with oil," a common form of healing remedy that has the sense of soothing pain and infusing life and movement. Its significance as a spiritual healing is given by the words spoken.

This actual form of the sacrament is also preceded by brief Scriptural passages that can be expanded. This is in keeping with the general principle of the new rites that each sacrament should begin with a proclamation of the Word of faith, since it is faith that opens the person to God's work and is the beginning of God's gifts.

Although the sacrament is valid with only the priest and the recipient present, this is not the ideal way to perform it. A study made in several public hospitals shows that the physicians and nurses frequently resent the visit of the priest to perform "the Last Rites" (Nolin, 1972). There are several reasons for this. One is the notion, now out of date, that these rites seal the fate of the patient and therefore mark the failure of the medical profession, something that healthcare professionals hate to face. Again, professionals think the rites may frighten and depress the patient. Another reason, however, is that the priest seems to be a medicine man who has been brought in as competition to the medical profession because the family has given up on the physician's efforts. An additional reason is the exclusive character of the rite. Even in Catholic hospitals when the priest arrives, the physicians, nurses, and family often leave the room. Finally, there is sometimes a simple objection to an outsider coming in to do something for the person, as if the hospital were not all-sufficient.

These misunderstandings can be traced to what is really poor pastoral theology and practice. If the purpose of the sacrament is to help patients escape their sense of isolation, it is best if family and friends can be present, which would include if possible the nurse and physician. Furthermore, if the sacrament is not to mark the end of life, but to help in the healing process, both physical and spiritual, it is certainly not separated from or in competition with the medical work of the hospital. Rather, it is part of that healing process. In fact, it is a celebration of God's healing work, which God performs not only through the ritual, but also through the *ministry* of the physicians, nurses, and administration. Priests are not the only ministers of health; they are part of a healing *team*, every member of which is called by God to a healing work and empowered by him through their natural gifts and education. The priest's special role on this team is to make explicit and eucharistic (thankful) the work of all.

It is essential to realize that the sacraments are not performed merely in the ritual moment. Rather, they are the celebration of a culminating moment (not necessarily the last) of the saving work of God that has gone on for some time through what are apparently merely secular events. Therefore, it is fitting not only that physicians and nurses be present at the anointing, but also that they participate in it by reading the Scriptures or saying some of the prayers and by imposing hands on the patient or making the sign of the cross. Priests, in their instruction and commentary and by additions to some of the prayers, if necessary, should thank God for the healing gifts and work of the medical staff. It would be very appropriate for patients also at this time to express their thanks to the physicians and nurses.

This expansion of the ritual can best be done when the sacrament takes place at mass in the hospital chapel, but it can also be done in the hospital room or ward when the physician can be present. The patient's confession when this is necessary would, of course, be done privately before the ceremony begins.

The proper rite for the dying patient is not the Anointing of the Sick but the reception of *Viaticum*, or final communion (Gusmer, 1984). This is the expression of the sick person's communion and unity with the Church on earth, which prays for his or her swift passage to the eternal banquet. Thus this communion should be shared with others present if possible.

When an emergency arises and someone must be anointed who has not yet received the sacrament in an illness, it is necessary to perform it quickly; but if the patient recovers consciousness, it is possible to hold a healing service of prayer so that the patient can more fully participate in the fruits of the sacrament. In the case of a person who is doubtfully alive, the Sacrament of Anointing should be administered, but the new ritual forbids it to be given to someone who has already died.

Previously priests were advised to administer the sacrament to someone who had recently died—up to two or three hours—if the death had been sudden. The ritual no longer prescribes this. In the present liturgical transition, however, when many people are still poorly instructed with regard to the Sacrament of Anointing, a Catholic family may be very disconsolate to hear that the sacrament was not received. Priests, therefore, may prudently judge in given circumstances whether they might better administer the anointing conditionally, where there is still some doubt (even minimal) that life still remains, for the sake of the family. Perhaps a better procedure is to assure the family that the patient received the proper rites of the Church, meaning by this that the priest has prayed for the departed and blessed the body, since these are the proper rites according to the present discipline. It is important to instruct people that the Church prays daily for all its members and that no one departs this life without the powerful intercession of the Church. In these ecumenical times, chaplains should not hesitate to administer anointing to non-Catholics who might present themselves at a general anointing service, since they probably are baptized and of good faith. If not, the sacrament still constitutes a prayer for their healing.

What should ministers who are not priests do? Today religious sisters and brothers and laypeople share in the sacramental ministry (Wicks, 1986). It is theologically disputed whether it might be possible for the Church to delegate to a deacon the Anointing of the Sick, as confirmation has been delegated by bishops to priests (Palmer, 1974). At present, this is not legal or valid. However, it is possible for deacons and nonordained persons, sisters, and laypersons to hold a service of healing (U.S. Catholic Conference, 1979). This can consist of Scripture readings, prayers, and the laying on of hands for the sick. It can even make use of blessed oil as a sacramental. It would seem, however, that in such services it should be made clear to all that what is taking place is not a sacrament in the strict sense. This does not mean, however, that the prayer is inefficacious (all true prayer is efficacious), but rather that it is *preparatory* to the full public visit of the priest to the sick as a representative of the Christian community. Just as the physician's arrival completes the care given to patients by nurses, although the physician does nothing additional except to approve and confirm what has already been done, so the priest approves and confirms the healing prayer of a local group and of auxiliary ministry. This is not a mere formality but an expression of the unity and public witness of the Church.

The Sacrament of Reconciliation, the *Rite of Penance,* (Helwig, 1983) for the sick can also take place in the form of a penance service in the hospital chapel or even in the ward, with the invitation to all who wish to make individual confession and receive absolution. Such a service is an opportunity for the priest to deal with the question of sin and guilt and the meaning of suffering and to alleviate *neurotic guilt*. When confession is made in a ward, it should be remembered that if it is difficult to achieve sufficient privacy, the penitent can be instructed simply to make a general acknowledgment of sins and to speak of them in detail in a future confession.

It should be remembered, too, that deacons, sisters, brothers, and other visitors, although they cannot give absolution, can truly help a sick person to conversion and reconciliation with God and neighbor in an efficacious way. We are not proposing revival of the "confession to a layman," which was common in the Middle Ages when a priest was not available, but are emphasizing that today in pastoral counseling such confession often takes place spontaneously. When it does, the ministers who are not priests should help such patients make an act of contrition and then encourage them to have a priest hear their confession when it becomes possible. They should also assure patients that here and now the mercy of God is truly present in prayer and that with this trust in God's mercy they should be at peace. The reason for confession later is to ratify and complete by the public acknowledgment of the priest as a representative of the Church a conversion that has already taken place. There is no reason for nonordained ministers to believe that because they are not ordained, they cannot help patients achieve this reconciliation here and now.

Baptism and Eucharist

If the patient is unbaptized and wishes to become a Catholic Christian, the new ritual should be followed (Duffy, 1984). When patients have been baptized as Protestants but wish to be Catholic, they should be received as members of the Catholic community and confirmed (Kiesling, 1974). What about the infant in danger of death or the unconscious dying person?

Today some Catholics are raising doubts about infant baptism. This, however, seems to have Pelagian overtones because it implies that the grace of God can only be received on one's initiative. Baptism, however, is a sign of the pure gift of God, the gift of faith and justification that comes to people without any merit on their part merely because they do not reject it. Before the infant is born, he or she is already subject to the grace of God through the prayers of the Church. Infant baptism is the public ratification of accepting the infant, alienated from God through no fault of his or her own by the sins of society (original sin), into the Church and into union with the Three Persons of the Trinity. The act of incorporating the infant into the life of the human community begins biologically and sociologically from the moment of conception and birth. Why, then, should not the infant also be incorporated into the redeemed community of the Church? Consequently, it is certain that baptism can be validly conferred on the child from the moment of conception and probable that it can be conferred on any unconscious adult (although not certain, since the person may have positively rejected the grace of God).

From this some theologians in the past concluded that it is essential that all children in danger of death, even in utero, should be baptized and encouraged the baptism of all doubtfully baptized adults who had not actually refused baptism. This was based on the idea that salvation without baptism (at least *in voto*, i.e., "baptism of desire") was impossible, since it is a matter of faith that persons can only be saved through Christ and thus through his Church. Augustinian theologians came to the inescapable but embarrassing conclusion (to a Christian believing in God's mercy as Augustine strongly did) that unbaptized children are damned. St. Thomas found a way out of this embarrassment by pointing out that it is possible (1) for unbaptized children to enjoy a natural happiness (Limbo) even if they are not admitted to the inner mystery of God, the existence of which they have never been aware, and (2) for unbaptized adults to be saved by an implicit desire for baptism if they have conscientiously followed what light God has given them.

Today theologians still maintain the principle that persons can only be saved by Christ through the Church, but they see the *prayer* of the Church as efficacious even when it cannot be ritually expressed in the sacraments (see 1 Co 7:14). Thus the infant dying before baptism probably has already been justified through the prayer of the Church (especially of the child's family) and will enter into the intimate mystery of God. The Sacred Congregation for the Doctrine of the Faith (SCDF, 1980b) says in its "Instruction on Infant Baptism," "As for infants who have died without baptism, the Church can do nothing but commend them to the mercy of God, as in fact she does in the funeral rite designed for them" (*Rite of Funerals*, 1969, n. 82). Nevertheless, it still is important to administer baptism to manifest the concern of the Church and thus to keep alive the consciousness of the dignity of the human person from the first moments of existence (SCDF, 1980b; *Rite of Baptism for Children*, 1971). Consequently, nurses and physicians should baptize infants who are in danger of death and even miscarried fetuses who exhibit human form and some sign of life. They should pour water on the child (on the head, if possible) so as actually to touch the skin and should say, "I baptize you in the name of the Father, Son, and Holy Spirit." In this way they have expressed Christian reverence and fellowship with this little person who will forever be part of the Trinitarian community. If the infant is surely dead, baptism should not be administered, but the family of the infant may be assured of God's mercy having been implored through the prayers of the Church.

For the dying unconscious person, it is permissible also to perform such a baptism with the condition, "If you are not baptized, I baptize you." Clearly this is not a grave obligation unless the person has asked to be baptized before lapsing into unconsciousness. This should not be done in a merely mechanical manner (trying to baptize everyone in the hospital, etc.) but as part of the nurses' care for particular persons in their charge whom they believe have given some indication that they might wish such an administration. Again, the reason is to show the Church's concern for a person who has providentially come under the care of the Catholic community.

The Eucharist is the supreme sacrament and sign of the Christian community, indicating that such patients remain a part of that community, even when absent from the public worship assembly, and that they are destined for eternal life with the community (Keifer, 1983). It is a life-giving, health-giving sacrament, since the eating of bread and drinking of wine are the basic symbols of the power to live. After Jesus raised the daughter of Jairus, "He told them to give her something to eat" (Lk 8:55). Again, St. Paul believed (1 Co 11:27-31) the unworthy reception of the Eucharist leads to sickness and death because this hyprocrisy cuts a person off from the God of the living.

Today the Eucharist is often distributed by auxiliary ministers, not by the priest. This is not inappropriate, since in the earliest days communion was taken from the public assembly to the homes of the sick. In a hospital it would be appropriate when possible (and the current practice with regard to the fast before communion makes this easy) to have the patients who wish to listen to the mass in the chapel on closed-circuit radio or television then to be brought communion immediately before the mass. Ambulatory patients who attended the mass could be the auxiliary ministers. In this way the union between mass and communion would be emphasized. It is essential in any case that communion in the healthcare facility should not be reduced to a routine in which someone pops in and out of a room to place a wafer in a sleepy patient's mouth. We would suggest at least a card containing Scripture reading and prayers that a patient can use while preparing for communion.

What we have been saying may sound liturgical rather than ethical, but it sums up the ethical message of this book. That is, medical ethics has to do not with certain rules about forbidden procedures, but with a healing process by which the dignity of every human person in all its dimensions is respected by the community and the sick person is restored to full life in community. Unethical behavior tends to exclude persons from the deepest sharing of communal life centered in the Trinity. Ethical behavior fosters this communion. This ethical vision with its perception of the true scale of values is summed up and expressed in the sacraments, especially in the Eucharist. A Catholic health facility that really understands the healing character of the sacraments will have a perfect model for an ethical treatment of the patients. The sacraments represent for us how Jesus went about treating sick people.

What makes a Catholic hospital different from all other hospitals? Its vision of the sick is a eucharistic vision, carried out in all details of the treatment of the patient and the mission of the healing team.

14.5 ETHICAL COUNSELING AND PASTORAL CARE

Respecting the Patient's Value System

Don Browning, in *The Moral Context of Pastoral Care* (1976), ably argues for renewed stress on the ethical dimension of pastoral care. He believes that the Christian emphasis on spiritual relation to God by grace must never be allowed to eradicate the memory of its Jewish origins in the Torah, in the law understood not as a death-dealing formalism but as a true discipline of life through which the seeds of grace can be cultivated. A Christian spirituality that neglects moral obligation, or that speaks of love but forgets justice, is foreign to the teaching of Jesus, who came not to destroy the law but to fulfill it (Mt 5:17-19). Systematic theologians have the task of relating and balancing law and grace, but pastoral care counselors have to live with the tension, neglecting neither grace nor discipline.

We have been arguing in this chapter that the primary task of pastoral care is *spiritual* guidance and celebration, yet the purpose of this book has been to deal with *ethical* questions confronted by healthcare professionals and their patients. Certainly, ministers frequently have to be of help to professionals and patients in their struggles to make such ethical decisions. What is the relation between *spiritual* and *ethical* guidance? Section 2.3 shows that the spiritual and ethical dimensions of the human person, although interrelated, are not identical. Spiritual counseling deals with the ultimate, existential questions, the problems of commitment to certain fundamental values or life goals. Ethical counseling in the strict sense, on the other hand, deals with the decisions that must be made about actions that have to be taken to achieve these goals. In brief, the former deals with *ends;* the latter, with the *means.*

Some theologians, especially of the Lutheran tradition (Thielicke, 1969), question whether ethics in this sense is relevant for a Christian. Are Christians not in danger of self-righteousness and legalism the moment they begin to measure their actions by some ethical system? For such theologians, Christian life is a spontaneous grateful response to God's gracious forgiveness, a loving response that can only be distorted by any ethical calculation of ends and means. Nevertheless, other Protestant theologians such as Gustafson (1983) recognize that although our ethical decisions must be motivated by faith and love, they also require a rational decision-making process. Thus, although the main task of pastoral care is spiritual, it must also extend to assisting professionals and patients to live out their spiritual commitments by prudent decisions about concrete actions.

This book has been devoted to providing ethical guidance for healthcare decisions, but in concluding we still have to ask, What is the responsibility of a minister or a pastoral care department in medical-moral decisions?

In answering this question, the first difficulty to consider is, How can a minister be an ethical counselor to persons who, in a pluralistic culture, are committed to such different value systems? As spiritual counselor, a minister may have to deal with someone who is struggling with a strictly spiritual problem that involves commitment to a value system, but as ethical counselor, the client's value system is not in question. The problem is its application. How are counselors to help if they do not share the client's value system?

Chapter 7 argues that different value systems cannot be simply reduced to some common denominator, but rather are *analogous* to each other, that is, fundamentally different yet having much in common. Consequently, we believe that in pastoral care it is possible to proceed ecumenically to find a common ground for ethical decisions between different value systems, whether these differences separate pastor and patient or members of the health team. Such an ecumenical method depends on (1) clarity about one's own values and fidelity to them, (2) respect for the values of others and their fidelity to these, and (3) a common effort to find a basis for mutual dialogue and action. Since at a time of sickness patients are seldom in any condition to rethink their whole outlook on life, an ethical counselor should in general not disturb the patient's basic commitment unless it becomes apparent that such issues at the spiritual level have to be faced because the patient is already struggling with them. Consequently, the counselor must deal with a Jew within the Jewish ethical tradition, a Baptist within the Baptist tradition, a humanist within a humanistic set of values. Efforts to proselytize patients to one's own faith are an unfair exploitation of the sick (Browning, 1983).

Next we must ask: What is the goal of ethical counseling? How can patients be helped within the context of their value system to achieve a free and informed conscience and to arrive at prudent ethical decisions? Human decisions to be ethical first must be free. The sick suffer from various limitations of their psychological freedom. When their illness is mental, this freedom is severely restricted or even eliminated by neurosis or psychosis. When it is physical, however, the sick still suffer some degree of unfreedom because of the weakness, mental confusion, depression, and so forth, consequent on their physical condition, and also because they are confined to a narrow and unfamiliar social situation. Thus the sick patient is often not able to think clearly and realistically.

Ethical counseling, therefore, must first aim at creating an atmosphere in which the patient's freedom is maximized. Until some area of genuine freedom opens up for the patient, ethical discussion is useless. When such an opening is achieved, the counselor must strive to keep ethical discussion confined to just that area of freedom and not waste time with what seem to be ethical arguments but that are in fact only the expression of emotional conflict. The means to achieving

409

this increased freedom are essentially the techniques of psychotherapy, which the minister needs to understand and use in a modest way, referring more difficult problems to members of the health team who are professionally skilled in such therapy. Religious ministers have something special to contribute to this freeing process, however, because they can help to lift the burden of existential fear or hopelessness that may be one of the chief obstacles to freedom. Patients who are confident of God's loving and forgiving care have a peace of mind even in the face of suffering and death that makes it possible for them to face difficult decisions with serenity and sanity.

Subjective and Objective Morality

Once the counselor is assured that the patient is sufficiently free to deal with an ethical decision, the counselor's next objective should be to help the patient arrive at a decision that is prudent and thus at least *subjectively* good, that is, according to the patient's honest conscience, even when the counselor is not convinced that this decision is *objectively* good. There are three reasons why such a gap between subjective and objective morality may occur or may seem to the counselor to exist (see 3.4): (1) the patient may have a different value system than the counselor; (2) the patient's decision may appear inconsistent with the patient's own value system; and (3) the patient's decision may be inconsistent with the facts of the situation as the counselor perceives these facts.

In the first case, as already said, the counselor generally should not attempt to convert the patient to the counselor's own value system but should help the patient to make decisions consistent with the patient's own values. In the second case, the counselor should do what is possible to help the patient to make a self-consistent decision, since only then will the decision be conscientious and subjectively right. In the third case, the counselor should try to help the patient perceive the facts of the situation correctly. Nevertheless, in this last case the counselor should remember that one's perception and interpretation of facts is influenced by one's value system and personal experience, so that it may not be possible for patient and counselor to come to an agreement on the facts.

The reason that the counselor first should be concerned to help the patient come to a subjectively honest decision is twofold: (1) because the patient always retains primary responsibility for health decisions (3.1) and, (2) because the proximate norm of all moral decisions is the conscience of the agent (3.4, 8.1). Ethically it is more important that persons do what they sincerely believe to be right at a given stage of their moral development than that they do what is objectively right. Because we live in a sinful world, and each of us suffers from the darkness of mind and hardness of heart resulting from our own sins, the Word of God is received by us in obscurity. Only little by little do we move forward into the light, as is so eloquently witnessed in the Old Testament by the history of the Chosen People. What is most essential is that we keep moving forward, even if our steps are frequently missteps. For those who make mistakes in good faith, experience is self-corrective. The New Testament shows how Jesus (unlike the Pharisees) is more concerned with the faith and goodwill of sinners than he is with their conformity with a law of which they are often ignorant and to which they do not know how to comply. St. Paul (1 Co 8) also urges respect for the conscience of others, even when they are mistaken and immature in their moral understanding.

The task of the counselor, however, does not stop with helping a patient arrive at a subjectively prudent and conscientious decision. The fact that a decision is honest does not prevent it from being harmful to others or even to the one who makes the decision when actually it is an *objectively* wrong decision. Honest mistakes do not injure moral integrity, destroy spiritual relations to God and neighbor, or prevent spiritual growth, but they do have consequences from which we and others suffer. Moreover, Christian morality is creative; it is a response to God's call to move forward toward him and to share in his redemptive work. This divine call is often present in the crisis of sickness and dying. Consequently, the counselor cannot be content simply to ratify, as it were, decisions made by a patient within the narrow limits of the patient's routine morality.

On the one hand, if the counselor sees that the patient's decision may in fact be clearly injurious to the patient or to others (e.g., if the patient is thinking of suicide or abortion), the counselor has to do what is possible to prevent this harm, even when the counselor is convinced of the subjective honesty of the decision (5.2). On the other hand, the counselor may judge that it is necessary in particular cases to confront the patient with the challenge inherent in the decision that has to be made. Thus the counselor must raise disturbing questions that ultimately go beyond the ethical level to the spiritual level of the patient's value system. Obviously, counselors must be very cautious about disturbing sick people in this manner, yet they should have the courage to do so when the patient's own behavior signals that such probing and confrontation are necessary. The wonderful scene of Jesus and the Samaritan woman (Jn 4:4-30) shows how the Spirit of God can be at work in the human conscience, revealing itself by the uneasiness, the denial, the defiance, and the disguised cries for help that a spiritually sensitive and experienced counselor can recognize. In these cases the apparent subjective honesty of the client masks a hidden conflict of conscience that cannot be resolved without probing that goes beyond the subjective to a new and deeper perception of reality.

It is no simple matter for a counselor to balance these two counseling aims of subjective and objective conscience. Formerly, it would seem that the clergy were too quick to impose objective moral standards on the people, with little sensitivity to the moral development or experience of different individuals. Today, with the growth in psychological understanding of individual differences and of the developmental aspects of morality, it would seem that the opposite temptation prevails. The axiom *people must make their own conscientious decisions* has often been pushed so far that ministers have lost interest in objective morality.

A disturbing example of this was provided by the way in which many clergymen who had been active as draft counselors during the Vietnam War then went on to become "abortion counselors" (Moody, 1971; Nathanson and Ostling, 1979). In both cases they believed they were serving the cause of human rights, and they probably contributed significantly by reason of their clerical prestige both to ending the war and to liberalizing the antiabortion laws. However, the accounts of some of them concerning their experience as counselors in the latter cause show that they seemed to have thought that compassion for the woman was the only ethical issue involved in abortion. They saw no inconsistency in their concern for the napalmed children of Vietnam and their lack of concern for the salined fetuses of the United States.

Why this apparent inconsistency was discussed so little was because these counselors saw their task purely in terms of the individual subjective conscience of the client. When the client was a conscientious objector, the counselors supported his decision to refuse service in the war. When the client was a pregnant woman who honestly believed it would be wrong for her to bear her child, they supported her decision and were ready to help her find a good clinic and to help her overcome any sense of guilt. The concern for the subjective conscience of the client in both cases was certainly proper, but we have to ask whether it was enough. Does not the counselor also have to face the question of the objective justice or injustice of the war and also the question of the rights of the unborn child? Although counselors cannot impose their personal judgment about the objective justice in either instance, they cannot simply avoid the issue. Rather, the minister must do what is possible to prevent objective harm and to challenge the judgment of the patient when signs indicate that such challenge may be an opportunity for successful moral growth.

Christian Discernment

An important aspect of this moral growth for the Christian is the deepening of the vital relation between the conscience of the individual and the conscience of the Christian community. The Holy Spirit guides us not merely privately, but also through dialogue within the historical Christian Church. Ethical counselors frequently find great immaturity in Catholic clients with regard to the relation between personal conscience and what they understand to be the official teaching of their Church. What is a counselor to do when confronted by patients who express such dilemmas as the following? (1) I know the Church condemns this, but I don't think God will condemn me. (2) I think I have to do this, but I am afraid I will have to go to hell for doing it. (3) I know this is supposed to be wrong, but why can't you as a priest give me permission to do it? (4) I have made up my mind, but I want to know what you think. (5) I am not going to confess this because I know the confessor will argue with me. (6) I guess I will just have to go ahead and do this and then go to confession afterward. (7) I am going to do what I think is right, but I guess this means I will have to leave the Church. (8) I did what I thought was right, but I still feel guilty about it.

Moreover, counselors find such difficulties not only in patients, but also in dealing with the professional staff who:

1. May separate their professional opinions and their obedience to Church teachings into mental compartments, making no effort to reconcile their professional and their Christian lives
2. Complain that the bishops and priests are ignorant of medical problems and always behind the times in the ethical regulations they impose on the medical profession
3. Complain that there is too much variation in the guidance given by different priests or different dioceses and there is a lack of clear enforcement of Church teachings
4. Object to taking time from their work to discuss moral issues because such discussions come to no clear conclusions

Finally, such difficulties are compounded by the fact that the members of the pastoral care department itself may have widely different ethical views and may themselves be struggling with the tension between official Church teaching, the diverse views of theologians, and their own pastoral experience.

We have argued previously (3.4) that such difficulties are not abnormal in the Christian community, since it is a historical, catholic, pilgrim people in which the pastors must struggle to keep the flock unified and continuously on its march; yet the diversity of experiences and talents must play their complementary and sometimes conflictual roles. The pastoral role in the situation of a healthcare facility is not to deny tension and conflict, but to help the persons involved make a contribution to the growth of all. Jesus welcomes into his following a great variety of people at various levels of moral growth, providing for the weak and challenging the strong. St. Paul followed this pattern, with special emphasis on helping the Christians of each community mature in conscience.

In carrying out this educative task, ministers should first emphasize, as we have attempted to do in this book, the primary values and principles of Christian living as they apply to the healing process. These principles should not be presented as rules, but as goals to be creatively achieved in a loving and generous response to the grace of God, after the pattern of the Good Samaritan (Lk 10:25-37), who saw in the injured man in the ditch the call of God. The professional or the patient who has these goals at heart and uses the knowledge and imagination available to reach these goals will act in a truly humane and Christian way, enlightened by the Holy Spirit.

Christians open to the Spirit in this way are not negligent of or ungrateful for the guidance given by the pastors of the Church, whether that guidance has the certitude of the Gospel or simply the authority of pastors doing what they can to apply the Gospel in a given time or place according to the lights they possess. On the other hand, mature Christians know that God requires of them personal decisions based not only on pastoral guidance, but also on their own gifts and experience.

The final task of ethical counselors, therefore, is to help those they counsel mature in conscience and live in peace with the responsibility for their own decisions, content with the assurance which God calls us to share in his own task of healing a wounded world.

BIBLIOGRAPHY

A

AAMC: Association of American Medical Colleges, *GPEP Report*, Panel on the General Professional Education of the Physician and College Preparation for Medicine, Washington DC, 1984.

AAN: American Academy of Neurology, "Care and Management of Persistent Vegetative State Patients," *Neurology* 39, Jan. 1989, 125-127.

ABA: American Bar Association, "Lawyers Reject AMA Solution to Crisis," *Medical World News* 27 (5), March 10, 1986, 24.

Abramowitz, Stephen, "Psychosocial Outcomes of Sex Reassignment Surgery," *Journal of Consulting and Clinical Psychology* 54 (2), 1986, 183-189.

Abrams, Richard, and Essman, Walter B., eds., *Electroconvulsive Therapy: Biological Foundations and Clinical Applications*, New York, Spectrum Publications, 1982.

Ackerknecht, Erwin, *A Short History of Medicine*, Baltimore: Johns Hopkins University Press, 1982.

Ackerman, Terrence F., "Fooling Ourselves with Child Autonomy and Assent in Non-Therapeutic Clinical Research," *Clinical Research*, 1979, 345-348.

ACOG: American College of Obstetricians and Gynecologists, "Professional Liability Implications of AFP Tests," *Alert*, May 1985.

Aday, Luann; Fleming, Gretchen; and Andersen, Ronald, *Access to Medical Care in the U.S.: Who Has It, Who Doesn't*, Chicago: Pluribus Press, 1984.

Adler, Mortimer J., *The Time of Our Lives: The Ethics of Common Sense*, New York: Holt, Rinehart and Winston, 1970, ch. 17, 185ff.

Agich, George, "Roles and Responsibilities in the Definition of Consultation Liaison Psychiatry," *Journal of Medicine and Philosophy* 10 (2), May 10, 1985, 105-126.

Agich, George, and Besley, C.E., "Some Problems With Pro-Competition Reforms," *Social Science Medicine* 21 (6), 1985, 623-630.

Agich, George, and Jones, Royce, "Theological Status of Brain Death Criteria," *Journal of Medicine and Philosophy* 10 (4), Nov. 10, 1985, 387-395.

Agras, W. Stewart, and Berkowitz, Robert, "Behavior Therapy," in *Textbook of Psychiatry*, John Talbott; Robert Hales; and Stuart Yudofsky, eds. Washington, DC, American Psychiatric Press, 1988, 891-905

AHA: American Hospital Association
    1972   "Patient's Bill of Rights," Chicago: American Hospital Association Press.
    1977   *Hospital Regulation*, Chicago: American Hospital Association.
    1986a   "Cost and Compassion," Chicago: American Hospital Association.
    1986b   "Hospital Responsibility Is in Requesting Organ Donations," *Technical Advisor Bulletin*, Sept. 15.

Aiken, Linda; and Mechanic, David, *Applications of Social Science to Clinical Medicine and Health Policy*, Newark: Rutgers University Press, 1986.

Alexander, Leo, "Medical Science Under Dictatorship," *New England Journal of Medicine* 241, 1949, 39-47. Reprinted in *Child and Family* 10, 1971, 40-57.

Alford, Robert R., *Health Care Politics: Ideological and Interest Group Barriers to Reform*, Chicago: University of Chicago Press, 1975.

Allport, Gordon W.
    1937   *Personality: A Psychological Interpretation*, New York: Henry Holt, 24-50.
    1961   *Pattern and Growth in Personality*, New York: Holt, Rinehart, and Winston.

Aloming, Phillip Clayton, *Mystical Experience: An Investigation of the Study of Mysticism in World Religions*, New York: Mouton Publishing, 1982.

Alpert, Joseph S., *A Clinician's Companion: A Study Guide for Effective and Humane Patient Care*, Boston: Little Brown, 1986.

Altman, Lawrence
    1987   *Who Goes First: The Story of Self-Experimentation in Medicine*, New York: Random House.

1988   "Sharp Drop in Autopsies Stirs Fear that Quality of Care May Also Fall," *New York Times,* July 21, 1988.

AMA: American Medical Association

1973   "Report of the Judicial Council on Death," adopted by the American Medical Association House of Delegates, Dec.

1981   "Opinions on Social Policy Issues," *Current Opinions of the Judicial Council of the American Medical Association,* Chicago: AMA.

1984   *Socioeconomic Characteristics of Medical Practice,* Chicago: American Medical Association.

1986a   *Health Plan for America,* Chicago: AMA.

1986b   "Closing the Gaps in Health Insurance Coverage," *Journal of the American Medical Association,* 225 (6), Feb. 14, 790-793.

1986c   Report of Judicial Council, "Treatment of Patients in Irreversible Coma," March 15.

1987a   AMA Special Task Force on Professional Liability and Insurance, *Journal of the American Medical Association* 257 (6), Feb. 13, 810-812.

1987b   *Health Policy Agenda for the American People,* Chicago: AMA.

1988a   Report of the Council on Ethical and Judicial Affairs, "Ethical Issues Involved in Growing AIDS Crisis," *Journal of the American Medical Association* 259, 1360.

1988b   "AMA House Delegates Reject Euthanasia," *New York Times,* June 28.

1988c   "News at Deadline: AMA Accepts Registered Care Technologist," *Hospitals* 14, July 10.

1988d   *Director of Graduate Medical Education Programs, 1988-89,* Chicago: AMA.

American Academy of Neurology: see AAN

American Bar Association: see ABA

American College of Obstetricians and Gyneocologists: see ACOG

American Hospital Association: see AHA

American Medical Association: see AMA

American Nurses' Association: see ANA

American Psychiatric Association: see APA

American Society of Neurosurgeons, in *Patricia Brophy v. New England Sinai Hospital,* (Mass. sup. court, jud. ct. Sept. 11, 1986), cited p. 12.

Amulree, Lord, et al., *On Dying Well: An Anglican Contribution to the Debate on Euthanasia,* London: Church Information Service, 1975.

ANA: American Nurses' Association, *Profession and the Empowerment of Nursing,* Kansas City: American Nurses' Association, 1982.

Anderson, Frank; and Rubenstein, A., "Frequency of Sexual Dysfunction in Normal Couples," *New England Journal of Medicine* 299, 1978, 111-115.

Anderson, W. French, "Human Gene Therapy: Scientific and Ethical Considerations," *Journal of Medicine and Philosophy* 3, Aug 10, 1985, 275-291.

Andrews, Lori, *State Laws and Regulations Governing Newborn Screening,* Chicago: American Bar Foundation, 1985.

Andrusko, Dave; and Bond, Leslie, "Harvesting the Living," *Call to Conscience,* ch. 9, Washington: National Right to Life Conference, 1988.

Annas, George

1973   "The Patients Have Rights: How Can We Protect Them?" *Hastings Center Report* 9, 8-9.

1976   "Confidentiality and the Duty to Warn," *Hastings Center Report* 6, 6-8.

1979   "Denying the Rights of the Retarded: The Phillip Becker Case," *Hastings Center Report* 9, 18-20.

1980   "Refusing Medication in Mental Hospitals," *Hastings Center Report* 10, 21-22.

1983   "Refusal of Life-Saving Treatment for Minors," *Journal of Family Law* 23 (2), 1983, 217-240.

1985a   "Is Genetic Screening Test Ready When the Lawyers Say It Is?" *Hastings Center Report* 6, Dec. 15.

1985b   "The Phoenix Heart, What We Have to Lose," *Hastings Center Report* 3, June 15, 1985, 15-16.

1985c   "Fashion and Freedom: When Artificial Feeding Should Be Withdrawn," *American Journal of Public Health* 75 (6), 685-688.

Annas, George, et al., "Guidelines for the Determination of Brain Death in Children," *Archives of Neurology* 44 (6), June 1987, 587-88.

Annas, George; Glantz, Leonard; and Katz, Barbara, "Rights in the Provider-Patient Relationship," in their *The Right of Doctors, Nurses and Allied Health Professionals: A Health Law Primer*, New York: Avon Books, 1981.

Ansabel, D.P., "Methadone Maintainance Treatment: The Other Side of the Coin," *International Journal of Addiction* 18, 1983, 851-862.

APA: American Psychiatric Association

1980   *Diagnostic and Statistical Manual of Mental Disorders* (DSM III), 3rd ed, Washington, DC: American Psychiatric Association.

1981   *The Principles of Medical Ethics with Annotations Especially Applicable to Psychiatry*, Washington: APA.

1985   Task Force, *Seclusion and Restraint: The Psychiatric Uses*, Washington, DC, APA.

1986a   "Unethical Behavior, Incompetency, and Impairment in the Ethical Decision Process," *Ethics Newsletter, APA* 2 (1), Jan.-Feb.

1986   "Sexual Involvement Between Psychiatrists, Their Students, Supervisors, Colleagues, and Employees," *Ethics Newsletter, APA* 2 (2), Apr.-May.

Applebaum, Paul, "The Cautious Advance on the Right to Treatment," *Hospital and Community Psychiatry* 33 (11), Nov. 1982, 895-896.

Applebaum, Paul, et al., "Researcher's Access to Patient Records: An Analysis of the Ethical Problems," *Clinical Research* 32 (4), Oct. 1984.

Applebaum, Paul, et al., "False Hopes and Best Data: Consent to Research and Therapeutic Misconceptions," *Hastings Center Report* 17 (2), April 1987, 16-30.

Applebaum, Paul; Lidz, Charles; and Meisel, Alan, *Informed Consent, Legal Theory and Clinical Practice*, New York: Oxford Press, 1987, 12.

Appleton, William S., "The Importance of Psychiatrists' Telling Patients the Truth," *American Journal of Psychiatry* 129, 1972, 742-745.

Aquinas, Saint Thomas, *Summa Theologiae*. Gilby, Thomas, OP, ed., New York: McGraw-Hill, 1976; On the body: vol. 11, I, 75, 4, ad. 2, 76, 1 ad. 6; *Principles of morality*, vol. 18, 1-11; 18-21; *Law and political theory*, vol. 28, 1-11, q. 90-97; On the principle of totality: vol. 38, II-II, q. 65, 1 c.

Areen, Judith. et al., "Death and Dying," in *Law, Science, and Medicine*, Mineola, NY: Foundation Press, 1984, 1063-1235.

Aries, Philippe, *The Hour of Our Death*, New York: Alfred A. Knopf, 1981.

Armstrong, David, *An Outline of Sociology as Applied to Medicine*, Bristol: Wright, 1980.

Arney, William Ray, and Berger, Bernard, *Medicine and the Management of Living; Taming the Last Great Beast*, Chicago: University of Chicago Press, 1984.

Arnold, William, *Introduction to Pastoral Care*, Louisville, KY: Westminster Press, 1982.

Arnstein, Robert, "Divided Loyalties in Adolescent Psychiatry: Late Adolescence," *Social Science and Medicine* 23 (8), 1986, 797-802.

Arraj, James, and Arraj, Tyra, *St. John of the Cross and Dr. C.G. Jung*, Chiloquin, OR: Tools for Inner Growth, 1984.

Arras, John, and Shinnar, Shlomo, "Anencephalic Newborns as Organ Donors: A Critique," *Journal of the American Medical Association* 259 (15), Apr. 15, 1988, 2284.

Aristotle, *Politics*, Richard McKeon, ed., Chicago: University of Chicago Press, 1950.

Ashley, Benedict, OP

1972   "A Psychological Model with a Spiritual Dimension," *Pastoral Psychology* 23, 31-40.

1976   "A Critique of the Theory of Delayed Hominization," in *An Ethical Evaluation of Fetal Experimentation: An Interdisciplinary Study*, Donald G. McCarthy and Albert S. Moraczewski, OP, eds., St. Louis: Pope John XXIII Medical-Moral

Research and Education Center, 113-133.

1981   "The Use of Moral Theory by the Church," in *Human Sexuality and Personhood*, St. Louis: Pope John XXIII Medical-Moral Research and Education Center, 223-242.

1985   *Theologies of the Body*, Braintree, MA: Pope John XXIII Medical-Moral Reserach and Education Center.

1987   "How the Roman Catholic Position on Euthanasia Developed," Report to the Catholic-Methodist Dialogue.

Ashley, Joann, *Hospitals Paternalism and the Role of the Nurse*, New York: Teacher's College Press, 1976.

Association of American Medical Colleges: see AAMC

Atkinson, Gary M., "Historical Perspective on the Duty to Preserve Life," research essay for the Pope John XXIII Medical-Moral Research and Education Center, St. Louis, 1979.

Atkinson, Gary M., and Moraczewski, Albert S., OP, *Genetic Counseling: The Church and the Law*, St. Louis: Pope John XXIII Medical-Moral Research and Education Center, 1980.

Australian Research Commission, *Human Embryo Experimentation in Australia*, Senate Select Committee on Human Experimentation Bill, Australian Government Printing Office, 1985, p. 25.

Auxter, Thomas, *Kant's Moral Theology*, Macon, GA: Mercer University Press, 1982.

Aviram, Uri, and Shnit, Dan, "Psychiatric Treatment and Civil Liberties in Israel: The Need for Reform" *Israel Journal of Psychiatry and Related Sciences* 21 (1), 1984, 3-18.

Axelrod, David, "Axelrod Faults MD's for Failure to Self-Regulate," *Medical Staff News* 2, May 1988.

Axelrod, David, et al., "Physician Competence: Whose Responsibility?" *Medical Staff News* 3 May 1988.

Axelrod, Saul, and Apsche, Jack, eds., *The Effects of Punishment on Human Behavior*, Orlando: Academic Press, 1983.

Ayer, A.J., *Language, Truth and Logic*, London: Gollancz, 1936.

B

Baker, Robert, and Elliston, Frederick, *Philosophy and Sex*, New York: Prometheus Books, 1984.

Bakken, Kenneth L., *The Call to Wholeness: Health as a Spiritual Journey*, New York: Crossroad Publishing Co., 1985.

Baldessarini, R., *Chemotherapy in Psychiatry*, Cambridge, MA: Harvard University Press, 1985.

Bandura, A., *Social Foundation of Thought and Action*, Englewood Cliffs, NJ: Prentice-Hall, 1986.

Barber, Bernard
    1965   "Some Problems of the Sociology of Professions," in *The Professions in America*, Kenneth S. Lynn, ed., Boston: Houghton Mifflin, Daedalus, 647-865.

    1967   *Drugs and Society*, New York: Russell Sage Foundation.

    1980   *Informed Consent in Medical Therapy and Research*, New Brunswick, NJ: Rutgers University Press.

Barger-Lux, Janet, and Heaney, Robert, "For Better or Worse: Technological Imperative in Healthcare," *Social Science and Medicine* 22 (12), 1986, 1313-1320.

Barlow, George W., and Silverberg, James, eds., *Sociobiology: Beyond Nature/Nurture? Reports, Definitions, and Debates*, Boulder, CO: Westview Press, Inc., 1980.

Barnard, Christian, *Good Life/Good Death: A Doctor's Case for Euthanasia and Suicide*, Englewood Cliffs, NJ: Prentice-Hall, 1980.

Barnlund, Dean C., "The Mystification of Meaning: Doctor-Patient Encounters," *Journal of Medical Education* 51, 1976, 716-725.

Baron, Charles H., "Fetal Research: The Question in the States," *Hastings Center Report* 15 (2), Apr. 15, 1985, 12-16.

Baron, Charles H., "The Case for the Courts," *Journal of American Geriatric Society* 32 (1), Oct. 1984, 734-38.

Baron, Richard J., "Bridging Clinical Distance: An Empathic Rediscovery of the Known," *Journal of Medicine and Philosophy* 16, 1981, 5-24.

Barry, Robert, "Withholding and Withdrawing Treatment," *Journal of the American Medical Association* 256 (4), Jul. 25, 1986, 469-71.

Barry, William A., and Connolly, William J., *The Practice of Spiritual Direction*, New York: Seabury Press, Inc., 1982.

Bashim, Yvonne, "Doctoring The Genes," *Science* 84 (10), Dec. 5, 1984, 52-60.

Basson, Marc; Caplan, Arthur; and Abrams, Gerald, "The Right to Privacy When Lives Are at Stake," in *Troubling Problems in Medical Ethics*, M. Basson, et al., eds., New York, Alan R. Liss, 1988.

Battin, Margaret P., "Suicide and Ethical Theory," *Suicide and Life Threatening Behavior* 13 (4), Winter, 1983, 231-239.

Battin, M. Pabst, and Mayo, David J., eds., *Suicide: The Philosophical Issues*, New York: St. Martin's Press, 1980.

Baumiller, Robert, "Genetic Counseling" in *Genetic Medicine and Engineering: Ethical and Social Dimensions*, St. Louis: Catholic Health Association of the United States, 1983, 31-44.

Bayer, Edward
    1982   *Oppression Within Marriage and Prevention of Pregnancy by Artificial Means*, Rome: St. Thomas University.
    1985   *Rape within Marriage: A Moral Analysis Delayed*, Lanham, MD: University Press of America.

Bayer, Ronald, *Homosexuality and American Psychiatry: The Politics of Diagnosis*, Princeton, NJ, Princeton University Press, 1987.

Bayer, Ronald, et al., "Guidelines for Confidentiality in Research on AIDS," *I.R.B.: A Review of Human Subject Research* 6 (6), Nov.-Dec. 1984, 1-7.

Bayer, Ronald, and Callahan, Daniel, "Medicare Reform: Social and Ethical Perspectives," *Journal of Health Politics* 10 (3), Policy and Law, Fall, 1985, 533-547.

Bayer, Ronald, and Moreno, Jonathan, "Ethical and Social Dilemmas of Government Policy," *Health Affairs* 5 (2), 1986, 72-85.

Bayer, Ronald; Levine, Carol; and Wolt, Susan, "HIV Antibody Screening: An Ethical Framework for Evaluation," *Journal of the American Medical Association* 256 (13), Oct. 3, 1986.

Bayley, Corrine, and McCormick, Richard A., SJ, "Sterilization: The Dilemma of Catholic Hospitals," *America* 143, Oct. 18, 1980, 222-225.

Beauchamp, Tom L., and Childress, James, *Principles of Biomedical Ethics*, New York: Oxford University Press, 1983, 43.

Beauchamp, Tom L., and McCullough, Lawrence B., *Medical Ethics: The Moral Responsibilities of Physicians*, Englewood Cliffs, NJ: Prentice-Hall, 1984.

Beck, Aaron, et al., *The Prediction of Suicide*, Philadelphia: Charles Press, 1986.

Becker, Ernest, *The Denial of Death*. New York: Free Press, 1973.

Becker, Howard S., "The Nature of a Profession," in *Education for the Professions*, Nelson B. Henry, ed., 61st Yearbook of the National Society for the Study of Education, 2nd ed., Chicago: University of Chicago Press, 1960, 27-46.

Becker, Judith, and Kavoussi, Richard, "Sexual Disorders," in *Textbook of Psychiatry*, John Talbott; Robert Hales; and Stuart Yudofsky, eds., Washington, DC: American Psychiatric Press, 1988, 587-604.

Bedau, Hugo Adam, "Soundness of Mind and 'Mental Setting'," a review of Fingarette and Hasse's "Mental Disabilities and Criminal Responsibility," *Hastings Center Report* 10 1980, 46-49.

Beis, Richard, "Some Contributions of Anthropology to Ethics," *The Thomist* 28, 1964, 174-190.

Bellah, Robert, et al., *Habits of the Heart: Individualism and Commitment in American Life*, New York: Harper & Row, 1986.

Belli, Melvin, "Warning of the Dangerous Patient: A Practical Approach," *American Journal of Forensic Psychiatry* 2 (2), 1982, 2-6.

The Belmont Report: Ethical Principles and Guidelines for the Protection of Human Subjects of Research, 2 vols., U.S. National Commission for the Protection of Human Subjects of Biomedical and Behavioral Research. Washington, DC: U.S. Government Printing Office, 1978.

Benjamin, Harry, *Standards of Care: The Hormonal and Surgical Sex Reassignment of Gender Dysphoric Persons*, Galveston: The Harry Benjamin International Gender Dysphoria Association, Inc., 1980.

Benjamin, Martin
    1985   "Lay Obligation in Professional Relations," *Journal of Medicine and Philosophy* 1, Feb. 10, 1985, 85-103.
    1988   "Medical Ethics and Economics of Organ Transplantation," *Health Progress*, March, 47.

Benton, Arthur, "Historical Development of the Concept of Hemispheric Cerebral Dominance," in *Philosophical Dimensions of the Neuro-Medical Sciences*, 2 vols., Stuart F. Spiker and H. Tristram Engelhardt, Jr., eds., Boston: Reidel, 1976, Vol 2, 35-38.

Berger, Brigette and Berger, Peter, *The War Over The Family*, New York: Anchor Press, 1983.

Berger, Peter, and Luckmann, Thomas, *The Social Construction of Reality: A Treatise in the Sociology of Knowledge*, Garden City, NJ: Doubleday, 1966.

Beriman, Daniel, and Navarro, Vincente, *Health and Work Under Capitalism: An Alternative Perspective*, Amityville, NY: Baywood Publishing, 1983.

Berlant, Jeffrey Lionel, *Profession and Monopoly: A Study of Medicine in the United States and Great Britain*, Berkeley: University of California Press, 1975.

Berlin, Fred, "Ethical Use of Psychiatric Diagnosis," *Psychiatric Annals* 13 (4), Apr. 1983, 321-331.

Bermel, Joyce, "Organs for Sale: From Marketplace to Jungle," *Hastings Center Report* 16 (1), Feb. 1986, 3.

Bernadine, Joseph, "The Consistent Ethic of Life," *Health Progress* 67 (6), July 1986, 48-51.

Bernstein, Dorothy M., and Simmons, Roberta G., "The Adolescent Kidney Donor: The Right to Give," *American Journal of Psychiatry* 131, 1975, 1338-1343.

Bertalanffy, Ludwig von, *General System Theory: Foundations, Development, Applications*. New York: Dover Publications, 1968.

Biggers, John, "In Vitro Fertilization and Embryo Transfer in Human Beings," *New England Journal of Medicine* 304 (6),Feb. 5, 1981, 336.

Billings, Evelyn, and Westmore, Ann, *The Billings Method: Controlling Fertility without Drugs or Devices*, 5th ed., Victoria, Australia: Gorbon and Gotch, 1985.

Billings, John, *The Ovulation Method*, 7th ed., Melbourne: Advocate Press, 1983.

Birch, Charles, *The Liberation of Life: From the Cell to the Community*, New York: Cambridge University Press, 1981.

Birmingham, William, *What Modern Catholics Think About Birth Control*, New York: New American Library, Signet Books, 1964.

Bissell, LeClair, and Royce, James, *Ethics for Addiction Professionals*, Center City, MN: Hazelden Foundation, 1987.

Black, Peter
    1983   "Clinical Problems in the Use of Brain-Death Standards," *Archives of Internal Medicine* 143 (1), Jan., 121-123.
    1984   "Declarations of Brain Death in Neurosurgical and Neurological Practice," *Neurosurgery* 15 (2), Aug., 170-174.

Black, Peter, and Szasz, Thomas, "The Ethics of Psychosurgery: Pro and Con," *The Humanist* 37, 1977, 6-11.

Blakeslee, Sandra, "A Baby Born Without Her Brain Is Kept Alive to Donate Her Heart," *New York Times*, Nov. 18, 1987.

Blendon, Robert J., "Uncompensated Care by Hospitals or Public Insurance for the Poor: Does it Make a Difference?" *New England Journal of Medicine* 314 (18), May 1, 1986, 1160-1163.

Blendon, Robert J., and Donelan, Karen, "Discrimination Against People with AIDS," *New England Journal of Medicine* 319 (15), Oct. 13, 1988, 1022.

Block, Sidney and Chodoff, Paul, eds. *Psychiatric Ethics*, New York: Oxford University Press 1981.

Bloom, Alan, *The Closing of the American Mind: Education and the Crisis of Reason*, New York: Simon and Schuster, 1987.

Blum, Henrick L.
   1974   *Planning for Health: Development and Application of Social Change*, New York: Behavioral Publishers.
   1983   *Expanding Health Care Horizons: From General Systems Concept of Health Care to a National Policy*, Oakland: Third Party Publications.

Blum, Richard H., *A Commonsense Guide to Doctors, Hospitals and Medical Care*, New York: Macmillan, 1964.

Boff, Leonardo, *Liberation Theology: From Dialogue to Confrontation*, San Francisco: Harper and Row, 1986.

Boffey, Philip M., "Organ Transplants Grow in Number and in Success," *New York Times*, Nov. 4, 1984, 8e.

Boisen, Anton T.
   1936   *Exploration of the Inner World*, New York: Harper & Row, Torchbooks.
   1945   *Religion in Crisis and Custom*, New York: Harper.

Bok, Derek, "Needed: A New Way to Train Doctors," *Connecticut Medicine* 48 (11), Nov. 1984, 741-48.

Bok, Sissela, *Secrets: On the Ethics of Concealment and Revelation*, New York: Pantheon Books, 1982, 116ff.

Boorse, C., "On the Distinction Between Disease and Illness," in *Concepts of Health and Disease Interdisciplinary Perspectives*, Reading, MA: Addison-Wesley, 1981.

Bopp, James, "Protection of Disabled Newborns: Are There Constitutional Limitations?" *Issues in Law and Medicine* 1 (3), Nov. 1985, 173-200.

Boros, SJ, Ladislaus, *The Mystery of Death*, New York: Herder & Herder, 1965.

Bosk, Charles
   1979   *Forgive and Remember, Managing Medical Failures*, Chicago: University of Chicago Press.
   1986   "The Health Care System: Overview," in James Childress, et al., *Biolaw* vol. 1, Frederick, MD: University Publications of America, 9-27.

Bourke, Vernon J., *History of Ethics*, 2 vols., New York: Doubleday, Image Books, 1970, Vol. 1: On Voluntarism, 147ff.

Bower, Robert, and de Gaspanis, Priscilla, *Ethics in Social Research: Protecting the Interests of Human Subjects*, New York: Praeger Publications, 1978.

Bowker, John, *Problems of Suffering in the Religions of the World*, New York: Cambridge University Press, 1970.

Bowman, Harold, "Benefits of Autopsies," *AMA News*, Nov. 11, 1983.

Boyle, Joseph, Jr.
   1980   "Toward Understanding the Principle of Double Effect," *Ethics* 90, 527-538.
   1985   "The Developing Consensus on the Right to Health Care, in *Justice and Health Care*, M. Kelly, ed., St. Louis: Catholic Health Association.

Boyle, Patrick, *Parvitas Material in Sexto in Contemporary Catholic Thought*, Lanhan, MD: University Press of America, 1987.

Boyle, Philip, and O'Rourke, Kevin, "Presumed Consent for Organ Donation," *America* 155 (15), Nov. 22, 1986, 326-332.

Boyle, Philip, "Access to Health Care," *Ethical Essays*, Dec. 1986.

Braen, C. Richard, "Sexual Assault," in *Emergency Medical Textbook*, Peter Rosen, et al., St.

Louis, C.V. Mosby, 1988.

Brahms, Diana, "Doctor's Duty to Answer Patients' Inquiries," *The Lancet* 1 (8538), Apr. 18, 1987, 932.

Braunstein, P., et al., "Evaluation of the Critical Deficit of Cerebral Circulation using Radioactive Tracers," in *Brain Death: Interrelated Medical and Social Issues*, J. Korein, ed., New York: New York Academy of Sciences, 1978, 143-167.

Breggin, Peter R.
    1972   "New Information in the Debate Over Psychosurgery," *Congressional Record*, March 30, E3380-86.
    1979   *Electroshock: Its Brain-Disabling Effects*, New York: Springer Publishing Co., 1979.

Brewin, Thurstan, "Voluntary Euthanasia," *The Lancet* 1 (8489), May 10, 1986, 1085-86.

Brodeur, Dennis, "Toward a Clear Definition of Ethics Committees," *Linacre Quarterly* 51 (3), Aug. 1984, 233-247.

Brody, Baruch A.
    1975   *Abortion and the Sanctity of Human Life: A Philosophical View*, Cambridge, MA: MIT Press.
    1983a "Autonomy and Paternalism: Some Value Problems; A Utilitarian Perspective, A Deontological Perspective," ch. 12-14 in his *Ethics and its Applications*, New York: Harcourt Brace Jovanovich, 159-198.
    1983b *Ethics and its Applications*, New York: Harcourt Brace Jovanovich.

Brody, Baruch A., and Engelhardt, H. Tristram, Jr., eds., "Mental Illness: Law and Public Policy," in *Philosophy and Medicine*, vol. 5, Boston: Reidel, 1980.

Brody, Baruch, A., et al., "Morality and Sex Change," *Hastings Center Report* 11, 1981, 8-13.

Brody, Howard, *Ethical Decisions in Medicine*, 2nd ed., Boston: Little, Brown, 1981, 37-72.

Brogan, Michael, "Recent Developments in Behavior Modification," *Nebraska Law Review* 60 (2), 1981, 363-399.

Bromley, Dorothy Dunbar, *Catholics and Birth Control: Contemporary Views on Doctrine*, Old Greenwich, CT: Devin-Adair Publications, Inc., 1965.

Brooks, Simon A., "Dignity and Cost Effectiveness: A Rejection of the Utilitarian Approach to Death," *Journal of Medical Ethics* 10 (3), Sept. 10, 1984, 148-151.

Brophy, Patricia v. New England Sinai Hospital, Inc., (Mass. sup. jud. ct., Sept. 11, 1986).

Brower, Leslie A., "The Health Care Team: Who Calls the Plays?" in *Biomedical Ethics: A Community Forum*, Henry M. Sondheimer, ed., Syracuse: SUNY Medical Center, 1985, 135-142.

Brown, Delwin, *To Set at Liberty, Christian Faith and Human Freedom*, Maryknoll, NY: Orbis Books, 1981.

Brown, N. Miller, "On Defining Disease," *The Journal of Medicine and Philosophy*, Nov. 1985.

Brown, J.B., et al., "Natural Family Planning," *American Journal of Obstetrics and Gynecology* 157, Oct. 1987, 1082.

Browning, Don
    1976   *The Moral Context of Pastoral Care*, Philadelphia: Westminster Press.
    1983   *Religious Ethics & Pastoral Care*, Philadelphia: Fortress Press.
    1987   *Religious Thought and the Modern Psychologies: A Critical Conversation in the Theology of Culture*, Philadelphia: Fortress Press.

Bruce, JoAnne, "Patient Access to Medical Records," in her *Privacy and Confidentiality of Health Care Information*, Chicago: American Hospital Publishing, 1984, 125-136.

Bryce, Edmund, and Wyschogord, Michael, *Principles of Treatment for Handicapped Newborns*, Washington, DC: National Conference of Catholic Bishops, 1985.

Bultmann, Rudolf, *Jesus and the Word*, New York: Charles Scribner's Sons, 1958.

Burtchaell, James T.
    1980 ed., *Abortion Parley*, Kansas City: Andrews and McMeel, 1980.
    1988 "University Policy on Experimental Use of Aborted Fetal Tissue," *IRB* 10 (4), July 1988, 8.

Byrne, Paul, et al., "Brain Death, An Opposing Viewpoint," *Journal of the American Medical Association* 242, 1979, 1985-1990.

C

Caffara, Carlo, "The Ecclesial Identity and Mission of the Family," in *The Family Today and Tomorrow*, St. Louis: Pope John XXIII Medical-Moral Research and Education Center, 1985.

Cahill, Lisa Sowle
- 1981 "Teleology, Utilitarianism, and Christian Ethics," *Theological Studies* 42, Dec. 1981, 601-629.
- 1985 *Between the Sexes: Foundations for a Christian Ethics of Sexuality*, Philadelphia: Fortress Press.

Cahn, Steven, *Saints and Scamps: Ethics in Academia*, Totowa: NJ: Rowman & Littlefield, 1986.

Califano, Joseph, *America's Health Care Revolution*, New York: Random House, 1985.

Callahan, Daniel
- 1973a *The Tyranny of Survival and Other Pathologies of Civilized Life*, New York: Macmillan.
- 1973b "The WHO Definition of Health," *Hastings Center Studies* 1 (3), 77-87.
- 1980 ed., "Will Biology Transform the Humanities?" *Hastings Center Report* 10, 1980, 27-39.
- 1981 "Arguing the Morality of Genetic Engineering," in *Medical Ethics and the Law: Implications for Public Policy*, Marc Hiller, ed., Cambridge, MA: Ballinger, 441-449.
- 1986 Technology Is Reframing the Abortion Debate," *Hasting Center Report* 1, Feb. 16, 1986, 33-42.
- 1987a "Surrogate Motherhood: A Bad Idea," *New York Times*, Jan. 20.
- 1987b *Setting Limits: Medical Goals in an Aging Society*, New York: Simon and Schuster.

Canada Law Reform Commission. *Criteria for the Determination of Death*, Ottowa: The Commission, 1981.

Canadian Medical Association Journal, "Confidentiality, Ownership, and Transfer of Medical Records," 133 (10), Nov. 15, 1985.

Cannon, David, "Abortion and Infanticide: Is There a Difference?" *Policy Review* 32, Spring 1985, 12-17.

Caplan, Arthur L., "Ethical Issues Raised by Research Involving Xenographs," *Journal of the American Medical Association* 254 (23), Dec. 20, 1985, 3339-3343.

Capps, Walter H., ed., *The Future of Hope: Essays by Block, Fackenheim, Motlmann, Metz, and Capps*, Philadelphia: Fortress Press, 1970.

Capron, Alexander M.
- 1984 "Current Issues in Genetic Screening," in Humber James, et al., ed., *Biomedical Ethics Review 1984*, Clifton, NJ: Humana Press, 121-149.
- 1986 "Determination of Death," in Katherine Benesch, et al., eds., *Medicolegal Aspects of Critical Care*, Rockville, MD: Aspen Publishers, 109-132.

Carmi, Ammon, "Genetic Engineering," *Medicine and Law* 3, Aug. 2, 1983, 181-192.

Carnes, Patrick, *Sexual Addiction*, Minneapolis: Comp-Care Publications, 1983.

Carney, Frederick, "On McCormick and Teleological Morality," *Journal of Religious Ethics* 6, 1978, 81-107.

Carrick, Paul, *Medical Ethics in Antiquity: Philosophical Perspectives on Abortion and Euthanasia*, Boston: D. Riedl, 1985.

Carroll, Douglas, and O'Callaghan, Mark, "Regulating Pychosurgery: Ethical, Social, and Scientific Considerations," *Medicine and Law* 3 (2), 1984, 193-203.

Cassel, Christine, "Ethical Issues in Mental Health Care of the Elderly," in *Geriatric Mental Health*, J.P. Abrahams, ed., New York: Grune and Stratton, 1984, 229-241.

Cassell, Eric
- 1976 *The Healer's Art*, New York: Lippincott.
- 1984 *The Place of Humanities in Medicare*, Hastings-on-Hudson: Hastings Center.

Cassell, Eric, et al., "Refinements in Criteria for the Determination of Death: An Appraisal," *Journal of the American Medical Association* 221, 1972, 48-53.

Cassens, Brett, "Social Consequences of the Acquired Immune Deficiency Syndrome," *Annals of Internal Medicine* 103 (5), Nov. 1985, 768-771.

Cassirer, Ernst, *The Philosophy of Symbolic Forms,* vol.1, New Haven: Yale University Press, 1953, 86-93.

Casswell, Donald, "Limitations in Canadian Law on the Right of a Prisoner to Refuse Medical Treatment," *Journal of Contemporary Health and Law Policy* (2), Spring 1986, 155-167.

Cavanaugh, John R., *The Popes, The Pill and The People,* Milwaukee: Bruce Books, 1964.

CCHCM: Commission for Catholic Health Care Ministry, "A New Vision for a New Century," Livonia, MI: Commission Control Office, 1988, 62.

CDC: Centers for Disease Control, "Update: Human Immunodeficiency Virus Infection in Health Care Workers Exposed to Blood of Infected Patients," *Morbidity and Morality Weekly Report* 36, 1987, 285-289.

Centers for Disease Control: see CDC

CHA: The Catholic Health Association of the United States

    1980   *Evaluative Criteria for Catholic Health Care Facilities,* St. Louis: The Catholic Health Association of the United States.

    1981   *National Health Insurance: Why CHA Is Taking Another Look,* St. Louis: The Catholic Health Association of the United States, 43.

    1983   *Health Care Ministry Assessment,* St. Louis: The Catholic Health Association of the United States.

    1986   *No Room in the Marketplace: The Health Care of the Poor,* St. Louis: The Catholic Health Association of the United States.

Chalkley, D.T., "Panel Discussion," in *Experiments and Research with Humans: Values in Conflict,* Washington, DC: National Academy of Sciences, 1975, 161-163.

Chaska, Norma L., *The Nursing Profession: A Time to Speak,* New York: McGraw-Hill, 1983.

Chayet, Neil L., "Confidentiality and Privileged Communication," *New England Journal of Medicine* 275, 1966, 1009-1010.

Chervenak, F.A., Farley, Margaret, Walters, Leroy, et al., "When is Termination of Pregnancy During the Third Trimester Justifiable," *New England Journal of Medicine* 310, 1984, 501-504.

Childress, James

    1982   *Who Should Decide: Paternalism in Health Care,* New York: Oxford University Press.

    1984   "Rights to Health Care in a Democratic Society," in *Biomedical Ethics Review,* Humber and Almeder, eds., Clifton, NJ: Humane Press, 47-70.

Choron, Jacques, *Suicide,* New York: Charles Scribner Sons, 1972.

CIC, Code of Canon Law, 1983, Canon 1055, Canon 1398.

Clark, Henry, *Altering Behavior: The Ethics of Controlled Experience,* Newbury Park, CA: Sage Publications, Inc., 1987.

Clark, Keith, *Being Sexual and Celibate,* Notre Dame, IN: Ave Maria Press, 1986.

Clark, W.H., "Ethics and LSD," *Journal of Psychiatric Drugs* 17 (4), Oct.-Dec. 1985, 229-34.

Clebsch, William A., and Jaekle, Charles R., *Pastoral Care in Historical Perspective,* New York: Jason Aronson, 1964.

Clements, Colleen

    1983   "Common Psychiatric Problems and Uncommon Ethical Solutions," *Psychiatric Annals* 13 (4), April 1983, 289-301.

    1985   "Therefore Choose Life: Reconciling Medical and Environmental Ethics," *Perspectives in Biology and Medicine* 28 (3), Spring 1985, 407-425.

Clinebell, John Howard, *Basic Types of Pastoral Care and Counseling Resources for the Ministry of Healing and Growth,* Nashville: Abingdon Press, 1984.

Clouser, K. Danner, *Teaching Bioethics: Strategies, Problems, and Resources,* New York: The Hastings Center Monograph: Plenum Press, 1980, 77.

Clouser, K. Danner; Culver, Charles M.; and Gert, Bernard, "Malady: A New Treatment of Disease," *Hastings Center Report* 11, 1981, 29-37.

Cobb, John B., *Theology and Pastoral Care,* Philadelphia: Fortress Press, 1977.

Coe, Rodney M., *Sociology of Medicine,* New York: McGraw-Hill, 1978.

College of Healthcare Executives, *The Future of Healthcare: Changes and Choices,* Chicago: Arthur Andersen Co., 1987.

College of Physicians Health and Public Policy Committee, "Acquired Immunodeficiency Syndrome," *Annals of Internal Medicine* 104 (4), Apr. 1986, 575-581.

Colombotos, John, and Kirchner, Corrine, *Physicians and Social Change,* New York: Oxford University Press, 1986.

Commission for Catholic Health Care Ministry: see CCHCM

Committee on Bioethical Issues of the Bishops of Great Britain and Ireland: see GBI

Congar, Yves
    1967   *Tradition and Traditions.* New York: Macmillan.
    1977   "The Magisterium and Theologians—A Short History," *Theology Digest* 25, 15-21.

Connell, Francis J., Articles in *New Catholic Encyclopedia,* New York: McGraw-Hill, 1968, vol. 4, "Principle of Double Effect," "Moral Doubt"; vol 9, "Systems of Morality"; vol 12, "Reflex Principles."

Connell, R.J., "A Defense of 'HV,'" *Laval Theologique et Philosophique* 26, 1970 57-88. Criticism by W.R. Albury, and reply by L. Connell, *Laval Theologique et Philosophique* 27, 1971, 135-149.

Connery, John, SJ
    1973   "Morality of Consequences: A Critical Appraisal," *Theological Studies* 34, 396-414.
    1977   *Abortion: The Development of the Roman Catholic Perspective,* Chicago: Loyola University Press.
    1980   "Prolonging Life: The Duty and Its Limits," *Catholic Mind,* Oct. 11, 43-57.
    1981   "Catholic Ethics: Has the Norm for Rule Making Changed?" *Theological Studies* 42, 1981, 232-250.

Connors, Edward, "Catholic Health Care: Future Blueprint," *Health Progress,* Nov. 1986, 31-35.

Conrad, Peter, and Kern, Rochelle, eds., *The Sociology of Health and Illness,* New York: St. Martin's Press, 1981.

Consensus Conference, "Electro-Convulsive Therapy," *Journal of the American Medical Association* 254 (15), Oct. 18, 1985, 210-08.

Cooper, David, "Trust," *Journal of Medical Ethics* 11 (2), June 1985, 92-93.

Cooper, Eugene J., "The Fundamental Option," *Irish Theological Quarterly,* 1972, 382-392.

Cope, Oliver, *Man, Mind and Medicine,* Philadelphia: Lippencott, 1968.

Copp, David, and Zimmerman, David, eds., *Morality, Reason and Truth: New Essays on the Foundations of Ethics,* Totowa, NJ: Rowan and Allanheld, 1985.

Couch, Nathen, et al., "The High Cost of Low Frequency Events: The Anatomy of Surgical Mishaps," *New England Journal of Medicine* 304, 1981, 634-637.

Council of Europe
    1982   "Artificial Insemination of Human Beings," *Medicine and Law* 1 (1), June, 3-10.
    1985   "Opinions on the Use of Dead Human Embryos for Industrial and Commercial Purposes," in *Council of Europe,* 37th Session, Strasbourg: The Council, 1-9.

Cousins, Norman
    1984   *The Healing Heart,* New York: Avon Publishers, 1984.
    1985   "How Patients Appraise Physicians," *New England Journal of Medicine* 313 (22), Nov. 28, 1985, 1422-1424.

Cox, Harvey, ed., *The Situation Ethics Debate,* Philadelphia: Westminster Press, 1968.

Cramer, D.W., et al., "Tubal Infertility and the Interuterine Device," *New England Journal of Medicine* 312, 1985, 941-947.

Cranford, Ronald, "Termination of Treatment in the Persistent Vegetative State," *Seminars in Neurology* 4(1), March 1984, 36-44.

Cranford, Ronald, "Life, Death, Awareness, and Suffering," in *Social Responsibility: Business, Journalism, Law, Medicine,* Louis Hodges, ed., Lexington, VA: Washington & Lee University, 1985, 41-50.

Crauford, D., and Harris, R., "Ethics of Predictive Testing for Huntington's Chorea: The Need for More Information," *British Medical Journal* 293 (6541), July 26, 1986, 249-251.

Creusen, I., SJ, "L'Onanisme Conjugal," *Nouvelle Revise Theologique* 59, 1932, 132-142.

Crisp, Roger, "A Good Death, Who Best to Bring it?" *Bioethics* 1 (1), Jan. 1987, 7479

Crissman, Susan, and Betz, Linda, "Education and Image: Critical Issues Confronting the Nursing Profession," *Journal of Contemporary Health Law & Policy* 3, Spring 1987, 174-184.

Cronin, John, *Catholic Social Principles,* Milwaukee: Bruce Books, 1950.

Crosby, John, *Sexual Autology Toward a Humanistic Ethic,* Springfield, IL: Charles C. Thomas Publications, 1981.

Cruchland, Paul, *Matter and Consciousness: A Comtemporary Introduction to the Philosophy of the Mind,* Cambridge: MIT Press, 1984.

Crufurd, D., and Harris, R., "Ethics of Predictive Testing for Huntington's Chorea," *British Medical Journal* 293, Jul. 26, 1986, 6541.

Culligan, Kevin, "The Counseling Ministry and Spiritual Direction," in *Pastoral Counseling,* Barry Estadt, ed., Englewood Cliffs, NJ: Prentice-Hall, 1983.

Culver, Charles et al., "Basic Curricular Goals in Medical Ethics," *New England Journal of Medicine* 312 (4), Jan. 24, 1985, 253-256.

Culver, C.M., and Gert, B, *Philosophy in Medicine: Conceptual and Ethical Issues in Medicine and Psychiatry,* New York: Oxford University Press, 1982.

Cunningham, Bert, *The Morality of Organic Transplantation,* Washington, DC: Catholic University of America Press, 1944.

Cuomo, Mario, "Religious Belief and Public Morality," *The Human Life Review* 11 (1-2), Spring 1985, 26-40.

Cupples, Brian, and Cochnauer, Myron, "The Investigator's Duty Not to Deceive," *I.R.B.: A Review of Human Subjects Research* 7 (5), Oct. 1985.

Curran, Charles E.

    1968   *A New Look at Catholic Morality,* Notre Dame: Fides Publishers.

    1973   "Sterilization, Roman Catholic Theory and Practice," *Linacre Quarterly,* May, 103.

    1975   *Ongoing Revision: Studies in Moral Theology,* Notre Dame: Fides Publishers, "On specificity of Christian ethics," pp. 1-37; "Theology of compromise," pp. 187-190; "Principle of double effect," pp. 173-209; "Cooperation," pp. 210-228.

    1977a   *Themes in Fundamental Moral Theology,* Notre Dame: University of Notre Dame Press.

    1977b   *Issues in Sexual and Medical Ethics,* Notre Dame: University of Notre Dame Press.

    1979   *Transition and Tradition in Moral Theology,* Notre Dame: University of Notre Dame Press.

    1982   *American Catholic Social Ethics: Twentieth Century Approaches,* Notre Dame: University of Notre Dame Press.

    1984   *Critical Concerns in Moral Theology,* Notre Dame: University of Notre Dame Press.

    1985   *Directions in a Fundamental Moral Theology,* Notre Dame: University of Notre Dame Press.

    1988   *Tensions in Moral Theology,* Notre Dame: Notre Dame Press.

Curran, Charles E., and Hunt, Robert E., *Dissent in and for the Church: Theologians and "Humanae Vitae,"* New York: Sheed & Ward, 1969.

Curran, Charles E., and McCormick, Richard A., SJ, "Moral Norms and Catholic Tradition," *Readings in Moral Theology* No. 1, New York: Paulist Press, 1979.

Curran, Charles E., and McCormick, Richard A., SJ, eds., "The Distinctiveness of Christian Ethics," *Readings in Moral Theology* No. 2., New York: Paulist Press, 1980.

Curran, Charles, and McCormick, Richard, SJ, *Official Catholic Social Teaching*, Mahwah, NJ: Paulist Press, 1986.

Curran, Charles, and McCormick, Richard, SJ, *Dissent in the Church*, New York: Paulist Press, 1988.

Curran, William J., "Medical Peer Review of Physician Competence and Performance: Legal Immunity and the Anti-Trust Laws," *New England Journal of Medicine* 316 (10), March 5, 1987, 597-598.

Curran, William J., and Cassells, W., "The Ethics of Medical Participation in Capital Punishment with Intravenous Drug Injection," *New England Journal of Medicine* 302, 1980, 226-230.

D

Daling, Janet et al., "Primary Tubal Infertility in Relation to the Use of an Intrauterine Device," *New England Journal of Medicine* 312, 1985, 937-91.

Daly, Robert, et al., *Christian Biblical Ethics*, New York: Paulist Press, 1984.

D'Amato, Debra, "Acknowledging the Need for Ethics in the Nursing Curriculum," *Imprint* 32 (4), Nov. 1985, 40-41

D'Arcy, Martin, *Humanism and Christianity*, New York: World Publishing Co., 1969.

Davis, Anne J, and Mahou, Kathleen A., "Research with Retarded and Mentally Ill: Rights and Duties versus Compelling State Interest," *Journal of Advanced Nursing* (1), Jan. 9, 1984, 15-21

Davis, Bernard D., "Prospects for Genetic Intervention in Man," *Science* 170, 1970),1279-1283.

Davis, John Jefferson
>   1984   *Abortion and the Christian*, Phillipsburg, NJ: Presbyterian Reformed Publishing.
>   1985   *Evangelical Ethics Issues Facing the Church Today*, Phillipsburg, NJ: Reformed Publishing Co.

Davis, Michael, "Foetuses, Famous Violinists, and the Right to Continued Aid," *Philosophical Quarterly* 33 (132), Jul. 1983, 259-278.

Dedek, John F.
>   1972   *Human Life: Some Moral Issues*, New York: Sheed & Ward.
>   1979   "Intrinsically Evil Acts: An Historical Study of the Mind of St. Thomas," *The Thomist* 43, 385-413.

Deeken, Alfons, *Process and Permanence in Ethics*, New York: Paulist Press, 1974.

DeKraai, Mark, and Sales, Braaj, "Confidential Communications of Psychotherapists," *Psychotherapy* 21 (3), Fall 1984, 293-318.

DeLancy, John, "The Role of the Guardian Ad Litem," in *By No Extrordinary Means*, Joanne Lynn, ed., Bloomington, IN: Indiana Press, 1986, 249-255.

Delgado, Jose, *Physical Control of the Mind: Toward a Psychocivilized Society*, New York: Harper & Row, 1969.

Delhaye, Phillipe
>   1968   *The Christian Conscience*, New York: Desclee.
>   1970   "Declarations episcopales du monde entier," Jan Grootaers, and Gustave Thils, eds., in *Pour Relire Humanae Vitae*, with commentaries by eds., Paris: Duculot.
>   1975   "Fecondite et Paternite Responsable," *Esprit et Vie* 85, 337-344.
>   1976   "La Masturbation," *Esprit et Vie* 86, 230-254.

Delhaye, Phillipe, et al., "A Symposium on *Humanae Vitae* and Natural Law," *Louvain Studies* 2, Spring 1969, 211-253.

Dellapenna, Joseph W., "Abortion and the Law: Blackman's Distortion of the Historical Record," in *Abortion and The Constitution*, Dennis Horan, Edward Grant, and Paige C. Cunningham, eds., Georgetown: Georgetown University Press, 1987.

427

Denes, Magda, *Necessity and Sorrow: Life and Death in an Abortion Hospital*, New York: Basic Books, 1976.

Denham, M. J., "The Ethics of Research With the Elderly," *Age and Aging* (6), Nov. 13, 1984, 321-327.

Derrickson, Paul, and Ebersolo, Myron, "Lasting Effects of CPE, A Five Year Review," *Pastoral Care* 30, March 1986, 5.

Devereux, George, *A Study of Abortion in Primitive Societies*, New York: International Universities Press, 1976 [1955].

deVries, Martin, ed., *The Use and Abuse of Medicine*, New York: Praeger Publications, 1982.

Dewey, John, *Reconstruction in Philosophy*, Boston: Beacon Press, 1948 [1920], ch. 7.

Diamond, Eugene, "Commentary on the A.M.A. Statement on Tube Feeding," *Linacre Quarterly* 54 (2), May 1973, 73-77.

Diamond, James J., "Abortion, Animation, and Biological Hominization," *Theological Studies* 36, 1975, 305-324.

Dickens, Bernard, "Abortion, Amniocentesis and the Law," *American Journal of Comparative Law* 34 (2), Spring 1986, 249-270.

Dickson, David, "Europe Split on Embryo Research," *Science* 242, Nov. 25, 1988, 1117.

Dickstein, Morris, "Columbia Recovered," *New York Times Magazine*, May 15, 1988, 32ff.

Dominian, Jacob, "*Humanae Vitae* Revisited: The Argument Goes On," *Tablet* 238, Oct. and Nov. 1984.

Doms, Herbert, *The Meaning of Marriage*, New York: Sheed & Ward, 1939.

Donceel, Joseph
    1970   "Immediate Animation and Delayed Hominization," *Theological Studies* 31, 76-105.
    1985   "Catholic Politicians and Abortion," *America*, Feb. 2, 81-83.
    1986   "A Liberal Catholic's View," in *The Problem of Abortion*, Joel Fienkers, ed., Belmont, CA: Wadsworth Publications.

Donnelly, Paul, et al., *One Approach to a Religious Sponsored Health Corporation*, St. Louis: Catholic Hospital Association, 1978.

Donnelly, Paul, and Williams, Ken, *Medical Care Quality, and the Public Trust*, Chicago: Pluribus Press, 1982.

Doubilet, Peter; Weinstein, Milton G; and McNeil, Barbara J., "Use and Misuse of the Term 'Cost Effective' in Medicare," *New England Journal of Medicine* 314 (4), Jan. 23, 1986, 253-256.

Dougherty, Charles, *Ideal, Fact, and Medicine*, Lanham, MD: University Press, 1985.

Drake, James, "Ethical Theory for Catholic Professionals," *Linacre Quarterly* 53 (1), Feb. 1986, 36-41.

Drucker, Peter F., "Freudian Myths and Freudian Realities," in *Adventures of a Bystander*, New York: Harper and Row, 1978, 83-99.

Dube, Leela, "Amniocentesis Debate Continued," *Economic and Political Weekly* 18 (38), Sept. 17, 1983, 1633-35.

Dubler, Nancy, "The Right to Privacy and the Right to Refuse Care for the Imperiled Newborn," in *Humanistic Dimension in the Care for Imperiled Newborn*, Thomas Murray and Arthur Captry, eds., Clifton, NJ: Humana Press, 1985, 137-148.

Duff, Raymond, and Hollingshead, August, *Sickness and Society*, New York: Harper and Row, 1968.

Duffy, Regis, *A Roman Catholic Theology of Pastoral Care*, Philadelphia: Fortress Press, 1983.

Duffy, Regis, *On Becoming a Catholic: The Challenge of Christian Invitation*, San Francisco: Harper & Row, 1984.

Dulles, Avery, "What is the Role of a Bishops' Conference," *Origins* 17 (46), Apr. 28, 1988, 789-796.

Durkheim, E., *Suicide*, Glencoe, IL: Free Press, 1951.

Dworkin, Gerland, "Autonomy and Behavior Control," *Hastings Center Report* 6, 1976, 23-28.

Dych, Arthur, "Ethics of Population Control," in *International Encyclopedia of Population,* John Ross, ed., New York, Free Press, 1982, 183.

E

Eastaugh, Stephen, *Medical Economics and Health Finance,* Boston: Auburn House, 1981.

Easthope, Gary, *Healers and Alternative Medicine: A Sociological Explanation,* Brookfield, VT: Gower Publishing, 1986.

Ebert, Robert, and Ginzberg, Eli, et al., "The Case for Medical Education Reform," in *Health Affairs Supplement,* 1988.

Echstein, Gustav, *The Body Has a Head,* New York: Harper & Row, 1970.

Eckholm, Erik, "AIDS Drug is Raising Host of Thorny Issues," *New York Times,* September 28, 1986.

Edelman, D.A., "IUD Complications in Perspective," *Contraception* 36 (1), 1987, 159-67.

Edelman, D.A.; McIntyre, S.; and Harper, J., "A Comparative Trial of the Today Contraceptive Sponge and Diaphragm," *American Journal of Obstetrics and Gynecology* 150, 1984, 869.

Edelman, Gerald, *Neural Darwinism: The Theory of Neuronal Group Selection,* New York: Basic Books, 1987.

Edelstein, Ludwig, *Ancient Medicine: Selected Papers,* O. and C. Tembia, eds., Baltimore: Johns Hopkins Press, 1967.

Edwards, R.B., "Mental Health as Rational Autonomy," *Journal of Medicine and Philosophy* 6 (3), 1981.

Egan, Gerard, *The Skilled Helper,* 3rd ed., Monterrey, CA: Brooks-Cole, 1986.

Egan, Harvey, *Christian Mysticism: The Future of a Tradition,* New York: Pueblo, 1984.

Ehrenfeld, David W., *The Arrogance of Humanism,* New York: Oxford University Press, 1978.

Ehrman, Lee, et al., "The Supreme Court and Patenting Life," *Hastings Center Report* 10, 1980, 1-15.

Eichna, Ludwig, "Medical Education 1975-1979: A Student's Perspective," *New England Journal of Medicine* 303, 1980, 727-732.

Eisenberg, John, *Doctors, Decisions and the Cost of Medical Care,* Ann Arbor: Health Administration Press, 1986.

Eisenberg, Leon, "Health Care for Patients or For Profit?" *American Journal of Psychiatry* 143 (8), Aug. 1986, 1015-1019.

Elinson, Jack, and Siegman, Athilia, ed., *Socio-Medical Health Indicators,* Amityville, NY; Baywood Publishing Co., 1984.

Ellul, Jacques
   1965   *The Technological Society,* New York: Alfred A. Knopf.
   1980   *The Technological System,* New York: Continuum Publishing Co.

Ellwood, Paul M., "Models for Organizing Health Services and Implications of Legislative Proposals," in *Organizational Issues in the Delivery of Health Care Services,* Irving K. Zole and John B. McKinlay, eds., New York: Milbank Memorial Fund, 1974, 67-90.

Ely, John, "The Wages of Crying Wolf," *The Yale Law Journal,* Apr. 1973, 935.

Emanuel, Ezekial, "Do Physicians Have an Obligation to Treat Patients with AIDS?" *New England Journal of Medicine* 318 (25), June 23, 1988, 1686-1690.

Emerson, James, *Suffering: Its Meaning and Ministry,* Nashville: Abingdon Press, 1986, ch. 5.

Empereur, James, *Prophetic Anointing,* Wilmington, DE: Michael Glazier Inc., 1982.

Engel, G.L., "The Clinical Application of the Biopsychosocial Model," *Journal of Medicine and Philosophy* 6 (2), 1981.

Engelhardt, H. Tristram, Jr.
   1977   "Some Persons Are Humans, Some Humans Are Persons, and the World Is What We Persons Make It," in *Philosophical Medical Ethics,* Stuart C. Spicker and H. Tristram Engelhardt, Jr., eds., Boston: Reidel, 183-194.

1979   "Is Death a Disease," in *Life-Span: Values and Life-Extending Technologies*, Robert Veatch, ed., New York: Harper & Row, 184-194.

1980   "Personal Health Care or Preventive Care: Distributing Scarce Medical Resources," *Soundings* 63, Fall, 234-56.

1982   "Bioethics in Pluralist Societies," *Perspectives in Biological Medicine* 26 (1), 64-78.

1986a   "Endings and Beginnings of Persons' Death: Abortion and Infanticide," in *The Foundations of Bioethics*, New York: Oxford University Press, 202-249.

1986b   *The Foundation of Bioethics*, New York: Oxford University Press, 107-110.

1986c   "Suicide and the Cancer Patient," *CA Cancer Journal for Clinicians* 36 (2), Mar.-Apr., 105-109

Engelhardt, Tristram, and Malloy, Michele, "Suicide and Assisting Suicide: A Critique of Legal Sanctions," *Southwestern Law Journal* 36 (4), Nov. 1982, 1003-1037.

Engler, R.L., et al., "Misrepresentation and Responsibility in Medical Research," *New England Journal of Medicine* 317, 1987, 1383-389.

Enthoven, Alain, *Health Plan: The Only Soaring Cost of Medical Care*, Menlo Park, CA: Addison-Wesley Publications Co., 1980.

Erde, Edmund, "Defining Health, Disease and Their Bearing on Medical Practice," *Ethics in Science and Medicine* 6, 1979, 31-48.

Erikson, Erik, *Identity: Youth and Crisis*, New York: W.W. Norton and Co., 1968.

Erwin, Richard, *Behavior Therapy: Scientific, Philosophical, and Moral Foundations*, New York: Cambridge University Press, 1978.

Esbjornson, Robert, ed., *The Manipulation of Life*, New York: Harper & Row, 1984.

Estadt, Barry, *Pastoral Counseling*, Englewood Cliffs, NJ: Prentice-Hall, 1983, ch. 7.

Eth, Spencer; Levine, Martin; and Lyon-Levine, Martha, "Ethical Conflicts at the Interface of Advocacy and Psychiatry," *Hospital and Community Psychiatry* 35 (7), Jul. 1984, 665-666

Ethical and Religious Directives for Catholic Health Facilities, Washington, DC: United States Catholic Conference, 1971, revised 1975.

Evans, Robert G., "Illusions of Necessity: Evading Responsibility for Choice in Health Care," *Journal of Health: Politics, Policy and Law 1985* 10 (3), Fall, 439-467.

Evans, Robert W., et. al., "Donor Availability as the Primary Determinant of the Future of Heart Transplantation," *Journal of the American Medical Association* 255 (14), Apr. 11, 1986, 1892-1898.

Ewan, Christine, "Teaching Ethics in Medical Schools," *Medical Teacher* 8 (2), 1986.

F

Fabrega, Horacio, Jr., ed., "Social and Cultural Perspectives on Disease," a special issue, *Journal of Medicine and Philosophy* 5, 1980, 146-168.

Facklam, Margery, and Facklam, Howard, *Brain: Magnificent Mind Machine*, New York: Harcourt Brace Jovanovich, 1982.

Faden, Ruth, and Beauchamp, Thomas, *A History and Theory of Informed Consent*, New York: Oxford Press, 1986, 161.

Falcone, David, and Hartwig, Lynn, "Congressional Process and Health Policy," in *Health Politics and Policy*, Theodore Liman, ed., New York: New York Weekly, 1984, 126-144.

Fath, Gerald, OP
1980   *Health Care Ministries*, St. Louis: Catholic Health Association of the United States.

1985   "Pastoral Counseling in the Hospital Setting," in *Clinical Handbook of Pastoral Counseling*, ed., Robert Wicks; Donald Parsons; and Donald Capps, eds., New York: Paulist Press, 349-360.

Feder, Judith; Holahan, John; and Marmor, Theodore, eds., *National Health Insurance: Conflicting Goals and Policy Choices*, Washington, DC: Urban Institute, 1980.

Federal Register, "Nondiscrimination on the Basis of Handicap Relating to Health Care for

Handicapped Infants." July 5, 1983, Vol. 48, 129, 30846.

Fein, Rashi, *Medical Costs: The Search for a Health Insurance Policy,* Cambridge: Harvard University Press, 1986.

Feinstein, Alvan, "The State of the Art," *Journal of the American Medical Association* 255 (11), Mar. 21, 1986, 1988.

Feldman, David

    1986a   *Health and Medicine in the Jewish Tradition,* New York: Crossroad Publishing Co., 1986.

    1986b   "The Matter of Abortion," in his *Health and Medicine in the Jewish Tradition,* New York: Crossroad Publishing Co., 1986.

Fersch, Ellsworth A., *Law, Psychology and the Courts: Rethinking Treatment of the Young and the Disturbed,* Springfield, IL: Charles C. Thomas, 1979.

Fichter, Joseph H, *Religion and Poor: The Spiritual Dimensions of Health Care,* New York: Crossroad Publishing Co., 1981.

Fingarette, Herbert, and Hasse, Ann Fingarette, *Mental Disabilities and Criminal Responsibility,* Berkeley: University of California Press, 1979.

Finnis, John

    1980   *Natural Law and Natural Rights,* Oxford: Oxford University Press.

    1983   *Fundamentals of Ethics,* Washington, DC: Georgetown University Press.

    1985   "Personal Integrity, Sexual Morality and Responsible Parenthood," *Anthropos,* 1985, 46-55.

Fisk, N., "Gender Dysphoria Syndrome," *Interdisciplinary Symposium on Transsexualism,* Palo Alto: Stanford University Press, 1973.

Fitzgerald, Frances, *Cities on a Hill,* New York: Simon & Shuster, 1986.

Fitzpatrick, Annelle, and Gaylor, Christine, "Catholic Institutions: Mirror or Model for Society," *Health Progress* 68 (3), Apr. 1987, 74-78.

Flannery, Austin, "Hierarchies Give Pastoral Advice on *Humanae Vitae,*" *Doctrine and Life* 19 (2), Feb. 1969.

Flannery, Ellen, "Should It Be Easier or Harder to Use Unapproved Drugs and Devices," *Hastings Center Report* 16 (1), Feb. 1986.

Fletcher, John

    1982   *Coping With Genetic Disorders: A Guide for Clergy and Parents,* San Francisco: Harper and Row.

    1983a   "The Evolution of the Ethics of Informed Consent," in Kare Berg and Erik Knat, eds., *Research Ethics,* New York: Alan R. Liss.

    1983b   "Maternal Bonding in Early Fetal Ultrasound Examinations," *New England Journal of Medicine* 308 (7), Feb. 17, 392.

    1985   "Ethical Issues in and Beyond Prospective Clinical Trials of Human Gene Therapy," *Journal of Medicine & Philosophy* 3, Aug. 10, 293-309.

Fletcher, John; Berg, Kare; and Tranoy, Kant, "Ethical Aspects of Medical Genetics: A Proposal for Guidelines in Genetic Counseling, Prenatal Diagnosis and Screening," in Kare Berg, ed., *Medical Genetics, Past, Present, Future,* New York: Alan R. Liss, 1985.

Fletcher, John, and Schulman, Joseph D., "Fetal Research: The State of the Question," *Hastings Center Report* 2, Apr. 15, 1985, 6-12.

Fletcher, Joseph

    1954   *Morals and Medicine,* Boston: Beacon Press.

    1960   "The Patient's Right to Die," *Harpers,* Oct., 138-143.

    1974   "Four Indicators of Humanhood: The Enquiry Matures," *Hastings Center Report* 4, 4-7. With replies in *Correspondence* 5 (4), 43-45.

    1975   "Triage and Lifeboat Ethics," in *Triage in Medicine and Society: Inquiries into Medical Ethics,* George R. Lucas, Jr., ed., Houston: Institute of Religion and Human Development, vol. 3, 23-34.

    1979   *Humanhood: Essays in Biomedical Ethics,* Buffalo: Prometheus Press.

    1982   "Situation Ethics Revisited," *Religious Humanism* 16, Winter, 9-13.

1988   *The Ethics of Genetic Control: Ending Reproductive Roulette,* Buffalo: Prometheus Books.

Flexner, Abraham, *Medical Education in The United States and Canada,* Carnegie Foundation for the Advancement of Teaching, Bulletin 4, Boston: Marymount Press, 1910. Reprinted Washington, DC: Science and Health Publications, 1960.

Fleyner, John, "Dying, Death, and the Front Line Physician," in *Dying and Death: A Clinical,* David Barton, ed., Baltimore: Williams and Wilkins, 1977.

Flickinger, Charles, "The Effects of Vasectomy on the Testis," *New England Journal of Medicine* 313 (20), Nov. 14, 1985, 1283-1285.

Ford, Amasa B., et al., *The Doctor's Perspective: Physicians View Their Patients and Their Practice,* Cleveland: Case Western Reserve University, 1967, 139ff.

Ford, John C., and Grisez, Germain, "Contraception and the Infallibility of the Ordinary Magisterium," *Theological Studies* 39 (2), June 1978, 258-312.

Ford, John C., and Kelly, Gerald, SJ, *Contemporary Moral Theology,* 2 vols., Westminster, MD: Newman Press, 1964, (on contraception, vol. 2, 245-275).

Fordney-Settlage, Diane S.; Motoshima, Masanabu; and Tredway, Donald S., "Sperm Transport From the External Cervical Os to the Fallopian Tubes in Woman: A Time and Quantitation Study," *Fertility and Sterility* 24, Sept. 1973, 655-661.

Forer, Lois G., "Medical Services in Prisons: Rights and Remedies," *American Bar Association Journal* 68, May 1982, 562-565.

Foucault, Michael, *The Birth of the Clinic: An Archaeology of Medical Perception,* New York: Pantheon, 1973.

Fox, Renee, *Essays in Medical Sociology,* Philadelphia: University of Pennsylvania, 1988.

Fox, Renee, and Swazy, Judith P., *The Courage to Fail: A Social View of Organ Transplant and Dialysis,* 2nd ed., Chicago: University of Chicago Press, 1978.

Frager, Robert, and Fadiman, James, *Maslow's Motivation and Personality,* 3rd ed., New York: Harper and Row, 1985.

Francis, Richard, and Franklin, John, "Alcohol and Other Psychoactive Substance Use Disorders," in *Textbook of Psychiatry,* John Talbott, et al., eds., Washington DC, American Psychiatric Press, 1988, 313-356.

Francke, Linda Bird, *The Ambivalence of Abortion,* New York: Random House, 1978.

Francoeur, Robert
    1972   "We Can — We Must: Reflections on the Technological Imperative," *Theological Studies* 33, 428-439.
    1976   *Perspectives in Evolution,* Baltimore: Helicon Press.
    1983   *Biomedical Ethics: A Guide to Decision Making,* New York: John Wiley and Sons.
    1988   "Two Different Worlds, Two Different Moralities," in *The Vatican and Homosexuality,* Jeane Gramich, and Pat Fruey, eds., New York: Crossroad Publishing Co., 189-200.

Frankena, William
    1980   *Thinking About Morality,* Ann Arbor: University of Michigan Press.
    1985   "The Potential of Theology for Ethics," in *Theology and Bioethics: Exploring the Foundations and Frontiers,* E. Shelp, ed., Boston: D. Reidel, 49-64.

Freedman, Benjamin, "Competence, Marginal and Otherwise: Concepts and Ethics," *International Journal of Law and Psychiatry* 4 (1-2), 1981, 53-72

Freeman, Harrop A., *Counseling in the United States,* San Francisco: Jossey-Bass, 1967.

Freeman, John, "Making Decisions for the Severly Handicapped Newborn," *Journal of Health Politics, Policy and Law* 11 (2), 1986, 285-294.

Freidson, Eliot, *Profession of Medicine: A Study of the Sociology of Applied Knowledge,* New York: Dodd, Mead, and Co., 1971.

Freud, Sigmund
    1920   *Beyond the Pleasure Principle,* in Complete Works, vol. 18, London: Hogarth and Institute of Psychoanalysis, 1958.
    1930   *Civilization and Its Discontents,* London: Hogarth Publishing.

Freund, Paul A., "The Legal Profession," in *The Profession in America,* Kenneth S. Lynn, ed., Boston: Houghton Mifflin, Daedalus, 1965, 35-46.

Freymann, John Gordon, *The American Health Care System: Its Genesis and Trajectory,* New York: Medcom, 1974.

Friedman, Emily, "The 'Dumping' Dilemma: Finding What's Fair," *Hospitals* 56 (18), Sept. 16, 1982, 75-84.

Fromm, Erich, *Crisis of Psychoanalysis,* New York: Fawcett World Library, 1975.

Fuchs, Josef, SJ
    1971   "The Absoluteness of Moral Terms," *Gregorianum* 52, 415-458.
    1980   "Sin of the World and Norinative Morality," *Gregorianum* 61, 67.
    1984   *Christian Ethics In A Secular Arena,* Washington, DC: Georgetown University Press.

Fuchs, Victor, *The Health Economy,* Cambridge, MA: Harvard University Press, 1986.

G

Gabriel, Trip, "Why Wed: The Ambivalent American Bachelor," *New York Times Magazine,* Nov. 15, 1987, 24.

Gaddes, William, *Learning Disabilities and Brain Function,* New York: Springer-Verlag, 1985.

Gadow, Sally, "Caring for the Dying: Advocacy or Paternalism," *Health Education* 3, 1980, 387-398.

Galdston, Iago, *Social and Historical Foundations of Modern Medicine,* New York: Brunner-Mazel, 1981.

Gallagher, John, "Magisterial Teaching from 1918 to the Present," in *Human Sexuality and Personhood,* St. Louis: Pope John XXIII Medical-Moral Research and Education Center, 1981.

Gallant, D., "The Right to Refuse Psychotropic Medications," *Progress in Clinical Biological Research* 139, 1983, 31-38.

Gallon, Michael, "*Humanae Vitae:* A Pastoral Priest's Viewpoint," *Clergy Review* 53, 1968, 874-878.

Gardell, Mary Ann, "June, Bioethics, and the Supreme Court," *Journal of Medicine and Philosophy* 3, Aug. 11, 1986, 285-290.

Garfield, Jay L., and Hennessey, Patricia, eds., *Abortion, Moral and Legal Perspectives,* Amherst: University of Massachusetts Press, 1984.

Garrison, Fielding H., *An Introduction to the History of Medicine,* 4th ed., Philadelphia: W.D. Saunders Co., 1960 [1929].

Gartrell, Nanette, "Psychiatrist-Patient Sexual Contact: Results of a National Survey," *American Journal of Psychiatry* 153 (9), Sept. 1986, 1126-1131.

Garver, Kenneth, and Marchese, Sandra, *Genetic Counseling For Clinicians,* Chicago: Medical Year Book, Medical Publishers, 1986.

Gatch, Milton M., *Death: Meaning and Morality in Christian Thought and Contemporary Culture,* New York: Seabury Press, 1969.

Gaylin, Willard, "Skinner Redux," *Harpers,* Oct. 1973, 48-56.

GBI: Committee on Bioethical Issues of the Bishops of Great Britain and Ireland
    1986a   "Use of the Morning After Pill in Cases of Rape," *Origins* 15 (39), Mar. 13, 633-638.
    1986b   "A Reply: Use of the Morning After Pill in Cases of Rape," *Origins* 16 (13), Sept. 11, 237-238.

Gebhard, P.H., "Incidence of Overt Homosexuality in the United States and Western Europe," *N.I.H. Task Force on Homosexuality,* Washington, DC: Department of Health, Education, and Welfare, 1972.

Gellman, Robert, "Divided Loyalties: A Physician's Responsibilities in an Information Age," *Social Science and Medicine* 23 (8), 1986, 817-826.

Gemuth, Saul, "The Reproductive Glands," in *Physiology,* Robert Berne, and Matthew Levy, eds., St. Louis: C.V. Mosby Co., 1988.

Gervais, Karen Grunstand, *Redefining Death,* New Haven: Yale University Press, 1986.

Gilbert, Daniel, "Shock Therapy and Informed Consent," *Illinois Bar Journal* 69 (5), Jan. 1981, 272-287.

Gilder, George, *Wealth & Poverty,* New York: Bantam, 1982.

Giles, James, *Medical Ethics: A Patient-Catered Approach,* Rochester, VT: Schenkmam, 1983.

Gilleman, Gerard, *The Primacy of Charity in Moral Theology,* Westminster, MD: Newman Press, 1961.

Gillon, Louis B., *Christ and Moral Theology,* Staten Island, NY: Alba House, 1967.

Gillon, Raanan
    1985a   "To What Do We Have Moral Obligations and Why?" *British Medical Journal,* Jan. 8, 290, (6483) 1734-1736.
    1985b   "Telling the Truth and Medical Ethics," *British Medical Journal* 29 (6508), Nov. 30, 1556-1557.
    1986a   "The Principle of Double Effect and Medical Ethics," *British Medical Journal* 292 (6514), Jan. 18, 193-194.
    1986b   The Patient's Interest Always Comes First," *British Medical Journal* 292 (6517), Feb. 8, 398-400.
    1986c   "Doctors and Patients," *British Medical Journal* 292 (6518), Feb. 15, 466-469.
    1987   "AIDS and Medical Confidentiality," *British Medical Journal* 294 (6588), June 27, 1675-1677.

Ginsberg, Eli, ed., *From Physician Shortage to Patient Shortage,* Boulder: Westview Press, 1986.

Ginsberg, Eli, et al., *The Coming Physician Surplus,* Totowa, NJ: Rowman and Allanheld, 1984.

Gish, Oscar, "Values in Health Care," *Social Science and Medicine* 19 (4), 1984, 333.

Glaser, William A., *Social Settings and Medical Organization: A Cross-National Study of the Hospital,* New York: Atherton, 1970.

Glass, Bentley
    1972   "Human Heredity and Ethical Problems," *Perspective in Biology and Medicine* 15, Winter 1972, 237-253.
    1975   *Human Heredity and Ethical Problems,* Philadelphia: Philadelphia Society for Health and Human Values.

Glick, Paul, "Social Change and the Family," *The Family Today and Tomorrow,* St. Louis: Pope John XXIII Medical-Moral Research and Education Center, 1985.

Glover, Jonathan, *What Sort of People Should There Be? Genetic Engineering, Brain Control and Their Impact on Our Future World,* New York: Free Press, 1985.

Glymour, Clark, and Stalker, Douglas, "Engineers, Cranks, Physicians, Magicians," *New England Journal of Medicine* 16, April 21, 1983, 308.

Godden, B., "How Wrong is Contraception," *Clergy Review* 53, 1968, 816-817.

Goffman, Erving, *Asylums: Essays on the Social Situation of Mental Patients and Other Inmates,* Chicago: Aldine, 1962.

Goldberg, Abbot, "The Peer Review Privilege: A Law in Search of A Valid Policy," *American Journal of Law* 10 (2), Summer 1984, 151-167.

Goldberg, Richard, and Tull, Robert, "Information Disclosure and Treatment Refusals: The Clinical Dimensions of Potential Ethical Conflicts," in *The Psychosocial Dimensions of Cancer,* New York: Free Press, 1983.

Goldenring, John M., "The Brain-Life Theory: Toward a Consistent Biological Definition of Humanness," *Journal of Medical Ethics* 4, Dec. 11, 1985, 185-204.

Goldman, Alan H., *The Moral Foundation of Professional Ethics,* Totowa, NJ: Rowman and Littlefield, 1980. See review by David Luban in *Hastings Center Report* 11, 1981, 38-40.

Goldsmith, Jeff, *Can Hospitals Survive? The New Competitive Health Care Market,* Homewood, IL: Dow Jones-Irwin, 1981.

Goode, William J., "The Theoretical Limits of Professionalization," in *The Semi-Professions and Their Organization,* Amitai Etzioni, ed., New York: Free Press, 1969, 266-313.

Goodman, Lenn E., and Goodman, Madeleine J., "Prevention: How Misuse of a Concept Undercuts its Worth," *Hasting Center Report* 2, Apr. 16, 1986, 26-38.

Gordis, Leon, and Gold, Ellen, "Privacy, Confidentiality, and the Use of Medical Records in Research," *Science* 207, 1980, 153-156.

Gorovitz, Samuel, "Buying and Selling Organs," in James Humber, ed., *Biomedical Ethics Review*, Clifton, NJ: Humana Press, 1985.

Gostin, L., "Ethical Considerations of Psychosurgery: The Unhappy Legacy of the Pre-Frontal Lobotomy, *Journal of Medical Ethics*, 6 (3), Sept. 1980, 149-154.

Granfield, Patrick, *The Limits of the Papacy*, New York: Crossroad Publishing Co., 1987.

Gray, R.H., "Aged Gametes, Adverse Pregnancy Outcomes and Natural Family Planning," *Contraception* 30 (4), Oct. 1984, 297-309.

Greeley, Andrew
    1973   "The Sexual Revolution among Catholic Clergy," *Review of Religious Research* 14, 91-101.
    1976   "Council or Encyclical," *Review of Religious Research* 18, Fall, 3-24.

Green, Judith, et al., "Reproduction and the New Genetics," in *Law Science and Medicine*, Mineola, NY: Foundation Press, 1984.

Green, Ronald M., "Conferred Rights and the Fetus," *Journal of Religious Ethics* 2, Spring 1974, 55-76. Reply by James Childress, "A Response," *Journal of Religious Ethics* 2, Spring 1974, 77-84.

Greenberg, Roger P., et al., "The Psychological Evaluation of Patients for a Kidney Transplant and Hemodialysis Program," *American Journal of Psychiatry* 130, 1973, 247-277.

Greene, Marjorie, *Dimensions of Darwinism: Themes & Counter Themes in Twentieth Century Evolutionary Theory*, New York: Cambridge University Press, 1983.

Greer, Germaine, *Sex and Destiny, The Politics of Human Fertility*, New York: Harper and Row, 1984.

Gregorek, Joseph, "Guide for Treating Rape Victims Emphasizes Compassion, Respect," *Health Progress* 69 (7), Sept. 1988, 71-72.

Griese, Orville, *Catholic Identity in Health Care: Principles and Practice*, Braintree, MA: Pope John XXIII Medical-Moral Reseach and Education Center, 1987, 46.

Griffin, Donald R., *Animal Thinking*, Cambridge, MA: Harvard University Press, 1984.

Grimes, Charlotte, "Cost of Care at Issue," *St. Louis Post-Dispatch*, May 15, 1988.

Grisez, Germain G.
    1964   *Contraception and the Natural Law*. Milwaukee: Bruce Books.
    1970   *Abortion: The Myths, the Realities, the Arguments*, Washington, DC: Corpus Books.
    1977   "Suicide and Euthanasia," in *Death, Dying and Euthanasia*, Dennis J. Horan and David Mall, eds., Washington, DC: University Publications, 742-818.
    1983   *The Way of the Lord Jesus*, Chicago: Franciscan Press.

Grisez, Germain G., and Boyle, Joseph M., Jr., *Life and Death with Liberty and Justice: A Contribution to the Euthanasia Debate*, Notre Dame: University of Notre Dame Press, 1979.

Gross, B.A., "Natural Family Planning Indicators of Ovulation," *Clinics in Reproductive Fertility* 3, Jan. 1987, 91-117.

Guerrero, Rodrigo, "Possible Effects of the Periodic Abstinence Method," in *Proceedings of a Research Conference on Natural Family Planning*, W.A. Uricchio, ed., Washington, DC: Human Life Foundation, 1973, 84-96.

Gula, Richard, "Euthanasia: A Catholic Perspective," *Health Progress*, Dec. 1987, 28-34.

Gusmer, Charles, *And You Visited Me: Sacramental Ministry to the Sick and Dying*, New York: Pueblo Publications Co., 1984.

Gustafson, James M.
    1973   "Genetic Engineering and the Normative View of the Human," in *Ethical Issues in Biology and Medicine*, Preston N. Williams, ed. Rochester, VT: Schenkman.

1975   *Can Ethics be Christian?* Chicago: University of Chicago Press.

1976   *Christ and the Moral Life,* Reissue (1968), Chicago: University of Chicago.

1978   *Protestant and Roman Catholic Ethics: Prospects for Rapprochement,* Chicago: University of Chicago Press.

1983   *Ethics from a Theocentric Perspective,* vol. 1 (1983), vol. 2 (1984), Chicago: University of Chicago Press.

Gutheil, Thomas, and Applebaum, Paul S., "The Substituted Judgment Approach: Its Difficulties and Paradoxes in Mental Health Settings," *Law, Medicine and Health Care* 2, Apr. 13, 1985, 61-64.

Gutierrez, Gustavo, *Liberation and Change,* Atlanta: John Knox Press, 1977.

Guttmacher, Sally, "Whole in Body, Mind and Spirit: Holistic Health and the Limits of Medicine," *Hastings Center Report* 9, 1979, 15-21.

Guydish, J., and Kramer, J.J., "Behavior Modification: Doing Battle in the Ethical Arena," *Journal of Behavior Therapy and Experimental Psychiatry* 4, Dec. 13, 1982, 315-320.

H

Haafhems, J.; Nijhof, G.; and Vander Pool, E., "Mental Health Care and the Opposition Movement in the Netherlands," *Social Science and Medicine* 22 (2), 1986.

Haan, Norma, et al., *On Moral Grounds,* New York: New York University Press, 1985.

Halleck, Seymour, "The Ethical Dilemmas of Forensic Psychiatry: A Utilitarian Approach," *Bulletin of the American Academy of Psychiatry and Law* 12 1984 (3), 279-288.

Hammet, Theodore, *AIDS in Correctional Facilities: Issues and Options,* Washington, DC: U.S. Department of Justice, 1986.

Hancock, Roger N., *Twentieth Century Ethics,* New York: Columbia University Press, 1974.

Hardin, Garrett

1974   "Living on a Lifeboat," *Bioscience* 24, 561-568.

1980   *Promethean Ethics: Living with Death, Competition, and Triage,* Seattle: University of Washington Press.

Hare, R.M.

1952   *Language of Morals.* Oxford: Oxford University Press.

1987   "Moral Reasoning About the Environment," *Journal of Applied Philosophy* 4 (1), 3-14.

Haring, Bernard, CSSR

1966   *The Law of Christ,* 3 vols., Philadelphia: Westminster Press.

1968   *The Christian Existentialist: The Philosophy and Theology of Self-Fulfillment in Modern Society,* New York: New York University Press.

1969   "The Inseparability of the Unitive-Procreative Functions in the Marital Act," in *Contraception: Authority and Dissent,* Charles E. Curran, ed., New York: Herder & Herder.

1973   *Medical Ethics,* Notre Dame: Fides Publishers.

1975   *Ethics of Manipulation: Issues in Medicine, Behavior Control and Genetics,* New York: Seabury Press.

1976   "New Dimensions of Responsible Parenthood," *Theological Studies* 37, 120-132.

Harolds, Louis R., and Block, Melvin, eds., *Medical Malpractice—The ATL Seminar,* Rochester, NY: Lawyers Co-operative Publishing Co., 1966.

Harper, P.S., *Practical Genetic Counseling,* Baltimore: University Park Press, 1981.

Harper, Robert A., *Psychoanalysis and Psychotherapy: 36 Systems* Englewood Cliffs, NJ: Prentice-Hall, 1959, 152-155.

Harris, John, *The Value of Human Life,* London: Routledge, and Kegan Publications, 1985.

Harrison, Beverly Wildung, *Our Right to Choose Toward A New Ethic of Abortion,* Boston: Beacon Press, 1984.

Harrison, Michael R.; Golbus, Michael S.; and Filly, Roy A., "Management of the Fetus with a Correctable Congenital Defect," *Journal of the American Medical Association* 246, 1981, 773-774.

Hart, Thomas, N., "Sin in the Concept of the Fundamental Option," *Homiletic and Pastoral Review* 71, 1970, 47-50.

Hastings Center Institute of Society, Ethics, and the Life Sciences: Research Group on Ethical, Social, and Legal Issues in Genetic Counseling and Genetic Engineering, "Ethical and Social Issues in Screening for Genetic Disease," *New England Journal of Medicine* 286, 1972, 1129-1132.

Hatcher, Robert A., et al., *Contraceptive Technology, 1986-1987*, 13th ed., New York: Irvington Publications, 1987.

Hauerwas, Stanley
> 1981 *A Community of Character: Toward a Contructive Christian Social Ethic*, Notre Dame: University of Notre Dame Press.
>
> 1986 *Suffering Presence: Theological Reflections on Medicine, The Mentally Handicapped and the Church*, New Orleans: University of New Orleans Press.

HCFA: Health Care Financing Agency, Review 1987, Washington, DC: Government Printing Office, 1987.

Health Care Financing Agency: see HCFA

Health Plus 1987, *Report to Trustees*, Indianapolis, IN:

Hecker, Konned, "Jansenism," in *Encyclopedia of Theology*, K. Rahner, ed., New York: Seabury Press Inc., 1975, 727-730.

Healy, Edwin, SJ, *Medical Ethics*, Chicago: Loyola University Press, 1956, On cooperation, 102-108.

Helwig, Monica, *Sign of Reconciliation and Conversion: The Sacrament of Penance for Our Times*, Wilmington: Michael Glazier Inc., 1983.

Hendren, Hardy, and Lillehi, Craig, "Pediatric Surgery," *New England Journal of Medicine* 319 (2), Jul. 14, 1988, 89-96.

Hendry, George S., *The Theology of Nature*, Philadelphia: Westminster Press, 1980.

Henry, William E; Sims, John; and Spray, Lee, *The Fifth Profession: Becoming a Psycho-therapist*, San Francisco: Josey-Bass, 1971.

Hilfaker, David, *Healang the Wounded*, New York: Parthenon Books, 1985.

Hilgers, Thomas W.
> 1980 "The New Technologies of Birth," in *The New Technologies of Birth and Death*, St. Louis: Pope John XXIII Medical-Moral Research and Education Center, 29-55.
>
> 1977 "Human Reproduction: Three Issues," *Theological Studies* 38, 136-152.

Hill, Carole E., ed., *Current Health Policy Issues and Alternatives*, Athens: University of Georgia Press, 1986.

Hill, John, "The Debate Between McCormick and Frankena," *Irish Theological Quarterly*, 49, 1982, 121-133.

Hiller, Marc D., and Beyda, V., "Computers, Medical Records, and the Right to Privacy," *Journal of Health Politics Policy and Law*, Fall 1981, 463-487.

Hiltner, Seward, *Pastoral Counseling*, Nashville, TN: Abingdon Press, 1969.

Hinds, Stuart W., "Triage in Medicine," in *Triage in Medicine and Society: Inquiries into Medical Ethics*, Houston: Institute of Religion and Human Development, vol. 3, 1975, 6-22.

Hitchcock, James
> 1982 *What is Secular Humanism*, Ann Arbor: Servant Books.
>
> 1984 "The Seamless Garment Unfolds," *The Human Life Review* 4, 15-30.

Hite, Shere
> 1976 *Hite Report on Female Sexuality*, New York: MacMillan.
>
> 1981 *Hite Report on Male Sexuality*, New York: Alfred A. Knopf.

Hoenig, J., *Etiology of Transexualism in Gender Dysphoria: Development, Research, Management*, New York: Plenum Press, 1985.

Hoff, Lee Ann, *People in Crisis: Understanding and Helping*, Menlo Park, CA: Addison-Wesley Publcations, 1984, ch. 2.

Holbrook, David, "Medicare Ethics and the Potentialities of the Living Being," *British*

Medical Journal 291 (6493), Aug. 17, 1985, 459-462.

Holck, Frederick H., ed., *Death and Eastern Thought,* Nashville: Abingdon Press, 1974.

Holden, C., "Sex Change Operations of Dubious Value," *Science* 205, 1979, 1235.

Holder, Angela Roddy, "Amniocentesis, Genetics, Counseling, and Genetic Screening," in her *Legal Issues in Pediatrics and Adolescent Medicine,* New Haven, CT: Yale University Press, 1985.

Holifield, E. Brooks, *A History of Pastoral Care in America from Salvation to Self-Realization,* Nashville: Abingdon Press, 1983.

Holmes, Helen, "Sex Preselection: Eugenics for Everyone?" in *Biomedical Ethics Review,* James Humber, ed., Clifton, NJ: Humana Press, 1985, 39-71.

Holst, Lawrence, ed., *Hospital Ministry: The Role of the Chaplain Today,* New York: Crossroad Publishing Co., 1985.

Holt, Robert T., "Freud's Impact on Modern Morality," *Hastings Center Report* 10, 1980, 38-45.

Holzgreve, H., et al., "Kidney Transplantation from Anencephalic Donors," *New England Journal of Medicine* 316 (17), Apr. 23, 1987, 1069-1070.

Hoose, Bernard, *Proportionalis: The American Debate and Its European Roots,* Washington, DC: Georgetown University Press, 1987.

Horan, Dennis J., and Grant, E.P., "The Legal Aspects of Withdrawing Nourishment," *Journal of Legal Medicine* 5 (4), 1984, 595-632.

Horan, Dennis J., Grant, Edward R., and Cunningham, Paige C. *Abortion and the Constitution, Reversing Roe vs. Wade Through the Courts,* Washington, D.C.: Georgetown University Press, 1987.

Horan, Dennis J., and Halligan, Patrick, "Informed Consent," *Linacre Quarterly* 49 (4), Nov. 1982, 358-369.

Horgan, John, and Flannery, Austin, *Humanae Vitae and the Bishops: The Encyclical and Statements of National Hierarchies,* Shannon: Irish University Press, 1972.

Horowitz, L.C., *Taking Charge of Your Medical Fate,* New York: Random House, 1988.

Horrobin, David F., *Medical Hubris: A Reply to Ivan Illich,* Quebec: Eden Press, 1980.

Hoyt, Robert, ed., *The Birth Control Debate: Interim History from the Pages of the National Catholic Reporter,* Kansas City: National Catholic Reporter, 1969.

Hsiao, William, *Cost-Based Relative Social Values,* Washington, DC: DHHW, 1988.

Hull, Richard T., "Involuntary Commitment and Treatment of Persons Diagnosed as Mentally Ill," in *Biomedical Ethics Review,* James Humber, et al., eds., 1983, Clifton, NJ: Humert Press, 1983.

"Humanist Manifesto," *The New Humanist* 6, May-June 1933. Reprinted in *The Humanist* 33, Jan.-Feb. 1973, 13-14.

"Humanist Manifesto II," *The Humanist* 33, Sept.-Oct. 1973, 4-9.

Hume, Kevin, "Latest Research Findings: The Pill and IUD," *Proceedings First International Congress for the Family,* Madras Congress, 1983

Humphrey, Derek, *Assisted Suicide: The Compassionate Crime,* Los Angeles: Hemlock Society, 1982.

Hunt, Morton, *Sexual Behavior in the 70s,* Chicago: Playboy Press, 1974.

Hussey, Edmund, "Needed: A Theology of Priesthood," *Origins* 17 (34), Feb 4, 1988, 517-583.

Hyde, Margaret, and Hyde, Lawrence, *Cloning and the New Genetics,* Hillside, NJ: Enslow Publishing, 1984.

I

Idziak, Anine M., *Divine Command Morality,* Lewiston, NY: Edwin Mellen Press, 1986.

Iglesias, Teresa
    1984a "In Vitro Fertilization: The Major Issues," *Journal of Medical Ethics* 1, March 10, 32-37.
    1984b ed., *Euthanasia and Clinical Trends, Principles and Alternatives,* London: Linacre Center.

Illich, Ivan D.
> 1972   "Technology and Conviviality," in *To Create a Different Future: Religious Hope and Technology*, Kenneth Vaux, ed., New York: Friendship Press, 40-66.
> 1976   *Medical Nemesis: The Expropriation of Health*, New York: Pantheon Books.

Illich, Ivan D., et al., *Disabling Professions*, Boston: Marion Boyars Publications, Ltd., 1978.

Ingelfinger, Franz, "Bedside Ethics in Hopeless Cases," *New England Journal of Medicine*, 289 (1973) 914-915.

Ingleby, David, ed., *Critical Psychiatry: The Politics of Mental Health*, New York: Pantheon Books, 1980.

Institute for Theological Encounter with Science and Technology: see ITEST

ITEST, 1968-1983, Institute for Theological Encounter with Science and Technology, *Contemporary Issues in Science and Theology*, P. Keilholz, ed., St. Louis: ITEST Publications, 1976, 1984, 30ff.

ITEST, 1975, Institute for Theological Encounter with Science and Technology, *Brain Research: Human Consciousness*, St. Louis: ITEST Publications, 1976.

J

Jackson, Jesse, "Political Campaign Speech," *Des Moines Register*, Jan. 16, 1988.

Jacobs, Seth, "Determination of Medical Necessity: Medicaid Funding for Sex Reassignment Surgery," *Case Western Reserve Law Review*, vol. 31, 1980, 179.

Janssens, Louis, "Ontic Evil and Moral Evil," *Louvain Studies* 4, 1972, 115-156.

Jeanson, Francis, *Sartre and the Problem of Morality*, Bloomington: Indiana University Press, 1980.

Johanson, Donald, and Edey, Maitland, *Lucy: The Beginnings of Humankind*, New York: Simon & Schuster, 1981.

John XXIII, *Mater et Magistra*, Washington, DC: National Catholic Welfare Conference, May 15, 1961.

John Paul II
> 1980a   Encyclical Letters, in *Dives in Misericordia Origins* 10 (26), Dec. 11.
> 1980b   "The Patient is a Person," (Oct. 23, 1980) *The Pope Speaks* 26 (1).
> 1980c   "Lust and Personal Dignity," *Origins* 10 (19), Oct. 23, 303.
> 1981a   Encyclical Letter: "On Human Work," *Origins* 11 (15), Sept. 24, 255.
> 1981b   *Familiaris Consortio*, "On the Human Family," *Origins* 11 (28-29), Dec. 24.
> 1984a   "On Reconciliation and Penance," *Origins* 74 (27), Dec. 20, 442.
> 1984b   *Reflections on Humanae Vitae*, Boston: St. Paul Editions.
> 1984c   "The Priest in an Indifferent World," *Origins* 14 (8), July 12, 1984, 122-130.
> 1985   "To the Council of European Episcopal Conferences," *Osservatore Romano* 42, Oct. 21, 908.
> 1986   "Medicines at the Service of Man" (Oct. 24, 1986), *Health Progress*, Apr. 1987.
> 1987a   *Sollicitudo Rei Socialis*, *Origins* 17 (38), March 3.
> 1987b   "The Catholic Schools in the 80s," *Origins* 17 (17), Oct. 8, 279-282.
> 1988   On U.N. Bill of Rights, "Serving the Cause of Human Rights," *Origins*, Jan. 26, 1989, 18, 33, 541-544.

Johnson, Gale D., *Population Growth and Economic Development Policy Questions*, Washington, DC: National Academy Press, 1986.

Johnson, Sandra, "Living Wills and Refusal of Treatment," *Health Progress* 1, Jan. 1987, 100-104.

Jonas, Hans
> 1979   "Toward a Philosophy of Technology," *Hastings Center Report* 9, 34-43.
> 1984   *The Importance of Responsibility: In Search of an Ethics for the Technological Age*, Chicago: Chicago University Press, 1984.

Jonas, Stephen, *Medical Mystery, The Training of Doctors in the United States*, New York: W.W. Norton and Co., 1978.

Jones, James, *Bad Blood: The Tuskegee Syphilis Experiment*, New York: Free Press, 1982.

Jonsen, Albert R.
    1968   *Responsibility in Modern Religious Ethics*, Washington, DC: Corpus Books, 1968.
    1984   "Public Policy and Human Research," in *Biomedical Ethics Review*, James Humber, and Robert Almeder, eds., Clifton, NJ: Humana Press, 1984, 3-20.
    1985   "Organ Transplants and the Principle of Fairness," *Law, Medical and Health Care* 1, Feb. 13, 37.
Jonsen, Albert R.; Cooke, Molly; and Koenigh, Barbara, "AIDS and Ethics," *Issues in Science and Technology* 2 (2), Winter 1986, 56-65.
Jung, Carl, et al., *Man and His Symbols*, London: Aldus Books, 1964, rev. ed. 1984.

K

Kagle, Jill D., "Privacy versus Accountability: A Health Care Dilemma," *Social Work in Health Care* 9 (3), Spring 1984, 25-36.
Kahn, Eva, *Clinical Genetics Handbook*, Orabell, NJ: National Genetics Foundation, 1987.
Kaiser, Irwin, "Fertilization and the Physiology and Development of Fetus and Placenta," in *Obstetrics and Gynecology*, David Danforth, and James Scott, eds., Philadelphia: J.B. Lippincott, 1986.
Kaiser, Robert Blair, *The Politics of Sex and Religion*, Kansas City: Leaven Press, 1985.
Kamisar, Yale, "The Real Quinlan Issue," *New York Times*, June 17, 1985, A19.
Kanigel, Robert, "Uncertain of Our Gods," *Notre Dame Magazine* 17 (2), Summer 1988, 34-42.
Kaplan, Helen Singer, *The New Sex Therapy*, New York: Brunner/Mazel, 1974, 86.
Karasu, Toksoz, "Psychotherapy and Pharmocotherapy: Toward an Integretive Model," *American Journal of Psychiatry* 139, 1982, 106-112.
Kass, Leon
    1985   *Toward A More Natural Science, Biology and Human Affairs*, New York: Free Press, 65ff.
    1987   "The Limits of Genetic Inquiry," *Hastings Center Report* 17 (4), August 1987, 5-11.
Katz, Jay, *The Silent World of Doctor and Patient*, New York: Macmillan, 1984.
Katz, Jay; Capron, Alexander M.; and Swift-Glass, Elenor, *Experimentation with Human Beings*, New York: Russell Sage Foundation, 1972.
Kaufman, David M., *Clinical Neurology for Psychiatrists*, New York: Grame and Stratton, 1985, 24.
Kauffmann, Christopher
    1976   *Tamers of Death*, New York: Crossroad Publishing Co.
    1978   *The Ministry of Healing*, New York: Crossroad Publishing Co.
Keane, Philip, *Sexual Morality: A Catholic Perspective*, New York: Paulist Press, 1977.
Kegley, Jacquelyn A., "Genetics and Mental Retardation," in *Moral Issues in Mental Retardation*, Ronald Laura, et al., ed., London: Croom Helm, 1985, 161-183.
Keifer, Ralph A., *Blessed and Broken, The Contemporary Experience of God in Eucharistic Celebration*, Wilmington, DE: Michael Glazier Inc., 1983.
Kelagham, J. et al., "Barrier-Method Contraceptives and Pelvic Inflammatory Disease," *Journal of American Medical Association* 248, 1982, 185.
Kelen, G.D., et al., "Unrecognized Human Immunodeficiency Virus Infection in Emergency Department Patients," *New England Journal of Medicine* 318, 1988, 1645-1650.
Kelly, David F., *The Emergence of Roman Catholic Medical Ethics in North America*, New York: Edwin Mellen Press, 1979.
Kelly, Gerald, SJ
    1951   "The Duty to Preserve Life," *Theological Studies* 12, 550-556.
    1956   "The Morality of Mutilation: Toward a Revision of the Treatise," *Theological Studies* 17, 322-344.

1958   *Medico-Moral Problems*, St. Louis: Catholic Hospital Association, "On Cooperation," 322-325.

Kelly, James, "Residual or Prophetic: The Cultural Fate of Roman Catholic Sexual Ethics of Abortion and Contraception," *Social Thought* 12, Spring 1986, 3-18.

Kelly, Margaret John, and McCarthy, Donald, *Ethics Committees: A Challenge for Catholic Health Care*, St. Louis: Catholic Health Association of the United States, 1984.

Kelman, Sander, "Social Organization and the Meaning of Health," *Journal of Medicine and Philosophy* 5, 1980, 133-144.

Kelsey, Morton, *Prophetic Ministry: The Psychology and Spirit of Pastoral Care*, New York: Crossroad Publishing Co., 1982.

Kerlanger, Fred, *Foundations of Behavioral Research*, New York: CBS College Publishing, 1986.

Kervasdoue, Jean; Kimberly, John F; and Rodwin, Victor G., eds., *The End of an Illusion: The Future Health Policy in Western Industrialized Nations*, Berkeley: University of California Press, 1984.

Kesey, Ken, *One Flew Over the Cuckoo's Nest*, New York: Viking Penguin, Inc., 1962.

Kesset, Ross, "Triage: Philosophical and Cross Cultural Perspectives," in *Ethics and Critical Care Medicine*, John Moskop, and Loretta Koppleman, eds., Boston: D. Reidel, 1985.

Khantzian, E.J., "The Self-Medication Hypotheses of Addiction Disorders: Focus on Heroin and Cocaine Dependence," *American Journal of Psychiatry* 142, 1985, 1259-1264.

Kiesling, Christopher, OP

    1970   *The Future of the Christian Sunday*. New York: Sheed & Ward.

    1974   *Confirmation and Full Life in the Spirit*, Cincinnati: St. Anthony's Messenger Press.

    1977   *Celibacy, Friendship and Prayer*, Staten Island, NY: Alba House.

    1986   "On Relating to the Persons of the Trinity," *Theological Studies* 47, 1986, 599-612.

Kindred, Michael, "The Legal Rights of Mentally Retarded Persons in Twentieth Centntury America," in *Ethics and Mental Retardation*, Loretta Koppleman, and John Moskop, eds., Boston: D. Riedel, 1984.

King, J. Charles, "The Inadequacy of Situation Ethics," *Thomist* 34, 1970, 423-427.

Kinsey, A.C., et al., *Sexual Behavior in the Human Male*, Philadelphia: W.B. Saunders, 1948.

Kinsey, A.C., *Sexual Behavoir in the Human Female*, Philadelphia: Saunders, 1953.

Kinzer, David, "The Decline and Fall of Deregulation," *New England Journal of Medicine* 318 (2), Jan. 14, 1988, 112-116.

Kippley, John F., "Catholic Sexual Ethics: The Continuing Debate on Birth Control," *Linacre Quarterly* 41, 1974, 8-25.

Kirwan, William, *Biblical Concepts for Christian Counseling*, Grand Rapids: Baber Book House, 1984.

Klaus, Hanna, "Natural Family Planning: The Contribution of Fertility Awareness to Body-Person Integration," *Social Thought*, Winter 1979, 35-42.

Klaus, Hanna, and Brennan, J., "Terminology and Care Curricula in Natural Family Planning," Los Angeles: Natural Family Planning Physicians' Conference, 1981.

Kleber, Karl Heinz, *De Parvitate Materiae in Sexto*, Regensburg: F. Pustet, 1971.

Kleinig, John I., *Ethical Issues in Psychosurgery*, Boston: Allen and Unwin, 1985.

Klerman, Gerald, "Ethical Aspects of Drug Treatment," in *Psychiatric Ethics*, Sidney Black, and Paul Chadoff, eds., New York: Oxford University Press, 1981, 117-130.

Kliman, Gilbert, and Rosenfeld, Albert, *Responsible Parenthood: The Child's Psyche Through the Six-Year Pregnancy*, New York: Holt, Rinehart and Winston, 1980.

Kluge, Eike-Henner, "Nursing Vocation or Profession," *Canadian Nurse* 78 (2), Feb. 1982, 34-36.

Knapp, Samuel, and Vandercreek, Leon, "Tarasoff: Five Years Later," *Professional Psychology* 4, Aug. 13, 1982, 511-515.

Knauer, Peter, "The Hermeneutic Function of the Principle of Double Effect," *National Law Forum* 12, 1967, 132-162.

Knight, Many, and Field, David, "A Silent Conspiracy: Coping with Dying Cancer Patients on an Acute Surgical Ward," *Journal of Advanced Nursing* 6 (3), 1981, May 221-229.

Knight, R.P., "The Comparative Clinical Status of Conditioning Theories and Psychoanalysis," in *The Conditioning Theories,* Joseph Wolpe, Andrew Slater, and L.J. Reyna, eds., New York: Holt, Rinehart and Winston, 1966, 3-20.

Knox, Ronald, *Enthusiasm,* New York: Sheed & Ward, 1950, 231-318.

Koester, Helmut, "Nomos Physeos: The Concept of Natural Law in Greek Thought," in *Religions in Antiquity: Essays in Memory of Erwin Ramsdell Goodenough,* Jacob Neusner, ed., Leiden: E.J. Brill, 1968, 521-541.

Kohlberg, Lawrence
 1973 "Indoctrination Versus Relativity in Value Education," *Theology Digest* 21, Summer, 113-119. Reprinted from *Zygon* 6, 1971, 285-310.
 1981 *Essays on Moral Development,* San Francisco: Harper & Row.

Kohn, Robert, and White, Kerr L., eds., *Health Care: An International Study,* Report of WHO Collaborative Study of Medical Care Utilization, New York: Oxford University Press, 1976.

Kolata, Gina, "Use of Condoms Lags, Survey of Women Finds," *New York Times,* July 28, 1988, Report on Contraception: Guttmacher Institute, 1988.

Kolb, Lawrence, and Brodie, Keith, *Modern Clinical Psychiatry,* Philadelphia, W.B. Saunders, 1982, 752.

Koop, C. Everett
 1986 "Surgeon General's Report on Acquired Immune Deficiency Syndrome," *Journal of the American Medical Association* 20, Nov. 28, 1986, 256.
 1987 "Doctors Who Shun AIDS Patients are Assailed by Surgeon General," Phillip Boffey, *New York Times,* Sept. 9, 1987, A1.

Koppleman, Loretta, "Consent and Randomized Clinical Trials: Are They Moral or Design Problems?" *Journal of Medicine and Philosophy* 4, Nov. 22, 1986, 317-345.

Kosnik, Anthony R., et al., *Human Sexuality: New Directions in American Catholic Thought,* New York: Paulist Press, 1977.

Kosten, T.R.; Rounsaville, B.J.; and Kleber, H.D.
 1985a "Comparison of Clinician Ratings to Self-Reports of Curing Detoxification of Opiate Addicts," *American Journal of Alcohol Abuse* 11, 1-10.
 1985b "Ethnic and Gender Differences Among Opiate Addicts," *International Journal of Addiction* 20, 1143-1162.

Kotton, Michael H., "Medical Confidentiality: An Intransigent and Absolute Obligation," *Journal of Medical Ethics* 3, Sept. 12, 1986, 117-122.

Krakoff, Irwin, "The Hospice Movement and its Relationship to Active Treatment," in *Cancer Treatment and Research in Humanistic Perspective,* Steven Gross and Solomen Garbo, eds., New York: Springer Publishing Co., 1985.

Krason, Stephen, *The Supreme Court's Abortion Decision: A Critical Study of the Shaping of a Major American Public Policy and a Basis for Change,* Ann Arbor: University Microfilms International, 1983.

Kristof, Nicolas, "More Insurers Screen Applicants for AIDS," *New York Times,* Dec. 26, 1985, D1, D4.

Krugman, Saul, "The Willow Brook Hepatitis Studies Revisited: Ethical Aspects," *Review of Infectious Diseases,* Jan. 1986, 157-162.

Kübler-Ross, Elisabeth
 1969 *On Death and Dying,* New York: Macmillan.
 1978 *To Live Until We Say Good-By,* Englewood Cliffs, NJ: Prentice-Hall.
 1987 *AIDS: The Ultimate Challenge,* New York: Macmillan.

Kung, Hans, *Eternal Life: Life After Death As a Medical, Philosophical, and Theological Program,* Garden City, NY: Doubleday, 1984.

Kurtz, Paul
    1983   *In Defense of Secular Humanism,* Buffalo: Prometheus Books.
    1988   *Forbidden Fruit: The Ethics of Humanism,* Buffalo: Prometheus Books.

L

LaBar, Martin, "The Pros and Cons of Human Cloning," *Thought* 59 (234), Sept. 1984, 319-333.

Lain-Entralgo, P., *The Therapy of the World in Classical Antiquity,* Rather & Sharp, trans., New Haven: Yale University Press, 1970.

Laing, R.D., *The Politics of Experience,* New York: Ballantine Books, 1976.

Lako, C.J., "Privacy Protection and Population-Based Health Research," *Social Science and Medicine* 23 (3), 1986, 293-295.

Landau, Richard, and Gustafson, James, "Death is Not the Enemy," *Journal of the American Medical Association* 252 (17), Nov. 2, 1984, 2458.

Langan, John, "The Christian Difference in Ethics," *Theological Studies* 49 (1), Mar. 1988, 131.

Langemann, Ellen C., *Nursing History: New Perspectives, New Possibilities,* New York: Teacher's College Press, 1983.

Lappe, Marc
    1972   "Moral Obligations and the Fallacies of 'Genetic Control'," *Theological Studies* 33, 411-427.
    1984   "The Predicting Power of The New Genetics," *Hastings Center Report* 5, Oct, 14, 18-21.
    1985   "Virtue and Public Health: Societal Obligation and Individual Need," in *Explorations in the Character of Medicine,* E. Shelp, ed., Boston: D. Reidel.
    1987   "The Limits of Genetic Inquiry," *Hastings Center Report* 4 (17).

LaPuma, John, et al., "An Ethics Consultation Service in a Teaching Hospital," *Journal of the American Medical Association* 260 (6), Aug. 12, 1988, 808-811.

Laura, Ronald, "Mental Retardation and Genetic Engineering," in *Moral Issues in Retardation,* Ronald Laura, ed., London: Croom Helius, 1985.

Lavin, Michael, "Mutilation, Deception, and Sex Changes," *Journal of Medical Ethics* 13, 1987, 86-91.

Lawler, Ronald; Boyle, Joseph; and May, William E., *Catholic Sexual Ethics,* Huntington, IN: Our Sunday Visitor, 1985, "On Sterilization," 10-44.

Lawrence, Susan, "Heart Transplants: Blessing or Boondoggle," *Forum on Medicine* 3 (7), July 1980, 441.

Lebacqz, Karen
    1977   "Commentary 'On Natural Death'" (California Natural Death Act), *Hastings Center Report* 7, 14.
    1985   "The Virtuous Patient," in *Virtue and Medicine: Explorations in the Character of Medicine,* E. Shelp, ed., Boston: D. Reidel, 275-288.

Lederberg, Joshua, "A Geneticist Looks at Contraception and Abortion," *Annals of Internal Medicine* 67, 1967, 26-27.

Lee, Patrick, "Permanence of the Ten Commandments: St. Thomas and His Commentators," *Theological Studies* 42, 1981, 422-433.

Lee, Phillip, et al., "Physicians' Competence: Whose Responsibility," *Medical Staff News,* May 1988.

Lee, Phillip, and Brown, Nancy, *The Nation's Health,* San Francisco: Boyd & Fraser Publishing Co., 1981.

Leech, Kenneth, *Experiencing God: Theology as Spirituality* San Francisco: Harper & Row, 1985.

Lehmann, H.E., "Problems with Ethical Aspects of Psychotropic Drug Use," *Progress Inc.,* 1979.

Lehrman, Dorothy, ed., *Fetal Research and Fetal Tissue Research*, Washington, DC: Association of American Medical Colleges, June 1988.

Lejeune, Jerome; Ramsey, Paul; and Wright, Gerard, "The Question of In Vitro Fertilization," *Studies in Law, Ethics and Medicine*, London: Society for Protection of Unborn Children, 1984.

Leo XIII, *Rights and Duties of Capital and Labor (Rerum Novarum) 1981*, in *The Social Teachings of the Church*, Anne Fremantle, ed., New York: New American Library, 1963.

Lepp, Ignace, *The Depth of the Soul: A Christian Approach to Psychoanalysis*, New York: Alba House, 1965.

Leslie, Gerald, and Korman, Shiela, *The Family in Social Context*, 6th ed., New York: Oxford Press, 1985, 54-55, 75.

Levin, Arthur, *Talk Back to Your Doctor: How to Demand (and Recognize) High Quality Health Care*, Garden City, NY: Doubleday, 1975.

Levine, Robert
  1981   *Ethics and Regulations of Clinical Research*, Baltimore: Orban and Schwartzenberg, 2nd ed. 1986.
  1983   "Informed Consent in Research and Practice: Similarities and Differences," *Archives of Internal Medicine* 143 (6), June, 1229-1231.
  1985   "Institutional Review Boards and Collaborations Between Academia and Industry: Some Counter Productive Policies and Practices," *Circulation* 72 (2), Aug., 148-150.

Levine, Stephen, F., and Lothstein, Leslie, "Transsexualism or the Gender Dysphoria Syndromes," *Journal of Sex and Marital Therapy* 12, 1981, 69-82.

Levinson, A-J Rock, "Termination of Life-Support Systems in the Elderly: Ethical Issues," *Journal of Geriatric Psychiatry* 14 (1), 1981, 71-85.

Levy, Charlotte, *The Human Body and the Law: Legal and Ethical Considerations*, New York: Oceana Publications, 1983, 90.

Levy, David, et al., "Differences in Cerebral Blood Flow and Glucose Utilization in Vegetative versus Locked-in Patients," *Annals of Neurology*, 1987, 673-682.

Lew, Myer S., *The Humanity of Jewish Law*, New York: Sancino Press, 1985.

Lewis, C.S., *The Problem of Pain*, New York: Macmillan, 1943.

Lewis, H. David, *The Elusive Self*, Philadelphia: Westminster Press, 1982.

Lewontia, R.C.; Rose, Steven; and Kamin, Leon, *Not in Our Genes*, New York: Pantheon Books, 1984

Lidz, Charles, et al., "Barriers to Informed Consent," *Annals of Internal Medicine* 99 (4), Oct. 1983, 539-543.

Lifshitz, Samuel, "Rape," in *Principles and Practice of Emergency Medicine*, George Schwartz, et al., eds., Philadelphia: Saunders, 1986.

Lifton, Robert Jay
  1986   *The Nazi Doctors*, New York: Free Press.
  1982   "Medicalized Killing in Auschwitz," *Psychiatry* 45 (4), Nov., 283-297.

Light, Donald, *Becoming Psychiatrists*, New York: W.W. Norton and Co., 1980.

Linacre Center for the Study of the Ethics of Health Care, Paper 3, "Ordinary and Extraordinary Means of Prolonging Life," London: Linacre Center, July 13, 1979.

Lind, Stuart, "Fee for Service Research," *New England Journal of Medicine* 314 (5), Jan. 30, 1986, 312-315.

Linzer, N., "Ethical Issues in Professional Behavior," *Forum* 22, Spring 1986.

Lipp, Martin, *The Bitter Pill, Doctors, Patients and Failed Expectations*, New York: Harper & Row, 1980.

Llewelyn, Susan, and Fielding, Gugi, "Am I Dying, Nurse?" *Nursing Mirror* 156 (16), Apr. 20, 1983, 30-31.

Llewellyn-Thomas, H., "The Measurement of Patients' Values in Medicine," *Medical Decision Making* 2 (4), Winter 1982, 449-462.

Lo, Bernard, et al., "Behind Closed Doors: Promises and Pitfalls of Ethics Committees," *New England Journal of Medicine* 317 (46), July 2, 1987.

Lock, S., "Fraud in Medicine," *British Medical Journal* 296, 1988, 376-77.

Loewy, Erich, "Physicians and Patients: Moral Agency in a Pluralistic World," *Journal of Medical Humanities and Bioethics* 1 (1), 1986, 57-68.

London, Perry, *The Modes and Morals of Psychotherapy*, New York: Holt, Rinehart and Winston, 1964.

 1969 *Behavior Control*, New York: Harper and Row.

Lothstein, L.M., "Sex Reassignment Surgery: Historical, Bioethical, and Theoretical Issues," *American Journal of Psychiatry* 139, 1982, 417-426.

Lotstra, Hans, *Abortion: The Catholic Debate in America*, New York: Irvington Publishers, 1985.

Louis, Thomas A., and Shapiro, Stanley H., "Critical Issues in the Conduct and Interpretation of Clinical Trials," *Annual Review of Public Health* 4, 1983, 25-46.

Ludmerer, Kenneth M., *Learning to Heal: The Development of American Medical Education*, New York: Basic Books, 1985.

Lurie, Nicole, et al., "Termination of Medi-Cal Benefits, A Follow-Up Study One Year Later," *New England Journal of Medicine* 314 (19), May 8, 1986, 1266-1268.

Lynn, Joanne, ed., *By No Extraordinary Means: The Choice to Forego Life-Sustaining Food and Water*, Bloomington, IN: Indiana University Press, 1986.

M

MacDonald, S., "The Meaning of Abortion," *American Ecclesiastical Review* 169, 1975, 219-236.

Machan, Tibor R., *The Pseudo-Science of B.F. Skinner*, New York: Arlington House, 1974.

MacIntyre, Alisdair

 1967 *A Short History of Ethics*, New York: Routledge and Kegan Publishing, (1987 ed.).

 1979 "Seven Traits for Designing Our Descendants," *Hastings Center Report* 9, 5-17.

 1981 *After Virtue*, Notre Dame, IN: Notre Dame University Press, 1981.

Mack, Arien, *Death in American Experience*, New York: Schocken Books, 1973.

Mack, Eric, "Bad Samaritanism and the Causation of Harm," *Philosophy and Public Affairs* 9 (1980) 230-259.

Mack, Robert, "Lessons From Living With Cancer," *New England Journal of Medicine* 311 (25), Dec. 20, 1984, 30-35.

Mackie, J.L., *Reasons and Values*, Oxford: Clarendon Press, 1985, esp. ch. 1 and 2.

Macklin, Ruth

 1982 *Man, Mind and Morality: The Ethics of Behavior Control*, Englewood Cliffs, NJ: Prenctice Hall.

 1983 "Philosophical Conceptions of Rationality and Psychiatric Notions of Competency," *Synthese* 57 (2), Nov., 205-225.

 1985 "Mapping the Human Genome: Problems of Privacy and Free Choice," in *Genetics and the Law*," Aubrey Milunsky and George Annas, eds., New York: Plenum University Press, 107-114.

MacNamara, Vincent, *Faith & Ethics*, Washington, DC: Georgetown University Press, 1986.

Macquarrie, John, *Three Ethical Issues*, New York: Harper & Row, 1970, Ch. 4, "Rethinking the Natural Law," 82-110.

Maguire, Daniel

 1974 *Death by Choice*, Garden City: Image Books, rev. 1984.

 1986 *The Moral Revolution: A Christian Humanist Vision*, New York: Harper & Row.

Maguire, P., "Barriers to Psychological Care for the Dying," *British Medical Journal* 291 (6510), Dec. 14, 1985, 1711-1713.

Mahkorn, S., and Dolan, W., "Sexual Assault and Pregnancy," in *New Perspectives on Human Abortion*, Thomas Hilers, D. Horan, and D. Mall, eds., Frederick, MD: University Publications of America, 1981.

Mahoney, John, et al., *Euthanasia and Clinical Practice*, London: Linacre Center, 1982.

Mahowald, Mary; Silver, Jerry; and Racheson, Robert, "The Ethical Options in Transplanting Fetal Tissue," *Hastings Center Report* 7 (1), Feb. 1987, 9-15.

Maida, Adam, ed. *Issues in Labor Management Dialogue: Church Perspectives*, St. Louis: Catholic Health Association of the United States, 1982.

Malone, Patrick, "Death Row and the Medical Model," *Hastings Center Report* 9, 1979, 5-7.

Mangan, J., "An Historical Analysis of the Principle of Double Effect," *Theological Studies* 10, 1949, 40-61.

Many, Seth, "Psychiatrists, State Hospitals, and Civil Rights," *New York State Journal of Medicine* 80 (12), Nov. 1980.

Marco, G.J.; Hollingworth, R.M.; and Durham, W.F., *Silent Spring Revisited*, Washington, DC: American Chemical Society, 1987.

Marcos, Luis, and Cohen, Neal, "Taking the Suspected Mentally Ill Off the Streets," *New England Journal of Medicine* 315 (19), Oct. 30, 1986, 1158-1161.

Marcus, Ruthanne, and CDC Surveillance Group, "Surveillance of Health Care Workers Exposed to Blood from Patients Infected with the Human Immunodeficiency Virus," *New England Journal of Medicine* 319 (17), Oct. 27, 1988, 1119.

Marcuse, Herbert
    1964   *One-Dimensional Man: Studies in the Ideology of Advanced Industrial Society*, Boston: Beacon Press.
    1972   *Counter Revolution and Revolution*, Boston: Beacon Press.

Margo, Curtis, "Selling Surgery," *New England Journal of Medicine* 314 (24), June 12, 1986, 1575-76.

Margolis, Joseph
    1985   "Triage and Critical Care," in *Ethics and Critical Care Medicine*, John C. Moskop and Loretta Koppleman, eds., Boston: Riedel, 141-190.
    1986   "Thoughts on Definitions of Disease," *The Journal of Medicine and Philosophy*, 11 (3), 233-236.

Maritain, Jacques, *Three Reformers: Luther, Descartes, Rousseau*, rev. ed., London: Sheed & Ward, 1929, 54ff.

Markland, Colin, "Transsexual Surgery," *Obstetrics & Gynecology Annual* 4, 1975, 309-330.

Marks, Joan H., *Advocacy in Health Care: The Power of a Silent Constituency*, Clifton, NJ: Humana Press, 1986.

Marmer, Stephen, "Theories of the Mind and Psychopathology," *Textbook of Psychiatry*, John Talbott, Robert John, and Stuart Hales-Yudofsky, eds., Washington, DC: American Psychiatric Press, 1988, 123-162.

Marmoc, Judd, ed., *Homosexual Behavior: A Modern Reappraisal*, New York: Basic Books, 1980.

Marquis, Don, "An Argument that All Prerandomized Clinical Trials Are Unethical," *Journal of Medicine and Philosophy* 11 (4), Nov. 1986, 367-383.

Martelet, Gustave, SJ
    1969   *L'Existence Humaine et L'Amour, Pour Mieux Comprendre L' Encyclicque Humanae Vitae*, Paris: Desclee, 1969.
    1981   "A Prophetic Text Under Challenge: The Message of *Humanae Vitae*," in *Natural Family Planning: Nature's Way/God's Way*, Anthony Zimmerman, SVD, ed., Collegeville, MN: DeRance Inc. and Human Life Center, 1981, 153-167.

Martorano, Joseph, "Ethics and Psychopharmacology: Revolution or War?" in *Ethics and Values in Psychotherapy A Guidebook*, Max Rosenbau, ed., New York: Free Press, 1982, 328-359.

Marty, Martin, and Vaux, Kenneth, ed., *Health, Medicine, and the Faith Traditions: An Inquiry into Religion and Medicine*, Philadelphia: Fortress Press, 1982.

Marx, Karl, *The Economic and Philosophic Manuscripts of 1844*, introduction by D.J. Struik, translated by Martin Milligan, New York: International Publishers, 1964, 179ff.

Marzen, Thomas, "The Uniform Rights of the Terminally Ill Act: A Critical Analysis," *Issues in Law and Medicine* 1 (6), May 1986, 441-475.

Maslow, Abraham J., *Motivation and Personality*, 2nd ed., New York: Harper & Row, 1970.

Masters, William H., and Johnson, Virginia
> 1966   *Human Sexual Response,* Boston: Little, Brown, 1966.
> 1970   *Human Sexual Inadequacy,* Boston: Little, Brown.
> 1976   *The Pleasure Bond,* New York: Bantam Books, paperback edition.

Masters, William H., et al., *Ethical Issues in Sex Research and Therapy,* Boston: Little, Brown, vol. 1 1977, vol. 2 1980.

Masters, William H.; Johnson, Virginia E.; and Kolodny, Robert, *Masters and Johnson on Sex and Human Loving,* Boston: Little, Brown, 1986.

May, Rollo, *Freedom and Destiny,* New York: Dell Books, 1983.

May, William E.
> 1976   "Proxy Consent to Human Experimentation," *Linacre Quarterly* 43, 73-84.
> 1977a "Situationism and Contemporary Roman Catholic Moral Theology," unpublished paper, courtesy of author.
> 1977b "Sterilization: Catholic Teaching and Catholic Practice," *Homeletic and Pastoral Review* 77, Aug,-Sept., 9-22.
> 1983   *Contraception and Catholicism,* Front Royal, VA: Christendom Publishing.
> 1984   "Aquinas and Janssens: On the Moral Meaning of Human Acts," *The Thomist* 48, 566-606.
> 1987b "Sexual Ethics and Human Dignity," in *Persona Verita e Morale,* Rome: Citta Nuova Edditrice, 477-494.

May, William E., et al., "Feeding and Hydrating the Permanently Unconscious and Other Vulnerable Persons," *Issues in Law and Medicine* 3 (3), 203-210.

May, William F., *The Physician's Covenant Images of the Healer in Medical Ethics,* Philadelphia: Westminster Press, 1983.

Mayo, David, "The Concept of Rational Suicide," *Journal of Medicine and Philosophy* 11 (2), May 1986, 143-155.

McBrien, Richard, *Ministry a Theological, Pastoral Handbook,* New York: Harper & Row, 1987.

McCabe, Herbert, OP, *What Is Ethics All About?* Washington, DC: Corpus Books, 1969.

McCarthy, Charles, "Experience with Boards and Commissions Concerned with Research Ethics in the United States," in *Research Ethics,* Kolb Berg, ed., New York: Alan R. Liss, 1983, 111-122.

McCarthy, Donald G.
> 1977   "Medication to Prevent Pregnancy after Rape," *Linacre Quarterly* 44, 210-222.
> 1983   "Infertility Bypass," *Ethics and Medics* 8 (10), Oct.
> 1988   "TOTS is for Kids," *Ethics and Medics* 13 (12), Dec.

McCartney, James, *Unborn Persons, Pope John Paul II and the Abortion Debate,* New York: Peter Lang, 1987.

McClendon, James, *Ethics,* Nashville: Abingdon Press, 1986.

McCloskey, Joanne, and Grace, Helen, *Current Issues in Nursing,* Boston: Blackwell Scientific Publications, 1985.

McCombie, S.C., "The Cultural Impact of the AIDS Test: The American Experience," *Social Science and Medicine I* 23 (5), 1986.

McCormick, Richard A., SJ
> 1973a *Ambiguity in Moral Choice,* 1973 Pere Marquette Theology Lecture, Milwaukee: Marquette University.
> 1973b "The Silence Since *Humanae Vitae,*" *America* 21, 30-33.
> 1974a "Proxy Consent in the Experimentation Situation," *Perspectives in Biology and Medicine* 118, Autumn, 2-20.
> 1974b "To Save or Let Die: The Dilemma of Modern Medicine," *Journal of the American Medical Association* 229, 172-176.
> 1976   "Experimentation in Children: Sharing in Sociality," *Hastings Center Report* 6, 41-46.
> 1977   "Man's Moral Responsibility for Health," *Catholic Hospital* 5, 609.

1981   *Notes on Moral Theology*, Washington, DC: University Press.

1984a   *Health and Medicine in the Catholic Tradition*, New York: Crossroad Publishing Co., 140.

1984b   *Notes on Moral Theology*, Lanham, MD: University Press of America.

1987   "Begotten, Not Made," *Notre Dame Magazine* 15 (3), Autumn, 22-26.

McCormick, Richard A., SJ, and Ramsey, Paul, eds., *Doing Evil to Achieve Good*, Chicago: Loyola University Press, 1978.

McCullagh, Peter, *The Foetus as Transplant Donor: Scientific, Social, Ethical Perspectives*, New York: John Wiley & Sons, 1987.

McCullough, Lawrence, "Methodological Concerns in Bioethics," *Journal of Medicine and Philosophy* 11 (1), Feb. 1986, 17-37.

McDonagh, Enda, *Doing the Truth: The Quest for Moral Theology*, Notre Dame, IN: University of Notre Dame Press, 1979.

McDonald, J.C., "The National Organ Procurement and Transplantation Network," *Journal of the American Medical Association* 259, 1988, 725-726.

McDowell, Jan, and Newell, Claire, *Measuring Health: A Guide to Rating Scales and Questionnaires*, New York: Oxford University Press, 1987.

McEllhenny, John Galen, *Cutting the Monkey Rope*, Valley Forge, PA: Judson Press, 1973.

McElhinney, Thomas F., ed., *Human Values Teaching Programs for Health Professionals*, Philadelphia: Society for Health and Human Values, 1981.

McFadden, Charles J.

1967   *Medical Ethics*, 6th ed., Philadelphia: F.A. Davis Co., "On cooperation," 357-372, "On truthfulness and professional secrecy," 389-414.

1976   *Dignity of Life: Moral Values in a Changing Society*, Huntington, IN: Our Sunday Visitor, 186ff.

McGill, Arthur Chute, ed., *Death and Life: An American Theology*, Philadelphia: Fortress Press, 1987.

McGrath, Patrick J.

1969   *The Nature of Moral Judgment*, Notre Dame: University of Notre Dame Press, 1969.

1976   "On Not Re-interpreting *Humanae Vitae*," *Irish Theological Quarterly* 38, 130-143.

McInerny, Ralph, "Fundamental Option," in *Persona Verita Morale*, Rome: Citta Nuova Edditrice, 1987, 427-434.

McIntyre, Neil, and Popper, Karl, "The Critical Attitude in Medicine: The Need for a New Ethics," *British Medical Journal* 287 (6409), Dec. 24-31, 1983, 1919-1923.

McIntyre, Russell, "The Conroy Decision" in *By No Extrordinary Means*, Joanne Lynn, ed., Bloomington, IN: Indiana University Press, 1986, 260-266.

McKeown, Thomas, *The Role of Medicine: Dream, Mirage, or Nemesis*, Princeton: Princeton University Press, 1980.

McLane, David, "The Diagnosis, Prognosis, and Outcome for the Handicapped Newborn: A Neonatal View," *Issues in Law and Medicine* 12 (11), July 1986, 15-24.

McNeill, D.R.; Morrison, P.A.; and Nouwen, H.J., *Compassion*, Garden City: Doubleday, 1982.

McNeill, John J., SJ, *The Church and the Homosexual*, Mission, KS: Sheed, Andrews & McMeel, 1976.

McNeill T.; Dolan, J.; and Watson, W., "What the Book Forgot," *Humane Medicine* 2 (2), Nov. 1986, 165-169.

Meadows, Donella H., et al., *The Limits to Growth*, New York: Universe Books, 1972.

Mechanic, David, "Physicians and Patients in Transition," *Hastings Center Report* 15 (6), Dec. 1985, 9-12.

Medical News 37, "Arizona M.D.'s Refuse AIDS Patients," Nov. 6, 1987.

Medical Review Bulletin, "Physician Competence: Whose Problem Is It?" Chicago: American Hospital Association, June 1988.

Medvedev, Roy A., and Medvedev, Zhores A., *A Question of Madness*, New York: Alfred A. Knopf, 1971.

Mehl, Roger, *Catholic Ethics and Protestant Ethics*, Philadelphia: Westminster Press, 1971.

Meier, Anton Meinrad, *Das Peccatum Mortale Ex Toto Genere Suo*, Regensburg: Pustet, 1966.

Meier, Levi, ed., *Jewish Values in Bioethics*, New York: Human Services Press, 1986.

Meilander, Gilbert, "Euthanasia and Christian Vision," *Thought* 57 (227), Dec. 1982, 465-475.

Meisel, Alan, "The Rights of the Mentally Ill Under State Constitutions," *Law and Contemporary Problems* 45 (3), 1982, 7-40.

Mendelhoff, John, "Politics and Bioethical Commissions, Muddling through and the Slippery Slope," *Journal of Health Politics, Policy and Law* 10 (1), Spring 1985, 81-92.

Mendelsohn, John, ed., *Medical Experiments on Jewish Inmates of Concentration Camps, The Holocaust*, New York: Garland Publishing, Inc., 1982.

Mendelsohn, John, ed., *The Holocaust 9: Medical Experiments on Jewish Inmates of Concentration Camps*, New York: Garland Publishing, Inc., 1982.

Mendelson, Jack, and Mello, Nancy, ed., *The Diagnosis and Treatment of Alcoholism*, New York: McGraw-Hill, 1985.

Menninger, Karl
   1938   *Man Against Himself*, New York: Harcourt Brace.
   1942   *Love Against Hate*, New York: Harcourt Brace.
   1958   *Theory of Psychoanalytic Technique*, New York: Basic Books, "On transference," 77-98.
   1968   *Crime of Punishment*, New York: Viking Penguin.

Merkelbach, Benedictus, OP, *Summa Theologiae Moralis*, 10th ed., 3 vols., Burge, Belgium: Desclee de Brouwer, 1959, vol. 1, "On cooperation," 487-492.

Mershey, Harold, "Variable Meanings for the Definition of Disease," *The Journal of Medicine and Philosophy*, 1986, 215-232.

Merton, Robert K., *Some Thoughts on the Professions in American Society* (address), Brown University, 1960.

Meyer, J.K., "Psychiatric Considerations in the Sexual Reassignment of Non-Intersex Individuals," *Clinics in Plastic Surgery* 1, 1974, 275-283.

Meyer, J.K., et al., "Sex Reassignment: Follow Up," *Archives of General Psychiatry* 36 (9), Aug. 1979, 1010-1015.

Meyers, John E.B., "Legal Issues Surrounding Therapy With Minors," *Clinical Social Work Journal* 10 (4), Winter 1982, 303-314.

Milewski, Elizabeth, "Points to Consider in the Design and Submission of Human Somatic-Cell Gene Therapy Protocals," *Recombinant DNA Bulletin* 8 (4), Dec. 1985, 176-180.

Milhaven, John Giles, "Thomas Aquinas on Sexual Pleasure," *Journal of Religous Ethics* 5, 1977, 1576-181.

Milkman, Harvey, and Shaffer, Howard, *The Addictions: Multidisciplinary Perspectives and Treatments*, Boston: Lexington Books, 1984.

Mill, John Stuart, *Utilitarianism and Other Writings*, Cleveland: New American Library, Meridian Books, 1962 [1863].

Miller, Bruce, "Autonomy and Proxy Consent," *IRB: A Review of Human Subjects Research*, Dec. 1982, 4(10).

Miller, J.D., *National Survey on Drug Abuse: Main Findings* Rockville, MD: National Institute of Drug Abuse, 1983.

Mills, Mark; Sullivan, Greer; and Eth, Spencer, "Protecting Third Parties: A Decade After Tarasoff," *American Journal of Psychiatry* 144 (1), Jan. 1987, 68-74.

Mills, Michael; Wofsy, Constana; and Mills, John, "The Acquired Immune Deficiency Syndrome Infection Control and Public Law," *New England Journal of Medicine* 314 (14), Apr. 3, 1986, 931-926.

Mishell, Daniel, "Control of Human Reproduction, Contraception, and Pregnancy," in *Obstetrics and Gynecology*, Daniel Danforth, and James Scott, Philadelphia: J.B. Lippincott Co., 1986, 231-283.

Mitchell, Leon, *Access to Health Care in the United States: Results of a 1986 Survey*, Princeton, NJ: Robert Wood Johnson Foundation, 1987.

Mitford, Jessica, *The American Way of Death,* 2nd ed., New York: Simon & Schuster, 1975.

Mizratti, Terry, *Getting Rid of Patients,* New Brunswick: Rutgers University Press, 1986.

Modde, Margaret, "The Christian Faithful and the Health Care Ministry," *Health Progress* 66 (7), Sept. 1985, 75-82.

Modell, Bernadette, "Social Aspects of Prenatal Monitoring for Genetic Disease," *The Future of Prenatal Diagnosis,* Edinburgh: Churchill Livingston, 1982.

Modgil, Celia, and Kohlberg, Lawrence, *Consensus and Controversy,* Philadelphia: Palmer Press, 1986.

Mohr, James, *Abortion in America: The Origins and Evolution of National Policy 1800-1900,* New York: Oxford University Press, 1978.

Molinari, G., "Review of Clinical Criteria of Brain Death," in *Brain Death: Interrelated Medical and Social Issues,* J. Korein, ed., New York: New York Academy of Sciences, 1978, 62-69.

Moline, Jon, "Professionals and Professions: A Philosophical Examination of an Ideal," *Social Science and Medicine* 22 (5), 1986, 501-508.

Moltmann, Jurgen, *Theology of Hope.* New York: Harper & Row, 1967.

Monahan, John, ed., *Who is the Client? The Ethics of Psychological Intervention in the Criminal Justice System,* Washington, DC: American Psychological Association, 1980.

Monod, Jacques, *Chance and Necessity: An Essay on the Natural Philosophy of Modern Biology,* New York: Alfred A. Knopf, 1971.

Monteleone, James A., "The Physiological Aspects of Sex," in *Human Sexuality and Personhood,* St. Louis: Pope John XXIII Medical-Moral Research and Education Center, 1981, 71-85.

Moody, Howard, "Abortion: Woman's Right and Legal Problem," *Christianity and Crisis* 31, 1971, 27-32.

Moore, G.E., *Ethics,* New York: Oxford Press, 1965 (original 1903).

Moore, Keith, *The Developing Human,* Philadelphia: W.B. Saunders, 1988.

Moore, Lorna, *The Biocultural Basis of Health: Expanding Views of Medical Anthropology,* Prospect Heights, IL: Waveland Press, 1987.

Moore, Maurice J., *Death of a Dogma? The American Catholic Clergy View on Contraception,* Chicago: University of Chicago Family Study Center, 1973.

Moore, Robert L.
    1978   "Ethics in the Practice of Psychiatry," *American Journal of Psychiatry* 135, 157-163.
    1985   "Ethics in the Practice of Psychiatry: Update on the Results of Enforcement of the Code," *American Journal of Psychiatry* 142 (7), Sept., 1043-1046.

Moore, Wilbert E., and Rosenblum, Gerald W., *The Professions: Roles and Rules,* New York: Russell Sage Foundation, 1970, 51-65, 174-186.

Morreim, E. Haau, "Philosophy Lessons From the Clinical Setting," *Theoretical Medicine* 7 (1), Feb. 1986, 47-63.

Morrison, James K.; Layton, Bruce D.; and Newman, Joan; "Ethical Conflict Among Clinical Psychologists and Other Mental Health Workers," *Psychological Reports* 51 (3), Dec. 1982, 703-715.

Mulstein, Suzanne, "The Uninsured and the Financing of Uncompensated Care: Scope, Costs and Policy Options," *Inquiry* 21 (3), Fall 1984, 214-229.

Mulvanney, Kieran, "The Other Side of Animal Rights," *New Scientist* 109 (1502), April 3, 1986, 52-53.

Mundinger, Mary O'Neill, "Health Services Funding Costs and the Declining Health of the Poor," *New England Journal of Medicine* 313 (1), July 4, 1985, 44-47.

Munetz, Mark R.; Lidz, Charles; and Meisel, Alan, "Informed Consent and Incompetent Patients," *Journal of Family Practice* 20 (3), Mar. 1985, 273-279.

Murnion, Philip, "A Sacramental Church in a Sacramental World," *Origins* 14 (6), June 21, 1984, 81-90, especially p. 88.

Murphy, Francis X., *Catholic Perspectives on Population Issues II,* vol. 35, Washington, DC: Population Reference Bureau, Feb. 1981.

Murray, J., et al. "Informed Consent for Research Publication of Patient Related Data," *Clinical Research* 32 (4), Oct. 1984, 404-408.

Murray, Joseph, E., "Decisions on the Frontlines of Surgery," *Harvard Medical,* 1986, 18-24.

Murray, Thomas, and Caplan, Arthur, eds., *Which Babies Shall Live? Humanistic Dimensions of the Care of Imperiled Newborns,* Clifton, NJ: Humana Press, 1985.

Myrich, J.A., "Competition in the Health Care Delivery System: Prescription for the 1980s," *Hospital Pharmacy Management* 3 (3), Nov. 1983, 1-11.

N

Nagel, Ernest, *Teleology Revisited,* New York: Columbia University Press, 1979.

Narveson, Jan, "Self-Ownership and the Ethics of Suicide," *Suicide and Life Threatening Behavior* 13 (4), Winter 1983, 240-253.

NAS: National Academy of Science, "Confronting AIDS, Update 1988," Washington, DC: 1988.

Nash, George H., *The Conservative Intellectual Movement in America Since 1945,* New York: Basic Books, 1976.

Natanson, Maurice, ed., "Suffering, Empathy and Compassion," a special issue of *Journal of Philosophy and Compassion* 6, Feb. 1981.

Nathanson, Bernard, *The Abortion Mentality,* New York: Frederich Fell, 1983.

Nathanson, Bernard, and Ostling, Richard, *Aborting America,* New York: Doubleday, 1979.

National Academy of Science: see NAS

National Catholic Reporter: see NCR

National Conference of Catholic Bishops: see NCCB

National Institute of Drug Abuse: see NIDA

National Institutes of Health: see NIH

Navarro, Vincente, *Crisis in Health and Medicine: A Social Critique,* New York: Tavistock Publications, 1986.

NCCB: National Conference of Catholic Bishops

    1974   *Documentation on the Right to Life and Abortion,* Washington, DC: United States Catholic Conference.

    1976   *To Live in Christ Jesus, A Pastoral Reflection on the Moral Life,* Washington, DC: United States Catholic Conference.

    1977a   *Commentary on Reply of Sacred Congregation for the Doctrine of the Faith on Sterilization in Catholic Hospitals,* Sept. 15, United States Catholic Conference.

    1977b   Statement in response to book on sexuality, *Origins,* 7 (24) Dec. 1, 376.

    1980   "Statement on Tubal Ligation," *Origins,* 10, 11, Aug. 28, 175.

    1984   "Political Responsibility: Choices for the 80s," *Origins* 13 (44), April 12, 1984, 732-736.

    1985   "Pastoral Plan for Prolife Activities: A Reaffirmation," *Origins* 15 (24), Nov. 28.

    1986   Committee for Prolife Activities, "Statement on Uniform Rights of the Terminally Ill Act" (June 26, 1986) *Origins* 16 (12), Sept. 4, 1986, 222-224.

    1988   Committee on Doctrine, "Announcing Revision of Ethical and Religious Directives for Catholic Health Facilities," July 16, private letter.

NCR: *National Catholic Reporter,* "Rome Document Sparks Firestorm of U.S. Reaction, Even Critics Advise It Should Not Be Ignored," Apr. 3, 1987.

Neumann, Erich, *The Origins and History of Consciousness,* Bollinger Series, New York: Pantheon Books, 1964, 318-320.

Neville, R., et al., "Should General Practioners Be Informed of Patient's Drug Conviction?" *British Medical Journal* 292 (6535), June 14, 1986, 1579-1580.

Newhouse, J.P., "Is Competition the Answer?" *Journal Health Economics* 1 (1), May 1982, 110-116.

New Jersey Catholic Conference, "Providing Food and Fluids to Severely Brain-Damaged Patients," *Origins* 16, 24, Jan. 22, 1987, 582.

New York Task Force on Medical Ethics, *The Determination of Death*, New York: The Task Force, 1986.

New York Times, "Surrogate Deals for Mothers Held Illegal in New Jersey," Feb. 3, 1988.

New York Times, "Pressure to Regulate *In Vitro* Fertilization Groups as Demand Rises," July 27, 1988.

New York Times, "Gallup Poll on Abortion Preference," Dec. 1, 1987.

Ngyan, William, and Sahat, Nadia, *Diagnostic Recognition of Genetic Disease*, Philadelphia: Lea and Debiger, 1987.

NIDA: National Institute of Drug Abuse, *Drug Use Among American High School Students and other Young Adults*, Washington, DC: U.S. Department of Health and Human Services, 1986.

Niebuhr, H. Richard, *The Responsible Self*, New York: Harper & Row, 1963.

NIH: National Institutes of Health
>   1985   "Consensus Conference: Electroconvulsive Therapy," *Journal of the American Medical Association* 254 (15), Oct. 18, 1985, 2105-08.
>   1987   *Human Somatic Cell Gene Therapy Prospects for Treating Inherited Diseases*, Washington, DC: NIH.

Nolan, Martin, "The Principle of Totality in Moral Theology," in *Absolutes in Moral Theology*, Charles E. Curran, ed., Washington, DC: Corpus Books, 1968.

Nolin, Kieran, OSB, "Attitudes of Medical Staff to Sacramental Ministry in Public Hospitals," paper read at Institute of Religious and Human Development, Texas Medical Center, Houston, 1972.

Noonan, John T.
>   1965   *Contraception: A History of Its Treatment by the Catholic Theologians and Canonists*, New York: Harvard University Press, "On zero population growth," 18-25, "On Church's middle course in sex ethics," 56-106, rev., 1987.
>   1967   "Abortion and the Catholic Church: A Summary History," *Natural Law Forum* 12, 85-131.
>   1970a   "An Almost Absolute Value in History," in *The Morality of Abortion: Legal and Historical Perspectives*, John T. Noonan, Jr., ed., Cambridge, MA: Harvard University Press, 1-59.
>   1970b   ed., *The Morality of Abortion: Legal and Historical Perspectives*, Cambridge, MA: Harvard University Press.
>   1979   *A Private Choice: Abortion in America in the Seventies*, New York: Free Press.
>   1985   "An Almost Absolute Value in History," *Human Life Review* 11 (1-2), Winter-Spring 1985, 125-178.

Nouwen, Henri J., *The Wounded Healer: Ministry in Contemporary Society*, Garden City, NY: Doubleday, 1972.

Novak, David
>   1971   *Suicide and Morality*, New York: Scholars Press.
>   1985   *Halakah in a Theological Dimension*, Chico, CA: Scholars Press.

Noyes, R., Jr., "Seneca on Death," *Journal of Religion and Health* 12, 1973, 223-240.

Nozick, Robert, *Philosophical Explanations*, Cambridge: Belknap Press, 1981.

Number, Ronald, ed., *Compulsory Health Insurance: The Continuing American Debate*, Westport, CT: Greenwood Press, 1982.

Nuremberg Code, 1946, see *Encyclopedia of Bioethics*, New York: Free Press, 1978, vol. 4, 1764.

O

Oakley, Deborah, "Reproductive Freedom and the Development of Population Policy," in *Medical Ethics and the Law: Implications for Public Policy*, Marc Hiller, ed., Cambridge: Ballinger, 1981, 327-343.

O'Callaghan, D.F., "Humanae Vitae in Perspective: Survey of Recent French Writing," *Irish Theological Quarterly* 37, 1970, 309-321

O'Connell, Timothy, *Changing Catholic Moral Theology: A Study of Josef Fuchs*, doctoral dissertation, Ann Arbor: University Microfilms, 1974.

O'Connor, Brian, ed., *The Pastoral in Caring for Dying and Bereaved: Pragmatic and Ecumenical*, New York: Praeger, 1986.

O'Donnell, Thomas

    1976   *Medicine and Christian Morality*, Boston: St. Paul Press, 66ff, (original ed. 1957).

    1986   "Professional Confidentiality," *Medical Moral Newsletter* 23 (6), June 21-22.

    1987   "Comment," *Medical Moral Newsletter*, 24, (2) Feb., 7

O'Donovan, Oliver, *Begotten or Made*, New York: Oxford University Press, 1984.

Office of Technology Assessment: see OTA

Oken, D., "What to Tell Cancer Patients: A Study of Medical Attitudes," *Journal of the American Medical Association* 175, 13 (Apr. 1, 1961), 1120-1128.

Olshansky, Ellen Francis, and Sammons, Lucy, "Artificial Insemination: An Overview," *Journal of Obstetric Gynocological and Neonatal Nursing* 14 (6), Nov. 1985, 49-54.

O'Meara, Thomas

    1973   *Loose in the World*, New York: Paulist Press.

    1983   *Theology of Ministry*, New York: Paulist Press

Oppenheimer, Gerald, and Padgug, Robert, "AIDS: The Risk to Insurers, The Threat to Equity," *Hastings Center Report* 16 (5), Oct. 1986, 18-22.

Ornstein, Paul, and Kay, Jerald, "Ethical Problems in the Psychotherapy of the Suicidal Patient," *Psychiatric Annals* 13 (4), Apr. 1983, 332-340.

O'Rourke, Kevin, OP

    1974   "The Christian Affirmation of Life," *Hospital Progress* 55, July, 65-72.

    1975   "Fetal Experimentation: An Evaluation of the New Federal Norms," *Hospital Progesss* 56, Sept., 60-69.

    1978   "Justice: A Goal of Coordinated Catholic Health Care," *Hospital Progress* 59, Nov.

    1983   *Reasons for Hope: Laity in Catholic Hospitals*, St. Louis: Catholic Health Association of the United States, 26ff.

    1986   "The A.M.A. Statement on Tube Feeding: An Ethical Analysis," *America* 155 (15), Nov. 22, 321-28.

    1987   "Medicine: Not an Exact Science," *Parameters* 12 (1), Winter.

    1988a   "Responsibility for Physician's Competence," *Ethical Essays*, St. Louis: St. Louis University Medical Center, June.

    1988b   "Developing in Younger Physicians an Ethical Perspective Toward Geriatric Patients," *Journal of the American Geriatrics Society* 36 (6), June, 555-568.

    1988c   *Development of Church Teaching on Prolonging Life*, Catholic Health Association of the United States.

    1988d   "Two Ethical Approaches to Research on Human Beings," *Health Progress*, 69, 8, October, 48.

    1989   "Ethics Committees in Catholic Health Care Facilities," *Critical Issues in Contemporary Health Care,* Braintree, MA: Pope John XXIII Medical-Moral Research and Education Center

O'Rourke, Kevin, and Boyle, Philip, *Medical Ethics: The Sources of Catholic Teachings*, St. Louis: Catholic Health Association of the United States, 1989.

O'Rourke, Kevin, and Brodeur, Dennis, *Medical Ethics: Common Ground for Understanding*, St. Louis: Catholic Health Association of the United States, 1986, 169.

Ory, H.W.; Forrest, J.D.; and Lincoln, R., *Making Choices: Evaluating the Health Risks and Benefits of Birth Control Methods*, New York: Guttmacher Institute, 1983.

Osmundsen, John A., "We Are All Mutants — Preventive Genetic Medicine: A Growing Clinical Field Troubled by a Confusion of Ethicists," *Medical Dimensions* 2, 1973, 5-7, 26-28.

OTA: Office of Technology Assessment

    1982   *Genetics Technology, A New Frontier*, Boston: Westminster Press, 1982.

1984   "Human Gene Therapy: Background Paper," Washington, DC: OTA, Dec. 1984.

Outka, Gene
    1968   *Norm and Context in Christian Ethics,* New York: Charles Scribner's Sons.
    1972   *Agape: An Ethical Analysis,* New Haven: Yale University Press.

Ozar, David T., "Social Ethics: The Philosophy of Medicine and Professional Responsibility," *Theoretical Medicine* 6 (3), Oct. 1985, 291-294.

P

Palmer, Paul, "Who Can Anoint the Sick?" *Worship* 48, 1974, 81-92.

Palmour, Jody, *On Moral Character: A Practical Guide to Aristotle's Virtues and Vices,* Washington, DC: Archon Institute, 1988.

Palouzie, Anne Marie, "Aspects of European Dying Process," *Social Science & Medicine* 26 (8), 1985, 851-853.

Paris, John, "When Burdens of Feeding Outweigh Benefits," *Hasting Center Report* 16 (1), Feb. 1986, 30-32.

Paris Statement of 1966, in *A Catholic/Humanist Dialogue,* Paul Kurtz and Albert Dondeyne, eds., Buffalo: Prometheus Books, 1972, 3ff.

Parsons, Talcott, *Essays in Sociological Theory,* New York: Free Press, 1964.

Parsons, Talcott, *The Social System,* Glencoe, IL: The Free Press, 1951.

Pastrana, Gabriel, OP, "Personhood and the Beginning of Human Life," *Thomist* 41, 1977, 247-294.

Patrick v. Burget, AHA News 24 (21), May 23, 1988.

Paul VI
    1967   *The Development of Peoples (Popolorum Progressio),* March 26, Washington, DC: United States Catholic Conference.
    1968   *Humanae Vitae: Encyclical Letter on the Regulation of Births,* Washington, DC: United States Catholic Conference.
    1971a   *A Call to Action: Apostolic Letter on Eightieth Anniversay of "Rerum Novarum,"* May 14, Washington, DC: United States Catholic Conference.
    1971b   "Justice in the World," issued by Synod of Bishops, *The Pope Speaks* 16, 377-384.
    1972   *Apostolic Constitution on the Sacrament of Anointing the Sick,* Washington, DC: United States Catholic Conference.
    1974   Message to President of United Nations General Assembly, Dec. 10, 1973, *The Pope Speaks* 18, 304-307.

Pellegrino, Edmund
    1981   "The Moral Foundations for Valid Consent," in *Proceedings of the Third National Conference on Human Values and Cancer,* Washington, DC: American Cancer Society.
    1985a   "Relevance and Utility of Courses in Medical Ethics: A Survey of Physicians' Perceptions," *Journal of the American Medical Association* 253 (1), Jan. 4, 49-53.
    1985b   "The Virtuous Physician, and the Ethics of Medicine" in *Virtue and Medicine Explorations in the Character of Medicine,* E. Shelp, ed., Boston: D. Reidel, 237-255.
    1987   "Altruism, Self-Interest and Medical Ethics," *Journal of the American Medical Association* 258 (14), Oct. 9, 1139-40.

Pellegrino, Edmund D., and Thomasma, David C.
    1981   *What is Medicine?: A Philosophical Basis of Medical Practice,* New York: Oxford University Press, 58-81.
    1988   *For the Patient's Good: The Restoration of Beneficence in Health Care,* New York: Oxford University Press.

Perkins, Harry, and Jonsen, Albert, "Dying Right in Theory and Practice: What Do We Really Know About Terminal Care?" *Archives of Internal Medicine* 5 (9), Aug. 14, 1985, 1460-1463.

Perl, Mark, and Shelp, Earl, "Psychiatric Consultation: Masking Moral Dilemmas in Medicine," *New England Journal of Medicine* 307 (14), 1982, 618-621.

Perry, Ralph, *General Theory of Value*, Cambridge: Harvard University Press, 1980.

Peters, David, "Advance Medical Directions: The Case for the Durable Power of Attorney for Health Care," *The Journal of Legal Medicine* 8 (3), 1987, 437-464.

Petersdorf, Robert G., "Medical Education for the Future: A Mandate for Change," *Internist* 27 (5), May 1986, 17-20.

Peterson, H.B., et al., "Deaths Attributable to Tubal Sterilization in the United States, 1977-1981," *American Journal of Obstetrics and Gynecology* 146, 1983, 131-6.

Peterson, Michael R., "Psychological Aspects of Human Sexual Behavior," in *Human Sexuality and Personhood*. St. Louis: Pope John XXIII Medical-Moral Research and Education Center, 1981.

Petrila, John, "Mental Health Therapies," in *Bio-Law Vol. 1*, Frederick, MD: University Publications of America, 1986, 177-215.

Physicians' Desk Reference, Oradell, NJ: Medical Economics Co., 1986.

Piaget, Jean, *The Moral Judgment of the Child*, New York: Free Press, 1965 [1929].

Pieper, Josef, *Leisure, the Basis of Culture*, New York: New American Library, 1964.

Pierce vs Swan Point Cemetary, 10 Rhode Island, 227, (1872)

Pietroferg, John, *Counseling: An Introduction*, New York: Houghton Mifflin, 1983.

Pincus, Jonathan, "Ethical Issues in Forensic Neurology," *Seminars in Neurology* 4 (1), 1984, 87-91.

Pinkus, Rosa Lynn, "Superman Meets Don Quixote: Stereotypes in Clinical Medicine," *Journal of Medical Humanities and Bioethics* 7 (1), Summer 1986, 17-32.

Pitts, F.N., et al., "Suicide by Women Physicians," and "Suicide by Male Physicians," *American Journal of Psychiatry* 136, 1979, 694-96, 1089-90.

Pius XI, "Casti Connubi," Dec. 31, 1930, *The Human Body: Papal Teachings*, Boston: St. Paul Editions, 1979 [1960], no. 4-12.

Pius XII

  1944 "Allocution to the Italian Medical-Biological Union of St. Luke" (Nov. 12), *The Human Body: Papal Teachings*, Boston: St. Paul Editions, 1979 [1960], no. 165-179.

  1949 "Allocution to Fourth International Conference of Catholic Doctors," *The Human Body: Papal Teachings*, Boston: St. Paul Editions, 1979, n. 165-179.

  1951 "Allocution to Italian Midwives" (Oct. 29) *The Human Body: Papal Teachings*, Boston: St. Paul Editions, 1979 [1960], no. 243-315.

  1952 "Allocution to the First International Congress of Histopathology" (Sept. 14), *The Human Body: Papal Teachings*, Boston: St. Paul Editions, 1979 [1960], no. 349-381.

  1954 "Allocution to World Medical Association," (Sept. 30), *The Human Body: Papal Teachings*, Boston: St. Paul Editions, 1979, n. 541-551.

  1956a "Allocution to a Group of Eye Specialists" (May 14), *The Human Body: Papal Teachings*, Boston: St. Paul Editions, 1979 [1960], no. 637-649.

  1956b "Allocution to Second World Congress on Fertility and Sterility," *The Human Body: Papal Teachings*, Boston: St. Paul Editions, 1979 [1960], no. 650-666.

  1957 "Prolongation of Life," (Nov. 24) *Issues in Ethical Decision Making*, Gary Atkinson, ed., St. Louis: Pope John XXIII Medical-Moral Research and Education Center, 1976.

Plato, *The Republic*, London: Penguin Books, 1970.

Pleak, Richard, and Appelbaum, Paul, "The Clinician's Role in Protecting Patients' Rights in Guardianship Proceedings," *Hospitals and Community Psychiatry* 36 (1), Jan. 1984, 77-79.

Plum, Fred, and Posner, Jerome, *The Diagnosis of Stupor and Coma*, Philadelphia: F.A. Davis Co., 1982, 315.

Pollner, Fran, "Abortion: Are Medicine and Law on a Collision Course?" *Medical World News* 26 (13), July 8, 1985, 96-68.

Polyani, Michael, *Personal Knowledge: Toward a Post-Critical Philosophy,* New York: Harper & Row Torchbooks, 1964.

Pontifical Academy of Sciences, *The Artificial Prolongation of Life, and the Exact Determination of the Moment of Death,* Oct. 31, 1985, *Origins,* 15, 25; Dec. 5, 1985, 415.

Pontifical Commission on Peace and Justice, "Church and Human Right," *Osservatore Romano* (Eng. ed.) 6, 1973; Oct. 23, 6-10; Oct. 30, 8-9; Nov. 6, 6-8; Nov. 13, 9-10.

Population Crisis Committee, "Issues in Contraceptive Development," *Population,* May 1985, 153.

Powsner, Rhoda, and Hemmersaith, Frances, "Medical Malpractice Crisis: The Second Time Around," *Journal of Legal Medicine* 8 (2), 1987, 283-304.

President's Commission for the Study of Ethical Problems in Medicine and Biomedical and Behavioral Research

    1981   "Report on the Definition of Death Legislation," Washington, DC: U.S. Government Printing Office.

    1982a   *Making Health Care Decisions: The Ethical and Legal Implications of Informed Consent in the Patient-Practitioner Relationship,* 3 vol., Oct.

    1982b   *Splicing Life: The Social and Ethical Issues of Genetic Engineering with Human Beings,* Nov.

    1982c   "Substantive and Procedural Principles of Decision Making for Incapacitated Patients," *Making Health Care Decisions,* Washington, DC: U.S. Government Printing Office.

    1983   *Screening and Counseling for Genetic Conditions: The Ethical, Social, and Legal Implications of Genetic Screening, Counseling, and Education Programs,* Feb.

    1983b   *Implementing Human Research Regulations: The Adequacy and Uniformity of Federal Rules and Their Implementation,* March.

    1983c   *Securing Access to Health Care: The Ethical Implications of Differences in the Availability of Health Services,* March.

    1983d   *Deciding to Forego Life-Sustaining Treatment: Ethical, Medical and Legal Issues in Treatment Decisions,* March.

    1983e   President's Commission I.R.B. Guidebook.

President's Commission on AIDS, *Final Report,* Washington, DC: Department of Health and Human Services, March 4, 1988.

Preston, Thomas, "Problems of Unrecognized Placebos," *Medical World News* 28 (11), June 1987.

Prottas, Jeffrey M., "Organ Procurement in Europe and the United States," *Health & Society, Milbank Quarterly* 63 (1), Winter 1985, 94-126.

Prucha, Milan, "Marxism and the Existential Problems of Man," in *Socialist Humanism: An International Symposium,* Erich Fromm, ed., Garden City, NY: Doubleday, 1965, 138-147.

Prummer, Dominicus M., OP, *Manuale Theologiae Moralis,* 14th ed., 3 vols., Barcelona: Herder, 1960, vol. 1, 340.

Q

Quay, Paul, *The Christian Meaning of Sexuality,* San Francisco: Ignatius Press, 1988, 3-10.

R

Rachels, James

    1983   "The Sanctity of Life," in *Biomedical Ethics Review,* James Humber and Robert Almeder, eds., Clifton, NJ: Humana Press, 29-42.

    1986   *The Elements of Moral Philosophy,* New York: Random House.

Rafferty, Frank, "The Case for Investor-Owned Hospitals," *Hospital and Community Psychiatry* 5 (10), Oct. 3, 1984, 1013-1016.

Rahner, Karl

    1963   "The Church and the Sacraments," in *Questiones Disputatoe,* no. 9. New York: Herder & Herder.

    1965   *On the Theology of Death*, New York: Herder & Herder.

    1975   *Theological Investigations*, Westminster, MD: Christian Classics.

Ramsey, Paul

    1965   *Deeds and Rules in Christian Ethics*, Edinburgh: Oliver & Boyd, 144ff.

    1970   *The Patient as Person*, New Haven: Yale University Press, 1980 (5th prtg.).

    1973   "Abortion: A Review Article," *Thomist* 37, 174-226.

    1975   *The Ethics of Fetal Research*, New Haven: Yale University Press.

    1983   *Basic Christian Ethics*, Chicago: University of Chicago Press, reprint of 1950 ed.

Rand, Ayn

    1964   *The Virtue of Selfishness: A New Concept of Egoism*, New York: New American Library, Signet Books.

    1967   *Capitalism: The Uncommon Ideal*, New York: New American Library.

Rankin, Sally H., and Duffy, Karen L., "Legal and Ethical Issues," in *Patient Education: Issues, Principals, Guidelines*, Philadelphia: J.B. Lippincott, 1983, 95-105.

Ratner, Herbert

    1977   "Biology and Biologism," *Child and Family* 16, 194-200.

    1981   "A Physician Speaks on the Right to Life," in *Natural Family Planning: Nature's Way/God's Way*, Anthony Zimmerman, SVD, ed., Collegeville, MN: De Rance, Inc. and Human Life Center, 44-47.

Ratzinger, Cardinal

    1984a "Bishops, Theologians, and Morality," *Origins* 13 (40), March 15; 657.

    1984b "Dissent and Proportionalism in Moral Theology," *Origins* 13 (40), March 15, 1984, 666-670.

    1986   "Letter to Father Charles Curran," *Origins* 16 (11), Aug. 23, 201-203.

    1987   *Principles of Catholic Theology: Building Stones for a Fundamental Theology*, San Francisco: Ignatius Press.

Ravich, Ruth, "Patient Advocacy," in *Advocacy in Health Care*, John H. Marks, ed., Clifton, NJ: Humana Press, 1986.

Rawls, John, *A Theory of Justice*, Cambridge, MA: Harvard University Press, 1971.

Reardon, David, *Aborted Women: Silent No Longer*, Chicago: Loyola University Press, 1987.

Reed, Michael, and Olson, Camille, "Proxy Decision Making for the Terminally Ill," *Bulletin of American College of Surgeons* 10 (6), June 1985, 25-29.

Reed, Sheldon, *Counseling in Medical Genetics*, 3rd ed., New York: Alan R. Liss, Inc., 1980.

Regan, Tom, ed., *Matter of Life and Death: New Introductory Essays in Moral Philosophy*, Newark: Random House, 1986.

Reich, Warren

    1984   "Moral Absurdities in Critical Care Medicine: Commentary on a Parable," *American Journal of Emergency Medicine* 2 (6), Nov./Dec., 554-558.

    1985   "Conceptual Construals v. Moral Experience: A Rejoinder," in *Ethics and Critical Care Medicine*, John Moskop and Loretta Koppleman, eds., 35-40.

Reichenbach, Bruce, "Euthanasia and the Active-Passive Distinction," *Bioethics* 1 (1), Jan. 1987, 51-73.

Reichley, A. James, *Religion in American Public Life*, Washington, DC: The Brookings Institution, 1985.

Reinhardt, Uwe

    1986   "An American Paradox," *Health Progress* 67 (9), Nov., 42-46.

    1988   "Perspectives from an Economist" in *Health Affairs Supplement*, 96-104.

Reiser, David, and Rosen, David, *Medicine as a Human Experience*, Baltimore: University Park Press, 1984.

Reiser, Stanley J., "Refusing Treatment for Mental Illness: Historical and Ethical Dimensions," in "Life, Liberty and the Pursuit of Madness—The Right to Refuse Treatment," special section of the *American Journal of Psychiatry* 137, 1980, 329-358.

Reiser, Stanley J., and Dyck, Arthur J., eds., *Ethics in Medicine: Historical Perspectives and Contemporary Problems*, Cambridge, MA: MIT Press, 1977, see Part 1 "Ethical Dimensions of the Physician-Patient Relationship through History,"

Rennie, Drummond, "Bubble Boy," *Journal of the American Medical Association* 253 (1), Jan. 4, 1985, 78-80.

Rescher, Nicholas, *Unpopular Essays on Technological Progress*, Pittsburgh: University of Pittsburgh Press, 1980.

Restak, Richard M., *Pre-Meditated Man: Bioethics and the Control of Future Human Life*, New York: Viking Press, 1975.

Rice, Charles E., *Beyond Abortion: The Theory and Practice of the Secular State*, Chicago: Franciscan Herald Press, 1979.

Rice, Nancy, and Doherty, Richard, "Reflections on Prenatal Diagnosis: The Consumer's View," *Social Work on Health Care* 8 (1), Fall 1982.

Richards, Larry, and Johnson, Paul, *Death and the Caring Community Ministering to the Terminally Ill*, Portland, OR: Multwomah Press, 1980.

Richardson, Herbert W., *Nun, Witch, Playmate*, New York: Harper & Row, 1971.

Rieff, Philip, *The Triumph of the Therapeutic: Uses of Faith After Freud*, New York: Harper & Row Torchbooks, 1968.

Rifkin, Jeremy, *Algeny: A New Word-A New World*, New York: Penguin Books, 1984.

Rigali, Norbert, "Artificial Birth Control: An Impasse Revisited," *Theological Studies* 47 (4), Dec. 1986, 681.

Riskin, Leonard L., "Sexual Relations Between Psychotherapists and Their Patients: Toward Research or Restraint," *California Law Review* 67, 1979, 1000-1027.

Rizzo, Robert, and Yonder, Paul, "Definition and Criteria of Clinical Death," *Linacre Quarterly* 40 (1973): 223-233.

Robbins, Christopher, "The Ethical Challenge of Health Care Rationing," in *The End of the Illusion: The Future of Health Policy in Western Industrialized Nations*, Jean Kervasdoue, ed., Berkeley: University of California Press, 1984.

Robertson, John, *The Rights of the Critically Ill*, New York: Bantam Books, 1983

Robertson, John A., "Genetic Alteration of Embryos: The Ethical Issues," in *Genetics and the Law III*, A. Milunsky, et al., eds., New York: Plenum Press, 1985.

Robinson, Jean, "Are We Teaching Students that Patients Don't Matter?" *Journal of Medical Ethics* 11 (1), March 1985, 19-21, 26.

Robinson, R.D., "Brain Death in Children," *Archives of Disease in Childhood* 56 (9), Sept. 1981.

Robitscher, Jonas, *The Powers of Psychiatry*, Boston: Houghton Mifflin, 1980.

Rodd, Rosemary, "Pacifism and Absolute Rights for Animals: A Comparison of Difficulties," *Journal of Applied Philosophy* 2 (1), March 1985, 53-61.

Rogers, Carl R., *Client-Centered Therapy*, Boston: Houghton Mifflin, 1951.

Rogers, William, and Barnard, David, *Nourishing the Humanistic in Medicine*, Pittsburgh: University of Pittsburgh Press, 1979.

Rokeach, Milton, *The Nature of Human Values*. New York: Free Press, 1973.

Rordorf, Willy, "Sunday: The Fullness of Christian Liturgical Time," Collegeville, MN: Liturgical Press, 1982, 90-96.

Rose, Stephen, "DNA in Medicine: Human Perfectibility," *Lancet* 2 (8416) Dec. 15, 1984, 1380-1383.

Rosenberg, Charles, *The Care of Strangers: The Rise of America's Hospital System*, New York: Basic Books, 1987.

Rosenberg, Jay, "Rational Suicide: The Question of Squandering Life," in *Thinking Clearly About Death*, Englewood Cliffs: NJ: Prentice-Hall, 1983.

Rosenberg, Jay, and Towers, Bernard, "The Practice of Empathy as a Prerequisite for Informed Consent" *Theoretical Medicine* 7 (2), June 1986, 181-194.

Rosenfield, Israel, *The Invention of Memory: A New View of the Brain*, New York: Basic Books, 1987.

Rosett, Richard, "Doing Well by Doing Good, Investor Owned Hospitals," *Frontiers of Health Service Management* (1), Sept. 1984, 2-10.

Rosner, Fred, *Modern Medicine and Jewish Ethics*, New York: Yashiva University Press, 1986.

Rosotti, Sidney, "Ethics of Life Support" (letter) *New England Journal of Medicine* 318 (26), June 30, 1988.

Ross, W.D., *The Right and the Good*, Oxford: Claredon Press, 1930.

Rostain, Anthony, "Deciding to Forego Life-Sustaining Treatment in the Intensive Care Nursery: A Sociologic Account," *Perspectives in Biology and Medicine* 30 (1), Autumn 1986, 117-123.

Rothman, David J.
    1975   "Behavior Modification in Total Institutions," *Hastings Center Report* 5, 17-24.
    1980   *Conscience and Convenience: The Asylum and Its Alternatives in Progressive America*, Boston: Little, Brown.

Rounsaville, B., and Kleber, H.D., "Psycotherapy Counseling for Opiate Addicts," *International Journal of Addiction* 20, 1985, 869-896.

Rousseau, Jean Jacques, *Discourse upon Origin and Foundations of Inequality among Mankind in Social Contract and Discourses*, New York: E.P. Dutton, 1976 [1753].

Rowland, Thomas, et al., "Brain Death in the Pediatric Intensive Care Unit: A Clinical Definition," *American Journal of Diseases of Children* 137 (6), June 1983, 547-550.

Roy, David, "Created Equal: The Moral Challenge of Prenatal Diagnosis," *Canadian Catholic Health Care Review*, Summer 1984, 13-18.

Ruark, J.E., and Raffin, T.A., "Initiating and Withdrawing Life Support: Principles in Adult Medicine," *New England Journal of Medicine* 318, 1988, 25-30.

Rubenstein, Leonard, "The American Psychiatric Association's Proposals on Civil Commitments, *Clearing House Review* 17 (5), Oct. 1983.

Rubin, Eva, *Abortion Politics and the Courts*, Westport, CT: Greenwood Press, 1987.

Rubin, Robert, et al., *Critical Condition: America's Health Care in Jeopardy*, Washington, DC: National Committee for Quality Health Care, 1988

Runciman, Steven, *The Medieval Manichee*, Cambridge: Cambridge University Press, 1982 [1947].

Rush, Vincent, *The Responsible Christian*, Chicago: Loyola University Press, 1984, especially chs. 1 and 2.

S

Sabbatini, Jean, "Ethics and Economic Appraisals in Health Care," *Social Science and Medicine* 21 (10), 1985, 1199-1202.

Sacred Congregation for the Doctrine of the Faith: see SCDF

Sacred Penitentiary, 1853/1880, "Responses on Infertile Period, March 2, 1853 and June 16, 1880," in *Natural Family Planning: Nature's Way/God's Way*, Anthony Zimmerman, SVD, ed., Collegeville, MN, DeRance Inc. and Human Life Center, 1981, 44-47.

Sadler, Alfred, et al., "The Uniform Anatomical Gift Act," *Journal of the American Medical Association* 206, 1968, 2501-2506.

Sahuc, Louis, J., *La Morale Catholique Est-elle Humaine?* Paris: Bloud et Gay, 1970.

St. John-Stevas, Norman
    1961   *Life, Death and the Law: Law and Christian Morals in England and the United States*, Bloomington, IN: Indiana University Press.
    1971   *The Agonizing Choice: Birth Control, Religion and the Law*, Bloomington, IN: Indiana University Press.

Sanders, John H., "Ethical Ingredients in Critical Care," *Bulletin of the American College of Surgeons*, May 1984, 69 (5), 14-15.

Sapolsky, Harvey, "A Solution to the Health Care Crisis," *Policy Analysis* 3, Winter 1977, 115-123.

Scarlett, B.C.; Singer, Peter; and Kuhse, Helga, "Singer and Kuhse on the Potential of Embryos," *Journal of Medical Ethics* 10 (40), Dec. 1984, 217-218.

SCDF: Sacred Congregation for the Doctrine of the Faith
    1963   "Cremation," in *Canon Law Digest* 6, Milwaukee: Bruce Books, 666ff.
    1974   *Declaration on Procured Abortion*, May, translated in *Osservatore Romano*, Dec. 5.
    1975a   "Declaration of Certain Problems of Sexual Ethics" (Dec. 29), in *Vatican Council II: More Postconciliar Documents*, vol. 2, Austin Flannery, OP, ed., Northport, NY: Costello Publishing Co., 1982, 486-499.

1975b   "Doctrinal Congregational Statement on Sterilization" (March 13), in *Commentary of National Conference of Catholic Bishop,* Washington, DC: United States Catholic Conference, 1978.

1979   "The Reality of Life After Death" (Mar. 11), in *Vatican Council II: More Postconciliar Documents,* vol. 2, Austin Flannery, OP, ed., Northport, NY: Costello Publishing Co., 1982, 500-504.

1980a   "Declaration on Euthanasia" (May 5), in *Vatican Council II: More Postconciliar Documents,* vol. 2, Austin Flannery, OP, ed., Northport, NY: Costello Publishing Co., 1982, 510-517.

1980b   "Instruction on Infant Baptism" (Oct. 20) in *Vatican Council II: More Postconciliar Documents,* vol. 2, Austin Flannery, OP, ed., Northport, NY: Costello Publishing Co., 1982, 103.

1986   "Pastoral Care of Homosexual Persons" (Oct. 1), *Origins* 16 (22), Nov. 13, 377-382.

1987   *Instruction on Respect for Human Life in Its Origin and on the Dignity of Procreation,* text published in U.S. by Pope John XXIII Medical-Moral Research and Education Center, Braintree, MA, 1987, also in *Origins* 16 (40), March 19, 697-709.

Schall, J.V., SJ, "The Long-Range Significance of the Encyclical HV," *Month* 40, 1968, 245-251.

Scherr, L., "AIDS: A Critical Test for Medicine," *American College of Physicians Journal* 7 (8), 1987, 2.

Schiff, Robert, et al., "Transfers to a Public Hospital," *New England Journal of Medicine* 314 (9), Feb 27, 1986, 552-560.

Schillebeeckx, Edward

     1981a   *Ministry,* New York: Crossroad Publishing Co.

     1981b   *Christ: The Experience of Jesus as Lord,* New York: Crossroad Publishing Co.

Schindler, Thomas, "Implications of Prolonging Life," *Health Progress,* Apr. 1988, 12.

Schlitz, Randy, *And the Band Played On,* New York: St. Martin's Press, 1987.

Schmid, Donald, et al., "Confidentiality in Psychiatry: A Study of Patients' Views," *Hospital and Community Psychiatry* 34 (4), Apr. 1983, 353-355.

Schnackenburg, Rudolf, *The Moral Teaching of the New Testament,* New York: Herder & Herder, 1965.

Schneller, Eugene, *The Physician's Assistant: Innovation in the Medical Division of Labor,* Lexington, MA: Lexington Books, 1978.

Schroeder, S., "Issues and Future Research Directions of Pharmaco-Therapy in Mental Retardation," *Psychopharmacology Bulletin* 21 (2), 1985, 323-326.

Schüller, Bruno, *Die Bergründung Sittlicher Urteile: Typen Ethiscer Argumentation in der Katholischen Moral Theologie,* Düsseldorf: Patmos Verlag, 1973.

Schwartz, H., and Gray, A., "Can You Say No? Can a Doctor Legally Withhold Treatment from a Patient with AIDS?" *Massachusetts Medical Society* 2 (5), 1987, 39-43.

Schwartz, Harold; Applebaum, Paul; and Kaplan, Richard, "Clinical Judgments in the Decision to Commit: Psychiatric Discretion and the Law," *Archives of General Psychiatry* 41 (8), Aug. 1984, 811-815.

Schwartz, Lee, "Involuntary Admission: A Century of Experience," *Journals of Clinical Psychiatry* 43 (1), Jan. 1982, 28-32.

Schwartz, Richard S., "Confidentiality and Secret Keeping on an In-Patient Unit," *Psychiatry* 17 (3), Aug. 1984, 279-284.

Schwartz, William, "The Inevitable Failure of Current Cost-Containment Strategies," *Journal of the American Medical Association* 257 (2), Jan. 9, 1987, 220-224.

Schwitzgebel, Robert L., and Schwitzgebel, Ralph K., eds., *Psychotechnology: Electronic Control of Mind and Behavior.* New York: Holt, Rinehart and Winston, 1973.

Scott, Gordon, "Merciful Release," *Transactions of the Medical Society of London 98, 1983,* 48-52.

Scott v. Casey, U.S. District Court, Atlanta Division, Apr. 29, 1983.

Scully, Diana, *Men Who Control Women's Health: The Miseducation of Obstetrician-Gynecologists,* Boston: Houghton Mifflin, 1980.

Second Vatican Council: see Vatican Council II

Seibel, Machelle, "A New Era in Reproductive Technology: In Vitro Fertilization, Gamete Intrafallopian Transfer, and Donated Gametes and Embryos," *New England Journal of Medicine* 318 (13), March 31, 1988, 838.

Senay, Patrick, "Biblical Teaching on Life and Death," in *Moral Responsibility in Prolonging Life Decisions,* Donald McCarthy and Albert Moraczewski, eds., St. Louis: Pope John XXIII Medical-Moral Research and Education Center, 1981.

Shaffer, Thomas, *Faith and the Professions,* Albany: State University of New York Press, 1987.

Shalom, Albert, *The Body/Mind Conceptual Framework and the Problem of Personal Identity,* Atlantic Highlands, NJ: Humanities Press International, 1985.

Shannon, M. Jordan, *Decision Making for Incompetent Persons: The Law and Morality of Who Shall Decide,* Springfield, IL: Charles C. Thomas, 1985.

Shannon, Thomas A., *Bioethics: Basic Writings on the Key Ethical Questions that Surround the Major Modern Biological Possibilities and Problems,* 3rd ed., Ramsey, NJ: Paulist Press, 1987.

Shannon, William H., *The Lively Debate: Response to "Humanae Vitae,"* New York: Sheed & Ward, 1970.

Shapiro, Larry, et al., "New Frontiers in Genetic Medicine," *Annals of Internal Medicine* 104 (4), Apr. 1986, 527-539.

Shapiro, Martin F., and Charron, Robert, "Scientific Misconduct in Investigational Drug Trials," *New England Journal of Medicine* 312 (11), Mar. 14, 1984, 731-736.

Shareef, R., "Restructuring the Health-Care Financing and Delivery System: National Health Insurance Through Market Competition," *Journal of Health Care Resources,* 7 (1), Summer 1984, 117-134.

Shaw, Margery, and Dondera, A. Edward, eds., *Defining Human Life: Medical, Legal and Ethical Implications,* Ann Arbor: ANAHA Press, 1983.

Shehan, Lawrence Cardinal, "Humanae Vitae: 1968-1973," *Homiletic and Pastoral Review* 74, 1973, 14-32 (Nov.), 20-32 (Dec.).

Shell, Susan Meld, *The Rights of Reason: A Study of Kant's Philosophy and Politics,* Toronto: University of Toronto Press, 1979.

Shelp, Earl, ed., *Sexuality and Medicine,* 2 vols., Boston: Reidel, 1987.

Shirm, M.C., et al., "Contraceptive Failure in the United States: The Impact of Social, Economic, and Demographic Factors," *Family Planning Perspective* 14, 1982, 68.

Showalter, Stuart, and Andrew, Brian, *To Treat or Not to Treat,* St. Louis: Catholic Health Association of the United States, 1984.

Sider, Roger C., "Mental Health Norms and Ethical Practice," *Psychiatric Annuals* 13 (4), April 1983, 302-309.

Sider, Roger C., and Clements, Colleen, "Patients' Ethical Obligation for Their Health," *Journal of Medical Ethics* 10 (3), Sept. 1984, 138-142.

Sidgwick, Henry, *The Methods of Ethics,* Indianapolis: Hackett Publishing, 1981, especially ch. 6.

Sieghart, Paul
    1984 "Medical Confidence, the Law, Computers," *Journal of the Royal Society of Medicine* 77 (8), Aug., 656-662.
    1985 "Professions and the Conscience of Society," *Journal of Medical Ethics,* 11, (3) Sept., 117-122.

Siegel, Karolyn, and Tuchel, Peter, "Rational Suicide and the Terminally Ill Cancer Patient," *Omega* 15 (3), 1985, 263-269.

Siegler, Mark, *Medical Innovations and Bad Outcomes: Legal, Social and Ethical Responses,* Ann Arbor: Health Administration Press, 1987.

Siegler, Miriam, and Osmond, Humphrey, *Models of Madness, Models of Medicine,* New York: Macmillan, 1974.

Sigerist, Henry E.
    1951   *History of Medicine,* New York: Oxford University Press.
    1960a "The Special Position of the Sick," in *Henry E. Sigerist on Medicine,* Milton E. Roemer and James M. MacKintosh, eds., New York: MD Publishers, 9-22.
    1960b "An Outline of the Development of the Hospital," in *Henry E. Sigerist on Medicine,* Milton E. Roemer and James M. MacKintosh, eds., New York: MD Publishers, 319-326.

Silber, Thomas J., "Amniocentesis and Selective Abortion," *Pediatric Annals* 10 (10), Oct. 1981, 397-400.

Silver, George, "Whom Do We Serve?" *Lancet* (1) 8476, Feb. 8, 1986, 315-316.

Silver, Jonathan, and Yudofsky, Stuart, "Pyschopharmocology and Electroconvulsive Therapy," in *Testbook on Psychiatry,* John Talbott, et al., ed., Washington, DC: American Psychiatric Association, 1988, 767-841.

Simmons, R., and Fulton, J., "Ethical Issues in Kidney Transplant," in *Is It Moral to Modify Man?* Claude A. Franzier, ed., Springfield, IL: Charles C Thomas, 1973.

Singer, Peter
    1980   *Practical Ethics,* New York: Cambridge University Press.
    1986   "Animals and the Value of Life," in *Matters of Life and Death,* Tom Regan, ed., New York: Random House.

Sinha, Ajit Kumar, *Philosophy of Health and Medical Sciences,* Ambala, India: Associated Publishers, 1983.

Skinner, B.F.
    1971   *Beyond Freedom and Dignity,* New York: Alfred A. Knopf.
    1976   *About Behaviorism,* New York: Random House.
    1985   *A Matter of Consequences,* New York: University Press.

Sloan, Frank A., "Statement before the Committee on Labor and Human Resources, U.S. Senate," *Health Care Cost: Defining the Issues,* Washington, DC: U.S. Government Printing Office, 1983, 325.

Smart, R.G., and Murray, G. F., "Narcotic Drug Abuse in 152 Countries: Social and Economic Factors as Predictors," *International Journal of Addiction* 20, 1985, 737-749.

Smart, Vivian, *The Religious Experience of Mankind,* New York: Charles Scribner's Sons, 1984.

Smith, Charles, "How Unacceptable is Research Involving Deception," *I.R.B. A Review of Human Subjects Research* 3 (8), Oct. 1981.

Smith, David, ed., *Respect and Care in Medical Ethics,* Lanham, MD: University Press of America, 1984.

Smith, David B., and Kaluzny, Arnold D., *The White Labyrinth: Understanding the Organization of Health Care,* Berkeley, CA: McCutchan Publishing, Corp., 1975.

Smith, William
    1977   "Catholic Hospitals and Sterilization," *Linacre Quarterly* 44, 107-116.
    1987   "The Question of Dissent in Moral Theology," *Persona Verita e Morale,* Roma: Citta Nuova Edditrice.

Snyder, Solomon
    1973   *Madness and the Brain,* New York: McGraw-Hill.
    1986   *Drugs and the Brain,* New York: Scientific Books.

Sobel, Alan, *Philosophy of Sex,* Totawa, NJ: Littlefield, Adams & Co., 1980.

Sorkin, Alan, *Health Care and the Changing Economic Environment,* Lexington, MA: Lexington Books, 1986.

Sparks, Anne, "Rape Crisis Programs Help Restore Dignity and Control," *Health Progress* 69 (7), Sept. 1988, 68-72.

Speedling, Edward J., and Rose, David N., "Building an Effective Doctor-Patient Relationship: From Patient Satisfaction to Patient Participation," *Social Science and Medicine* 21 (2), 1985, 115-120.

Speroff, L.; Glass, R.H.; and Kase, N.G., *Clinical Gynecologic Endocrinology and Infertility,* 3rd ed., Baltimore: Williams and Wilkins, 1983, 315ff.

Spicker, Stuart F., and Gadow, Sally, eds., *Nursing: Images and Ideals,* New York: Springer Publishing Co., 1980.

Spicq, Ceslaus, *Agape in the New Testament,* 3 vols., St. Louis: B. Herder, 1963.

Spiro, Howard, *Doctors, Patients, Placebos,* New Haven: Yale University Press, 1986.

Sprague, Robert, "Principles of Clinical Trials and Social Ethical and Legal Issues of Drug Use in Children," in *Pediatric Psychopharmacology: The Use of Behavior Modifying Drugs in Children,* John Inwerry, ed., New York: Brunner/Mazel, 1978.

Springer, Robert, "Transexual Surgery: Some Reflections on the Moral Issues," in *Sexuality and Medicine,* vol. 2, E. Shelp, ed., Boston: D. Riedel, 1987.

Stanley, Barbara Hrevnack, and Stanley, Michael, "Psychiatric Patients in Research: Protecting Their Autonomy," *Comprehensive Psychiatry* 22 (4), 1981, 450-457.

Stanley, Linda, "Dangerous Doctors: What to Do When the MD is Wrong?" *RN* 42 (3), Mar. 1979, 22-30.

Starr, Paul
    1981   "Voluntary Health Risks and Public Policy," *Hastings Center Report* 81, Oct. 18, 26-44.
    1982   *The Social Transformation of American Medicine,* New York: Basic Books.

Steel, Knight, et al., "Iatrogenic Illness on a General Medical Service at a University Hospital," *New England Journal of Medicine* 304, 1981, 636-642.

Steinbrook, Robert, and Lo, Bernard, "The Case of Elizabeth Bouvia: Starvation, Suicide, or Problem Patient?" *Archives of Internal Medicine* 6 (1), Jan. 14, 1986, 161-164.

Stenchever, Morton, "Rape, Incest, Abortion," in *Comprehensive Gynocology,* William Droegemueller, ed., St. Louis: C.V. Mosby Co., 1987.

Stephens, Ronald, "Do-Not-Resuscitate Orders: Ensuring the Patient's Participation," *Journal of the American Medical Association* 255 (2), Jan. 10, 1986, 240-24.

Stevens, Jay, *Storming Heaven: LSD and the American Dream,* New York: Atlantic Monthly Press, 1987.

Still, A.W., and Todd, C.J., "Role Ambiguity in General Practice: The Care of the Patient Dying at Home," *Social Science and Medicine* 23 (5), 1986, 519-525.

Stillman, Paula, et al., "Physician Competence: Whose Responsibility," *Medical Staff News,* May, 1988.

Storch, Janet, *Patient's Rights: Ethical and Legal Issues in Health Care and Nursing,* New York: McGraw-Hill, 1982.

Stover, Eric, and Nightengale, Elena, eds., *The Breaking of Bodies and Minds, Torture, Psychiatric Abuse, and The Health Professions.* New York: W.H. Freeman and Co., 1985

Strasburg-Cohen, T., "The Judicial Aspects of Artificial Insemination," *Medicine and Law* i (1), 1982, 71-80.

Strauss, Anselm, ed., *When Medicine Fails,* San Francisco: University of California, 1984.

Strickler, Ronald C.; Keller, P.W.; and Warren, J.C., "Artificial Insemination with Fresh Donor Semen," *New England Journal of Medicine* 289, 1975, 848-852.

Sullivan, Francis, *Magisterium and Teaching Authority in the Catholic Church,* Dublin: Gilland Macmillan, 1983.

Sullivan, Joseph V., *The Morality of Mercy Killing,* Westminster, JD: Newman Press, 1952.

Summers, Jim, "Take Patients' Rights Seriously to Improve Patient Care and Lower Cost," *Health Care Management Review* 10 (4), Fall 1985, 55-62.

Sumner, L.W., *Abortion and Moral Theory,* Princeton, NJ: Princeton University Press, 1981.

Sumner, William Graham, "A Defense of Cultural Relativism," in *Issues in Moral Philosophy,* Thomas Donaldsen, ed., New York: McGraw-Hill, 1986.

Swift, Francis W., "An Analysis of the American Theological Reaction to Janssens' Stand on 'The Pill'," *Louvain Studies* 1, Fall 1966, 19-53.

Szasz, Thomas
    1974   *The Myth of Mental Illness,* rev. ed., New York: Harper & Row (orig. pub. 1961).
    1977   *The Theology of Medicine: The Political-Philosophical Foundations of Medical Ethics,* New York: Harper & Row.

1982 "The Psychiatric Will: A New Mechanism for Protecting Persons Against 'Psychosis' and Psychiatry," *American Psychologist* 37 (7), July, 762-770.

1986 "The Case Against Suicide Prevention," *American Psychologist* 41 (7), July, 806-812.

1987 *Insanity, the Idea and Its Consequences*, New York: John Wiley and Sons.

Szasz, Thomas, and Hollender, Marc H., "The Basic Models of the Doctor-Patient Relationship," *American Medical Association Archives of Internal Medicine* 97, 1956, 585-592.

T

Tancredi, Lawrence, and Edlund, Matthew, "Are Conflicts of Interest Endemic to Psychiatric Consultation?" *International Journal of Law and Psychiatry* 6 (3-4), 1983, 293-316

Tancredi, Lawrence, and Slaby, Andrew, "Ethical Issues in Mental Health Care," in *Medical Ethics and the Law*, Mark Hillired, ed., Cambridge, MA: Ballinger Publishing, 1981, 283-302.

Tauer, Carol, "Personhood and Human Embryos and Fetuses," *Journal of Medicine and Philosophy* 10 (3), Aug. 1985, 253-266.

Taysi, Kutay, "Genetic Disorders," *Genetic Medicine and Engineering: Ethical and Social Dimensions*, St. Louis: Catholic Health Association of the United States, 1983.

Teilhard de Chardin, Pierre, *The Future of Man*, New York: Harper & Row, 1964.

Temkin, Owsei, "The Scientific Approach to Disease: Specific Entity and Individual Sickness," in *Scientific Change*, A.C. Crombie, ed., London: Heinemann, 1963, 629-660.

Texas Catholic Conference, "Labor Relations in Catholic Hospitals," *Origins* 13, June 2, 1983, 53-55.

Texas Medical Association, *Second Supplemental Report*, Nov. 20, 1987.

Thayer, Nelson, *Spirituality and Pastoral Care*, Philadelphia: Fortress Press, 1985.

Theis, Charlotte, "Ethical Issues: A Nursing Perspective," *New England Journal of Medicine* 315 (19), Nov. 6, 1986, 122N-125.

Theological Commission (International), *Thesis on the Relationship between the Ecclesiastical Magisterium and Theology*, Washington, DC: U.S. Catholic Conference, 1976.

Thielicke, Helmut

1964 *The Ethics of Sex*, New York: Harper & Row.

1969 "Moral Dilemmas," in *Theological Ethics* 2 vols., Philadelphia: Fortress Press, vol. 1, 609-668.

1983 *Living with Death*, Grand Rapids: Erdmans.

Thomasma, David

1983 "Beyond Medical Paternalism and Patient Autonomy: A Model of Physician Conscience for the Physician-Patient Relationship," *Annals of Internal Medicine* 98 (2), Feb., 243-248.

1984 "What Does Medicine Contribute to Ethics," *Theoretical Medicine* 5 (3), Oct., 267-277.

Thompson, James, and Thompson, Margaret, *Genetics in Medicine*, Philadelphia: W.B. Saunders Co., 1980, rev. ed. 1988, 309.

Thomson, Judith Jarvis, "A Defense of Abortion," *Philosophy and Public Affairs*, Fall 1971, 47-66, also in *Ethics and Public Policy: An Introduction to Ethics*, Tom Beauchamp and Terry Pinkard, eds., Englewood Cliffs, NJ: Prentice-Hall, 1983, 268-283.

Thorup, Oscar, et al., "High Tech Cardiology—Issues and Costs: A Panel Discussion," *Pharos* 48 (3), Summer 1985, 31-37.

Thundy, Zacharias, et al., *East and West Meet: Religions in Dialogue*, Lanham, MD: University Press of America, 1985.

Tillich, Paul, "The Meaning of Health," in *Religion and Medicine*, David Belgum, ed., Ames, IA: Iowa State University Press, 1967, 3-12.

Tomilson, T., and Brody, H., "Ethics and Communication in Do-Not-Resuscitate Orders" *New England Journal of Medicine* 318, 1988, 43-46.

Tooley, Michael, *Abortion and Infanticide,* Oxford: Clarendon Press, 1983.

Torrens, Paul, "Hospice Care: What Have We Learned?" in *Annual Review of Public Health,* Lester Breslow, et al., eds., 1985, Palo Alto: Annual Reviews.

Torrey, E. Fuller, *The Mind Game: Witchdoctors and Psychiatrists,* New York: Bantam Books, 1972.

Toulmin, Stephen, "Divided Loyalties and Ambiguous Relationships," *Social Science and Medicine* 23 (8), 1986, 783.

Transplantation Society, "Commercialization in Transplantation: The Problems and Some Guidelines for Practice," *Lancet* 2 (8457), Sept. 28, 1985, 715-716.

Turnquist, Arlynne, "The Issue of Informed Consent and the Use of Neuroleptic Medications," *International Journal of Nursing Studies* 20 (3), 1983, 181-186.

U

Ullmann, Manfred, *Islamic Medicine* (Islamic Surveys II), Edinburgh: Edinburgh University Press, 1978.

Underwood, Kenneth, *The Church, the University, and Social Policy,* 2 vols., Middletown, CT: Wesleyan University Press, 1972; vol. 1, 422-436.

United Nations, *Universal Declaration of Human Rights,* New York: United Nations Publications, 1948.

Ursano, Robert, and Silberman, Robert, "Individual Psychotherapies," in *Textbook of Psychiatry,* John Talbott; Robert Hales; and Stuart Yudofsky, eds., Washington, DC: American Psychiatric Press, 1988, 855-891.

United States Catholic Conference: see USCC

USCC: United States Catholic Conference

    1971   *Ethical and Religious Directives for Catholic Health Facilities,* approved by National Conference of Catholic Bishops and the United States Catholic Conference, Nov., as "the national code, subject to the approval of the bishop for use in the diocese," Washington, DC: United States Catholic Conference.

    1976   *To Live in Christ Jesus,* Washington, DC: USCC.

    1979   *The Deacon, Minister of Word and Sacrament,* Washington, DC: United States Catholic Conference.

    1981   *Pastoral Letter on Health and Health Care,* Washington, DC: United States Catholic Conference.

    1983   "The Challenge of Peace: God's Promise and Our Response," *Origins* 13 (1), May 19.

    1986   "Economic Justice for All: Catholic Social Teaching and the U.S. Economy," (3rd draft) *Origins* 16 (3), June 5.

    1987   "The Many Faces of AIDS: A Gospel Response," *Origins* 7 (28), Dec. 24, 481ff.

    1988   *Partners in the Mystery of Redemption: A Pastoral Response to Women's Concerns for Church and Society, Origins* 17 (45), Apr. 21, 97.

U.S. Congress 1984 Senate Committee on Labor and Human Resources, "Organ Transplantation: Examination of Problems Involved in Obtaining Organs for Transplant Surgery," Washington, DC: U.S. Government Printing Office, May 25, 1984

U.S. Department of Health, Education, and Welfare

    1973   Report of the Secretary's Commission on Medical Malpractice, Jan. 16.

    1975   The National Commission for the Protection of Human Subjects of Biomedical and Behavioral Research, *Research on the Fetus,* Washington, DC: U.S. Government Printing Office.

    1978   National Commission for Protection of Human Subjects of Biomedical and Behavioral Research, *Report and Recommendations, Institutional Review Boards,* DHEW (o.s.) 78-0008.

    1981   "Final Regulations for the Protection of Human Subjects," *Federal Register* 46 (16), Jan. 26, 8366-8392.

U.S. Department of Health and Human Services
  1983 "Nondiscrimination on the Basis of Handicap Relating to Health Care for the Handicapped Infant," *Federal Register*, 48, 129, July 5, 30846.
  1986 Task Force on Organ Transplantation, *Organ Transplantation, Issue and Recommendations*, Rochville, MD, April.
U.S. Select Committee on Aging, U.S. Congress, *Dying with Dignity: Difficult Times, Difficult Choices*, Washington, DC: U.S. Government Printing Office, 1965.

V

Vacek, Edward, "Vatican Instruction on Reproductive Technology," *Theological Studies* 49 (6), March 1988, 11-130.
Vaillant, G.E.
  1977 *Adaptation to Life*, Boston: Little Brown.
  1984 "Alcohol Abuse and Dependence," *American Psychiatric Association Annual Review*, Washington, DC: American Psychiatric Press.
Valenstein, Elliot
  1986 *Great and Desperate Cures: The Rise and Decline of Psychosurgery and other Radical Treatments for Mental Illness*, New York: Basic Books.
  1980 "Brain Disabling Therapies," in *The Psycho-Surgery Debate*, San Francisco: Witt, Freeman.
Valsecchi, Ambrogio, *Controversy: The Birth Control Debate, 1958-1968*, Washington, DC: Corpus Books, 1968.
Van der Haag, Ernest, and Conrad, John, *The Death Penalty, A Debate*, New York: Plenum Press, 1983.
Van der Sluis, I., "The Movement of Euthanasia 1875-1975," *Janus* LVI, 1979, 131-172.
Van Kaam, Adrian
  1983 *Fundamental Formation*, New York: Crossroad Publishing Co.
  1985 *Human Formation*, New York: Crossroad Publishing Co.
  1986 *Formation of the Human Heart: Formative Spirituality*, New York: Crossroad Publishing Co.
Vaporis, N.M., ed., *Orthodox Christians and Muslims*, Brookline, MA: Holy Cross Press, 1986.
Varga, Andrew
  1978 *On Being Human: Principles of Ethics*, Washington, DC: Paulist Press.
  1984 *The Main Issues in Bioethics*, 2nd ed., Mahwah, NJ: Paulist Press, 42, 81.
Vatican Council II Documents
  Quotations and citations are from *Vatican II: The Conciliar and Post Conciliar Documents*, Austin Flannery, OP, ed., Collegeville, MN: Liturgical Press, 1975. see also The Documents of Vatican II, Walter M. Abbott, SJ, ed., New York: Association Press, 1966.
  1964a *Dogmatic Constitution on the Church (Lumen Gentium,)* Nov. 21, 350-426.
  1964b *Decree on Ecumenism (Unitatis Redintegratio)*, Nov. 21, 452-470.
  1965a *Declaration on the Relation of the Church to Non-Christian Religious (Nostra Aetate)*, Oct. 28, 738-742.
  1965b *Declaration on Religious Liberty (Dignitatis Humanae,)* Dec. 7, 799-812.
  1965c *Pastoral Constitution on the Church in the Modern World (Guadium et Spes)*, Dec. 7, 903-1001.
  1984 *The Church*, 15-16.
Vaughan, Mary Ellen, "Mission Committee: Role Evolves From Operations to Oversight," *Health Progress* 68 (1), Jan. 1987, 74-80.
Vaux, Kenneth L., *This Mortal Coil: The Meaning of Health and Disease*, San Francisco: Harper & Row, 1978.
Veatch, Henry, *For an Ontology of Morals: A Critique of Contemporary Ethical Theory*, Evanston, IL: Northwestern University Press, 1971.

Veatch, Robert
    1975   "The Whole-Brain-Oriented Concept of Death: An Outmoded Philosophical Formulation," *Journal of Thanatology* 3 (1), 13-30.
    1981   *A Theory of Medical Ethics,* New York: Basic Books.
    1985   "The Relationship of the Professional to Society," *Journal of Dental Education* 49 (4), Apr., 207-213.
    1986   "DRG's and the Ethical Reallocation of Resources," *The Hastings Center Report* 16 (3), 32-40.

Vitz, Paul, *Psychology as Religion: The Cult of Self-Worship,* Grand Rapids: Erdmans, 1977.

Viviano, Benedict, *The Kingdom of God in History,* Wilmington, DE: Michael Glazier, Inc., 1988.

Vivieri, C., *Flexner, Seventy Five Years Later,* Lanham, MD: University Press of America, 1987.

Vogel, Morris J., *The Invention of the Modern Hospital: Boston 1870-1930,* Chicago: University of Chicago Press, 1980.

Von Hildebrand, Dietrich, *Marriage: The Mystery of Faithful Love,* Chicago: Franciscan Press, 1984.

Von Hildebrand, Dietrich, and Von Hildebrand, Alice, *The Art of Living,* Chicago: Franciscan Press, 1965.

W

Wahlberg, Rachel Conrad
    1971   "The Woman and the Fetus: 'One Flesh'?" *Christian Century* 88, 1045-1048.
    1973   "Abortion: Decisions to Live With," *Christian Century* 90, 1973, 691-693.

Waitzkin, Howard, *The Second Sickness: Contradiction of Capitalistic Health Care,* New York: Free Press, 1983.

Walgrave, John J., OP, *Person and Society: A Christian View,* Pittsburgh: Duquesne University Press, 1965, 94-116.

Walinder, Jan, "Outcome of Sex Reassingment Surgery," *Acta Psychiatry Scandanavia* 70, 1984, 289-294.

Walters, LeRoy
    1985   "Ethical Issues in Human *In Vitro* Fertilization and Embryo Transfer," in *Genetics and the Law III,* Ambroz Milunsky and George Annas, eds., New York: Plenum Press.
    1986   "The Ethics of Human Gene Therapy," *Nature* 320 (6059), March 20, 225-227.
    1988   "Ethical Issues in the Prevention and Treatment of HIV Infection and AIDS," *Science* 239, Feb. 5, 597-602.

Warnock, Mary, "Do Human Cells Have Rights," *Bioethics* 1 (1), Jan. 1987, 1-14.

Warnock *Report, Report of Inquiry into Human Fertilization and Embryology: Medical Research Council Response,* London: The Council, 1985.

Warren, James; Plumb, Diane; and Tazebiatouski, Gregory, "A Crisis in Medical Education," *Journal of the American Medical Association* 253 (16), Apr. 26, 1985, 2404-2407.

Warren, John W., et al., "Informed Consent by Proxy: An Issue in Research with Elderly Patients," *New England Journal of Medicine* 315 (18), Oct. 30, 1986, 1124-1128.

Wasserstrom, Richard, "The Status of the Fetus," *Hastings Center Report* 5, 1975, 18-22.

Watson, James D., "Moving Toward the Clonal Man: Is This What We Want?" *The Atlantic,* 245, 5 May 1971, 50-53.

Watson, James D., et al., *Molecular Biology of the Gene: General Principles,* Menlo Park, CA: Benjamin-Cummings, 1987.

Weichert, Carol, and Gerard, John W., "Breast Feeding: First and Second Thoughts," *Child and Family* 16, 1977, 203-208.

Weikel, M.K., "Competition: Hallmark of Health Care in the Decades Ahead," *American Pharmacology* 24 (11), Nov. 1984, 48-52.

Weiss, S.J., et al., "Risk of Human Immunodeficiency Virus (HIV-1) Infection Among Laboratory Workers," *Science* 239, 1988, 68-71.

Welch, Gilbert, and Larson, Eric, "Dealing With Limited Resources: The Oregon Decision to Curtail Funding for Organ Transplantation," *New England Journal of Medicine* 319 (3), July 21, 1988, 171-173.

Welsby, Phillip, "HILV-III Testing Without Consent," *British Medical Journal* 292 (652), Apr. 5, 1986.

Wertheimer, Michael, et al., "Ethics and Communication in the Surgeon-Patient Relationship," *Journal of Medical Education* 60 (10), Oct. 1985, 4-6.

White, Andrew Dickson, *A History of the Warfare of Science with Theology in Christendom* [1896], New York: Dover Publications, 1960, vol. 2, 55-63.

Whitehead, Alfred North, *Process and Reality* [1929]. New York: Free Press, 1957.

WHO: World Health Organization
    1957   "Geneva Declaration on Human Research," *Encyclopedia of Bioethics*, New York: Free Press, vol. 4, 1768.
    1964   "Helsinski Statement on Research on Human Subjects," World Health Association: see *Encyclopedia of Bioethics*, New York: Free Press, vol. 4, 1769.
    1981   "A Prospective Multicenter Trial of the Ovulation Method of Natural Family Planning: The Teaching Phase," *Fertility and Sterility* 36, 152.
    1984   "A Prospective Multicenter Trial of the Ovulation Method of Natural Family Planning, IV: The Outcome of Pregnancy," *Fertility and Sterility* 41, 573.
    1987   "A Prospective Multicenter Trial of the Ovulation Method of Natural Family Planning, V: Psychosexual Aspects," *Fertility and Sterility* 47, 765.

Wicks, Robert, "Lay Pastoral Care: Spiritual and Psychological Challenges," *Health Progress* 67, Sept. 1986, 26.

Wicks, Robert; Parson, Richard; and and Capps, Donald, eds., *Clinical Handbook of Pastoral Counseling*, Mahwah, NJ: Paulist Press, 1985.

Wilcox, Allen, et al., "Incidence of Early Loss of Pregnancy," *New England Journal of Medicine* 319 (4), July 28, 1988, 189-194.

Wilkinson, Greg; Shapiro, David; and Stewart, Harold, "Psychoanalysis and Analytic Psychotherapy in the NHS: A Process for Medical Ethics," *Journal of Medical Ethics* 12 (2), June 1986, 87-94.

Williams, Cornelius, "The Hedonism of Aquinas," *Thomist* 38, 1974, 257-290.

Williams, Oliver, and Houck, John, *The Common Good and U.S. Capitalism*, Lanham, MD: University Press of American, 1987.

Williams, Preston, et al., *Ethical Issues in Biology and Medicine*, Rochester, VT: Schenkman, 1973.

Wilson, Edward O., *On Human Nature*, Cambridge, MA: Harvard University Press, 1978.

Wilson, Edward O., and Lumsden, Charles J., *Genes, Mind: The Coevolutionary Process*, Cambridge, MA: The Harvard University Press, 1981.

Winslade, William, and Ross, Judith, *Choosing Life or Death: A Guide for Patients, Families, and Professionals*, New York: Free Press, 1986.

Winslow, Gerald R., *Triage and Justice*, Berkeley: University of California Press, 1982.

Wolinsky, Howard, "Transplants from the Unborn," *American Health*, Apr. 1988.

Wolpe, Joseph, "The Comparative Clinical Status of Conditioning Theories and Psychoanalysis," in *The Conditioning Therapies: The Challenge of Psychiatry*, Joseph Wolpe, Andrew Slater, and L.J. Reyna, eds., New York: Holt, Rinehart and Winston, 1966, 3-20.

Worden, J. William, "The Right to Die," *Pastoral Psychology* 23, 1972, 9-14.

World Health Organization: see WHO

World Population Conference, *Bucharest Report of the Symposium on Population and Human Rights*, Bucharest, Romania, Jan. 21-29, 1974, New York: Unipub, 1974.

World Synod of Catholic Bishops, "Message to Christian Families," and John Paul II, "Closing Homily to the Synod," 1980, in *Origins* 10, Nov. 6, 1980, 323-328, with commentary by the editors.

Y

Yamaguchi, K., and Kandel, D.B., "Patterns of Drug Use From Adolesence to Young Adulthood," *American Journal of Public Health* 74, 1984, 673-680

Younger, Stuart, and Bartlett, Edward, "Human Death and High Technology: The Failure of the Whole Brain Formulation," *Annals of Internal Medicine* 99 (2), Aug. 1983, 252-258.

Z

Zalba, M., "Applicato encyclicae 'Humanae Vitae' apud conferentias episcopales," *Periodica de re Morale, Cononica, et Liturgica* 59, 1970, 371-413.

Zaner, Richard, ed., *Death: Beyond Whole-Brain Criteria*, Norwell, CT: Kluwee Academic Publishers, 1988.

Ziegenfuss, James T., *Patients' Rights and Professional Practice*, New York: Van Nostrand Reinhold, 1983.

Zimmerman, Anthony, SVD, ed., *Natural Family Planning: Nature's Way/God's Way*, Collegeville, MN: De Rance Inc. and Human Life Center, 1981.

Zuger, Abigail, and Miles, Stephen, "Physicians, AIDS and Occupational Risk," *Journal of the American Medical Association* 258 (14), Oct. 8, 1987, 1924-1928.

NAME INDEX

Abbott, Walter W., 466
Abramowitz, Stephen, 315, 415
Abrams, Gerald, 419
Abrams, Richard, 346, 415
Ackerknecht, Erwin, 84, 415
Ackerman, Terrence F., 240, 415
Aday, Luann, 71, 415
Adler, Mortimer J., 163, 198, 415
Agich, George, 92, 102, 115, 366, 415
Agras, W. Stewart, 332, 345, 415
Aiken, Linda, 29, 113, 128, 415
Albert the Great, 212
Albury, W. R., 425
Alexander, Leo, 150, 415
Alexander the Great, 85
Alford, Robert R., 113, 115, 415
Allport, Gordon W., 17, 415
Aloming, Phillip Clayton, 36, 415
Alpert, Joseph S., 102, 415
Altman, Lawrence, 373, 415
Amulree, Lord, 386, 416
Andersen, Ronald, 415
Anderson, Frank, 355, 416
Anderson, W. French, 316, 318, 320, 416
Andrew, Brian, 461
Andrews, Lori, 322, 416
Andrusko, Dave, 312, 416
Annas, George, 72, 73, 105, 234, 311, 324, 350, 383, 385, 416, 417, 445, 467
Ansabel, D. P., 353, 417
Applebaum, Paul S., 103, 104, 106, 235, 239, 385, 340, 341, 417, 436, 455, 460
Appleton, William S., 103, 417
Apsche, Jack, 339, 349, 418
Aquinas, Saint Thomas, 36, 37, 67, 155, 164, 165, 181, 198, 212, 213, 217, 417
Areen, Judith, 366, 417
Aries, Philippe, 361, 417
Aristotle, 33, 85, 150, 155, 161, 213, 217, 417
Armstrong, David, 30, 417
Arney, William Ray, 417
Arnold, William, 393, 417
Arnstein, Robert, 351, 417
Arraj, James, 332, 417
Arraj, Tyra, 332, 417
Arras, John, 311, 417
Asclepius, 84
Ashley, Benedict, xii, 17, 44, 212, 245, 297, 379, 417

Ashley, Joann, 89, 133, 418
Atkinson, Gary M., 213, 323, 418
Atoka, 128
Augustine, Saint, 247
Auxter, Thomas, 153, 418
Aviram, Uri, 339, 418
Axelrod, David, 71, 87, 418
Axelrod, Saul, 339, 349, 418
Ayer, A. J., 149, 418

Baker, Robert, 418
Bakken, Kenneth L., 23, 25, 418
Baldessarini, R., 348, 418
Bandura, Albert, 334, 418
Barber, Bernard, 78, 352, 418
Barden, 322
Barger-Lux, Janet, 82, 418
Barlow, George W., 170, 418
Barnard, Christian, 418
Barnard, David, 89, 458
Barnlund, Dean C., 100, 418
Baron, Charles H., 241, 385, 418, 419
Baron, Richard J., 103, 150, 419
Barry, Robert, 382, 419
Barry, William A., 400, 419
Bartlett, Edward, 367, 469
Barton, David, 432
Bashim, Yvonne, 318, 419
Basson, Marc, 105, 419
Battin, M. Pabst, 106, 376, 419
Baue, Arthur, xii
Baumiller, Robert, 323, 419
Bayer, Edward, 286, 419
Bayer, Ronald, 30, 68, 104, 106, 114, 115, 419
Bayley, Corrine, 276, 419
Beauchamp, Thomas L., 68, 92, 157, 203, 232, 235, 419, 430
Beck, Aaron, 106, 419
Becker, Ernest, 199, 361, 419
Becker, Howard S., 78, 419
Becker, Judith, 248, 419
Bedau, Hugo Adam, 338, 419
Beis, Richard, 419
Bellah, Robert, 6, 14, 419
Belli, Melvin, 97, 420
Benesch, Katherine, 423
Benjamin, Harry, 313, 420
Benjamin, Martin, 98, 309, 420
Benton, Arthur, 368, 420
Berg, Kare, 220, 431
Berg, Kolb, 447
Berger, Bernard, 417

Berger, Brigette, 420
Berger, Peter, 29, 420
Bergson, Henri, 208
Beriman, Daniel, 78, 420
Berkowitz, Robert, 332, 345, 415
Berlant, Jeffrey Lionel, 83, 420
Berlin, Fred, 338, 420
Bermel, Joyce, 308, 420
Bernadine, Joseph, 230, 420
Berne, Robert, 433
Bernstein, Dorothy M., 307, 420
Bertalanffy, Ludwig von, 23, 28, 420
Besley, C. E., 115, 415
Betz, Linda, 82, 89, 426
Beyda, V., 106, 437
Biggers, John, 281, 420
Billings, Evelyn, 269, 420
Billings, John, 269, 420
Birch, Charles, 24, 420
Birmingham, William, 255, 260, 420
Bissell, LeClair, 353, 354, 420
Black, Peter, 305, 346, 364, 420
Blakeslee, Sandra, 311, 420
Blendon, Robert J., 69, 118, 421
Block, Melvin, 109, 436
Block, Sidney, 342, 421
Bloom, Alan, 14, 199, 344, 421
Blum, Henrick L., 21, 22, 23, 116, 421
Blum, Richard H., 70, 421
Boff, Leonardo, 12, 123, 175, 249, 421
Boffey, Philip M., 308, 421
Boisen, Anton T., 392, 421
Bok, Derek, 88, 421
Bok, Sissela, 103, 104, 421
Bond, Leslie, 312, 416
Boorse, C., 25, 421
Bopp, James, 385, 421
Boros, Ladislaus, 361, 421
Bosk, Charles, 72, 362, 421
Bourke, Vernon J., 147, 175, 421
Bower, Robert, 358, 421
Bowker, John, 187, 421
Bowman, Harold, 373, 421
Boyle, Joseph M., Jr., 223, 224, 421, 435, 443
Boyle, Patrick, 293, 421
Boyle, Philip, xii, 42, 58, 310, 372, 421, 453
Braen, C. Richard, 288, 421
Brahms, Diana, 99, 422
Braunstein, P., 367, 422
Breggin, Peter R., 347, 422
Brennan, J., 269, 441
Breslow, Lester, 465
Brewin, Thurstan, 378, 422
Brodeur, Dennis, 109, 138, 422, 453

Brodie, Keith, 97, 334, 442
Brody, Baruch A., 17, 147, 148, 211, 313, 328, 422
Brody, Howard, 147, 370, 384, 422, 464
Brogan, Michael, 422
Bromley, Dorothy Dunbar, 260, 422
Brooks, Simon A., 92, 422
Brophy, Paul, 381
Brower, Leslie A., 131, 422
Brown, Delwin, 66, 422
Brown, J. B., 269, 270, 422
Brown, Nancy, 114, 443
Brown, N. Miller, 23, 422
Browning, Don, 34, 399, 408, 409, 422
Bruce, JoAnne, 73, 422
Bryce, Edmund, 384, 422
Bultmann, Rudolf, 154, 422
Burtchaell, James T., 188, 207, 312, 422
Byrne, Paul, 366, 367, 422

Caffara, Carlo, 254, 423
Cahill, Lisa Sowle, 159, 254, 423
Cahn, Steven, 78, 423
Califano, Joseph, 114, 123, 423
Callahan, Daniel, 2, 114, 126, 127, 170, 211, 227, 232, 284, 309, 310, 318, 319, 419, 423
Callis, Donna, xii
Cannon, David, 214, 423
Caplan, Arthur L., 234, 310, 419, 423, 451
Capps, Donald, 468
Capps, Walter H., 196, 423
Capron, Alexander M., 320, 323, 364, 423, 440
Carmi, Ammon, 320, 423
Carnes, Patrick, 50, 252, 423
Carney, Frederick, 164, 423
Carrick, Paul, 215, 423
Carroll, Douglas, 347, 423
Cassel, Christine, 385, 423
Cassell, Eric, 92, 361, 365, 370, 423
Cassells, W., 339, 427
Cassens, Brett, 69, 424
Cassirer, Ernst, 24, 424
Casswell, Donald, 331, 424
Catherine of Siena, Saint, 60
Cavanaugh, John R., 256, 424
Chalkley, D. T., 235, 424
Charron, Robert, 235, 461
Chaska, Norma L., 89, 128, 424
Chayet, Neil L., 104, 424
Chervenak, F. A., 367, 424
Childress, James, 42, 87, 113, 157, 203, 232, 419, 424, 435
Chodoff, Paul, 342, 421

Choron, Jacques, 375, 424
Clark, Henry, 346, 424
Clark, Keith, 41, 424
Clark, W. H., 348, 424
Clebsch, William A., 390, 424
Clements, Colleen, 49, 233, 334, 340,
        343, 424, 461
Clinebell, John Howard, 397, 424
Clouser, K. Danner, 25, 92, 424
Cobb, John B., 392, 424
Cochnauer, Myron, 242, 426
Coe, Rodney M., xii, 23, 425
Cohen, Neal, 331, 446
Colombotos, John, 90, 425
Comas, Manual, xii
Congar, Yves, 59, 60, 425
Connell, Francis Y., 185, 425
Connell, L., 425
Connell, R. J., 258, 425
Connery, John, 164, 166, 167, 185, 186,
        215, 217, 219, 294, 382, 425
Connolly, William J., 400, 419
Connors, Edward, 138, 425
Conrad, John, 37, 466
Conrad, Peter, 29, 128, 129, 425
Cooke, Molly, 440
Cooper, David, 99, 425
Cooper, Eugene J., 179, 425
Cope, Oliver, 369, 425
Copp, David, 425
Couch, Nathen, 72, 425
Cousins, Norman, 45, 73, 425
Cox, Harvey, 157, 425
Cramer, D. W., 279, 425
Cranford, Ronald, 361, 383, 425, 426
Crauford, D., 321, 326, 426
Creusen, I., 291, 426
Crisp, Roger, 379, 426
Crissman, Susan, 82, 89, 426
Crombie, A. C., 464
Cronin, John, 123, 426
Crosby, John, 426
Cruchland, Paul, 52, 426
Culligan, Kevin, 399, 426
Culver, Charles M., 89, 331, 424, 426
Cunningham, Bert, 305, 426
Cunningham, Paige C., 427, 438
Cuomo, Mario, 229, 426
Cupples, Brian, 242, 426
Curran, Charles E., 32, 36, 60, 66-67,
        104, 108, 117, 160, 168, 173,
        184, 187, 189, 211, 217, 219,
        220, 229-30, 257, 266, 274-75,
        426, 427, 436, 452
Curran, William J., 339, 427

Daling, Janet, 279, 427
Daly, Robert, 427
D'Amato, Debra, 90, 427
Danforth, Daniel, 449
D'Arcy, Martin, 11, 427
Darwin, Charles, 84
Davis, Anne J., 238, 240, 242, 427
Davis, Bernard D., 318, 427
Davis, John Jefferson, 217, 228, 427
Davis, Michael, 224, 427
Dedek, John F., 164, 211, 427
Deeken, Alfons, 158, 427
de Gaspanis, Priscilla, 358, 421
DeKraai, Mark, 97, 351, 427
DeLancy, John, 385, 427
Delgado, Jose, 347, 427
Delhaye, Phillipe, 178, 291, 292, 295,
        296, 427
Dellapenna, Joseph W., 227, 427
Democritus, 27
Denes, Magda, 220, 428
Denham, M. J., 238, 428
Derrickson, Paul, 392, 428
Descartes, Rene, 35, 262
Devereux, George, 428
deVries, Martin, 113, 114, 428
Dewey, John, 11, 161, 177, 196, 208, 428
Diamond, Eugene, 428
Diamond, James J., 211, 428
Dickens, Bernard, 324, 428
Dickson, David, 241, 428
Dickstein, Morris, 123, 428
Diehl, Betty, xii
Doherty, Richard, 326, 458
Dolan, J., 448
Dolan, W., 287, 445
Dominian, Jacob, 295, 428
Doms, Herbert, 252, 428
Donaldsen, Thomas, 463
Donceel, Joseph, 212, 213, 229, 428
Dondera, A. Edward, 213, 461
Donelan, Karen, 69, 421
Donnelly, Paul, 128, 138, 428
Donovan, Peggy, xii
Doubilet, Peter, 114, 428
Dougherty, Charles, 214, 428
Doyle, John, xii
Drake, James, 90, 428
Drucker, Peter F., 101, 428
D'Souza, Noreen, xii
Dube, Leela, 321, 428
Dubler, Nancy, 385, 428
Duff, Raymond, 99, 428
Duffy, Karen L., 130, 457
Duffy, Regis, 392, 405, 428

Dulles, Avery, 60, 428
Durham, W. F., 446
Durkheim, E., 375, 428
Dworkin, Gerland, 336, 428
Dych, Arthur, 267, 429
Dyck, Arthur J., 83, 457

Eastaugh, Stephen, 114, 429
Easthope, Gary, 84, 429
Ebersolo, Myron, 392, 428
Ebert, Robert, 88, 90, 429
Echstein, Gustav, 5, 429
Eckholm, Erik, 231, 429
Edelman, D. A., 279, 429
Edelman, Gerald, 52, 303, 429
Edelstein, Ludwig, 49, 84, 429
Edey, Maitland, 439
Edlund, Matthew, 464
Edwards, R. B., 335, 429
Egan, Gerard, 400, 429
Egan, Harvey, 399, 429
Ehrenfeld, David W., 12, 429
Ehrman, Lee, 319, 429
Eichna, Ludwig, 88, 429
Einstein, Albert, 157
Eisenberg, John, 115, 429
Eisenberg, Leon, 101, 429
Eisenhower, Dwight David, 123
Elinson, Jack, 50, 429
Elliston, Frederick, 418
Ellul, Jacques, 53, 302, 429
Ellwood, Paul M., 114, 429
Ely, John, 227, 429
Emanuel, Ezekial, 81, 429
Emerson, James, 396, 429
Emerson, Ralph Waldo, 14
Empereur, James, 402, 429
Engel, G. L., 332, 429
Engelhardt, H. Tristram, Jr., 4-5, 8, 26,
    49, 56, 119, 147, 157, 207, 211,
    213, 328, 340, 375, 376, 420,
    422, 429, 430
Engler, R. L., 87, 430
Enthoven, Alain, 126, 430
Erde, Edmund, 20, 430
Erikson, Erik, 251, 344, 430
Erwin, Richard, 329, 430
Esbjornson, Robert, 52, 430
Essman, Walter B., 346, 415
Estadt, Barry, 399, 430
Eth, Spencer, 350, 430, 449
Etzioni, Amitai, 434
Evans, Robert G., 124, 430
Evans, Robert W., 310, 430
Ewan, Christine, 89, 430

Fabrega, Horacio, Jr., 29, 430
Facklam, Howard, 52, 430
Facklam, Margery, 52, 430
Faden, Ruth, 68, 235, 430
Fadiman, James, 36, 432
Falcone, David, 113, 430
Farley, Margaret, 424
Fath, Gerald, 394, 396, 430
Feder, Judith, 118, 430
Fein, Rashi, 118, 431
Feinstein, Alvan, 379, 431
Feldman, David, 10, 216, 431
Fersch, Ellsworth A., 339, 431
Fichter, Joseph A., 399, 431
Field, David, 369, 442
Fielding, Gugi, 370, 444
Filly, Roy A., 436
Fingarette, Herbert, 338, 431
Finnis, John, 152, 155, 175, 248, 431
Fisk, N., 313, 431
Fitch, Coy, xii
Fitzgerald, Frances, 15, 431
Fitzpatrick, Annelle, 140, 431
Flannery, Austin, 257, 291, 292, 295, 431,
    438, 466
Flannery, Ellen, 57, 431
Fleming, Gretchen, 415
Fletcher, John, 54, 57, 68, 156-57, 163,
    220, 241, 250, 318, 320, 321,
    322, 323, 324, 375, 393, 431
Fletcher, Joseph, xiv, 233, 272, 431
Flexner, Abraham, 88, 89, 432
Fleyner, John, 362, 432
Flickinger, Charles, 272, 432
Ford, Amasa B., 90, 92, 432
Ford, John C., 63, 257, 258, 432
Fordney-Settlage, Diane S., 288, 432
Forer, Lois G., 72, 432
Forrest, J. D., 453
Foucault, Michael, 83, 86, 432
Fox, Renee, 88, 305, 432
Fox, Richard, xii
Fra Angelico, 60
Frager, Robert, 36, 432
Francis, Richard, 351, 354, 432
Francke, Linda Bird, 220, 432
Francoeur, Robert, 51, 301, 432
Frankena, William, 153, 156, 432
Franklin, John, 351, 354, 432
Freedman, Benjamin, 350, 432
Freeman, Harrop A., 77, 432
Freeman, John, 385, 432
Freidson, Eliot, 29, 30, 54, 77, 83, 432
Fremantle, Anne, 444
Freud, Sigmund, 32, 46, 48, 84, 101, 150,
    332, 334, 343, 344, 345, 432

Freund, Paul A., 77, 432
Freymann, John Gordon, 23, 77, 82, 84, 433
Friedman, Emily, 131, 433
Fromm, Erich, 11, 344, 433
Fuchs, Josef, 158, 433
Fuchs, Victor, 126, 433
Fulton, J., 305, 462
Furnish, 174

Gabriel, Trip, 249, 433
Gaddes, William, 368, 433
Gadow, Sally, 89, 362, 433, 463
Galdston, Iago, 10, 49, 83, 433
Galen, 85
Gallagher, John, 254, 433
Gallant, D., 350, 433
Gallon, Michael, 291, 433
Galofre, Alberto, xii
Gandhi, Indira, 273
Gardell, Mary Ann, 106, 433
Garfield, Jay L., 228, 433
Garrison, Fielding H., 83, 433
Gartrell, Nanette, 341, 357, 433
Garver, Kenneth, 323, 433
Gatch, Milton M., 199, 433
Gaylin, Willard, 336, 349, 433
Gaylor, Christine, 140, 431
Gebhard, P. H., 248, 433
Gellman, Robert, 106, 433
Gemuth, Saul, 314, 433
Gerard, John W., 280, 467
Gert, Bernard, 331, 424, 426
Gervais, Karen Grunstand, 434
Gilbert, Daniel, 350, 434
Gilby, Thomas, 417
Gilder, George, 14, 434
Giles, James, 98, 434
Gilleman, Gerard, 191-92, 434
Gillon, Louis B., 434
Gillon, Raanan, 3, 103, 105, 185, 236, 369, 384, 434
Ginsberg, Eli, 109, 132, 434
Ginzberg, Eli, 88, 90, 429
Gish, Oscar, 21, 434
Glantz, Leonard, 417
Glaser, William A., 85, 434
Glass, Bentley, 321, 325, 434
Glass, R. H., 462
Glick, Paul, 251, 434
Glover, Jonathan, 316, 434
Glymour, Clark, 328, 434
Godden, B., 291, 434
Goffman, Erving, 128, 129, 329, 434
Golbus, Michael S., 436

Gold, Ellen, 105, 435
Goldberg, Abbot, 108, 434
Goldberg, Richard, 369, 434
Goldenring, John M., 208, 213, 434
Goldman, John M., 88, 434
Goldsmith, Jeff, 127, 434
Goode, William J., 79, 434
Goodman, Lenn E., 50, 435
Goodman, Madeleine J., 50, 435
Gordis, Leon, 105, 435
Gorovitz, Samuel, 307, 435
Gostin, L., 347, 435
Grace, Helen, 89, 133, 447
Granfield, Patrick, 59, 435
Grant, Edward, 384, 427, 438
Gray, A., 81, 460
Gray, R. H., 270, 435
Greeley, Andrew, 257, 291, 435
Green, Judith, 435
Green, Ronald M., 8, 435
Greenberg, Roger, 307, 435
Greene, Marjorie, 32, 435
Greer, Germaine, 254, 435
Gregorek, Joseph, 289, 435
Griese, Orville, 282, 285, 435
Griffin, Donald R., 3, 435
Grimes, Charlotte, 309, 435
Grisez, Germain G., 17, 33, 58, 59, 63, 152, 166, 177, 186, 187, 223, 224, 257, 258, 378, 432, 435
Gross, B. A., 269, 435
Grundstrand, 365
Guerrero, Rodrigo, 270, 435
Gula, Richard, 379, 435
Gusmer, Charles, 401, 404, 435
Gustafson, James M., 151, 173, 177, 318, 361, 408, 435, 443
Gutheil, Thomas, 385, 436
Gutierrez, Gustavo, 12, 175, 436
Guttmacher, Sally, 84, 436
Guydish, J., 350, 436

Haafhems, J., 329, 436
Haan, Norma, 35, 436
Hales, Robert, 419
Hales-Yudofsky, Stuart, 446
Halleck, Seymour, 339, 349, 436
Halligan, Patrick, 369, 438
Hammet, Theodore, 69, 436
Hancock, Roger N., 16, 436
Hardin, Garrett, 232, 233, 234, 436
Hare, R. M., 17, 52, 436
Haring, Bernard, 39, 151, 159, 211, 259, 274, 282, 349, 436
Harolds, Louis R., 109, 436

Harper, J., 429
Harper, P. S., 323, 436
Harper, Robert A., 335, 436
Harris, John, 368, 436
Harris, R., 200, 244, 321, 326, 426
Harrison, Beverly Wildung, 220, 436
Harrison, Michael R., 302, 436
Hart, Thomas N., 179, 437
Hartwig, Lynn, 113, 430
Harvey, William, 83, 85
Hasse, Ann Fingarette, 338, 431
Hatcher, Robert A., 272, 278, 279, 437
Hauchal, 120
Hauerwas, Stanley, 150, 437
Healy, Edwin, 288, 437
Heaney, Robert, 82, 418
Hecker, Konned, 437
Hegel, Georg Wilhelm Friedrich, 161,
    208
Heidegger, Martin, 166
Helwig, Monica, 405, 437
Hemmersaith, Frances, 108, 456
Hendren, Hardy, 241, 321, 324, 437
Hendry, George S., 51, 302, 437
Hennessey, Patricia, 228, 433
Henry, Nelson B., 77, 419
Henry, William E., 437
Hilers, Thomas, 445
Hilfaker, David, 361, 437
Hilgers, Thomas W., xii, 269, 270, 279,
    437
Hill, Carole E., 113, 437
Hill, John, 437
Hiller, Marc D., 106, 437, 452
Hillired, Mark, 464
Hiltner, Seward, 392, 437
Hinds, Stuart W., 437
Hippocrates, 26, 49, 85, 123
Hitchcock, James, 230, 437
Hite, Shere, 247, 437
Hitler, Adolf, 10, 123, 150
Hobbes, Thomas, 13
Hoenig, J., 314, 437
Hoff, Lee Ann, 399, 437
Holahan, John, 430
Holbrook, David, 209, 437
Holck, Frederick H., 375, 438
Holden, C., 315, 438
Holder, Angela Roddy, 320, 324, 438
Holifield, E. Broods, 390, 438
Hollender, Marc H., 94, 464
Hollingshead, August, 99, 428
Hollingsworth, R. M., 446
Holmes, Helen, 317, 438
Holst, Lawrence, 401, 438

Holt, Robert T., 337, 438
Holzgreve, H., 311, 367, 438
Hoose, Bernard, 438
Horan, Dennis J., 213, 369, 384, 427,
    435, 438, 445
Horgan, John, 291, 292, 295, 438
Horowitz, L. C., 73, 438
Horrobin, David F., 127, 438
Houck, John, 120, 468
Hoyt, Robert, 256, 263, 438
Hsiao, William, 86, 438
Hull, Richard T., 330, 438
Humber, James, 423, 435, 438
Hume, David, 162
Hume, Kevin, 255, 279, 438
Humphrey, Derek, 379, 438
Hunt, Morton, 438
Hunt, Robert E., 257, 426
Hussey, Edmund, 77, 438
Hyde, Lawrence, 212, 438
Hyde, Margaret, 212, 438

Idziak, Anine M., 151, 438
Iglesias, Teresa, 9, 379, 438
Illich, Ivan D., 71, 76, 77, 78, 126-27, 439
Ingelfinger, Franz, 362, 439
Ingleby, David, 330, 349, 439

Jackson, Jesse, 228, 439
Jacobs, Seth, 315, 439
Jaekle, Charles R., 390, 424
Janssens, Louis, 159, 166, 255, 439
Jeanson, Francis, 154, 439
Johanson, Donald, 7, 439
John, Robert, 446
John Paul II, Pope, 10, 12, 15, 48, 60, 61,
    78, 117, 159, 183, 201, 233,
    237, 240, 244, 246, 252, 254,
    257, 258, 259, 260, 262, 264,
    266, 267, 268, 272, 273, 282,
    286, 291, 293, 297, 298, 439,
    468
Johnson, Gale D., 233, 439
Johnson, Paul, 391, 458
Johnson, Sandra, 379, 439
Johnson, Virginia E., 197, 247, 337, 355,
    356, 447
John XXIII, Pope, 117, 233, 256, 439
Jonas, Hans, 301, 439
Jonas, Stephen, 89, 439
Jones, James, 142, 235, 439
Jones, Royce, 415
Jonsen, Albert R., 57, 106, 160, 305, 308,
    387, 440, 454
Jung, Carl, 35, 332, 337, 440

Kagle, Jill D., 104, 440
Kahn, Eva, 320, 321, 440
Kaiser, Irwin, 210, 440
Kaiser, Robert Blair, 256, 258, 440
Kaluzny, Arnold D., 116, 462
Kamin, Leon, 444
Kamisar, Yale, 385, 440
Kandel, D. B., 352, 469
Kanigel, Robert, 80, 440
Kant, Immanuel, 153, 154, 155-56, 160, 262, 375
Kaplan, Helen Singer, 355, 357, 440
Kaplan, Richard, 460
Karasu, Toksoz, 334, 440
Kase, N. G., 462
Kass, Leon, 88, 214, 318, 440
Katz, Barbara, 234, 239, 417
Katz, Jay, 71, 235, 440
Kauffmann, Christopher, 128, 440
Kaufman, David M., 330, 440
Kavoussi, Richard, 248, 419
Kay, Jerald, 342, 453
Keane, Philip, 165, 247, 440
Kegley, Jacquelyn A., 330, 440
Keifer, Ralph A., 407, 440
Kelagham, J., 279, 440
Kelen, G. D., 81, 440
Keller, P. W., 463
Kelly, David F., 158, 175, 440
Kelly, Gerald, 188, 258, 305-6, 307, 380, 432, 440
Kelly, James, 254, 441
Kelly, Margaret John, 140, 441
Kelman, Sander, 119, 441
Kelsey, Morton, 398, 441
Kerlanger, Fred, 345, 441
Kern, Rochelle, 29, 128, 129, 425
Kervasdoue, Jean, 113, 126, 441, 458
Kesey, Ken, 329, 441
Kesset, Ross, 231, 441
Khantzian, E. J., 352, 441
Kiesling, Christopher, 7, 41, 49, 160, 165, 406, 441
Kimberly, John F., 441
Kindred, Michael, 131, 441
King, J. Charles, 157, 441
Kinsey, A. C., 247, 441
Kinzer, David, 115, 441
Kippley, John F., 258, 260, 270, 441
Kirchner, Corrine, 90, 425
Kirwan, William, 402, 441
Kitchen, Alice, xii
Klaus, Hanna, xii, 269, 270, 441
Kleber, H. D., 353, 459
Kleber, Karl Heinz, 293, 441

Kleinig, John I., 346, 441
Klerman, Gerald, 348, 441
Kliman, Gilbert, 441
Kluge, Eike-Henner, 82, 441
Knapp, Samuel, 105, 441
Knat, Erik, 431
Knauer, Peter, 104, 158, 167, 184, 187, 376, 442
Knaus, 254-55
Knight, Many, 369, 442
Knight, R. P., 334, 442
Knox, Ronald, 156, 442
Koenigh, Barbara, 440
Koester, Helmut, 155, 442
Kohlberg, Lawrence, 146, 442, 450
Kohn, Robert, 113, 442
Kolata, Gina, 248, 442
Kolb, Lawrence, 97, 334, 442
Kolodny, Robert, 197, 447
Koop, C. Everett, 69, 80, 442
Koppleman, Loretta, 237, 238, 441, 442, 446, 457
Korein, J., 422, 450
Korman, Shiela, 249, 251, 444
Kosnik, Anthony R., 32, 247, 250, 258, 266, 295, 442
Kosten, T. R., 352, 353, 442
Kotton, Michael H., 104, 442
Krakoff, Irwin, 387, 442
Kramer, J. J., 350, 436
Krason, Stephen, 220, 227, 442
Kristof, Nicolas, 69, 442
Krugman, Saul, 235, 442
Kubler-Ross, Elisabeth, 363, 370, 371, 387, 442
Kung, Hans, 364, 442
Kurtz, Paul, 11, 156, 200, 244, 249, 443

LaBar, Martin, 302, 443
Lain-Entralgo, P., 25, 26, 443
Laing, R. D., 328, 443
Lako, C. J., 106, 443
Landau, Richard, 361, 443
Langan, John, 173, 443
Langemann, Ellen C., 89, 443
Lappe, Marc, 49, 52, 54, 320, 321-22, 443
LaPuma, John, 140, 443
Larrey, Jean, 231
Larson, Eric, 309, 468
Laura, Ronald, 318, 440, 443
Lavin, Michael, 315, 443
Lawler, Ronald, 244, 272, 296, 443
Lawrence, Susan, 305, 443
Layton, Bruce D., 450
Lebacqz, Karen, 98, 387, 443

Lederberg, Joshua, 8, 443
Lee, Patrick, 164, 443
Lee, Phillip, 71, 114, 443
Leech, Kenneth, 401, 443
Lehmann, H. E., 350, 443
Lehrman, Dorothy, 312, 372, 444
Lejeune, Jerome, 60, 241, 318, 444
Leo XIII, Pope, 117, 444
Lepp, Ignace, 47, 444
Leslie, Gerald, 249, 251, 444
Levin, Arthur, 72, 444
Levine, Carol, 68, 419
Levine, Martin, 430
Levine, Robert, 236, 237, 350, 444
Levine, Stephen F., 314, 315, 444
Levinson, A.-J. Rock, 444
Levy, Charlotte, 367, 444
Levy, David, 444
Levy, Matthew, 234, 433
Lew, Myer S., 444
Lewis, C. S., 359, 444
Lewis, H. David, 32, 444
Lewis, Larry, xii
Lewontia, R. C., 330, 348, 444
Lidz, Charles, 239, 417, 444, 450
Lifshitz, Samuel, 286, 444
Lifton, Robert Jay, 150, 207, 235, 349, 444
Light, Donald, 92, 343, 444
Lillehi, Craig, 241, 321, 324, 437
Lincoln, R., 453
Lind, Stuart, 77, 444
Linzer, N., 86, 444
Lipp, Martin, 72, 444
Llewellyn-Thomas, H., 70, 444
Llewelyn, Susan, 370, 444
Lo, Bernard, 139, 385, 444, 463
Lock, S., 87, 445
Locke, John, 13
Loewy, Erich, 100, 130, 445
London, Perry, 332, 445
Lothstein, Leslie M., 314, 315, 444, 445
Lotstra, Hans, 217, 445
Louis, Thomas A., 238, 445
Luban, David, 434
Lucas, George R., Jr., 431
Luckmann, Thomas, 29, 420
Ludmerer, Kenneth M., 88, 445
Lumsden, Charles L., 3, 27, 468
Lurie, Nicole, 114, 310, 445
Luther, Martin, 66, 90
Lynn, Joanne, 445
Lynn, Kenneth S., 382, 432
Lyon-Levine, Martha, 430

MacDonald, S., 293, 445
Machan, Tibor R., 336, 445
MacIntyre, Alisdair, 11, 149, 161, 303, 445
Mack, Arien, 199, 445
Mack, Eric, 307, 445
Mack, Robert, 362, 445
Mackie, J. L., 207, 445
MacKintosh, James M., 462
Macklin, Ruth, 235, 242, 320, 445
MacNamara, Vincent, 173, 445
Macquarrie, John, 155, 173, 445
Maguire, Daniel, 217, 219, 247, 249, 376, 391, 445
Maguire, P., 362, 445
Mahkorn, S., 287, 445
Mahon, Kathleen A., 238, 240, 242, 427
Mahoney, John, 445
Mahowald, Mary, 312, 445
Maida, Adam, 138, 446
Mall, David, 435, 445
Malloy, Michele, 430
Malone, Patrick, 339, 446
Mangan, J., 185, 380, 446
Many, Seth, 330, 446
Marcel, Gabriel, 60
Marchese, Sandra, 323, 433
Marco, G. J., 77, 446
Marcos, Luis, 331, 446
Marcus, Ruthanne, 80, 446
Marcuse, Herbert, 53, 244, 446
Margo, Curtis, 72, 446
Margolis, Joseph, 25, 232, 446
Maritain, Jacques, 60, 446
Markland, Colin, 313, 446
Marks, Joan H., 135, 446
Marmer, Stephen, 198, 341, 446
Marmoc, Judd, 30, 446
Marmor, Theodore, 430
Marquis, Don, 237, 238, 446
Martelet, Gustave, 262, 291, 446
Martorano, Joseph, 348, 446
Marty, Martin, 134, 446
Marx, Karl, 51-52, 126, 208, 446
Marzen, Thomas, 379, 446
Maslow, Abraham J., 3, 17, 18, 25, 36, 446
Masters, William H., 197, 247, 337, 355, 356, 357, 447
May, Rollo, 50, 335, 344, 447
May, William, xii
May, William E., 33, 164, 166, 240, 258, 272, 381, 382, 383, 443, 447
May, William F., 82, 95, 447
Mayo, David J., 375, 376, 419, 447

McBrien, Richard, 398, 447
McCabe, Herbert, 150, 165, 447
McCarrick, Patricia Milmoe, xi
McCarthy, Charles, 235, 285, 447
McCarthy, Donald G., 140, 288, 417, 441, 447, 461
McCartney, James, 217, 447
McClendon, James, 228, 447
McCloskey, Joanne, 89, 133, 447
McCombie, S. C., 69, 447
McCormick, Richard A., 60, 117, 157, 158, 159, 173, 175, 184, 220, 222, 240, 266, 276, 284, 292, 325, 382, 384, 419, 426, 427, 447, 448
McCullagh, Peter, 312, 448
McCullough, Lawrence B., 92, 148, 419, 448
McDonagh, Enda, 170, 180, 448
McDonald, J. C., 308, 312, 373, 448
McDowell, Jan, 22, 448
McElhinney, Thomas F., 89, 448
McEllhenney, John Galen, 376, 448
McFadden, Charles J., 38, 188, 306, 448
McGill, Arthur Chute, 448
McGrath, Patrick J., 257, 448
McInerny, Ralph, 164, 179, 448
McIntyre, Neil, 108, 448
McIntyre, Russell, 385, 448
McIntyre, S., 429
McKeon, Richard, 417
McKeown, Thomas, 86, 448
McKinlay, John B., 429
McLane, David, 385, 448
McNeil, Barbara J., 428
McNeill, D. R., 400, 448
McNeill, John J., 32, 448
McNeill, T., 89, 208, 448
Meadows, Donella H., 77, 448
Mechanic, David, 83, 113, 128, 415, 448
Medvedev, Roy A., 329, 448
Medvedev, Zhores A., 329, 448
Mehl, Roger, 151, 449
Meier, Anton Meinrad, 293, 449
Meier, Levi, 214, 216, 449
Meilander, Gilbert, 379, 449
Meisel, Alan, 72, 417, 449, 450
Mello, Nancy, 353, 449
Mendel, Gregor, 320
Mendelhoff, John, 241, 449
Mendelsohn, John, 235, 449
Mendelson, Jack, 353, 449
Menninger, Karl, 45-46, 244, 330, 336, 341, 375, 449
Merkelbach, Benedictus, 188, 449

Mershey, Harold, 23, 449
Merton, Robert K., 78, 79, 449
Metz, Johannes, 196
Meyer, J. K., 313, 315, 449
Meyers, John E. B., 105, 449
Michelangelo, 60
Mikhail, Girgis, xii
Miles, Stephen, 81, 469
Milewski, Elizabeth, 449
Milhaven, John Giles, 198, 449
Milkman, Harvey, 50, 449
Mill, John Stuart, 157, 449
Miller, Bruce, 240, 449
Miller, J. D., 355, 449
Milligan, Martin, 446
Mills, John, 449
Mills, Mark, 105, 449
Mills, Michael, 69, 449
Milunsky, A., 458
Milunsky, Ambroz, 467
Milunsky, Aubrey, 445
Mishell, Daniel, 272, 449
Mitchell, Leon, 114, 449
Mitford, Jessica, 371, 450
Mizratti, Terry, 72, 450
Modde, Margaret, 136, 450
Modell, Bernadette, 321, 450
Modgil, Celia, 450
Mohr, James, 226, 450
Molinari, G., 366, 450
Moline, Jon, 77, 78, 450
Moltmann, Jurgen, 175, 196, 450
Monahan, John, 339, 450
Monod, Jacques, 177, 450
Monteleone, James A., xii, 313, 314, 450
Monteleone, Patricia, xii
Moody, Howard, 411, 450
Moore, G. E., 155, 450
Moore, Keith, 212, 450
Moore, Lorna, 10, 86, 450
Moore, Maurice J., 291, 450
Moore, Robert L., 108, 341, 450
Moore, Wilbert E., 79, 450
Moraczewski, Albert S., xii, 323, 417, 418, 461
Moreno, Jonathan, 115, 419
Morreim, E. Haau, 100, 450
Morrison, James K., 450
Morrison, P. A., 242, 448
Moskop, John C., 441, 446, 457
Motoshima, Masanabu, 432
Mulstein, Suzanne, 113, 450
Mulvanney, Kieran, 207, 450
Mundinger, Mary O'Neill, 115, 450
Munetz, Mark R., 68, 450

Murnion, Philip, 345, 450
Murphy, Francis X., 256, 258, 260, 261, 262, 263, 450
Murray, G. F., 352, 462
Murray, J., 106, 305, 320, 451
Murray, Joseph E., 451
Murray, Thomas, 428, 451
Mussolini, Benito, 10, 123
Myrich, J. A., 115, 451

Nagel, Ernest, 28, 451
Napoleon Bonaparte, 231
Narveson, Jan, 376, 451
Nash, George H., 121, 451
Natanson, Maurice, 208, 451
Nathanson, Bernard, 226, 411, 451
Navarro, Vincente, 9, 78, 116, 119, 420, 451
Neumann, Erich, 31, 451
Neusner, Jacob, 442
Neville, R., 106, 451
Newell, Claire, 22, 448
Newhouse, J. P., 115, 451
Newman, Joan, 450
Newton, Isaac, 157
Ngyan, William, 320, 452
Niebuhr, H. Richard, 452
Niebuhr, N., 160
Nietzche, Friedrich Wilhelm, 13
Nightengale, Elena, 329, 463
Nightingale, Florence, 391
Nijhof, G., 436
Nolan, Martin, 274, 307, 452
Nolin, Kieran, 403, 452
Noonan, John T., xvi, 201, 214, 215, 217, 227, 247, 294, 452
Nouwen, Henri J., 359, 396, 448, 452
Novak, David, 168, 374, 452
Noyes, R., Jr., 375, 452
Nozick, Robert, 14, 452
Number, Ronald, 118, 452

Oakley, Deborah, 32, 452
O'Callaghan, 295
O'Callaghan, D. F., 452
O'Callaghan, Mark, 347, 423
O'Connell, Timothy, 158, 453
O'Connor, Brian, 393, 453
O'Donnell, Thomas, 38, 105, 223, 288, 378, 384, 453
O'Donovan, Oliver, 211, 453
Oken, D., 369, 453
Olshansky, Ellen Francis, 280, 453
Olson, Camille, 239, 457
O'Meara, Thomas, xii, 59, 136, 174, 360, 396, 453

Oppenheimer, Gerald, 69, 453
Origino, 254-55
Ornstein, Paul, 342, 453
O'Rourke, Kevin, xii, 58, 68, 87, 109, 138, 139, 141, 236, 240, 310, 372, 381, 382, 383, 387, 421, 453
Ory, H. W., 279, 453
Osmond, Humphrey, 95, 461
Osmundsen, John A., 320, 321, 453
Ostling, Richard, 226, 411, 451
Outka, Gene, 156, 157, 454
Ozar, David T., 100, 454

Padgug, Robert, 69, 453
Pagon, 106
Palmer, Paul, 405, 454
Palmour, Jody, 150, 454
Palouzie, Anne Marie, 369, 454
Pannenburg, Wolfhart, 196
Paris, John, 385, 454
Parson, Richard, 468
Parsons, Talcott, 29, 98, 454
Pasteur, Louis, 84
Pastrana, Gabriel, 212, 213, 454
Paul VI, Pope, 12, 15, 59, 60, 117, 201, 233, 252, 257, 259, 261, 262, 266, 267, 291, 293, 297, 402, 454
Pellegrino, Edmund D., xiv, 25, 54, 68, 81, 82, 87, 89, 92, 98, 116, 147, 182, 239, 384, 454
Pepper, Anita, xii
Perkins, Harry, 387, 454
Perl, Mark, 328, 340, 455
Perry, Ralph, 16, 455
Peters, David, 379, 455
Petersdorf, Robert G., 88, 455
Peterson, H. B., 272, 455
Peterson, Michael R., 314, 455
Petrila, John, 332, 335, 455
Philo, 155
Piaget, Jean, 146, 455
Pieper, Josef, 198, 455
Pietroferg, John, 81, 455
Pincus, Jonathan, 339, 455
Pinkus, Rosa Lynn, 89, 455
Pitts, F. N., 374, 455
Pius XI, Pope, 254, 293, 455
Pius XII, Pope, xv, 36, 37, 39, 237, 254, 255, 256, 274, 275, 282, 284, 293, 305, 349-50, 360, 372-73, 380-81, 382, 383, 385, 386, 455
Plato, 5, 16, 33, 35, 40, 121, 161, 201, 251, 375, 455
Pleak, Richard, 340, 455

Plum, Fred, 455
Plumb, Diane, 467
Polanyi, Michael, 178, 456
Pollner, Fran, 211, 455
Popper, Karl, 108, 448
Posner, Jerome, 455
Powsner, Rhoda, 108, 456
Preston, Thomas, 99, 456
Prottas, Jeffrey M., 310, 372, 456
Prucha, Milan, 11, 456
Prummer, Dominicus M., 219, 456

Quay, Paul, 254, 456
Quinlan, Karen, 381
Quinn, John, 260

Rachels, James, 16, 170, 378, 391, 456
Racheson, Robert, 445
Rafferty, Frank, 100, 456
Raffin, T. A., 384, 459
Rahner, Karl, 55, 162, 361, 371, 403, 456
Ramsey, Paul, xiv, 40, 82, 99, 154, 157,
            158, 159, 217, 240, 305, 306,
            307, 319, 373, 382, 444, 448,
            457
Rand, Ayn, 14, 155, 457
Rankin, Sally H., 130, 457
Ratner, Herbert, 168, 258, 457
Ratzinger, Cardinal, 60, 258, 285, 457
Ravich, Ruth, 135, 457
Rawls, John, 8, 153, 233, 457
Reardon, David, 220, 457
Reed, Michael, 239, 457
Reed, Sheldon, 320, 457
Regan, Tom, 391, 457
Reich, Warren, 233, 457
Reichenbach, Bruce, 378, 457
Reichley, A. James, 228, 457
Reinhardt, Uwe, 116, 457
Reiser, David, 71, 83, 457
Reiser, Stanley J., 83, 457
Rennie, Drummond, 40, 458
Rescher, Nicholas, 52, 458
Restak, Richard M., 330, 458
Reter, 315
Reyna, L. J., 442, 468
Rice, Charles E., 230, 458
Rice, Nancy, 326, 458
Richards, Larry, 391, 458
Richardson, Herbert W., 32, 458
Rieckelman, Maria, xii
Rieff, Philip, 50, 343-44, 345, 458
Rifkin, Jeremy, 318, 458
Rigali, Norbert, 254, 458
Riskin, Leonard L., 358, 458
Rizzo, Robert, 367, 458

Robbins, Christopher, 114, 458
Robertson, John A., 302, 316, 385, 458
Robinson, Jean, 89, 458
Robinson, R. D., 311, 458
Robitscher, Jonas, 330, 458
Rodd, Rosemary, 207, 458
Rodwin, Victor G., 441
Roemer, Milton E., 462
Rogers, Carl R., 96, 458
Rogers, William, 89, 458
Rokeach, Milton, 342, 458
Rordorf, Willy, 49, 458
Rose, David N., 103, 462
Rose, Stephen, 319, 444, 458
Rosen, David, 71, 83, 457
Rosenberg, Charles, 128, 458
Rosenberg, Jay, 70, 375, 385, 458
Rosenblum, Gerald W., 79, 450
Rosenfeld, Albert, 441
Rosenfield, Israel, 52, 303, 458
Rosett, Richard, 100, 458
Rosner, Fred, 214, 216, 458
Rosoff, 383
Rosotti, Sidney, 458
Ross, Judith, 72, 468
Ross, W. D., 157, 176, 459
Rostain, Anthony, 384, 459
Rothman, David J., 329, 340, 459
Rounsaville, B., 353, 459
Rousseau, Jean Jacques, 150, 153, 459
Rowland, Thomas, 311, 459
Roy, David, 321, 459
Royce, James, 353, 354, 420
Royce, Josiah, 161
Ruark, J. E., 384, 459
Rubenstein, A., 355, 416
Rubenstein, Leonard, 331, 459
Rubin, Eva, 224, 227, 459
Rubin, Robert, 72, 113, 459
Runciman, Steven, 32, 459
Rush, Vincent, 207, 459

Sabbatini, Jean, 114, 459
Sadler, Alfred, 310, 372, 459
Sahat, Nadia, 320, 452
Sahuc, Louis J., 295, 459
St. Augustine. *See* Augustine, Saint
St. Catherine of Siena. *See* Catherine of
            Siena, Saint
St. John-Stevas, Norman, 226, 459
St. Teresa of Avila. *See* Teresa of Avila,
            Saint
Sales, Braaj, 97, 351, 427
Sammons, Lucy, 280, 453
Sanders, John H., 132, 459
Sapolsky, Harvey, 114, 459

Sartre, Jean Paul, 154
Scarlett, B. C., 211, 459
Schaffer, Howard, 50, 449
Schall, J. V., 293, 460
Scheler, Max, 158, 166
Scherr, L., 81, 460
Schiff, Robert, 131, 460
Schillebeeckx, Edward, 361, 401, 460
Schindler, Thomas, 381, 460
Schlitz, Randy, 87, 460
Schmid, Donald, 104, 338, 341, 351, 460
Schnackenburg, Rudolf, 177, 245, 460
Schneller, Eugene, 135, 460
Schroeder, S., 349, 460
Schuller, Bruno, 158, 460
Schulman, Joseph D., 241, 431
Schwartz, George, 444
Schwartz, Harold, 81, 329, 460
Schwartz, Lee, 329, 460
Schwartz, Richard S., 104, 460
Schwartz, William, 116, 460
Schwitzgebel, Ralph K., 347, 460
Schwitzgebel, Robert L., 347, 460
Scott, Gordon, 379, 460
Scott, James, 449
Scully, Diana, 92, 461
Seibel, Machelle, 281, 285, 461
Senay, Patrick, 380, 461
Sgarlata, Carmelo, xii
Shaffer, Thomas, 77, 80, 461
Shalom, Albert, 44, 461
Shannon, M. Jordan, 240, 461
Shannon, Thomas A., 147, 461
Shannon, William H., 255, 262, 292, 461
Shapiro, David, 468
Shapiro, Larry, 235, 302, 461
Shapiro, Martin F., 235, 461
Shapiro, Stanley H., 238, 445
Shareef, R., 118, 461
Shaw, Margery, 213, 461
Shehan, Lawrence Cardinal, 296, 461
Shell, Susan Meld, 153, 461
Shelp, Earl, 328, 340, 432, 443, 454, 455, 461, 463
Shinnar, Shlomo, 311, 417
Shirm, M. C., 279, 461
Shnit, Dan, 339, 418
Showalter, Stuart, 382, 461
Sider, Roger C., 49, 242, 331, 334, 461
Sidgwick, Henry, 461
Siegel, Karolyn, 461
Sieghart, Paul, 76, 79, 104, 461
Siegler, Mark, 109, 377, 461
Siegler, Miriam, 95, 461
Siegman, Athilia, 429
Sigerist, Henry E., 48, 83, 128, 462

Silber, Thomas J., 324, 462
Silberman, Robert, 331, 332, 465
Silver, George, 100, 462
Silver, Jerry, 445
Silver, Jonathan, 347, 462
Silverberg, James, 170, 418
Simmons, Roberta G., 305, 307, 420, 462
Sims, John, 437
Singer, Peter, 156, 168, 207, 462
Sinha, Ajit Kumar, 27, 462
Skinner, B. F., 334, 336, 349, 462
Slaby, Andrew, 46, 464
Slater, Andrew, 442, 468
Sloan, Frank A., 114, 462
Sluis, Van der. See Van der Sluis, I.
Smart, R. G., 352, 462
Smart, Vivian, 11, 462
Smith, Adam, 121
Smith, Charles, 242, 462
Smith, David B., 108, 116, 462
Smith, Dermott, xii
Smith, Kenneth, xii
Smith, William, 59, 60, 277, 462
Snyder, Solomon, 330, 348, 462
Sobel, Alan, 462
Sondheimer, Henry M., 422
Sorkin, Alan, 114, 115, 127, 462
Sparks, Anne, 286, 462
Speedling, Edward J., 103, 462
Speroff, L., 279, 462
Spicker, Stuart C., 429
Spicker, Stuart F., 89, 463
Spicq, Ceslaus, 174, 463
Spiker, Stuart F., 420
Spillane, Edward, xii
Spiro, Howard, 49, 463
Sprague, Robert, 350, 463
Spray, Lee, 437
Springer, Robert, 314, 463
Stalin, Joseph, 10, 37
Stalker, Douglas, 328, 434
Stanley, Barbara Hrevnack, 240, 463
Stanley, Linda, 89, 463
Stanley, Michael, 240, 463
Starr, Paul, 50, 114, 463
Steel, Knight, 72, 463
Steinbrook, Robert, 385, 463
Stenchever, Morton, 288, 463
Stephens, Ronald, 387, 463
Stevens, Jay, 348, 463
Stewart, Harold, 468
Still, A. W., 371, 463
Stillman, Paula, 71, 463
Stoneman, William, xii
Storch, Janet, 72, 135, 463
Stover, Eric, 329, 463

Strasburg-Cohen, T., 281, 463
Strauss, Anselm, 72, 133, 463
Strickler, Ronald C., 280, 463
Struik, D. J., 446
Sullivan, Francis, 59, 63, 463
Sullivan, Greer, 449
Sullivan, Joseph V., 379, 463
Summers, Jim, 72, 463
Sumner, L. W., 213, 463
Sumner, William Graham, 152, 463
Swazy, Judith P., 305, 432
Swift, Francis W., 255, 463
Swift-Glass, Elenor, 440
Szasz, Thomas, 14, 30, 94, 106, 242,
    328-29, 330, 346, 353, 420, 463,
    464

Talbott, John, 419, 432, 446
Tancredi, Lawrence, 46, 339, 464
Tauer, Carol, 4, 464
Taysi, Kutay, 320, 464
Tazebiatouski, Gregory, 467
Teilhard de Chardin, Pierre, 24, 60, 208,
    464
Tembia, C., 429
Tembia, O., 429
Temkin, Owsei, 25, 26, 464
Teresa of Avila, Saint, 60
Tertullian, 218
Thayer, Nelson, 399, 464
Theis, Charlotte, 90, 464
Thielicke, Helmut, 66, 408, 464
Thomasma, David C., xiv, 17, 25, 54, 82,
    98, 116, 147, 182, 454, 464
Thompson, James, 212, 322, 464
Thompson, Margaret, 212, 322, 464
Thomson, Judith Jarvis, 224, 464
Thorup, Oscar, 305, 464
Thundy, Zacharias, 10, 464
Tillich, Paul, 30, 464
Todd, C. J., 371, 463
Tomilson, T., 384, 464
Tooley, Michael, 213, 223, 465
Torrens, Paul, 387, 465
Torrey, E. Fuller, 328, 465
Toulmin, Stephen, 116, 465
Towers, Bernard, 70, 385, 458
Tranoy, Kant, 431
Tredway, Donald S., 432
Tuchel, Peter, 377, 461
Tull, Robert, 369, 434
Turnquist, Arlynne, 350, 465

Ullmann, Manfred, 10, 465
Ulpian, 155
Underwood, Kenneth, 79, 465

Uricchio, W. A., 435
Ursano, Robert, 331, 332, 465

Vacek, Edward, 284, 466
Vaillant, G. E., 17, 352, 466
Valenstein, Elliot, 346, 466
Valsecchi, Ambrogio, 255, 256, 293, 466
Vandercreek, Leon, 441
Van der Haag, Ernest, 37, 466
Vander Pool, E., 436
Van der Sluis, I., 375, 466
Van Kaam, Adrian, 33, 50, 344, 345, 466
Vaporis, N. M., 10, 466
Varga, Andrew, 152, 273, 466
Vaughan, Mary Ellen, 140, 466
Vaux, Kenneth L., 20, 134, 446, 466
Veatch, Henry, 150, 169, 466
Veatch, Robert, 77, 95, 99, 115, 147, 368,
    467
Vesalius, Andreas, 83
Vitz, Paul, 34, 467
Viviano, Benedict, 12, 120, 467
Vivieri, C., 89, 467
Vogel, Morris J., 86, 467
Von Hildebrand, Alice, 252, 467
Von Hildebrand, Dietrich, 252, 467

Wahlberg, Rachel Conrad, 212, 220, 467
Waitzhib, 78, 124
Waitzkin, Howard, 467
Walgrave, John J., 6, 467
Walinder, Jan, 315, 467
Walters, LeRoy, 424, 467
Warnock, Mary, 467
Warren, James, 88, 467
Warren, J. C., 385, 463
Warren, John W., 240, 467
Wasserstrom, Richard, 212, 467
Watson, James D., 320, 467
Watson, W., 318, 448
Weichert, Carol, 280, 467
Weikel, M. K., 114, 467
Weinstein, Milton G., 428
Weiss, S. J., 81, 468
Welch, Gilbert, 309, 468
Welsby, Phillip, 68, 468
Wertheimer, Michael, 73, 468
Westmore, Ann, 269, 420
White, Andrew Dickson, 85, 468
White, Kerr L., 113, 442
Whitehead, Alfred North, 24, 208, 468
Wicks, Robert, 399, 405, 468
Wilcox, Allen, 211, 468
Wilkinson, Greg, 335, 468
Williams, Cornelius, 198, 468
Williams, Ken, 128, 428

Williams, Oliver, 120, 468
Williams, Preston N., 305, 435, 468
Willman, Val, xii
Wilson, Edward O., 3, 27, 251, 468
Winslade, William, 72, 468
Winslow, Gerald R., 231, 468
Wofsy, Constana, 449
Wolinsky, Howard, 312, 468
Wolpe, Joseph, 334, 335, 442, 468
Wolt, Susan, 419
Worden, J. William, 468
Wright, Gerard, 444
Wyschogord, Michael, 422

Yamaguchi, K., 352, 469
Yonder, Paul, 367, 458
Younger, Stuart, 367, 469
Yudofsky, Stuart, 347, 419, 462

Zalba, M., 292, 469
Zaner, Richard, 368, 469
Ziegenfuss, James T., 109, 469
Zimmerman, Anthony, 260, 270, 457,
    459, 469
Zimmerman, David, 425
Zole, Irving K., 429
Zuger, Abigail, 81, 469
Zusy, Dennis R., xii

SUBJECT INDEX

AA. *See* Alcoholics Anonymous (AA)

AAMC. *See* Association of American Medical Colleges (AAMC)

AAN. *See* American Academy of Neurology (AAN)

AARP. *See* American Association of Retired Persons (AARP)

ABA. *See* American Bar Association (ABA)

Abortion, 206
    and Supreme Court, 226-28
    traditional views, 214-20
    and woman's rights, 220-24

Acceptance, 96
    and addiction, 353

ACOG. *See* American College of Obstetricians and Gynecologists (ACOG)

Acquired immunodeficiency syndrome (AIDS), xi, 67, 68-70, 80-81, 106-7, 231, 363, 401, 456

Act, and goal, 181-83

Action therapy, 332

Activity, and passivity, 210

Act utilitarianism, 156

Addiction
    and chemical dependency, 351-55
    physiological, 352

Advocacy, and personhood, 213-14

Advocates, patient, 133-35

Affirmation of life, 47-49, 387

Agape, 157

Age of Darwin and Freud, 84

Age of Pasteur, 84

Age of Reason, 160

Aggressiveness, 46

AHA. *See* American Hospital Association (AHA)

AID. *See* Artificial insemination by donor (AID)

AIDS. *See* Acquired immunodeficiency syndrome (AIDS)

AIH. *See* Artificial insemination by the husband (AIH)

Ailment, and disease, 25

Al-Anon, 354

Alcoholics Anonymous (AA), 354, 355

Alcoholism, 354

Alienation, direct and indirect, 183

"Allocution to Italian Midwives," 254

AMA. *See* American Medical Association (AMA)

American Academy of Neurology (AAN), 383, 415

American Association of Retired Persons (AARP), 113

American Bar Association (ABA), 415

American College of Obstetricians and Gynecologists (ACOG), 324, 415

American College of Physicians, 81

American Hospital Association (AHA), 109, 114, 115, 124, 310, 369, 415

American Medical Association (AMA), 81, 83, 89, 92, 107, 108, 113, 114, 116, 118, 133, 369, 379, 385, 416

American Nurses' Association (ANA), 416

American Psychiatric Association (APA), 108, 313, 329, 341, 342, 355, 357, 417

American Society of Neurosurgeons, 416

Amniocentesis, 320

ANA. *See* American Nurses' Association (ANA)

Analysis
    defined, xvi, 9
    responsible, 60

Anatomical Gift Act, 310

Anatomical integrity, 306

Angelicism, 35

Angiogram, 367

Anointing the sick, and reconciliation, 402-5

Antabuse, 346

Antifertility treatment, 288-90

Anxiety, neurotic, 333

APA. *See* American Psychiatric Association (APA)

Apostolic Constitution on the Sacrament of Anointing the Sick, 402

"Apostolic Exhortation on the Family," 298

Aquinas Institute of Theology, xii

Arbitrariness, 147

Artificial insemination by a donor (AID), 280-86

Artificial insemination by the husband (AIH), 280-86

Asexuality, 212

Association of American Medical Colleges (AAMC), 89, 109, 116, 415

Asylums, 128

Australian Research Commission, 213, 241, 311, 418

Autonomous person, 335

Autopsy, 373-74

Baptism, and eucharist, 405-8
Basic common needs, 162-64
Behavior control, 345-51
Behavior Control, 332
Behaviorism, 207
Behavior modification, and psycho-
  therapy, 328-58
*Belmont Report: Ethical Principles and Guide-
  lines for the Protection of Human
  Subjects of Research, The*, 239, 420
Beneficence, 153
Benefratelli, 84
Biases, and medical education, 88-93
Billings method, 269
Bioethical decision making, 145-204,
  205-387
  logic of, 146-72
Bioethics Line, The, 144
Biography, 5, 208, 209-11
Biological dimension, of personality, 17
Biological health, and biologism, 31-33,
  168-69, 262
Biological needs, 25
Biologism, and biological health, 31-33,
  168-69, 262
Biophysical events, 314
Birth of the Clinic, The, 83
*Bitter Pill; Doctors, Patients, and Failed Ex-
  pectations, The*, 72
Bodily being, 5
Brain, and lobotomy and ESB, 346-47
Brain death, 366-68
Breast feeding, 279
*Brophy, Patricia v. New England Sinai Hospi-
  tal, Inc.*, 383, 385, 422
Brotherhood, 15

Cadaver, care of, 371-74
Calendar rhythm, 255
Calling, 79
Callous conscience, 66-68
Canada Law Reform Commission, 365,
  423
Canadian Medical Association Journal, 73,
  423
Capitation, 113
Care, and cure, 127-29
Casti Connubii, 254, 255, 257
Catholic Health Association of the United
  States, The (CHA), xii, 118,
  119, 137, 140, 424
Catholic hospital, 136-38
Catholic identity, 136-38

Catholic Theological Society of America,
  The, 258
CCHCM. *See* Commission for Catholic
  Health Care Ministry (CCHCM)
CDC. *See* Centers for Disease Control
  (CDC)
Celebration, of healing process, 401-8
Celibacy, 41
Centers for Disease Control (CDC), 81,
  424, 446
Centralization, 114-15
Certitude, in ethical decision, 56-57
Cervical cap, 279
Chance and Necessity, 177
CHA. *See* Catholic Health Association of
  the United States, The (CHA)
Character, 150
Charity, 174
Chemical dependency, and addiction,
  351-55
Child Labor Amendment, 124
Choosing Life or Death, 72
Chorionic villi sampling, 320
Christian Affirmation of Life, 387
Christian decision making, 173-204
Christian ethics, 173-76
Christian faith, norms of, 176-91
Christian hope, 196-203
*Christianity and Social Progress (Mater et
  Magistra)*, 117
Christian love, norms of, 191-96
Christian physician, 86-88
Christian values, xiv
Church in the Modern World, The, 117
CIC. *See* Code of Canon Law (CIC)
Circumstantial intention, 182
Civilization and Its Discontents, 150
Classicist mentality, 158
Clients, 77
Clinical iatrogenesis, 127
Clinical pastoral education (PCE), 392,
  393, 401
Closed way, 180
Closing of the American Mind, The, 344
CMSM. *See* Conference of Major Su-
  periors of Men (CMSM)
Code of Canon Law (CIC), 424
College of Healthcare Executives, 72, 425
College of Physicians Health and Public
  Policy Committee, 425
"Commercialization in Transplantation:
  The Problems and Some Guide-
  lines for Practice," 465
Commission for Catholic Health Care
  Ministry (CCHCM), 136, 137,
  424

Commission for the Protection of Human Subjects of Biomedical and Behavioral Research (CPHS), 142, 143
Commission of Medical Malpractice, 108
Commitment, fundamental, 179
Committee on Bioethical Issues of the Bishops of Great Britain and Ireland (GBI), 289, 290, 433
Committees, ethics and mission effectiveness, 138-42
Common good, principle of, 116-21, 193-94, 203-4, 225, 308
Common needs, basic, 162-64
Communication, 100
 professional, 102-7, 190-91, 351
Communitarian, 162
Community, 15
 hospital as, 127-31
 and person, 39
 and personal health, 6-9
 and principles of human dignity, 19, 192-93, 203-4, 308, 349
Complaint, and disease, 25
Concern, 99
Conditioning, 332
 psychological, 349
Condom, 279
Conference of Major Superiors of Men (CMSM), 137
Confidentiality, 103-7
Congress. *See* United States Congress
Conroy (court case), 385
Conscience, 15
 and consent, 54-70, 179
 private, 156
 well-formed, 64-68, 70, 177-78, 184
Consent
 and conscience, 54-70, 179
 informed, 68-69, 179, 203-4
 vicarious, 239-41
Consequences, 197
Consequentialism, 148, 156
Conservative Intellectual Movement in America Since 1945, 121
Conservative movements, 15
Conspiratorial model of therapeutic relationships, 95
Consumer discipline, 110
Contemporary Issues in Science and Theology, 439
Contingent fee system, 109
Contraception
 controversy on, 253-67
 oral, 278-80

and sterilization, 271-73
"Contraception: Adverse Effects," 278
Control
 behavior, 345-51
 self-. *See* Self-control
Conventional phase, 146
Cooperation, legitimate, 188-90
Corporatism, 122
Corpse, care of, 371-74
Council of Europe, 425
Council of Trent, 159
Counseling
 ethical. *See* Ethical counseling
 genetic. *See* Genetic counseling
 healthcare, 81-83, 94-102
 spiritual. *See* Spiritual counseling
Counselor, 81
Countertransference, 97
Covenant, 82
Co-workers, and physicians, 131-33
CPE. *See* Clinical pastoral education (PCE)
CPHS. *See* Commission for the Protection of Human Subjects of Biomedical and Behavioral Research (CPHS)
Creative dimension, of personality, 18
Creative needs, 25
Creativity, and stewardship, 51-53, 197, 201-3, 304, 318
Criminals, 330
Crisis of limits, 126
Criticism, responsible, 60
Cultural iatrogenesis, 127
Cultural relativism, 30
Cure, and care, 127-29

D & C. *See* Dilation and curettage (D & C)
Death
 allowing, 380-87
 brain, 366-68
 defining, 364-68
 fear of, 361-64
 mystery of, 359-61
 and suffering, 359-87
 and truth telling, 368-71
Decision making
 bioethical, 145-204, 205-387
 Christian, 173-204
Declaration of Certain Problems of Sexual Ethics, 257, 291
Declaration of Religious Liberty, 189
Declaration on Euthanasia, 378, 379, 382, 384
Declaration on Procured Abortion, 218, 229

Declaration on Religious Liberty, 229
Delayed hominization, 213-13
Deontological ethical methodology, xiv, 147-54
Deoxyribonucleic acid (DNA), 51, 319, 320
Department of Health, Education, and Welfare (HEW). *See* United States Department of Health, Education, and Welfare (HEW)
Department of Health and Human Services. *See* United States Department of Health and Human Services (DHHS)
Dependency
    chemical, 351-55
    psychological, 352
Depersonalization, 76-83
DES. *See* Diethylstibestrol (DES)
De Somniis, 85
Development of Peoples, The, 117
DHHS. *See* United States Department of Health and Human Services (DHHS)
Diagnostic and Statistical Manual of Mental Disorders (DSM III), 313
Diamond v. Chakrabarty, 319
Diaphragm, 279
Didache, 217
Diethylstibestrol (DES), 288
Dignity, human, 19, 192-93, 203-4, 259, 308, 349
Dilation and curettage (D & C), 288
Dimensions, of personality, 17-18
Direct abortion, 214
Direct alienation, 183
Directives. *See Ethical and Religious Directives for Catholic Health Facilities*
Discernment
    and ethical counseling, 412-13
    moral, 183-84
    and spiritual counseling, 399-401
Discipline
    peer and consumer, 110
    professional, 107-11
Discrimination, moral, 179-81, 203-4
Disease
    concepts of, 25-27
    and health, 20-43
    iatrogenic, 126-27
Disorder, and disease, 25
Dissent, right to, 60
Disturbance, emotional. *See* Emotional disturbance
Disulfiram, 346
Disvalues, ontic, 166-68

Divine Command Morality, 151
Divorce, and marriage, 248
DNA. *See* Deoxyribonucleic acid (DNA)
DNR orders. *See* Do-not-resuscitate (DNR) orders
Doctor's Perspective: Physicians View Their Patients and Their Practice, The, 90
Doctrine, developing, 60-64
Documents of Vatican II, The, 466
Doe v. Bolton, 226
Do-not-resuscitate (DNR) orders, 140
Donum Vitae, 257
Double-blind control, 238
Double effect, principle of, 184-88, 189, 190, 203-4, 236, 288
Doubts
    scientific, 52-53
    solving, 57-59
Douche, postcoital, 279
Drugs, psychoactive, 347-48
DSM III. *See Diagnostic and Statistical Manual of Mental Disorders* (DSM III)
Dualism, 33
Duty methodology. *See* Deontological ethical methodology

EAB. *See* Ethics Advisory Board (EAB)
Economic Justice for All ,119
Economic model of health, 21
Education
    medical, 88-93
    for sexual future, 298-300
EEG. *See* Electroencephalogram (EEG)
Effect, double. *See* Double effect
Eichner (Brother Fox) (court case), 385
Electrical stimulation of the brain (ESB), 347
Electroencephalogram (EEG), 367
Emotional disturbance, 331
Emotivism, 149-51
Empathy, 207
Encyclopedia of Bioethics, 144, 452
Equal Rights Amendment, 124
ESB. *See* Electrical stimulation of the brain (ESB)
Eschatology, 196
ET. *See* Embryo transfer (ET)
Ethical and Religious Directives for Catholic Health Facilities, xv, 65, 136, 141, 215, 224, 273-75, 276, 278, 369, 386, 430
Ethical counseling, and pastoral care, 408-13
Ethical pluralism, 146-47
Ethical principles, 175-76

Ethics
    APA. *See Principles of Medical Ethics,*
        The (APA)
    Christian, 173-76
    healthcare, and public policy, 142-44
    intuitionist, 155
    natural law, 155
    and pastoral care, 390-413
Ethics Advisory Board (EAB), 142, 143
Ethics committees, 138-42
Eucharist, and baptism, 405-8
Eugenics, 321
European common market, 123
Euthanasia, and suicide, 374-80
Evaluative Criteria for Catholic Health Care
    Facilities, 137
Evil
    intrinsic, 158
    ontic, 166
Exceptionless norms, 148
Existentialism, 154
Experimentation
    and human subjects, 234-43
    psychological, 242-43
Explicit, 181
Extraordinary magisterium, 62

Faith, 59, 60, 174, 175
    norms of, 176-91
Falsehood, 104
Familiaris Consortio, 60, 201, 252, 259,
    264, 266, 268, 272
Family, 245, 246-47
Family-interaction model of therapeutic
    relationships, 95
Family living, 249
Family planning, natural, 270
Fear, of death, 361-64
Federal Register, 430
Feelings, 17
Fees, healthcare, 100-102
Fee system, contingent, 109
Fertilization, 280-81
Finis operantis, 182
Finis operis, 182
Foam, vaginal, 279
Formal cooperation, 188
Formalism, 153-54
"Fostering the Nobility of Marriage," 256
Freedom, 56
    intelligent, 15, 168-69, 202
French Revolution, 86, 121
Fully human, 2-19
Functional integrity, 306
Functionalism, 122-26, 193-94, 203-4,
    225

Fundamental commitment, 179
Fundamental option, 179

Gamete intrafallopian transfer (GIFT),
    284
GBI. *See* Committee on Bioethical Issues
    of the Bishops of Great Britain
    and Ireland (GBI)
Gender dysphoria syndrome, 314
Gender identity, 314
Gender role, 314
Genes, 320
Genetic counseling, and screening, 320-
    27
Genetic intervention, 316-19
Genetic screening, and counseling, 320-
    27
Geneva Declaration, The, 379
Genotype, 319
Georgetown University, xi, 144
Getting Rid of Patients, 72
GIFT. *See* Gamete intrafallopian transfer
    (GIFT)
GMENAC Report, 86
Gnostics, 247
GNP. *See* Gross national product (GNP)
Goal, and act, 181-83
Golden Rule, 208
Good, common, 116-21, 193-94, 203-4,
    225, 308
GPEP Report, 89
Great Depression, 123
Gregorian University, 158
Gross national product (GNP), 309
Group practice, 113
Group therapy, 338
Growing through suffering, principle of,
    197-99, 203-4
Guesthouses, 128
Guidance, by the Spirit, 59-60

Happiness, and growing through suffer-
    ing, 197
Hastings Center Institute of Society,
    Ethics, and the Life Sciences:
    Research Group on Ethical, So-
    cial, and Legal Issues in Genetic
    Counseling and Genetic En-
    gineering, 144, 322, 437
HCFA. *See* Health Care Financing
    Agency (HCFA)
Healing
    celebration of, 401-8
    defined, 20
    and person, 44-49
Healing profession, 75-144

Health
    biological, 31-33
    and community, 6-9
    concepts of, 20-25
    defined, 20
    and disease, 20-43
    higher levels of, 34-35
    and personal responsibility, 44-74
    and persons, 2-6
    and sociology, 29-30
Healthcare
    counseling, 81-83, 94-102
    ethics, and public policy, 142-44
    fees, 100-102
    limits of, 126-27
    pastoral ministry in, 389-413
    social organization of, 112-44
    and spiritual counseling, 396-401
Health Care Financing Agency (HCFA),
    114, 119, 437
Health Care Ministry Assessment, 137
Healthcare profession, xiii, 76-83, 94-111
Healthcare team, and pastoral ministry,
    390-94
Health maintenance organization (HMO),
    115, 278
Health planning model of health, 22
Health Plus, 437
Health seeker, 1-74
Health team, 131-35
Hedonism, and addiction, 351-52
Helsinki Statement, of WHO, 379
Hierarchical order, 23
Hierarchy of values, 173
Hippocratic Oath, 379
Historical mentality, 158
HMO. *See* Health maintenance organiza-
    tion (HMO)
Holiness, 20
Holistic medicine, 84
Hominization, delayed, 213-13
Hope, 174, 175
    Christian, 196-203
    theology of, 175, 196
Hospital
    Catholic, 136-38
    as community, 127-31
Hospital of the Benefratelli, 84
Hospital staff, and pastoral ministry,
    394-96
Hosts, 128
Human, fully, 2-19
Humanae Vitae, 59, 201, 252, 256, 257,
    258, 259, 260, 261, 262, 263,
    264, 267, 268, 271, 287, 290-92,
    295, 297

Human being, 207
    reconstructing, 301-27
Human body, modifying, 302-4
Human dignity, principles of, 19, 192-93,
    203-4, 308, 349
Humanism, 177
Humanist, The, 438
"Humanist Manifesto," 11, 438
Humanitarian model of health, 21
Human person, 207
Human rights, and individualism, 13-16
Human Sexuality, 258
Human subjects
    and experimentation or research,
        234-43
    and research, 206

Iatrogenic diseases, 126-27
Identity
    Catholic, 136-38
    gender, 314
Idolatry, 180
Ignorance, 55
Illness
    and disease, 25
    mental. *See* Mental illness
    and sociology, 29-30
Impaired model of therapeutic relation-
    ships, 95
Implicit, 181
Index Medicus, 278
Indirect abortion, 214
Indirect alienation, 183
Individualism, and human rights, 13-16
Industrial-military complex, 123
Industrial Revolution, 254
Infallibility, 59
Information, 190
Informed consent, 68-69, 179, 203-4
Innate power, 5
Inquisition, 329
Insight therapy, 332
Instinct, and Stoics, 156
Institute for Theological Encounter with
    Science and Technology, 3, 303,
    439
Institute of Religion, xii
Institutional review board (IRB), 235,
    237
*Instruction on Respect for Human Life in Its
    Origin and on the Dignity of Procre-
    ation,* 218
Integrity
    anatomical and functional, 306
    and principle of totality, 36-43,
        194-96, 203-4, 264, 274-75, 316

Integrity (continued)
  and totality, 41-43
Intellectualists, 147
Intelligent freedom, 15, 168-69, 202
Intention, 179, 182
Interdependence, mutual, 36
Intervention, genetic. *See* Genetic intervention
Intrauterine device (IUD), 279
Intrinsically evil, 158
Intuitionist ethics, 155
Intuitivism, 158
In vitro fertilization (IVF), 280-81
IRB. *See* Institutional review board (IRB)
ITEST. *See* Institute for Theological Encounter with Science and Technolog
IUD. *See* Intrauterine device (IUD)
IVF. *See* In vitro fertilization (IVF)

Jelly, vaginal, 279
Jesus, as model, 161-62
Jobes (court case), 385
Justice, 153

Kennedy Institute of Bioethics, 144
Knowing, 176
Knowledge, 203
  and medicine, 99-100
Ku Klux Klan, 337

Last Rites, 403
Law
  natural, 154-55
  and personhood, 225-31
LCWR. *See* Leadership Conference of Women Religious (LCWR)
Leadership Conference of Women Religious (LCWR), 137
Legalism, religious, 151-52
Legitimate cooperation, principle of, 188-90, 203-4
Letter on Health and Health Care, 119
Liberation, 175
Libertarianism, 155
Life
  affirmation of, 47-49, 387
  preservation of, 203
Lifestyle, and preventive medicine, 49-51
Limits
  crisis of, 126
  of medicine, 206-43
Linacre Center for the Study of the Ethics of Health Care, 380, 444
Listening, and truth telling, 102-3
Live in Christ Jesus, To, 161

Living Will, 387
Lobotomy, 346-47
Logic, of bioethical decisions, 146-72
Long term care facility, 136-38
Love, 175, 245, 246-47
  Christian, 191-96
Low tubal ovum transplant (LTOT), 284, 285
LSD. *See* Lysergic acid diethylamide (LSD)
LTOT. *See* Low tubal ovum transplant (LTOT)
Lying, 104
Lysergic acid diethylamide (LSD), 348

Magisterium, 59, 62
Maher v. Roe, 227
Malady, and disease, 25
Man
  therapeutic, 343
  virtuous, 335
Man Against Himself, 45
Manicheans, 247
Many Faces of AIDS, The, 67
Marriage, and divorce, 248
Marxism, 10
  and Christian values, xiv-xv, 177
Material cooperation, 188
Mature personality, 335
Maximum utility, principle of, 184
MD. *See* Medical doctor (MD)
Meaninglessness, 104
Means-ends methodology. *See* Teleological ethical methodology
Mediate material cooperation, 188
Medicaid, and Medicare, 115
Medical doctor (MD), 76, 132
Medical education, 88-93
Medical model of health, 21
Medical model of therapeutic relationships, 95, 98-100
Medical Nemesis, 126
Medical News, 81, 448
Medical profession, xiii
  and ideals, 83-88
Medical Review Bulletin, 109, 448
Medical sexual problems, pastoral approach to, 290-300
Medicare
  and Medicaid, 115
  and NHI, 113
Medicine
  holistic, 84
  and knowledge and skill, 99-100
  and limits, 206-43
  preventive, 49-51

Memoirs (Larrey), 231
Mental health model of health, 22
Mental illness, concept of, 328-32
"Message to Christian Families," 297
Ministry, pastoral, 389-413
Ministry of Healing, The, 128
Miscarriage, 214
Mission effectiveness committees, 138-42
Mixed systems, 148
Models of Madness, Models of Medicine, 95
Modification, behavior. *See* Behavior
　　modification
Moral action, 34
Moral Context of Pastoral Care, The, 408
Moral decision, in immoral world, 66-68
Moral discernment, principle of, 183-84
Moral discrimination, principle of,
　　179-81, 203-4
Morality
　　criteria of, 159-61
　　subjective and objective, 410-12
Moral model of therapeutic relationships,
　　95
Moral object, 181
Moral purism, 185
Moral relativism, 152
Mortal sin, 180
Motherhood, surrogate, 283-84
Motivation, 191-92
Mutual interdependence, 36
Myself, 6
Myth of Mental Illness, The, 328

NACC. *See* National Association of Catho-
　　lic Chaplains (NACC)
NAS. *See* National Academy of Science
　　(NAS)
National Academy of Science (NAS), 451
National Association of Catholic Chap-
　　lains (NACC), 392
National Catholic Reporter, 451
National Conference of Catholic Bishops
　　(NCCB), 60, 63, 65, 136, 224,
　　230, 273-74, 275-76, 296, 380,
　　451
National health insurance (NHI), 113
National Institute of Drug Abuse (NIDA),
　　355, 452
National Institutes of Health (NIH), 319,
　　321, 346, 350, 452
National Organ Transplant Act, 373
National Reference Center for Bioethics
　　Literature, xi, 144
Natural family planning, 270
Natural law, 148

ethics, 155
　　and teleology, 154-55
Nature, 26, 28
Nature religions, 10
NCCB. *See* National Conference of Cath-
　　olic Bishops (NCCB)
NCR. *See National Catholic Reporter*
Needs
　　common, 162-64
　　hierarchy, 25
　　and truth, 54-56
　　and values, 16-18
Negative eugenics, 321
Neoplatonists, 247
Neurotic anxiety, 333
New Humanist, The, 438
New Jersey Catholic Conference, 383,
　　451
New Vision for a New Century, A, 137
New York Task Force on Medical Ethics,
　　366, 452
New York Times, 228, 281, 283-84, 452
NHI. *See* National health insurance
　　(NHI)
Nichomachean Ethics, The, 150
NIDA. *See* National Institute of Drug
　　Abuse (NIDA)
NIH. *See* National Institutes of Health
　　(NIH)
Nonmoral object, 182
Norms
　　of Christian decision making, 173-
　　　204
　　of Christian faith, 176-91
　　of Christian hope, 196-203
　　of Christian love, 191-96
　　exceptionless, 148
　　pastoral, 387
*No Room in the Marketplace: The Health Care
　　of the Poor,* 137
Nuremberg Code, 236, 237, 452
Nurses, 133-35

Object
　　moral, 181
　　physical or nonmoral, 182
　　premoral, 158
Objective morality, 410-12
Office of Technology Assessment (OTA),
　　52, 319, 453-54
Ombudsman, 135
One Flew Over the Cuckoo's Nest, 329
Ontic values and disvalues, 166-68
Ontological concept of disease, 25-26
Open way, 180

Operant conditioning, 332
Optimal functioning, 23
Option, fundamental, 179
Oral contraception, 278-80
Organismic theory of disease, 27-29
Organizational models, 112-26
Organ transplantation, 304-12
OTA. *See* Office of Technology Assessment (OTA)
Ovral, 288
Ovulation method, 269

Pain, 386-87
Paranoia, 329
Parental responsibility, 325-27
Paris Statement, 11, 454
Passivity, and activity, 210
Pastoral approach, to medical sexual problems, 290-300
Pastoral care, xvi
    and ethical counseling, 408-13
    and ethical decisions, 390-413
    See also Pastoral ministry
Pastoral Care of Homosexual Persons, 257, 291
Pastoral Constitution on the Church in the Modern World, 53, 160, 218, 256 261, 268
Pastoral ministry
    in healthcare, 389-413
    and healthcare team, 390-94
    to hospital staff, 394-96
    See also Pastoral care
Pastoral norms, for allowing to die, 387
Paterfamilias, 215
Patient advocates, 133-35
Patient/professional relationships, 94-96
Patients, and AIDS, 80-81
"Patient's Bill of Rights," 369-70
Patient's rights, 70-74
Patrick v. Burget, 454
PCEMR. *See* President's Commission for the Study of Ethical Problems in Medicine and Biomedical and Behavioral Research (PCEMR)
Peer discipline, 110
Peer relations, and professional discipline, 107-11
Peer service review organization (PSRO), 113
Perlmutter (court case), 385
Perplexed conscience, 66
Person
    autonomous, 335
    and community, 39

and healing, 44-49
and health, 2-6
totality of, 37-41
Personalism, prudential, xiv, 159-65, 168-69, 186
Personalistic concept of profession, 78-80
Personality, 4, 5-6
    dimensions of, 17-18
    mature, 335
Personalization, and healthcare profession, 94-111
Personalized sexuality, principle of, 197, 199-201, 203-4, 244-53, 259, 356
Personal responsibility, and health, 44-74
Personhood
    advocacy of, 213-14
    and law, 225-31
    politics of, 9-16
Person profession, 76
Phenotype, 318
Phenylketonuria (PKU), 322, 323
Philosophical, defined, 175
Philosophical model of health, 22
Physicalism, 33, 168-69, 262
Physical object, 182
Physician
    and AIDS, 80-81
    choosing, 70-72
    Christian, 86-88
    and co-workers, 131-33
    and ideals of profession, 83-88
Physicians' Desk Reference, 279, 455
Physiological addiction, 352
Physiological concept of disease, 26
Pierce v. Swan Point Cemetary, 372, 455
PKU. *See* Phenylketonuria (PKU)
Placebo effect, 238
Pleasure, 245, 246-47
Pluralism, 228-31
    ethical, 146-47
Pluralist system, 113, 114
Policy, public. *See* Public policy, 142-44
Politics, of personhood, 9-16
Pontifical Academy of Sciences, 366, 383, 456
Pontifical Commission on Peace and Justice, 15, 263, 456
Pope John XXIII Medical-Moral Research and Education Center, 144
Population Crisis Committee, 456
Positivism, 152-53
Postcoital douche, 279
Postconventional phase, 146

Potentiality, 209
PPO. *See* Preferred provider organization (PPO)
Pragmatics, 91
Preconventional phase, 146
Preferred provider organization (PPO), 115
Prefrontal lobotomy, 346-47
Pre-Meditated Man, 330
Premoral object, 158
Preservation of life, 203
President's Commission for the Study of Ethical Problems in Medicine and Biomedical and Behavioral Research (PCEMR), 142, 143, 235, 236, 311, 364, 365, 366-67, 368, 380, 384, 456
President's Commission on AIDS, 456
President's Commission on Ethical Issues in Medicine and Research, 139
Preventive medicine, and lifestyle, 49-51
Preventive model of health, 21
Priest, and scientist, 83-86
Principle of common good, 116-21, 193-94, 203-4, 225, 308
Principle of double effect, 184-88, 189, 190, 203-4, 236, 288
Principle of free and informed conscience, 70, 179, 203-4
Principle of growing through suffering, 197-99, 203-4
Principle of human dignity in community, 19, 192-93, 203-4, 259, 308, 349
Principle of legitimate cooperation, 188-90, 203-4
Principle of maximum utility, 184
Principle of moral discernment, 183-84
Principle of moral discrimination, 179-81, 203-4
Principle of personalized sexuality, 197, 199-201, 203-4, 244-53, 259, 356
Principle of professional communication, 102-7, 190-91, 351
Principle of proportion, 185, 187, 203-4, 223, 224
Principle of prudent conscience and informed consent, 54-70
Principle of stewardship and creativity, 51-53, 197, 201-3, 304, 318
Principle of subsidiarity, 112-26, 193-94, 203-4, 225
Principle of totality, and integrity, 36-43, 194-96, 203-4, 264, 274-75, 316
Principle of well-formed conscience, 64-68, 70, 177-78, 184

Principles
   coordination of, 203-4
   ethical, 175-76
   reflex, 58
   of research, 236-39
Principles of Medical Ethics, The (APA), 357
Priorities, in needs and values, 16-18
Private, 13
Private conscience, 156
Probabilism, 58, 219
Procreation, 203, 245
Production funnels, 78
Profession
   depersonalizing trends, 76-83
   healing, 75-144
   healthcare, xiii, 76-83, 94-111
   and ideals, 83-88
   medical, xiii, 83-88
   person, 76
   personalistic concept of, 78-80
Professional communication, principle of, 102-7, 190-91, 351
Professional discipline, and peer relations, 107-11
Professional/patient relationships, 94-96
Profession of Medicine: A Study of the Sociology of Applied Knowledge, 29, 54
Proportion, principle of, 185, 187, 203-4, 223, 224
Proportionalism, 158-59, 164-65
Proxy, 239-41
Prudence, 176
Prudential personalism, xiv, 159-65, 168-69, 186
PSRO *See* Peer service review organization (PSRO)
Psychedelic model of therapeutic relationships, 95
Psychoactive drugs, 347-48
Psychoanalysis, 336
Psychoanalytical model of therapeutic relationships, 95
Psychological conditioning, 349
Psychological dependency, 352
Psychological dimension, of personality, 17
Psychological experimentation, 242-43
Psychological needs, 25
Psychologism, 34
Psychosurgery, 346
Psychotherapeutic models of therapeutic relationships, 96-97
Psychotherapy
   and behavior modification, 328-58
   ethical problems of, 338-45

Public health model of health, 21
Public policy, healthcare, and ethics, 142-44
Punishment, and therapy, 338-40
Purism, moral, 185
Purpose, moral, 181

Quinlan (court case), 385

Randomization, 238
Rape, treatment of victims, 286-90
Rationality, 6, 7
Reason, 15
Reassignment, sexual. *See* Sexual reassignment
Recombinant DNA, 319
Reconciliation, and anointing the sick, 402-5
Reconstructing human beings, 301-27
Reflex principles, 58
Regimen, 49
Relations, peer, 107-11
Relationships, therapeutic, 95-100
Relativism
    cultural, 30
    moral, 152
    and profession, 78-79
Religious legalism, 151-52
Report of Inquiry into Human Fertilization and Embryology: Medical Research Council Response, 467
Reproduction, and sexuality, 244-300
Republic, 121
Research
    and human subjects, 234-43
    involving human subjects, 206
    principles of, 236-39
    and sex therapy, 355-58
    therapeutic, 236
Researchers, 128
Research Group on Ethical, Social, and Legal Issues in Genetic Counseling and Genetic Engineering, 322, 437
Research staff, 128
Res ipsa loquitur, 109
Respect, 194
Responsibility
    parental, 325-27
    personal, 44-74
Rest, 49
Rights
    human, 13-16
    patient's, 70-74
    protection of, 72-74
    woman's, 220-24

Rights and Duties of Capital and Labor, 117
Rigid conscience, 65
Rigorism, 185
Risks, and therapy, 340-42
Rite of Baptism for Children, 406
Rite of Funerals, 406
Rite of Penance, 405
Roe v. Wade, 226, 228
Role, gender, 314
Rule utilitarianism, 157

Sacrament, and word, 401-2
Sacramentality, 245, 246-47
Sacrament of Reconciliation, 405
Sacred Congregation for the Doctrine of the Faith (SCDF), 168, 199, 218, 257, 258, 274, 282, 283, 284, 285, 298, 319, 361, 374, 378, 382, 384, 386, 387, 406, 459
Sacred Penitentiary, 255, 459
Sacrifice, 13
Sadism, 46
Saikewicz (court case), 385
SCDF. *See* Sacred Congregation for the Doctrine of the Faith (SCDF)
Scientific doubts, 52-53
Scientist, and priest, 83-86
Scott v. Casey, 239, 460
Screening, genetic. *See* Genetic screening
Secondary signs, 197
Self-conscious mind, 5
Self-control, 337
Self-development, 210
Self-respect, 194
Sensual pleasure, 245
Sensus fidelium, 59, 60
Sex, and education, 298-300
Sex therapy, and research, 355-58
Sexuality
    personalized, 197, 199-201, 203-4, 244-53, 259, 356
    and reproduction, 244-300
Sexual problems, pastoral approach to, 290-300
Sexual reassignment, 313-16
Sexual revolution, 254, 298
Shock therapy, 346
Sickness, and disease, 25
Signs, 197
Sin bravely, 66
Sins, mortal and venial, 180
Situationism, 156-57
Skill, and medicine, 99-100
Social contact theory, 8
Social Development, On, 117
Social dimension, of personality, 17-18

Social iatrogenesis, 127
Social model of therapeutic relationships, 95
Social needs, 25
Social organization, of healthcare, 112-44
Social workers, 133-35
Society
    living in, 203
    therapeutic, 343
Sociology, and health and illness, 29-30
"Some Persons Are Humans, Some Humans Are Persons, and the World Is What We Persons Make of It," 5
Song of Songs, The, 247
Species-survival model of health, 22
Spirit, guidance by, 59-60
Spiritual counseling, and healthcare, 396-401
Spiritual dimension, of personality, 18
Spiritual needs, 25
Sponge, vaginal, 279
Spring (court case), 385
Staff
    and pastoral ministry, 394-96
    research, 128
Sterilization, and contraception, 271-73
Stewardship, and creativity, 51-53, 197, 201-3, 304, 318
Stipend, 101
St. Louis University School of Medicine, xi-xii
Stoics, 247
    and instinct, 156
Stress, 49
Students, 128
Subjective morality, 410-12
Subsidiarity, principle of, 112-26, 193-94, 203-4, 225
Substantialist, 208
Suffering
    and death, 359-87
    growing through, 197-99, 203-4
Suicide, and euthanasia, 374-80
Summa Theologicae, 67, 155, 165, 181
Super biological systems model of health, 21-22
Supreme Court, 283, 319
    and abortion, 226-28
Surgery, 346
Surrogate motherhood, 283-84
Symbolic communication, 34
Sympto-thermal method, 269

Talk Back to Your Doctor, 72

Tamers of Death, 128
Tarasoff v. Regents of University of California, 105
Task Force on Organ Transplantation, 309
Tay-Sachs syndrome, 320
Teachers, 128
Team, healthcare, 131-35, 390-94
Technology, and values, 249-52
Teleological ethical methodology, xiv, 147-49, 154-59
Teleology, and natural law, 154-55
Telos, 28
Tendency, 17
Texas Catholic Conference, 138, 464
Texas Medical Association, 81, 464
Theological, defined, 175
Theological Commission (International), 60, 61, 464
Theology of hope, 175, 196
Therapeutic man, 343
Therapeutic relationships, models of, 95-100
Therapeutic research, 236
Therapeutic society, 343
Therapy
    action. *See* Action therapy
    group. *See* Group therapy
    insight. *See* Insight therapy
    psycho-. *See* Psychotherapy
    sex. *See* Sex therapy
Third World model of health, 22
TOT. *See* Tubal ovum transfer (TOT)
Totality
    and integrity, 41-43
    of person, 37-41
    principle of. *See* Principle of totality
TOTS. *See* Tubal ovum transfer with sperm (TOTS)
Transduction, 318
Transference, 97, 341
Transplantation, organ. *See* Organ transplantation
Transplantation Society, 373, 465
Transsexualism, 314
Transvestism, 314
Triage, 206
    and extending care, 231-34
Triumph of the Therapeutic, The, 343
Trust, 72
    and spiritual counseling, 396-99
Trusteeship, 82
Truth, need for, 54-56
Truth telling, 203
    and death, 368-71

Truth telling (continued)
and listening, 102-3
Tubal ovum transfer (TOT), 285
Tubal ovum transfer with sperm (TOTS), 285
Tuskegee Syphilis Study, 142, 235
Tutorism, 185

UN. *See* United Nations (UN)
Unconditional benign acceptance, 96
Unhealthy health, 30
Uniform Anatomical Gift Act, 372
United Nations (UN), 15, 16, 19, 119, 124, 173, 177, 214, 465
United States Catholic Conference (USCC), 65, 67, 119, 136, 137, 161, 294, 363, 369, 386, 405, 465
United States Congress, 308, 465, 466
United States Department of Health, Education, and Welfare (HEW), 108, 142, 465
United States Department of Health and Human Services (DHHS), 309, 466
United States National Commission for the Protection of Human Subjects of Biomedical and Behavioral Research, 235, 420
United States Select Committee on Aging, United States Congress, 466
Universal Declaration of Human Rights, 15, 16, 19, 119, 173, 176, 177, 214, 465
USCC. *See* United States Catholic Conference (USCC)
Utilitarianism, 155-57
Utility, maximum, 184

Vaginal foam, 279
Vaginal jelly, 279
Vaginal sponge, 279

Values
Christian, xiv
hierarchy of, 173
and needs, 16-18
ontic, 166-68
and technology, 249-52
Value systems, 342-45
Vatican Council II, xv, 9, 10, 11, 12, 54, 59, 63, 64, 117, 160, 174, 189, 225, 229, 252, 256, 257, 260, 261, 266, 392, 396, 466
Vatican II: The Conciliar and Post Conciliar Documents, 466
Venial sin, 180
Viaticum, 404
Vicarious consent, 239-41
Virtuous man, 335
Vocation, 90
Voluntarists, 147

Warnock Report, 281, 467
Washington University, 356
Way, open and closed, 180
Well-being model of health, 21
Well-formed conscience, principle of, 64-68, 70, 177-78, 184
WHO. *See* World Health Organization (WHO)
Wholeness, 20
Will, 191
Willowbrook experiments, 235
Woman's rights, and abortion, 220-24
Word, and sacrament, 401-2
World Health Organization (WHO), 2, 21, 24, 25, 236, 269, 270, 379, 468
World Population Conference, 267, 468
World Synod of Catholic Bishops, 258, 297-98, 468

Xenodochia, 128